Clinical Education for the Health Professions

Debra Nestel • Gabriel Reedy •
Lisa McKenna • Suzanne Gough
Editors

Clinical Education for the Health Professions

Theory and Practice

Volume 1

With 128 Figures and 94 Tables

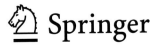

Editors
Debra Nestel
Monash University
School of Clinical Sciences
Clayton, VIC, Australia

University of Melbourne
Department of Surgery (Austin)
Melbourne, VIC, Australia

Lisa McKenna
La Trobe University
School of Nursing and Midwifery
Melbourne, VIC, Australia

Gabriel Reedy
King's College London
London, UK

Suzanne Gough
Bond University
Faculty of Health Sciences and Medicine
Gold Coast, QLD, Australia

ISBN 978-981-15-3343-3   ISBN 978-981-15-3344-0 (eBook)
https://doi.org/10.1007/978-981-15-3344-0

© Springer Nature Singapore Pte Ltd. 2023

This work is subject to copyright. All rights are reserved by the Publisher, whether the whole or part of the material is concerned, specifically the rights of translation, reprinting, reuse of illustrations, recitation, broadcasting, reproduction on microfilms or in any other physical way, and transmission or information storage and retrieval, electronic adaptation, computer software, or by similar or dissimilar methodology now known or hereafter developed.

The use of general descriptive names, registered names, trademarks, service marks, etc. in this publication does not imply, even in the absence of a specific statement, that such names are exempt from the relevant protective laws and regulations and therefore free for general use.

The publisher, the authors, and the editors are safe to assume that the advice and information in this book are believed to be true and accurate at the date of publication. Neither the publisher nor the authors or the editors give a warranty, expressed or implied, with respect to the material contained herein or for any errors or omissions that may have been made. The publisher remains neutral with regard to jurisdictional claims in published maps and institutional affiliations.

This Springer imprint is published by the registered company Springer Nature Singapore Pte Ltd.
The registered company address is: 152 Beach Road, #21-01/04 Gateway East, Singapore 189721, Singapore

Preface

The education and training of health professionals is fundamental to the success of health services. Philosophies, approaches, and practices vary internationally. We frame clinical education as any activities that prepare health professionals to learn and work effectively in clinical settings. We believe this major reference work, *Clinical Education for the Health Professions*, represents, supports, and advances scholarship and practice in this field. It assembles accessible and evidence-based content, on what is known about many facets of clinical education.

Clinical Education for the Health Professions is divided into eight parts. We start with the contemporary context of health professions education; shift focus to theoretical underpinnings, curriculum considerations, and approaches to supporting learning in clinical settings; a specific focus to assessment approaches; and then to evidence-based educational methods and content. Governance and other formal processes associated with the maturation of education programs are also considered, including the increasing professionalization of clinical education. Finally, we look to the future drawing upon much of what has surfaced in the past and present.

The development of multi-authored international work can be complex. We outline the development process in the introduction. We are grateful for the generosity of contributors – researchers, educators, and clinicians – who have given their time, especially coinciding with the COVID-19 pandemic.

Melbourne, Australia	Debra Nestel
London, UK	Gabriel Reedy
Melbourne, Australia	Lisa McKenna
Gold Coast, Australia	Suzanne Gough
July 2023	Editors

Acknowledgments

We are grateful to all the contributors to this major reference work.
We thank Ms. Shameem Aysha S. of Springer Nature for coordinating the editorial process.

Contents

Volume 1

Part I The Contemporary Context of Health Professions Education **1**

1 **Medical Education: Trends and Context** 3
   Jennene Greenhill

2 **Surgical Education: Context and Trends** 29
   David J. Coker

3 **General Practice Education: Context and Trends** 49
   Susan M. Wearne and James B. Brown

4 **Anesthesia Education: Trends and Context** 69
   S. D. Marshall and M. C. Turner

5 **Clinical Education in Nursing: Current Practices and Trends** ... 87
   Marilyn H. Oermann and Teresa Shellenbarger

6 **Nursing Education in Low and Lower-Middle Income Countries: Context and Trends** 107
   Christine Sommers and Carielle Joy Rio

7 **Obstetric and Midwifery Education: Context and Trends** 121
   Arunaz Kumar and Linda Sweet

8 **Allied Health Education: Current and Future Trends** 135
   Michelle Bissett, Neil Tuttle, and Elizabeth Cardell

9 **Dental Education: Context and Trends** 153
   Flora A. Smyth Zahra and Sang E. Park

10 **Interprofessional Education (IPE): Trends and Context** 167
   Lyn Gum and Jenn Salfi

11 Global Surgery and Its Trends and Context: The Case of Timor-Leste 181
Sean Stevens

12 Surgical Training: Impact of Decentralization and Guidelines for Improvement 201
Christine M. Cuthbertson

13 Mental Health Education: Contemporary Context and Future Directions 217
Christopher Kowalski and Chris Attoe

14 Dental Education: A Brief History 251
Andrew I. Spielman

15 Surgical Education and Training: Historical Perspectives 267
John P. Collins

16 Nursing and Midwifery Education: Historical Perspectives 285
Lisa McKenna, Jenny Davis, and Eloise Williams

17 Health Sciences and Medicine Education in Lockdown: Lessons Learned During the COVID-19 Global Pandemic 303
Suzanne Gough, Robin Orr, Allan Stirling, Athanasios Raikos, Ben Schram, and Wayne Hing

Part II Philosophical and Theoretical Underpinning of Health Professions Education **333**

18 Cognitive Neuroscience Foundations of Surgical and Procedural Expertise: Focus on Theory 335
Pamela Andreatta

19 Mastery Learning in Health Professions Education 347
Raymond Yap

20 Threshold Concepts and Troublesome Knowledge 361
Sarah E. M. Meek, Hilary Neve, and Andy Wearn

21 Social Semiotics: Theorizing Meaning Making 385
Jeff Bezemer

22 Communities of Practice and Medical Education 403
Claire Condron and Walter Eppich

23 Activity Theory in Health Professions Education Research and Practice 417
Richard L. Conn, Gerard J. Gormley, Sarah O'Hare, and Anu Kajamaa

24 Reflective Practice in Health Professions Education 441
Jennifer M. Weller-Newton and Michele Drummond-Young

Contents

25 Transformative Learning in Clinical Education: Using Theory to Inform Practice 463
Anna Jones

26 Self-Regulated Learning: Focus on Theory 481
Susan Irvine and Ian J. Irvine

27 Critical Theory 499
Nancy McNaughton and Maria Athina (Tina) Martimianakis

28 Focus on Theory: Emotions and Learning 521
Aubrey L. Samost-Williams and Rebecca D. Minehart

29 Ecological Systems Theory in Clinical Learning 537
Yang Yann Foo and Raymond Goy

30 Philosophy for Healthcare Professions Education: A Tool for Thinking and Practice 555
Kirsten Dalrymple and Roberto di Napoli

Part III Curriculum Considerations in Health Professions Education 573

31 Health Profession Curriculum and Public Engagement 575
Maree O'Keefe and Helena Ward

32 Teaching and Learning Ethics in Healthcare 587
Selena Knight and Andrew Papanikitas

33 Simulation as Clinical Replacement: Contemporary Approaches in Healthcare Professional Education 607
Suzie Kardong-Edgren, Sandra Swoboda, and Nancy Sullivan

34 Teaching Simple and Complex Psychomotor Skills 625
Delwyn Nicholls

35 Developing Professional Identity in Health Professional Students 645
Kathleen Leedham-Green, Alec Knight, and Rick Iedema

36 Hidden, Informal, and Formal Curricula in Health Professions Education 667
Lisa McKenna

37 Arts and Humanities in Health Professional Education 681
Pam Harvey, Neville Chiavaroli, and Giskin Day

38 Debriefing Practices in Simulation-Based Education 699
Peter Dieckmann, Rana Sharara-Chami, and Hege Langli Ersdal

39 Written Feedback in Health Sciences Education: "What You Write May Be Perceived as Banal" 717
Brian Jolly

40 Technology Considerations in Health Professions and Clinical Education 743
Christian Moro, Zane Stromberga, and James Birt

41 Role of Social Media in Health Professions Education 765
Victoria Brazil, Jessica Stokes-Parish, and Jesse Spurr

42 E-learning: Development of a Fully Online 4th Year Psychology Program 777
F. J. Garivaldis, S. P. McKenzie, and M. Mundy

43 Teaching Diversity in Healthcare Education: Conceptual Clarity and the Need for an Intersectional Transdisciplinary Approach 795
Helen Bintley and Riya E. George

44 Planetary Health: Educating the Current and Future Health Workforce 815
Michelle McLean, Lynne Madden, Janie Maxwell, Patricia Nanya Schwerdtle, Janet Richardson, Judith Singleton, Kristen MacKenzie-Shalders, Georgia Behrens, Nick Cooling, Richard Matthews, and Graeme Horton

Volume 2

Part IV   Supporting Learning in Clinical Settings 845

45 Learning and Teaching in Clinical Settings: Expert Commentary from an Interprofessional Perspective 847
Debra Kiegaldie

46 Learning and Teaching at the Bedside: Expert Commentary from a Nursing Perspective 869
Michelle A. Kelly and Jan Forber

47 Learning and Teaching in Clinical Settings: Expert Commentary from a Midwifery Perspective 891
Linda Sweet and Deborah Davis

48 Learning and Teaching in the Operating Room: A Surgical Perspective 909
V. Chao, C. Ong, Debra Kiegaldie, and Debra Nestel

Contents xiii

49 Learning and Teaching in the Operating Theatre: Expert Commentary from the Nursing Perspective 933
Rachel Cardwell, Emmalee Weston, and Jenny Davis

50 Learning and Teaching in Pediatrics 955
Ramesh Mark Nataraja, Simon C. Blackburn, and Robert Roseby

51 Optimizing the Role of Clinical Educators in Health Professional Education 985
Simone Gibson and Claire Palermo

52 Well-Being in Health Profession Training 999
Andrew Grant

53 Embedding a Simulation-Based Education Program in a Teaching Hospital 1017
Rebecca A. Szabo and Kirsty Forrest

54 Targeting Organizational Needs Through the Development of a Simulation-Based Communication Education Program 1039
J. Sokol and M. Heywood

55 Effective Feedback Conversations in Clinical Practice 1055
C. E. Johnson, C. J. Watling, J. L. Keating, and E. K. Molloy

56 Supervision in General Practice Settings 1073
James Brown and Susan M. Wearne

57 Conversational Learning in Health Professions Education: Learning Through Talk 1099
Walter J. Eppich, Jan Schmutz, and Pim Teunissen

58 Underperformance in Clinical Education: Challenges and Possibilities 1119
Margaret Bearman

Part V Assessment in Health Professions Education **1133**

59 Approaches to Assessment: A Perspective from Education 1135
Phillip Dawson and Colin R. McHenry

60 Measuring Attitudes: Current Practices in Health Professional Education 1149
Ted Brown, Stephen Isbel, Mong-Lin Yu, and Thomas Bevitt

61 Measuring Performance: Current Practices in Surgical Education 1177
Pamela Andreatta, Brenton Franklin, Matthew Bradley, Christopher Renninger, and John Armstrong

62 Programmatic Assessment in Health Professions Education 1203
Iris Lindemann, Julie Ash, and Janice Orrell

63 Entrustable Professional Activities: Focus on Assessment Methods 1221
Andrea Bramley and Lisa McKenna

64 Workplace-Based Assessment in Clinical Practice 1235
Victor Lee and Andrea Gingerich

65 Focus on Selection Methods: Evidence and Practice 1251
Louise Marjorie Allen, Catherine Green, and Margaret Hay

66 Practice Education in Occupational Therapy: Current Trends and Practices 1277
Stephen Isbel, Ted Brown, Mong-Lin Yu, Thomas Bevitt, Craig Greber, and Anne-Maree Caine

67 Practice Education in Lockdown: Lessons Learned During the COVID-19 Global Pandemic 1303
Luke Robinson, Ted Brown, Ellie Fossey, Mong-Lin Yu, Linda Barclay, Eli Chu, Annette Peart, and Libby Callaway

Part VI Evidence-Based Health Professions Education: Focus on Educational Methods and Content **1323**

68 Team-Based Learning (TBL): Theory, Planning, Practice, and Implementation 1325
Annette Burgess and Elie Matar

69 Learning with and from Peers in Clinical Education 1355
Joanna Tai, Merrolee Penman, Calvin Chou, and Arianne Teherani

70 Simulation for Procedural Skills Teaching and Learning 1375
Taylor Sawyer, Lisa Bergman, and Marjorie L. White

71 Simulation for Clinical Skills in Healthcare Education 1395
Guillaume Alinier, Ahmed Labib Shehatta, and Ratna Makker

72 Screen-Based Learning 1417
Damir Ljuhar

73 Artificial Intelligence in Surgical Education and Training 1435
Melanie Crispin

74 Coaching in Health Professions Education: The Case of Surgery 1447
Martin Richardson and Louise Richardson

Contents

xv

75 Developing Health Professional Teams 1463
John T. Paige

76 Developing Care and Compassion in Health Professional
Students and Clinicians 1485
Karen Livesay and Ruby Walter

77 Developing Patient Safety Through Education 1501
David Pinnock

78 Supporting the Development of Professionalism in the
Education of Health Professionals 1519
Anne Stephenson and Julie Bliss

79 Supporting the Development of Patient-Centred Communication
Skills 1535
Bernadette O'Neill

80 Contemporary Sociological Issues for Health Professions
Curricula 1553
Margaret Simmons

81 Developing Clinical Reasoning Capabilities 1571
Joy Higgs

**Part VII Governance, Quality Improvement, Scholarship and
Leadership in Health Professions Education** **1589**

82 Professional Bodies in Health Professions Education 1591
Julie Browne

83 Scholarship in Health Professions Education 1611
Lisa McKenna

84 Developing Educational Leadership in Health Professions
Education 1627
Margaret Hay, Leeroy William, Catherine Green, Eric Gantwerker,
and Louise Marjorie Allen

85 On "Being" Participants and a Researcher in a Longitudinal
Medical Professional Identity Study 1657
Michelle McLean, Charlotte Alexander, and Arjun Khaira

86 Health Care Practitioners 'Becoming' Doctors: Changing
Roles and Identities 1671
Michelle McLean and Carla Pecoraro

Part VIII Future Directions for Health Professions Education 1691

87 Health Professional Education in 2020: A Trainee Perspective ... 1693
Karen Muller and Savannah Morrison

88 Future of Health Professions Education Curricula 1705
Eric Gantwerker, Louise Marjorie Allen, and Margaret Hay

89 Competencies of Health Professions Educators of the Future 1727
Louise Marjorie Allen, Eric Gantwerker, and Margaret Hay

Index 1737

About the Editors

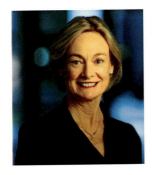

Debra Nestel has worked at the University of Hong Kong, China, Imperial College, United Kingdom, the University of Melbourne and Monash University, Australia, for over 35 years. Her first degree was in sociology, and her doctorate was in program evaluation and communication skills education in medicine and dentistry. Currently, her education and research activities focus on faculty development for health professional, surgical, and simulation educators. Dr. Debra is an experienced editor-in-chief (EIC) and has edited several books. She was the foundation EIC of *Advances in Simulation* and is EIC of the *International Journal for Healthcare Simulation*. Dr. Debra is a Fellow of the Academy of the Society for Simulation in Healthcare (United States) and is also a Fellow of the Academy of Medical Educators (United Kingdom). In 2021, Dr. Debra was appointed as Member of the Order of Australia for her service to medical education and simulation. She has received the Ray Page Lifetime Simulation Service Award and a Presidential Citation from the Society for Simulation in Healthcare.

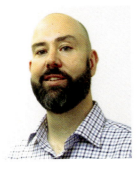

Gabriel Reedy has led the interprofessional postgraduate program in health professions education at King's College, London, the largest health sciences university in Europe, for most of his academic career. His research focuses on how healthcare professionals and emergency responders learn, how to support and train them more effectively, with a focus on the power of simulated environments, and how they can help train individuals, teams, departments, organizations, and inter-agency systems. He is a Principal Fellow of the Higher

Education Academy (United Kingdom), a Fellow of the Academy of Medical Educators (United Kingdom), and a Fellow of the Academy of the Society for Simulation in Healthcare (United States). He has served on the Scientific Committee of the Society for Simulation in Europe (SESAM) and the Research Committee for the Society for Simulation in Healthcare (United Kingdom). He is Editor-in-Chief of *Advances in Simulation.*

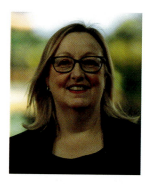

Lisa McKenna has worked at Monash University and La Trobe University, Australia, for over 30 years. Her initial qualifications were hospital-based nursing and midwifery certificates with her first degree in education. She has since completed postgraduate degrees in education, business administration, and history, and a PhD in nursing. Lisa is currently the Dean of the School of Nursing and Midwifery at La Trobe, and EIC of *Collegian: The Australian Journal of Nursing Practice, Scholarship and Research* from 2014 to 2022. Prof. Lisa has published extensively on nursing, midwifery, and health professions education. Her recent research has focused on health workforce development and competence. In 2022, Prof. Lisa was inducted into the Sigma International Nurse Researcher Hall of Fame.

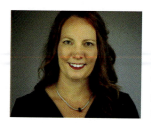

Suzanne Gough is an Associate Professor of Physiotherapy and Associate Dean of Learning and Teaching at Bond University, Australia. She is a member of the Bond Translational Simulation Collaborative team, with national and international experience in healthcare simulation education. Suzanne transitioned from clinical to academic practice in 2004, as a Senior Lecturer at Manchester Metropolitan University. She is a Principal Fellow of the Higher Education Academy (United Kingdom). As Principal Investigator, she has led international project teams to develop simulated patient governance frameworks and training resources for use across the United Kingdom, on behalf of Health Education England. Suzanne's current research interests include the use of virtual reality across diverse patient groups, simulation and technology-enhanced learning, stress and burnout, and curriculum design.

Contributors

Charlotte Alexander Emergency Department, Gold Coast University Hospital, Gold Coast, QLD, Australia

Guillaume Alinier Hamad Medical Corporation Ambulance Service, Doha, Qatar
School of Health and Social Work, University of Hertfordshire, Hatfield, UK
Weill Cornell Medicine Qatar, Doha, Qatar
Faculty of Health and Life Sciences, Northumbria University, Newcastle upon Tyne, UK

Louise Marjorie Allen Monash Centre for Professional Development and Monash Online Education, Monash University, Clayton, VIC, Australia

Pamela Andreatta The Norman M. Rich Department of Surgery, Uniformed Services University & the Walter Reed National Military Medical Center "America's Medical School", Bethesda, MD, USA

John Armstrong University of South Florida Morsani College of Medicine, Tampa, FL, USA

Julie Ash Prideaux Centre for Health Professions Education, Flinders University, Adelaide, SA, Australia

Chris Attoe Maudsley Learning, South London and Maudsley NHS Foundation Trust, London, UK

Linda Barclay Department of Occupational Therapy, Monash University – Peninsula Campus, Frankston, VIC, Australia

Margaret Bearman Centre for Research in Assessment and Digital Education (CRADLE), Deakin University, Melbourne, VIC, Australia

Georgia Behrens School of Medicine, Sydney, University of Notre Dame, Sydney, NSW, Australia

Lisa Bergman The Office of Interprofessional Simulation for Innovative Clinical Practice, University of Alabama at Birmingham, Birmingham, AL, USA

Thomas Bevitt Faculty of Health, The University of Canberra Hospital, Canberra, Bruce ACT, Australia

Jeff Bezemer Institute of Education, University College London, London, UK

Helen Bintley Barts and The London, School of Medicine and Dentistry, Queen Mary University of London, London, UK

James Birt Faculty of Society and Design, Bond University, Gold Coast, QLD, Australia

Michelle Bissett Discipline of Occupational Therapy, Griffith University, Gold Coast, QLD, Australia

Simon C. Blackburn The Learning Academy, Great Ormond Street Hospital for Children, London, UK

Julie Bliss Florence Nightingale Faculty of Nursing, Midwifery & Palliative Care, King's College London, London, UK

Matthew Bradley The Norman M. Rich Department of Surgery, Uniformed Services University & the Walter Reed National Military Medical Center "America's Medical School", Bethesda, MD, USA

Andrea Bramley Department of Dietetics and Human Nutrition, La Trobe University, Melbourne, VIC, Australia

Victoria Brazil Faculty of Health Sciences and Medicine, Bond University, Gold Coast, QLD, Australia

James B. Brown Eastern Victoria GP Training, Churchill, VIC, Australia
Gippsland Medical School, Monash University , Churchill, VIC, Australia

James Brown Royal Australian College of General Practice, East Melbourne, VIC, Australia
Gippsland Medical School, Monash University, Churchill, VIC, Australia

Ted Brown Department of Occupational Therapy, School of Primary and Allied Health Care, Faculty of Medicine, Nursing and Health Sciences, Monash University – Peninsula Campus, Frankston, VIC, Australia

Julie Browne Centre for Medical Education, Cardiff University School of Medicine, Cardiff, UK

Annette Burgess Faculty of Medicine and Health, Sydney Medical School, Education Office, The University of Sydney, Sydney, NSW, Australia
Faculty of Medicine and Health, Sydney Health Professional Education Research Network, The University of Sydney, Sydney, NSW, Australia

Anne-Maree Caine School of Allied Health Sciences – Occupational Therapy, Griffith University, Nathan, QLD, Australia

Libby Callaway Department of Occupational Therapy, Monash University – Peninsula Campus, Frankston, VIC, Australia

Elizabeth Cardell Discipline of Speech Pathology, Griffith University, Gold Coast, Australia

Rachel Cardwell Austin Health, La Trobe University, Melbourne, VIC, Australia

V. Chao National Heart Centre, Singapore, Singapore

Neville Chiavaroli Department of Medical Education, University of Melbourne, Melbourne, VIC, Australia

Calvin Chou Department of Medicine, University of California, San Francisco and Veterans Affairs Health System, San Francisco, CA, USA

Eli Chu Department of Occupational Therapy, Monash University – Peninsula Campus, Frankston, VIC, Australia

David J. Coker Department of Surgery, Royal Prince Alfred Hospital, Camperdown, NSW, Australia

Discipline of Surgery, University of Sydney, Camperdown, NSW, Australia

John P. Collins University Department of Surgery, University of Melbourne, Melbourne, Australia

Nuffield Department of Surgical Sciences, University of Oxford, Oxford, UK

Green Templeton College, Oxford, UK

Claire Condron RSCI University of Medicine and Health Sciences, Dublin, Ireland

Richard L. Conn Centre for Medical Education, Queen's University Belfast, Belfast, UK

Nick Cooling School of Medicine, College of Health & Medicine, University of Tasmania, Hobart, TAS, Australia

Melanie Crispin Monash Health & The University of Melbourne, Melbourne, Australia

Christine M. Cuthbertson Monash Rural Health, Bendigo, Monash University, North Bendigo, VIC, Australia

Kirsten Dalrymple Department of Surgery and Cancer, Imperial College London, London, UK

Deborah Davis University of Canberra and Canberra Hospital and Health Services, Canberra, ACT, Australia

Jenny Davis School of Nursing and Midwifery, La Trobe University, Melbourne, VIC, Australia

Phillip Dawson Centre for Research in Assessment and Digital Learning (CRADLE), Deakin University, Geelong, VIC, Australia

Giskin Day Imperial College London, London, UK

Roberto di Napoli Centre for Innovation and Development for Education, St. George's University of London, London, UK

Peter Dieckmann Copenhagen Academy for Medical Education and Simulation (CAMES), Center for Human Resources and Education, Herlev and Getofte Hospital, Herlev, Denmark

Department of Quality and Health Technology, Faculty of Health Sciences, University of Stavanger, Stavanger, Norway

Department of Clinical Medicine, University of Copenhagen, Copenhagen, Denmark

Michele Drummond-Young School of Nursing, McMaster University, Hamilton, ON, Canada

Walter J. Eppich RCSI SIM Centre for Simulation Education and Research, RCSI University of Medicine and Health Sciences, Dublin, Ireland

Hege Langli Ersdal Department of Quality and Health Technology, Faculty of Health Sciences, University of Stavanger, Stavanger, Norway

Department of Anaesthesiology and Intensive Care, Stavanger University Hospital, Stavanger, Norway

Yang Yann Foo Office of Education, Duke-NUS Medical School, Singapore, Singapore

Jan Forber School of Nursing and Midwifery, University of Technology Sydney, Sydney, NSW, Australia

Kirsty Forrest Faculty of Health Sciences and Medicine, Bond University, Gold Coast, QLD, Australia

Ellie Fossey Department of Occupational Therapy, Monash University – Peninsula Campus, Frankston, VIC, Australia

Brenton Franklin The Norman M. Rich Department of Surgery, Uniformed Services University & the Walter Reed National Military Medical Center "America's Medical School", Bethesda, MD, USA

Eric Gantwerker Northwell Health, Lake Success, NY, USA

Zucker School of Medicine at Northwell/Hofstra, Hempstead, NY, USA

F. J. Garivaldis School of Psychological Sciences, Monash University, Melbourne, VIC, Australia

Riya E. George Barts and The London, School of Medicine and Dentistry, Queen Mary University of London, London, UK

Contributors

Simone Gibson Deparment of Nutrition, Dietetics and Food, Medicine, Nursing and Health Sciences, Monash University, Clayton, VIC, Australia

School of Clinical Sciences, Medicine, Nursing and Health Sciences, Monash University, Clayton, VIC, Australia

Andrea Gingerich Northern Medical Program, University of Northern British Columbia, Prince George, BC, Canada

Gerard J. Gormley Centre for Medical Education, Queen's University Belfast, Belfast, UK

Suzanne Gough Faculty of Health Sciences and Medicine, Bond University, Gold Coast, QLD, Australia

Raymond Goy KKH Women and Children's Hospital, Singapore, Singapore

Andrew Grant Emeritus Professor Swansea University, Swansea, UK

Craig Greber Faculty of Health, University of Canberra, Canberra, ACT, Australia

Catherine Green Royal Victorian Eye and Ear Hospital, East Melbourne, VIC, Australia

Jennene Greenhill Rural Clinical School, University of Western Australia, Perth, WA, Australia

Lyn Gum College of Nursing and Health Sciences, Flinders University, Adelaide, SA, Australia

Pam Harvey La Trobe Rural Health School, La Trobe University, Bendigo, VIC, Australia

Margaret Hay Faculty of Education, Monash Centre for Professional Development and Monash Online Education, Monash University, Clayton, VIC, Australia

M. Heywood The Royal Children's Hospital Simulation Program, Department of Medical Education, The Royal Children's Hospital, Melbourne, VIC, Australia

Joy Higgs Professional Practice and Higher Education, Charles Sturt University, Sydney, NSW, Australia

Wayne Hing Faculty of Health Sciences and Medicine, Bond University, Gold Coast, QLD, Australia

Graeme Horton Faculty of Health and Medicine, University of Newcastle, Newcastle, NSW, Australia

Rick Iedema Centre for Team-Based Practice & Learning in Health Care, King's College London, London, UK

Ian J. Irvine University of Newcastle, Newcastle, NSW, Australia

Susan Irvine Victoria University, Melbourne, VIC, Australia

Stephen Isbel Faculty of Health, University of Canberra, Canberra, ACT, Australia

C. E. Johnson Monash Doctors Education, Monash Health and Faculty of Medicine, Nursing and Health Sciences, Monash University, Melbourne, VIC, Australia

Brian Jolly Faculty of Health and Medicine, University of Newcastle, Newcastle, NSW, Australia

School of Rural Medicine, University of New England, Armidale, NSW, Australia

Anna Jones School of Medical Education, King's College London, London, UK

Anu Kajamaa Faculty of Education, University of Oulu, Oulu, Finland

Suzie Kardong-Edgren Nursing Operations, Texas Health Resources Harris Methodist Hospital, Ft. Worth, TX, USA

J. L. Keating Department of Physiotherapy, School of Primary and Allied Health Care, Faculty of Medicine Nursing and Health Science, Monash University, Melbourne, VIC, Australia

Michelle A. Kelly Curtin School of Nursing, Curtin University, Perth, Australia

Arjun Khaira Psychiatry Department, Canberra Hospital, Canberra, ACT, Australia

Debra Kiegaldie Faculty of Medicine, Nursing and Health Sciences, Monash University; Faculty of Health Sciences and Community Studies, Holmesglen Institute and Healthscope Hospitals, Melbourne, VIC, Australia

Alec Knight School of Population Health and Environmental Sciences, King's College London, London, UK

Selena Knight School of Population Health and Environmental Sciences, King's College London, London, UK

Christopher Kowalski Oxford Health NHS Foundation Trust, Oxford, UK

Arunaz Kumar Monash University, Melbourne, VIC, Australia

Victor Lee Centre for Integrated Critical Care, The University of Melbourne, Melbourne, VIC, Australia

Austin Health, Melbourne, VIC, Australia

Kathleen Leedham-Green Medical Education Research Unit, Imperial College London, London, UK

Iris Lindemann Prideaux Centre for Health Professions Education, Flinders University, Adelaide, SA, Australia

Karen Livesay School of Health and Biomedical Sciences, College of Science, Engineering and Health, RMIT University, Melbourne, VIC, Australia

Damir Ljuhar Department of Surgical Simulation, Monash Children's Hospital, Clayton, VIC, Australia

Department of Paediatrics, School of Clinical Sciences, Faculty of Medicine, Nursing and Health Sciences, Monash University, Melbourne, VIC, Australia

Kristen MacKenzie-Shalders Master of Nutrition & Dietetic Practice, Faculty of Health Sciences & Medicine, Bond University, Gold Coast, QLD, Australia

Lynne Madden School of Medicine, Sydney, University of Notre Dame, Sydney, NSW, Australia

Ratna Makker Consultant Anaesthetist, Clinical Tutor, Clinical Director of the WISER (West Herts Initiative in Simulation Education and Research), West Herts Hospitals NHS Trust, Watford, Hertfordshire, UK

S. D. Marshall Department of Anaesthesia and Perioperative Medicine, Monash University, Melbourne, VIC, Australia

Maria Athina (Tina) Martimianakis Department of Paediatrics, Faculty of Medicine, University of Toronto, Toronto, Canada

Elie Matar Faculty of Medicine and Health, Sydney Medical School, Education Office, The University of Sydney, Sydney, NSW, Australia

Faculty of Medicine and Health, Sydney Medical School, Central Clinical School, The University of Sydney, Sydney, NSW, Australia

Richard Matthews Faculty of Health Sciences & Medicine, Bond University, Gold Coast, QLD, Australia

Janie Maxwell Nossal Institute of Global Health, University of Melbourne, Melbourne, VIC, Australia

Colin R. McHenry School of Medicine and Public Health, University of Newcastle, Newcastle, NSW, Australia

Lisa McKenna School of Nursing and Midwifery, La Trobe University, Melbourne, VIC, Australia

S. P. McKenzie School of Psychological Sciences, Monash University, Melbourne, VIC, Australia

Michelle McLean Faculty of Health Sciences & Medicine, Bond University, Gold Coast, QLD, Australia

Nancy McNaughton Wilson Centre for Research in Education, University of Toronto and University Health Network, Toronto, Canada

Sarah E. M. Meek School of Medicine, Dentistry and Nursing, University of Glasgow, Glasgow, UK

Rebecca D. Minehart Department of Anesthesia, Critical Care and Pain Medicine, Massachusetts General Hospital, Boston, MA, USA

Harvard Medical School, Boston, MA, USA

Center for Medical Simulation, Boston, MA, USA

E. K. Molloy Department of Medical Education, Melbourne Medical School, University of Melbourne, Melbourne, VIC, Australia

Christian Moro Faculty of Health Sciences and Medicine, Bond University, Gold Coast, QLD, Australia

Savannah Morrison General Medicine, John Hunter Hospital, Newcastle, NSW, Australia

Karen Muller Orthopaedic Surgery, John Hunter Hospital, Newcastle, NSW, Australia

M. Mundy School of Psychological Sciences, Monash University, Melbourne, VIC, Australia

Ramesh Mark Nataraja Monash Children's Hospital, Clayton, VIC, Australia

Department of Paediatrics, School of Clinical Sciences, Faculty of Medicine, Nursing and Health Sciences, Monash University, Clayton, VIC, Australia

Debra Nestel Monash University Institute for Health & Clinical Education, Monash University, Clayton, VIC, Australia

Department of Surgery (Austin), University of Melbourne, Parkville, VIC, Australia

Hilary Neve Peninsula Medical School, Faculty of Medicine and Dentistry, University of Plymouth, Plymouth, UK

Delwyn Nicholls College of Nursing and Health Sciences, Flinders University, Adelaide, SA, Australia

Sydney Ultrasound for Women, Sydney, NSW, Australia

Sarah O'Hare Centre for Medical Education, Queen's University Belfast, Belfast, UK

Maree O'Keefe Faculty of Health and Medical Sciences, The University of Adelaide, Adelaide, SA, Australia

Bernadette O'Neill GKT School of Medical Education, King's College London, London, UK

Marilyn H. Oermann Duke University School of Nursing, Durham, NC, USA

C. Ong KK Women's and Children's Hospital, Singapore, Singapore

Robin Orr Faculty of Health Sciences and Medicine, Bond University, Gold Coast, QLD, Australia

Janice Orrell Prideaux Centre for Health Professions Education, Flinders University, Adelaide, SA, Australia

John T. Paige Department of Surgery, Louisiana State University (LSU) Health New Orleans School of Medicine, New Orleans, LA, USA

Claire Palermo Deparment of Nutrition, Dietetics and Food, Medicine, Nursing and Health Sciences, Monash University, Clayton, VIC, Australia

Monash Centre for Scholarship in Health Education, Medicine, Nursing and Health Sciences, Monash University, Clayton, VIC, Australia

Andrew Papanikitas Nuffield Department of Primary Care Health Sciences, University of Oxford, Oxford, UK

Sang E. Park Office of Dental Education, Harvard School of Dental Medicine, Boston, MA, USA

Annette Peart Department of Occupational Therapy, Monash University – Peninsula Campus, Frankston, VIC, Australia

Carla Pecoraro Faculty of Health Sciences & Medicine, Bond University, Gold Coast, Australia

Merrolee Penman Work Integrated Learning, The University of Sydney, Camperdown, NSW, Australia

David Pinnock School of Health Sciences, University of Nottingham, Nottingham, UK

Athanasios Raikos Faculty of Health Sciences and Medicine, Bond University, Gold Coast, QLD, Australia

Christopher Renninger The Norman M. Rich Department of Surgery, Uniformed Services University & the Walter Reed National Military Medical Center "America's Medical School", Bethesda, MD, USA

Janet Richardson School of Nursing and Midwifery, University of Plymouth, Plymouth, UK

Louise Richardson Epworth Hospital, Melbourne, Australia

Martin Richardson Epworth Clinical School, University of Melbourne, Melbourne, Australia

Carielle Joy Rio Faculty of Nursing, Universitas Pelita Harapan, Karawaci, Tangerang, Indonesia

Luke Robinson Department of Occupational Therapy, Monash University – Peninsula Campus, Frankston, VIC, Australia

Robert Roseby Monash Children's Hospital, Clayton, VIC, Australia

Department of Paediatrics, School of Clinical Sciences, Faculty of Medicine, Nursing and Health Sciences, Monash University, Clayton, VIC, Australia

Jenn Salfi Nursing, Brock University, St. Catharines, ON, Canada

Aubrey L. Samost-Williams Department of Anesthesia, Critical Care and Pain Medicine, Massachusetts General Hospital, Boston, MA, USA

Harvard Medical School, Boston, MA, USA

Taylor Sawyer Division of Neonatology, Department of Pediatrics, Seattle Children's Hospital, University of Washington School of Medicine, Seattle, WA, USA

Jan Schmutz Department of Psychology, University of Zurich, Zurich, Switzerland

Ben Schram Faculty of Health Sciences and Medicine, Bond University, Gold Coast, QLD, Australia

Patricia Nanya Schwerdtle Nursing and Midwifery, Faculty of Medicine, Nursing and Health Sciences, Monash University Melbourne, Melbourne, VIC, Australia

Institute of Global Health, Heidelberg University, Heidelberg, Germany

Rana Sharara-Chami Department of Pediatrics and Adolescent Medicine, American University of Beirut, Beirut, Lebanon

Ahmed Labib Shehatta Medical Intensive Care Unit, Hamad General Hospital, Hamad Medical Corporation, Doha, Qatar

Clinical Anaesthesiology, Weill Cornell Medicine, Qatar, Doha, Qatar

Teresa Shellenbarger Department of Nursing and Allied Health Professions, Indiana University of Pennsylvania, Indiana, PA, USA

Margaret Simmons Monash Rural Health, Monash University, Churchill, VIC, Australia

Judith Singleton School of Clinical Sciences (Pharmacy), Faculty of Health, Queensland University of Technology, Brisbane, QLD, Australia

Flora A. Smyth Zahra Faculty of Dentistry, Oral & Craniofacial Sciences, King's College London, London, UK

J. Sokol The Royal Children's Hospital Simulation Program, Department of Medical Education, The Royal Children's Hospital, Melbourne, VIC, Australia

University of Melbourne Department of Paediatrics, Melbourne, VIC, Australia

Christine Sommers Universitas Pelita Harapan, Jakarta, Indonesia

Andrew I. Spielman New York University College of Dentistry, New York, NY, USA

Jesse Spurr Intensive Care Unit, Redcliffe Hospital, Redcliffe, QLD, Australia

Anne Stephenson School of Population Health & Environmental Sciences, Faculty of Life Sciences and Medicine, King's College London, London, UK

Sean Stevens Department of Surgery, Austin Health, University of Melbourne, Melbourne, VIC, Australia

Allan Stirling Faculty of Health Sciences and Medicine, Bond University, Gold Coast, QLD, Australia

Jessica Stokes-Parish Hunter Medical Research Institute, Hunter New England Local Health District, Newcastle, NSW, Australia

Zane Stromberga Faculty of Health Sciences and Medicine, Bond University, Gold Coast, QLD, Australia

Nancy Sullivan Johns Hopkins University School of Medicine and Nursing, Baltimore, MD, USA

Linda Sweet Deakin University and Western Health Partnership, Melbourne, VIC, Australia

Sandra Swoboda Johns Hopkins University School of Medicine and Nursing, Baltimore, MD, USA

Rebecca A. Szabo Department of Obstetrics & Gynaecology and Department of Medical Education, Gandel Simulation Service The Royal Women's Hospital, University of Melbourne, Melbourne, VIC, Australia

Joanna Tai Centre for Research in Assessment and Digital Learning, Deakin University, Geelong, VIC, Australia

Arianne Teherani Department of Medicine and Center for Faculty Educators, School of Medicine, University of California, San Francisco, CA, USA

Pim Teunissen Faculty of Health Medicine and Life Sciences (FHML), School of Health Professions Education (SHE), Maastricht University, Maastricht, The Netherlands

M. C. Turner School of Clinical Medicine, The University of Queensland, St Lucia, QLD, Australia

Neil Tuttle Discipline of Physiotherapy, Griffith University, Gold Coast, QLD, Australia

Ruby Walter School of Nursing and Midwifery, College of Science, Health and Engineering, LaTrobe University, Melbourne, VIC, Australia

Helena Ward Faculty of Health and Medical Sciences, The University of Adelaide, Adelaide, SA, Australia

C. J. Watling Centre for Education Research and Innovation, Schulich School of Medicine and Dentistry, Western University, London, ON, Canada

Andy Wearn Medical Programme Directorate, Faculty of Medical and Health Sciences, University of Auckland, Auckland, New Zealand

Susan M. Wearne Health Workforce Division, Commonwealth Department of Health, Canberra, ACT, Australia

Academic Unit of General Practice, Australian National University, Canberra, ACT, Australia

Jennifer M. Weller-Newton Department of Rural Health, Melbourne University, Melbourne, VIC, Australia

School of Nursing, McMaster University, Hamilton, ON, Canada

Nursing and Midwifery, Monash University, Melbourne, VIC, Australia

Emmalee Weston Austin Health, Melbourne, VIC, Australia

Marjorie L. White The Office of Interprofessional Simulation for Innovative Clinical Practice, University of Alabama at Birmingham, Birmingham, AL, USA

Departments of Pediatric Emergency Medicine and Medical Education School of Medicine, University of Alabama at Birmingham, Birmingham, AL, USA

Department of Health Services Administration School of Health Professions, University of Alabama at Birmingham, Birmingham, AL, USA

Leeroy William Eastern Health Clinical School, Monash University, Box Hill, VIC, Australia

Eloise Williams Northern Health, La Trobe University, Melbourne, VIC, Australia

Raymond Yap Department of Surgery, Cabrini Hospital, Cabrini Monash University, Malvern, Melbourne, VIC, Australia

Mong-Lin Yu Department of Occupational Therapy, School of Primary and Allied Health Care, Faculty of Medicine, Nursing and Health Sciences, Monash University, Frankston, VIC, Australia

Introduction

We believe *Clinical Education for the Health Professions* represents, supports, and advances scholarship and practice in the field of health professions education. The development process of this major reference work (MRW) is important to appreciate the contents. In this introduction, we outline the process of development, our editorial practices, and characteristics of the contributors and then provide an overview of each part.

The Development Process

One editor (Debra Nestel) was approached by the publisher to propose an MRW for clinical education. The Springer MRWs are intended to provide a "foundational starting point for students, researchers, and professionals needing authoritative, expertly validated summaries of a field, topic or concept." (1) The MRW concept is also attractive because it enables individual chapters to be updated by authors as required. Some fields move more quickly than others, and so we believe that the MRW gives authors more flexibility in revising their work to maintain currency, rather than the traditional single volume with one publication date.

One aim of the MRW was to present accessible and evidence-based content, on *what is known* about many facets of clinical education. While we acknowledged the proposed audience outlined in the Springer MRW, our main target audience was anticipated to be individuals involved in the design and delivery of educational activities for health professionals and students. Additionally, the likely audience will include researchers, policy makers, and others involved in any facet of health professional practice.

In initial development, DN identified a small editorial team with diverse experiences of working in clinical education. While a slightly daunting prospect, once the editorial team was assembled and the proposal and specific aims were outlined, the project quickly shifted to one of honor and excitement as the editorial team reached out to our networks for contributions.

The development process was fluid, with the initial proposal comprising 122 chapters across 9 parts. As we consulted with prospective authors, the proposal was adjusted to further reflect their expertise, and this meant some ideas initially

xxxi

proposed as independent chapters were combined (and, on some occasions, chapters were omitted). The COVID-19 pandemic also occurred during the commissioning process, which meant that some new chapters were added, and the entire project took longer than we had originally planned.

We were keen to promote chapters with multiple authors facilitating diverse perspectives and, sometimes even within a chapter, to have authors from different parts of the world. Our editorial team typically appointed a senior author and, with support and guidance, agreed that final decisions about author team were for the senior author to make.

We were also excited by the management of chapters through the Springer Meteor system, which is like online peer review systems for academic journals. This greatly assisted the management of the review process. All reviews were undertaken by the editorial team, with at least two reviewers for each chapter.

The depth of content varies across chapters. This was intentional, as it reflects the diversity of topics we selected for inclusion, as well as the dynamic nature of the field of health professions education. Some topics are already well established in both scholarship and practice (e.g., feedback, supervision), while others have a very wide scope (e.g., history and trends chapters), or are relatively new contributions to the field (e.g., ecological systems theory, planetary education, etc.). Among other things, these different reasons for inclusion accounted for the varying levels of depth.

The editorial team felt strongly that the final, published chapters in this MRW should reflect the professional and scholarly voices of the authors. While this is easy to claim, our experience as authors ourselves has been that editors can impose their own vision on the work so strongly that the voices of individual authors disappear. Instead, we saw our task as ensuring there was a consistent narrative to the overall MRW, as well as to each part within it, and to remind authors of what we thought would be valuable to the broad readership of the MRW. We hope that our editorial efforts have been successful, allowing authors' voices to come through in individual chapters that fit together across the work.

We are conscious of international differences in the terms used to describe health professions and their education and training. Rather than mandating language, or seeking to "standardize" terms, we left author teams to decide what was most appropriate. Our feedback encouraged authors to invite readers to consider how the terms might relate to their contexts, and to make connections across geographical, linguistic, and other contexts.

The Editorial Team

While as editors we had previously variously worked with each other, assembling as an editorial team was an exciting opportunity to bring our networks together. We have briefly sketched our profiles (see editor biographies). Our experiences are diverse, together with the places that we have worked. The institutions in which our networks have developed include large, long-established world-leading research-intensive universities associated with academic health sciences centers

Introduction

and teaching hospitals and those that are relatively new, privately funded, and vocationally focused.

Contributors to the MRW

As editors, we looked at this MRW as a chance to help broaden the diversity of voices represented in the literature, and to provide opportunities to a range of scholars at various stages in their careers and from both clinical and academic backgrounds. This is an effort that we as individuals are committed to continuing – it is never complete, of course, due to the dynamic nature of the field. We surveyed our authors near the completion of the project and found that, based on those who responded, we have contributions from scholars and researchers representing 13 countries, a near balance of clinical and other backgrounds, more than a dozen health professions, and a near balance of gender identification.

Within our author community are early-career scholars and long-time experts in their fields, and they are highly educated: over 80% of contributors reported having master's qualifications, and over 60% reported having doctoral qualifications.

While we sought a diverse mix of contributors, we had hoped to have an even more international group of authors. Especially missing were voices from the southern Americas, Africa, and Asia. This continues to be an area of weakness for the field, impoverishing our shared conversation and negatively impacting our work as educators.

About the Major Reference Work

The final version of the MRW is divided into eight parts, reflecting our attempts to meaningfully map the terrain of health professions education. Some chapters will only appear in an online version since they were unavailable at the time of publication. We focus first on the contemporary context of health professions education; shift focus to theoretical underpinnings, curriculum considerations, and approaches to supporting learning in clinical settings; a specific focus to assessment approaches; and then to evidence-based educational methods and content. Governance and other formal processes associated with the maturation of education programs are considered, including the increasing professionalization of clinical education. Finally, we look to the future drawing upon much of what has surfaced in the past and present.

Part I: The Contemporary Context of Health Professions Education

Part I comprises 17 chapters that examine the contemporary contexts of health professions education. Making meaning of contemporary practice is sometimes achieved by authors examining the origins of their practice, which is illustrated for education and training in surgery, nursing, midwifery, and dentistry. While there are similarities across professions, there are also many differences and particularities that justify the range of chapters offered. Even within medicine, the trends and contexts for specialties vary (e.g., general practice, surgery, anesthesia, etc.). We also wanted to promote health professions that are often less well represented in mainstream literature; this led to chapters on mental health and allied health. There are sometimes very specific drivers for change in the structure and process of professional education. One chapter addresses structural issues in the provision of specialty training (e.g., decentralization of surgical training), while another chapter describes the provision of education in low- and middle-income countries. Part I finishes with a chapter outlining what is likely to become mainstream in educational approaches that were developed in response to the COVID-19 pandemic.

Part II: Philosophical and Theoretical Underpinning of Health Professions Education

There are frequent calls to improve the theoretical underpinnings of health professions education. While there are many classifications of educational theories (or theories that inform educational design and practice), we sought here to include theories that are either commonly cited in educational design or research studies, and that were most likely to inform readers' practices. The theories vary in their focus on individuals or the settings in which the learning occurs and emphasize cognitive, behavioral, or constructivist approaches to learning. Each theory is likely to have most relevance to educational design and practice. From the 13 chapters, selected examples include: *mastery learning*, which has been popularized in simulation-based education for supporting the development of procedural skills; *threshold concepts and troublesome knowledge*, which has become a powerful influence in framing curriculum content; a framework from *social semiotics*, which fosters reflection of the ways in which clinicians make sense of, and the meanings they ascribe to, all facets of their work; the theoretical notion of *communities of practice*, including the role of professional identify development; *reflective practice*, such that it has become the essence of professional practice; and *ecological systems theory*, which that provides a lens to examine individuals' development within the complex and dynamic systems of clinical learning and practice. Part II ends with a critical reflection on the *philosophy of health professions education*, offering a tool for readers to deepen their thinking and practice about education.

Part III: Curriculum Considerations in Health Professions Education

Conceptually, *curriculum considerations* could cover any amount of content, so in this part of the MRW, we have had to be selective. There is also some overlap between Parts III, IV, and V, meaning that in some cases we had to make editorial decisions about where to locate the chapter content within the broader scope of the MRW. While authors developed their chapters based on our brief, we respected the authors' expertise to take the chapter in the directions they thought most appropriate. We have 14 chapters with an exciting range of considerations, such as: the role of public engagement in curricula; using simulation as substitution for clinical placements; how social media can inform curriculum design; exploring nuances in the educational design for teaching simple and complex psychomotor skills; debriefing practices in simulation-based education; and effective written feedback. Another important thread is the development of professional identity among students and trainees in the health professions. There are also explorations of contemporary issues, including the role of technology in health professions education; teaching

Introduction xxxv

about the role of diversity; and planetary health in health curricula. Other chapters cover diverse topics such as learning and teaching ethics in healthcare; the hidden curriculum and its variants; and the role of the arts and humanities.

Part IV: Supporting Learning in Clinical Settings

In Part IV, comprising 14 chapters, the authors explore ways in which learning can be supported in various settings. While principles to support learning may be similar, their application can manifest in different ways derived from many factors. A key factor is that learning in clinical settings usually takes place alongside, or as part of, healthcare service delivery. There is expert commentary provided from an interprofessional perspective, from a nursing perspective relative to learning "at the bedside" and in "the operating theater." Based on a scoping review, learning and teaching in the operating theater from a surgeon perspective is provided. The patient population can also influence opportunities to learn and teach, and we include an example from pediatrics. For clinical educators to function effectively, there are considerations for their development too. One chapter outlines the qualities of clinical educators, especially in their capacity to support learning in clinical settings, alongside care delivery. Another chapter considers well-being in health professions training. While simulation is not strictly a *clinical* setting, we have included it in this part, because the opportunity to learn using simulation often prepares healthcare professionals to optimize their learning in clinical practice. One chapter illustrates a process for setting up a simulation service in a healthcare institution, and another provides a specific example of a simulation program to promote the development of communication skills across a health service. Three chapters consider the role of interpersonal relationships and conversation in clinical settings – specifically, targeting feedback, supervision, and the ways in which trainees learn and develop through their telephone conversations. The final chapter considers underperformance, its recognition, and approaches to management.

Part V: Assessment in Health Professions Education

We have a focused part dedicated to assessment. We consider assessment as any form of measurement of individuals – and for purposes of entering, progressing, or completing professional training; final qualification within specialties; or ongoing professional registration. Nine chapters cover foundational and contemporary approaches to assessment in health professions education. There are specific examples from occupational therapy, surgery, and the impact of COVID-19 on assessment practices.

Part VI: Evidence-Based Health Professions Education: Focus on Educational Methods and Content

The 14 chapters in Part VI target evidence-based educational methods and content in health professions education. There is evidence of human-based strategies: team-based learning, peer learning, and coaching. Core practices for all health professionals are examined – patient-centered communication skills and clinical reasoning. Staying with the human focus, a chapter looks at key sociological concepts for health professions education. Contemporary technology-mediated educational methods are also explored and include examples from teaching procedural and other clinical skills, screen-based learning, and artificial intelligence.

Part VII: Governance, Quality Improvement, Scholarship, and Leadership on Health Professions Education

In Part VII, the eight chapters cover governance in health professions education. This necessarily includes considerations of quality and improvement. The role of professional bodies is explored, as well as that of scholarship in professional education. This part reflects the maturation of the profession of clinical education, and of clinical educators.

Part VIII: Future Direction for Health Professions Education

In our educational practice, we value the importance of being future-focused. Embedded in many of the earlier chapters are hints at future directions. However, in this part, it becomes the sole focus. The first chapter reflects a future world in which junior doctors will learn. The chapter offers two contrasting scenarios, and what is key to success is the importance of productive human relationships, of which one form is mentoring. While not a new concept itself, the authors describe its prominence, potentially shifting career directions for individuals based on single encounters. In an era of workforce shortages and maldistribution, human relationships become even more important to nurture trainees. If the authors' thoughtfulness reflects the future of the medical workforce, then we have much to look forward to. We also wish the authors success with their own specialty training. Two chapters are written by the same author team – first focusing on curriculums for healthcare professionals and the second on the competencies of those involved in education, in designing curriculums, and in their implementation. Technology is a focus in both chapters with implications for the curriculum itself and those who provide it.

In summary, this MRW consists of almost 90 chapters of research and scholarship, which we and the authors hope will inspire your practice, expand your thinking, support your learners and trainees, and help you to create the future of health professions education. We are already using the chapters in our own teaching, having been inspired and impressed by the quality of the authors' contributions.

When we took on this project, we had high hopes for the MRW. Those hopes have been exceeded, as we were astounded by the quality, breadth, and depth of the contributions from our colleagues around the world. Although it has been a challenge, and the project has taken longer than we originally planned, it has been our pleasure and privilege to curate this MRW.

Part I

The Contemporary Context of Health Professions Education

Medical Education: Trends and Context

1

Jennene Greenhill

Contents

Introduction	4
Growth and Changing Roles	5
Number and Distribution of Medical Schools	5
Regulation and Accreditation	5
The Changing Role of Medical Schools	6
Historical Overview	7
Trends Arising from North American Medical Education	8
Trends in Asia	9
Educational Theories and Trends in Curriculum Design	10
Teaching and Learning Trends	11
Socially Accountable Medical Schools	12
Changing Demographics of Students and Faculty	14
Future Curriculum Design Priorities and Challenges	16
Student Well-Being	16
Climate Change	17
Integration	17
Clinical Simulation	18
Interprofessional Education	19
Hidden Curriculum	19
Conclusions	20
References	22

Abstract

This chapter provides an understanding of historical trends in medical education. It begins with a discussion on recent rapid expansion of medical schools internationally. Trends in medical education are influenced by technology, specialties in clinical practice and changes in health care delivery. However, many medical schools have not addressed unmet needs for more doctors in disadvantaged

J. Greenhill (✉)
Rural Clinical School, University of Western Australia, Perth, WA, Australia

© Springer Nature Singapore Pte Ltd. 2023
D. Nestel et al. (eds.), *Clinical Education for the Health Professions*,
https://doi.org/10.1007/978-981-15-3344-0_2

communities. A critical theoretical perspective and transformative learning is needed to challenge the status quo. Socially accountable medical education has emerged as a trend that empowers communities to influence medical schools. Other related trends that take account of different contexts, can potentially transform future medical schools include: the changing demographics of students and faculty; a focus on student well-being, longitudinal integrated clerkships and experiential learning though clinical simulation, interprofessional education and climate change.

Keywords

Trends · Context · Medical · Education

Introduction

Medical education is on the rise internationally and healthcare is at the forefront in developing strong and sustainable communities. While the health status of the population in many countries is continuously improving, significant inequalities remain globally. Future challenges such as climate change, global pandemics and migrant health, the impact of new technologies and big data are rapidly changing the ways we work in health services across the spectrum from primary to acute care.

Medical studies such as history, philosophy, sociology, arts and humanities are often squeezed out of curriculum and replace by technocratic learning whereby the body is viewed as a machine, becoming ever more technical Medical schools continue to be very competitive and attract hard working, high achievers often from privileged backgrounds. After graduation, young doctors are seeking interesting, rewarding roles with work-life balance.

Accompanying the expansion of medical schools are large medical research institutes as medical research also expands. There is an insatiable appetite in the media for scientific breakthroughs and ongoing claims of innovation within institutions. However, most research investment is in pharmaceutical and biomedical research and transformative changes are rare.

There is a need for a critical theoretical approach to medical education and attention to the social processes in health and illness to reduce inequities and integrate scientific evidence with peoples' experiences. There has been exponential growth in the number of medical schools (Boulet et al. 2007) but how are medical schools responding and preparing graduates for the future?

This chapter outlines current trends in medical education and questions many of the approaches and traditional directions. Medical schools that are socially accountable have a vision for a more equitable, responsive, accessible, interprofessional health system that has practitioners who understand the local context and supports their local communities.

Growth and Changing Roles

Number and Distribution of Medical Schools

The World Health Organization (WHO) established a World Directory of Medical Schools in 1953. There were 567 medical schools in the original edition, which grew to 1,642 in the year 2000 when the directory was discontinued (Opalek and Gordon 2018). According to the World Federation for Medical Education (WFME) there are 2,919 medical schools with the highest numbers in India (392) Brazil (242) United States of America (184) and China (158) The highest growth since 2000 are in sub-Saharan Africa and the Caribbean, Southern Asia and South America (Rigby and Gururaja 2017). The highest number of graduates per population in OECD countries are in Belgium, Ireland, Latvia and Denmark (see https://data.oecd.org/healthres/medical-graduates.htm). Cuba has the highest proportion of doctors and Malawi has the lowest including most of the poorest countries in Africa such as Sierra Leone, Somalia, Liberia, Guinea and Senegal. Others include Papua New Guinea and Cambodia (see https://www.who.int/gho/health_workforce/physicians_density/en/).

There are also many private medical schools being established, with the largest numbers in India and Brazil. However, there is a global shortage of doctors. This large number of medical schools does not provide a good indication of the supply of medical graduates or the distribution of doctors. Even developed countries have underserved areas that continue to be a source of major concern internationally. Thirteen countries have no medical school and recruitment of international graduates is not a sustainable solution. However, the global trend towards expansion of medical schools may not meet the international demand for a medical workforce.

Regulation and Accreditation

The overarching goal of medical education is to provide improved health and therefore several organizations have been established to enhance the quality of medical education. The World Medical Association (WMA) and the WHO established the World Federation for Medical Education (WFME) in 1972. WFME works with member organizations in six regions to promote quality and new learning methods and teaching tools for medical education. One of their goals is to gain consensus for standards, competencies of doctors, and quality of educational institutions. WFME Global Standards cover three phases of medical education. These include basic medical education, postgraduate medical education and continuing professional development. The WFME promotes diversity to account for different contexts; changing community demands; a variety of educational needs; economic, social and cultural conditions; different disease patterns; and to encourage social responsibility. The World Directory of Medical Schools has been managed by WFME through a partnership with the Foundation for Advancement of International

Medical Education and Research (FAIMER). The quality of medical education and training is difficult to measure but through collaboration it is possible to report on significant accomplishments, harness complementary areas of strength to meet social needs (Javaid 2017).

In 2017, the USA-based National Academies of Sciences, Engineering, and Medicine (NASEM) conducted a workshop focused on graduate medical outcomes for the future. Participants reflected strong consensus in support of collecting and using outcomes data to develop better approaches to education and related policy. Although there are challenges to implementation including: identifying meaningful metrics, minimizing administrative burden, addressing privacy concerns, and recognizing variability in mission and capabilities of medical schools (Weinstein and Thibault 2018).

The curriculum and systems of medical education and entry to practice vary from place to place. Globalization and the growing mobility of health professionals has increased the need to develop processes to evaluate and authenticate medical qualifications from countries with differing systems of education, healthcare, and professional regulation. International medical graduates may not be able to practice until their qualifications are verified and they complete training and assessments. Some countries have medical training that commences after secondary school while others have mostly postgraduate courses; graduate clinical training differs in length; some require internships; and some have assessment and research requirements stipulated by medical colleges. Also, telemedicine and medical tourism raises concerns about health professionals providing care beyond the area they are licensed to practice. These trends highlight the need for shared information to gain an understanding of the different systems, knowledge, skills and competencies required for registration as a medical practitioner internationally (Opalek and Gordon 2018).

The Changing Role of Medical Schools

Traditionally, the role and purpose of medical schools in society has been to train doctors. Medical schools teach students to assess, diagnose and treat individuals who experience medical conditions and are seldom focused on population groups that have higher needs. This individualistic approach is predominant despite extensive critique of the medical model (Farre and Rapley 2017). The most significant achievements and improvements in healthcare have come from public health such as vaccinations and sanitation and primary healthcare but many courses do not have an emphasis on public health and medical graduates are less attracted to general practice than other specialties.

The United Kingdom's General Medical Council produced a curriculum framework for medical schools that outlines the standards for educating doctors and retains the medical model (Tomorrow's doctors UK General Medical Council 2009; Outcomes for graduates 2020). However, not all UK doctors progress through predicted training trajectories, and 50% leave the training pipeline following completion of foundation year one to take a break and work overseas. One fifth of those who leave do not return (Scanlan et al. 2018). The Association of American Medical Colleges similarly seeks to set a standardized approach for its 171 accredited medical schools in the USA and Canada and there is currently a push to increase diversity.

Historical Overview

Medicine practice in ancient times relied on an apprentice style of learning whereby teachers would pass forward their knowledge and skills in using instruments. For example, early Western medical schools were established in southern Italy in the ninth century (Della Monica et al. 2013). Medicine was learned though books and experimentation. This approach is inherent in the Hippocratic Oath (Fulton 1953). In Europe, from the middle ages until the mid-nineteenth century, medical practitioners were either academic doctors with theoretical knowledge or practical surgeons who may have belonged to a guild where they learnt their craft.

During the rise of the industrial revolution, scientific medicine formed the basis for growth in medical education and specialty disciplines emerged. Abraham Flexner revolutionized medical schools in the USA and visited European medical schools. There was an international movement towards standardized curricula, internships and examinations (Duffy 2011). By the 1920s, the standard curriculum was altered to include a holistic approach and students were offered the opportunity to plan and select electives and independent research. However, most undergraduate courses retain the foundations such as anatomy, physiology and biochemistry then introduce medical specialties. Students are taught predominately in laboratories and lecture format and assessed by disciplines such as surgery, obstetrics, psychiatry etc.

The problem is that as disciplines continue to create more and more sub-specialties, the curriculum becomes increasingly crowded. Moreover, medical education research demonstrated that didactic formats, whist efficient, are not effective in developing clinical reasoning and assessment of clinical skills and interprofessional practice are now vital graduate qualities. Norman (2005) states that "the most critical aspect of learning is not the acquisition of a particular strategy or skill, nor is it the availability of a particular kind of knowledge. Rather, the critical element may be deliberate practice with multiple examples which, on the hand, facilitates the availability of concepts and conceptual knowledge (i.e., transfer) and, on the other hand, adds to a storehouse of already solved problems."

There is considerable variability in medical training internationally. However, there are three dominant models: the British model, which influences Commonwealth countries; the North American model, which is being adopted by many emerging schools; and the European model, which requires European countries to comply with the European Union rules and regulations. All prospective medical students complete secondary school and then either directly enter medical school, or complete a bachelor's degree, followed by internship and residency (with sometimes mandatory service being required). Models differ by the courses required for training pathways and most countries require between 10 and 15 years of training (O'Brien et al. 2018).

Trends Arising from North American Medical Education

William Osler (1849–1919) was the first to establish structured postgraduate residency training at Johns Hopkins Hospital. This postgraduate training model spread internationally and became the standard following WWII. Courses were shortened during World War II, with pre-medical training being required for a 4-year course that encompassed the physical and mental treatment and prevention of disease and expanding research activity in most medical schools. Post-war saw many more medical schools established, and graduate medical education became more prevalent; also, conferences and journals were introduced to promote and improve medical education (Irby 2011). Field's paper (1957) also outlined the widespread use of small group learning beginning with a case presentation by students followed by discussion of the key concepts guided by the instructor.

As courses evolved during the twentieth century, the curriculum has become longer, procrustean, and not learner centered (Field 1957). Curriculum changes included more electives with a focus on social and economic health issues. One solution to a long, overcrowded curriculum was the requirement for pre-medical courses. Premedical education has been a source of much debate. Medical educators grapple with whether students are well prepared and have the cognitive ability and scientific knowledge to undertake medical studies. The integration of pre-clinical and clinical teaching has become increasingly important. Medical knowledge and clinical competencies is increasingly a focus, giving rise to the competency-based medicine education (CBME) movement (Custers and Ten Cate 2018).

CBME has become a dominant approach to medical education in many countries. CBME has a 50-year history originating in theories such as outcome-based education and mastery learning. Medical regulatory bodies in Canada, the USA, and other countries have embraced CBME. CBME focuses on specific domains of competence applicable in workplace training (McGaghie et al. 1978). CBME is now widely used in postgraduate training in Canada and the USA with the introduction of the *CanMEDS* framework, which is the Canadian Medical Education Directives for Specialists and of the ACGME Project (Accreditation Council for Graduate Medical Education in the USA). Critiques of the CBME movement are based on the varying interpretations of what it is, and how it is being applied (Ten Cate 2017).

Another trend during the 1960s to the 1990s to deal with overcrowded curricula was Problem-Based Learning (PBL). PBL involves using patient problems as the basis for educating doctors, and was pioneered at McMaster University in Canada, and continues to be popular internationally (Hillen et al. 2010; Barrows 1993).

The Carnegie Foundation for the Advancement of Teaching commissioned a report published in 2010. The authors made four recommendations for reform drawing on contemporary educational innovations and research: (1) standardize learning outcomes while individualizing the learning process, (2) integrate formal knowledge with clinical experience, (3) imbue habits of inquiry and improvement to achieve lifelong learning and excellence, and (4) explicitly cultivate the formation of professional identity (Irby 2011).

Contemporary medical schools have a strong focus on early exposure to clinical contexts and seek students with emotional intelligence, interpersonal, communication and social skills. Many schools have adapted their selection processes but most still predominately rely on high academic achievement. Some schools are using situational judgement tests that present job-related situations and possible responses to these situations or video scenarios. Applicants indicate the appropriate response. The origin of SJTs stems from civil service and military examinations (Lievens et al. 2008). The multiple mini interview (MMI), developed at McMaster University Medical School in the early 1990s, has also become popular as a selection process. They are said to be valid and reliable and do not bias against gender, race age or socioeconomic status. However, they do not correlate with personality inventories such as emotional intelligence, which are also being used for selection and assessment in some schools (Rees et al. 2016).

Emotional intelligence (EI) is a concept from organizational theory that has been adopted because EI is applicable to medical education. EI is defined as the ability to recognize, understand, and manage emotions in yourself and in others. EI aims to promote a culture of professionalism, improve interpersonal communications, and enable conflict resolution. Therefore, it is applicable to team-based healthcare. EI proponents suggest that this approach assists learners to build consensus among multidisciplinary teams and seeks to change attitudes and behaviors that may lead to improved patient safety and clinical outcomes (Roth et al. 2019).

Trends in Asia

Significant population growth in Asia during the late twentieth and early twenty-first centuries has resulted in an increasing gap in access to healthcare and economic development and has also led to an increased number of medical schools throughout Asia. However, there are variable standards of education and not all have salutogenic benefits for their countries (Shehnaz 2011).

Medical education throughout Asia was originally influenced by religions such as Buddhism, Hinduism and Muslim traditions. In India, western medicine was introduced by the Portuguese during the 1600s, then via English colonialism. Post-independence, some schools reintroduced traditional naturopathy and yoga and more recently competency-based curriculum has been introduced through national regulation (Anshu and Supe 2016).

Japan has approximately 79 medical schools and has been largely influenced by the American model of medical education. During the twentieth century, Japanese medical schools have undergone significant changes with the introduction of an integrated curriculum though PBL and clinical education followed by a national licensing examination (Tadahiko 2006). Similarly, Thailand has been influenced by the American model while Indonesia has Dutch influences. Since the 1960s, many countries in Southeast Asia have begun to redesign medical schools to suit national priorities because graduates tend to establish practices in major cities rather than where they are need in rural areas (Hani 1962). Bleakley et al. (2008) argue that this pot-colonialism is "unreflecting dissemination of conceptual frameworks and practices which assume that 'metropolitan West is best'."

In China during 2017, the State Council of China launched a plan to revolutionize medical education and promote collaboration between medical education and practice. The goal is to train more qualified medical professionals to improve public healthcare, for a "Healthy China 2030." However, with the low professional status of Chinese doctors, frequent incidents of violence against them, long working hours and a heavy workload, and an unsatisfactory income, attracting medical students has become a challenge. Studies have found that 78% of physicians work more than 8 h a day, and 7% of physicians work more than 12 h a day, but the average annual income of Chinese physicians in 2015 was 77,000 yuan (about $12,360). There is a mindset that medical technology is a priority and growing expectations among the public. The new medical education reform aims to "foster the humanistic spirt of medical students in order to improve public healthcare in China" (Song et al. 2017). A seminal paper in medical education by Frenk et al. (2010) challenged the dominant neoliberal approach to medical education highlighting the inequities in healthcare. They argue that fragmented, outdated, and static curricula and the predominant hospital orientation at the expense of primary care produce ill-equipped graduates. There is a need for a thorough re-examination of health professional education. This Lancet Commission involved 20 professional groups and academic leaders. The proposed changes are for transformative learning through instructional reforms and interdependence through institutional reforms (Frenk et al. 2010).

Educational Theories and Trends in Curriculum Design

Medical education has increasing emphasis on sociocultural theories that recognize it as a complex transformative process with the aim of preparing graduates who can work in a wide range of clinical contexts (Mann 2010). Medical education has been critiqued for its atheoretical approach to curriculum design (Prideaux 2008). More recently, there has been a shift to acknowledge the influences of learning theories such as Constructivism (Vygotsky 1978), that views learning is a socially constructed process that builds new knowledge on the foundations previous understandings. Cognitive and behavioral theories influence the way medical students are assessed and social learning theories (Bandura 1977) underpin the trends towards experiential learning (Kolb 1984) and the importance of contexts and clinical placements through situated learning and communities of practice (Lave and Wenger 1991; Wenger 1998).

Healthcare systems and the educational culture of medical schools tend to have an individualistic approach to competence. There is emphasis on the individual learner and their knowledge, abilities and values in teaching and assessment. In reality, an individual's competence is interdependent with the healthcare team and clinical context. A collectivist discourse of competence reflects the complex nature of the health system and includes share knowledge and teamwork. "Collective competence draws on social learning theory with its premise that knowledge is constructed through participation. This focus is particularly appropriate in apprenticeship or work-based learning settings like medicine, where what is 'learned' is not in the complete control of teacher or learner; it emerges as a consequence of the social interaction, which is shaped by the physical, social and organizational context" (Lingard 2009).

Professionalism and ethics have also become important fields in medical education and many students have activities that encourage reflective learning and practice (Schön 1983). Over the last five decades, medical ethics has become an increasingly important aspect of medical education. An ethical doctor is more likely to be trustworthy. In the UK, USA, and in Australia, guidelines for designing, implementing, and assessing ethics education in medical schools have been produced. Medical students often perceive ethics as a "fluffy" discipline (Lovy et al. 2010). However, ethics assessment and having the right role models is essential for the development of professionalism and leadership. Students need to demonstrate compassion, integrity, and respect for others; responsiveness to patient needs that supersedes self-interest; respect for patient privacy and autonomy; accountability to patients, society and the profession; sensitivity and responsiveness to a diverse patient (Giubilini et al. 2016).

Medical school assessments tend to focus on testing knowledge and skills. Students in most schools also develop their confidence and competence through clinical simulations and by being immersed in clinical practice. It has been suggested that many assessments used by medical schools have poor predictive measures of performance, however scores on national qualifying examinations are significant predictors of quality-of-care, problems based on regulatory, practice-based peer assessment. Nevertheless, medical schools need to assess students aligned with changing health care and workplace requirements. Therefore, it is important for schools to continuously improve assessment methods, so we can maximize the quality of graduates upon completion (Hamdy et al. 2006; Wenghofer et al. 2009).

Most medical courses are highly structured and continue to deliver content in didactic formats. Courses include development of clinical reasoning and have adopted experiential learning through clinical simulation and aspects of self-directed learning with the flipped class room approach and learning portfolios becoming the norm.

Medical education should be a transformative learning journey that fundamentally shift the perspective of medical students. Transformative learning theory is underpinned by a critical perspective that proposes that individuals must reflect on life events to change their beliefs or behaviours (Van Schalkwyk et al. 2019).

Teaching and Learning Trends

Most of the trends in teaching and learning have developed in response to changing knowledge and expectations and many changes have been underpinned by theoretical approaches. These include: *PBL, case-based learning, team-based learning,* and *e-learning* strategies. Assessment methods have been widely debated with varying combinations of *formative and summative assessment*. Exams continue to use *multiple-choice questions*, and some rely on short answer questions. Structured clinical assessments such as *objective structured clinical examination (OSCEs) and mini clinical evaluation exercise (mini-CEX)* have become common in medical courses (Thomas et al. 2016). Students learn *clinical skills in health services, and they are usually scaffolded through simulation* scenarios and *simulated patient interactions* (Lin and Hwang 2019). The majority of medical courses remain true to their traditional roots, but most adopt learning technologies to improve efficiency.

Learning technologies, online learning, and social media are prevalent in a digital era where students routinely explore and answer self-generated questions with information literally at their fingertips. Students enthusiastically embrace computer-based learning such as holographic anatomy to augment dissection of cadavers. The "flipped classroom" is beginning to be the new normal, with self-directed reading assignments completed before attending class so that classroom time can be devoted to interactive small group learning (Lin and Hwang 2019).

Learning technologies and the use of smartphones for teaching and learning among the medical community is increasing day by day and will continue to develop, because medical knowledge now exceeds the storage capacity of the human brain. Yet medical education still remains based on a model of information acquisition and application. This information overload for our learners is further complicated by the fact that skill sets now must include collaborating with and managing artificial intelligence (AI) applications (Wartman and Combs 2019). Clinical practice is being shaped by big data, whereby analytics can generate diagnostic and treatment recommendations, and assign confidence ratings to those recommendations. Medical curricula should focus on knowledge management rather than acquisition and recall, students need to understand how to use AI and synthesize information but the core skills are communication and empathy (Latif et al. 2019; Davis 2018).

Socially Accountable Medical Schools

It is time for medical schools to move beyond a narrow focus on a technocratic approach to training towards preparing a new generation of medical graduates with social values, knowledge and skills to work in areas of need. Enlightened medical schools have shifted towards a more person-centered and preventive approach whereby students gain an understanding of the local health needs of the population and make a genuine contribution as part of the healthcare team. There are rich learning opportunities in underserved urban and rural communities where students are welcomed and well supported to maximize their learning. Rather than just training doctors in hospitals or in large buildings next to these hospitals, medicine should also be learned in a range of contexts including disadvantaged communities. Only when students are immersed in these communities, can they gain an understanding of the health challenges that impact on the most vulnerable community members. Integration is a buzzword in medical education, there are many silos but a medical school without walls is a vision that has been brought to fruition in socially accountable medical schools (Boelen and Heck 1995).

A definition of social accountability for medical schools by the WHO in 1995 states, "The obligation to direct their education, research, and service activities towards addressing the priority health needs of the community, region, and/or nation they have a mandate to serve. The priority health needs are to be identified jointly by governments, healthcare organizations, health professionals, and the public" (Murray et al. 2012).

Social accountability has been attracting considerable attention and gathering momentum. It is becoming a focus for curriculum reform because it enables medical education to attract students from local communities and therefore reflects the local demographics. These students have a commitment to work in underserved communities and start with a good understanding of health needs, so they can be responsive to health priorities of communities (Woolley et al. 2018).

Socially accountable medical schools increase the health workforce in areas of need and can improve health outcomes. For example, medical graduates who graduated from socially accountable medical schools in communities in The Philippines significantly strengthened child and maternal health services resulting in positive child health outcomes (Larkins et al. 2018). The characteristics of students that are predictive of practice in a rural location are: those who come from a rural or low-income background, and medical school training in a rural area. A large study of socially accountable medical schools showed that respondents from the Philippines and Africa who have a high income and urban backgrounds are more likely to emigrate following graduation (Boelen and Woollard 2011).

Many medical schools have mission statements saying that they "serve communities" but they face the challenge of providing evidence that what they do actually leads to improved health outcomes (Larkins et al. 2013). Health professional schools that have a commitment to social accountability have developed an evaluation framework founded the Training for Health Equity Network (THEnet). This tool was developed collaboratively and is openly accessible, see https://thenetcommunity.org/the-framework/ (Global Consensus for Social Accountability of Medical Schools 2020).

A key to socially accountable medical education is the development of partnerships. Accountability requires community involvement in planning and implementing research projects, providing clinical service to the community through community-based placements and offer continuing medical education especially in rural and regional areas (Hennen 1997). Through partnerships medical schools have a major role to play in influencing the changes in the healthcare system. Social accountability is essential in shaping the future of medical education, research, and healthcare in response to present and future societal needs.

Rourke (2006) outlines the social accountability vision for Canadian medical schools:

- The development of a clear and shared vision of the healthcare system and of the healthcare providers (both individuals and institutions) of the twenty-first century, a vision that will have to be clearly articulated and constantly revised to respond to changing needs
- The optimal preparation of future practitioners to respond to population needs

- The establishment and promotion of innovative practice patterns to better meet individual and community needs
- The reinforcement of partnerships with other stakeholders, including academic health centers, governments, communities, and other relevant professional and lay organizations
- Advocacy for the services and resources needed for optimal patient care
- The definition and clarification of the concept of social accountability, and the dissemination of methods for measuring responsiveness to societal needs
- The inclusion of the concept of social accountability in the accreditation process of medical schools and other health institutions (Rourke 2006)

Recently, an increasing number of medical schools have developed a social accountability mandate seek students who have the and pro-social qualities and diverse characteristics such as self-efficacy, and with a passion to work in under-served communities as confirmed by the Global consensus for social accountability of medical schools (https://healthsocialaccountability.org/ 2020) (Global Consensus for Social Accountability of Medical Schools 2020).

Changing Demographics of Students and Faculty

The trend to increase gender, ethnic, and racial diversity in medical education is getting stronger, not least because of a drive to ensure that doctors are reflective of the populations they serve. However, the socioeconomic diversity gap continues to widen with more than 48% of medical students from the top income quintile and less than 6% from the bottom quintile. Medical school is unaffordable for most of the population and most students are from privileged backgrounds but fortunately some students who come from disadvantaged backgrounds persevere and succeed with scholarships and support (Le 2017).

There are consistent trends across medical schools internationally in the interplay between race and socioeconomic status. There are structural barriers to inter-generational socioeconomic mobility and subsequent impact on educational attainment. In the UK, students in the highest social stratum are 30 times more likely to gain access to medical school than those from low socioeconomic backgrounds (Baugh et al. 2019). This socioeconomic divide has a compounding effect as students seeking high incomes are interested in high status specialties rather than those were there in most need such as family medicine/general practice gerontology, and psychiatry (Wilkins et al. 2018).

While research has confirmed that growing up in a rural setting is a strong predictor of future rural practice, there has been little change in the recruitment of rural medical students internationally (Walker et al. 2012). One US study found a 15-year decline in the number of rural medical students, culminating in rural students' representing less than 5% of all incoming medical students in 2017 (Shipman et al. 2019). The Australian Government Rural Clinical School Program funds 18 clinical schools (RCSs) and requires them to have at least 25% of students

1 Medical Education: Trends and Context

from a rural background. A national study found that having a rural background and at least 12 months training in a rural area is strongly associated with rural location of practice (McGirr et al. 2019).

The most notable changes in medical education has been in gender balance. In the USA, the proportion of graduating women medical students has increased on average 0.5% per year from 1994 to 2014 and this trend is mirrored in other western countries. Women are attracted to particular specialties and fewer take up surgical training, but numbers are increasing. In the UK, for example, only 3% are of consultant surgeons are women (Skinner and Bhatti 2019). Moreover, in senior positions in specialty colleges women are significantly underrepresented (Silver et al. 2019).

In medical schools, women make up less than 10% of professors. Despite improvements over the past 20 years, there are still inequities for trainees and in academic leadership that require significant culture change (Abelson et al. 2016).

Cultural diversity among medical students is changing but is still not representative of cultural differences in communities. A recent cross-sectional study from 2002 to 2017 on race and ethnicity of medical schools in the USA found that the number of medical school applicants increased 53%, from 33,625 to 51,658, and the number of graduates increased 29.3%, from 16,488 to 21,326 between 2002 and 2017. However, African American, Hispanic, and American Indian and Alaskan students remain underrepresented in medical schools despite medical education diversity accreditation guidelines implemented in 2009. They recommend more robust policies and programs to create a physician workforce that is demographically representative of the population (Ahmed et al. 2018). Research shows that international medical graduates are more likely to enter primary care specialties and practice in underserved areas (Mian et al. 2019).

A key priority for medical schools internationally must be Indigenous medical student recruitment and support to graduation and beyond. One successful model based on social accountability is the Northern Ontario School of Medicine (NOSM), a Canadian medical school with the mandate to recruit students whose demographics reflect the service region's population. One of the major challenges in attracting First Nations students was their relatively low, Grade Point Average (GPA) but the MMI scores resulted in a higher proportion of mature female students. Community engagement is vitally important (Strasser et al. 2018).

Indigenous populations suffer from entrenched health inequities primarily due to the effects of colonization, racism, and marginalization. A process named "two-eyed seeing" from Canadian Mi'kmaw Elders, provides opportunity for medical educators to prioritize indigenous worldviews. Two-Eyed Seeing assists students to use both eyes to see western and indigenous knowledges and ways of knowing (see http://www.integrativescience.ca/Principles/TwoEyedSeeing/). The benefits of "two-eyed seeing" will be a future workforce who are prepared to meet the needs of vulnerable populations and become change agents for health equity (McKivett et al. 2020). Indigenous health also requires alternative ways of learning whereby students can be immersed in the community to gain a deep understanding of the culture and ways of knowing about healthcare (Henderson et al. 2015).

Medical education may be a relatively new field of research but there is good evidence emerging that the student body should be as diverse as the population they serve. Many potential benefits can be realized by changing the demographic to include students with lower socioeconomic status, gender balance, rural backgrounds, race, and ethnic differences in medical school cohorts. These benefits include: cultural awareness, advocacy, empathy and a deep understanding and willingness to work with people who come from underserved populations and their health challenges (Whitla et al. 2003).

Future Curriculum Design Priorities and Challenges

Student Well-Being

Mental health is a major issue for medical students and graduates. Some student may not disclose pre-existing mental health problems, while others succumb to the rigorous nature of medical education, which triggers depression and anxiety. This is further exacerbated by a low uptake of mental health services by medical students. Many students are resilient but even they rely on bravado. Research has found up to 45% of polled students perceived that their mental health worsened during medical school and 62% of students would not disclose their mental condition (Castle et al. 2019; Waheed-Ul-Rahman and Mills 2019).

Fatigue is often a factor that leads to burnout and medical errors. Research suggests that junior doctors perceive fatigue as a surmountable personal burden rather than an occupational hazard. Unprecedented levels of sleep deprivation combined with uncertainty and confusion can lead to significant fatigue during training. Trainees believe that fatigue contributes to three distinct threats that evoke different coping strategies: (i) threat to personal health, managed by perseverance; (ii) threat to patients, managed by faith in the system, and (iii) threat to professional reputation, managed by stoicism (Taylor et al. 2019).

Internationally, there is early deterioration of the psychosocial health of medical students. Students who find it difficult to distance themselves from work, have a lack of regular physical activity are particularly at risk. Therefore, medical schools need to implement interventions that prevent a harmful stressful curriculum and support for students as early as possible during medical education. Interventions should target individuals, the learning environment and the clinical setting. Such interventions will have a sustainable positive effect on the quality of patient care (Kötter 2019).

One potential solution is to offer part-time and more flexible medical courses that may lead to improved wellbeing of medical students. This has been demonstrated in the Netherlands where medical training has become increasingly individualized. Working hours are restricted by the European Working Time Directive. Trainees who choose part-time can simply extend the length of their program. The extension period can be used to develop specific competencies, complete an elective rotation or research, or explore a focus area. Flexible training is feasible and improving work–

life balance a necessity. However, attention must be paid to ensure they gain adequate experience and competencies and to maintain continuity of care to ensure that high-quality patient care is provided (Hoff et al. 2018).

Climate Change

Climate change has significant implications for medical education, and medical schools need to comprehensively address the topic of climate change as it pertains to human health in both the undergraduate and postgraduate curriculum. The WHO projects approximately 250,000 deaths annually due to climate change between 2030 and 2050 (Finkel 2019). The changing global climate poses major risks to the health of individuals and communities. Vulnerable groups such as rural, remote, and Indigenous populations suffer the health consequences of climate change. Climate change can have direct effects of on health with higher mortality and morbidity from extreme weather events, accidents and trauma, psychosocial stress, homelessness, or damage to housing and basic infrastructure. Increased incidence of vector-borne infectious disease; poor air quality can cause asthma, cardiovascular and respiratory illness and death. Noncommunicable diseases will rise due to retreating ice and rising sea levels leading to population displacement; increased risk of food and waterborne illnesses; and drought, fires and floods reduce food and water security. The integration of climate-change-related topics with training of essential physician skills in a rapidly changing environment is important and feasible because courses already address the social determinates of health so many health topic areas already exist in medical school curricula in which climate change education can be incorporated (Saraswat et al. 2016; Wellbery et al. 2018).

Integration

Clinical experience often now starts in the first week of medical school, with integrated basic and clinical science learning building toward longitudinal clerkships in later years. Longitudinal integrated clerkships (LICs) emphasize continuity with patients, preceptors, peers, and health systems. Research on students who undertake LICs demonstrate benefits for the community, patients, students, clinicians, and health services. Internationally the number of LICs is increasing (Mazotti et al. 2019; Poncelet and Hirsh 2016).

However, the uptake of LICS has not been rapid and recent curricular developments have embraced Entrustable Professional Activities (EPAs). EPAs enable educators to make competency-based decisions on the level of supervision required by trainees. EPAs are units of professional practice, defined as tasks or responsibilities that are entrusted to the unsupervised execution by a trainee once he or she has attained sufficient specific competence in specialist disciplines (Ten Cate et al. 2015).

Medical education should not be based solely upon a competency model. Current debates through a critical theoretical lens, contribute to a discourse of infallibility of

CBME that silences critique and reinforces traditional power structures in medical education. Competences may be a useful way to categorize simple, technical skills for deliberate practice, but they fail to accommodate the sophisticated clinical reasoning processes, discourse, and reflective practice that clinicians continuously rely upon. Researchers suggest that if CBME is not able to be questioned, only certain groups with power have the authority to determine competencies and there is a need to promote a broader understanding of CBME design, development, and implementation (Boyd et al. 2018). Evans et al. (2019) propose there are opportunities for medical schools to use longitudinal clerkships as a lens through which EPAs can be effectively evaluated.

Clinical Simulation

Clinical Simulation has been long used in medical education. Centuries ago, intricate models were used to help teach anatomy and physiology and in training in obstetrics and many surgical disciplines. There are beautiful wax models in Bologna and Pavia, and life size bronzes were used in China to teach acupuncture, and despite Flexner's recommendations to use simulation, there was a decline in medical schools during the twentieth century. Simulation is vital for training students about quality and safety and to prevent patents being used for students to practice on as they develop clinical skills (Owen 2012).

Many medical schools and hospitals have been investing in building simulation centers and in virtual reality simulators, serious games and high technology simulators such as mannequins. Additionally, part-task trainers have been rapidly adopted and simulated patients are largely embedded in curricula (Rosen 2008). These resources are not only expensive they need to be continuously updated to reflect current practice. Faculty development is also required so that they can keep abreast of medical education trends.

There is extensive research on the effectiveness of simulation (McGaghie et al. 2010). A systematic review reported that few simulation-based studies have reported the cost of simulation training compared with other instructional approaches is comparable although more research is needed (Zendejas et al. 2013). Internationally, there is increasing consensus on the way simulation is integrated in medical curricula. Simulation education has moved away from a technocratic approach, focused on emergency, surgical and critical care rather than primary care contexts and developing technical skills rather than non-technical skills and interprofessional teamwork. There has been some critique of the assumptions that underpin simulation challenging claims of authenticity because many scenarios ignore or avoid the messy contexts and complex relationships (Bleakley 2018). In simulations, scenarios presenting problems are often oversimplified and bodies are dehumanized and compartmentalized despite the high incidence of multi morbidities and goals of holistic care. This oversimplification is rationalized by claims of cognitive overload and providing a safe learning environment. Another critique of simulation-based education is that it perpetuates the socioeconomic inequalities. As an increasing number of new medical schools are established in developing countries, there are challenges including equipment costs, difficulty in procurement, lack of context-appropriate curricula, unreliable power, limited local teaching capacity, and lack of coordination (Bulamba et al. 2019).

Interprofessional Education

Interprofessional education (IPE) can result in transformative learning and is fundamental to an understanding of interprofessional practice in health services. Threshold concepts that were identified in one study included: broadening perspectives on healthcare practice; strengthening sense of professional self; gaining an appreciation of holistic patient care; and actioning holistic, patient-centered healthcare (Morgan et al. 2019).

There is a need to increase research on interprofessional education and to demonstrate that it improves healthcare delivery and patient outcomes (Reeves et al. 2013). Health professional educational programs find IPE difficult to implement and maintain. IPE is difficult to schedule and requires a commitment from more than individual champions towards a collaborative learning culture. Also, IPE requires resources to map and redesign the curricula of multiple courses and ongoing support for successful implementation. A common educational lexicon of competencies and learning outcomes for IPE is being worked on across faculties and accrediting bodies (Steven et al. 2017).

IPE is included in accreditation standards from several healthcare professions educational programs. A recent study suggests that there was little consistency in the terminology and learning outcomes, which are regulated by accreditation standards, conflict with implementation of IPE initiatives. Shared language and mental models for IPE are needed to normalize learning outcomes (Stoddard et al. 2019).

Health professionals usually work in collaborative teams and to be successful in interprofessional healthcare, medical students need to be exposed to interprofessional learning early in their education. However. IPE is not often a priority in medical courses. Interprofessional education is limited to some mere collaborative learning. A US study of medical schools found that 13 reported teaching IPE but there was significant variation. They found the most common collaboration is between medical and nursing schools (93%). Of those with a shared curriculum, the most prevalent included some integrated modules (57%). Small group IPE activities represented the majority (64%), and simulation-based learning, games and role-play (71%) were the most utilized learning methods (West et al. 2016).

Hidden Curriculum

Hafferty (1998) defined the hidden curriculum as "*a set of influences that function at the level of organizational structure and culture*." The hidden curriculum refers to the implicit norms, behaviors attitudes, and underlying values that are imbued in the culture of the medical school. A scoping review uncovered 3,747 articles relating to the hidden curriculum in medical education. This review found the term "hidden curriculum" remains ambiguous "shrouded in a fog of vague definitions and widespread application" (Lawrence et al. 2018).

The hidden curriculum permeates the learning environment such that students and postgraduate trainees learn not only skills and knowledge from teachers as part of an explicit and formal curriculum, they are socialized to become part of the culture of the learning and clinical contexts. The hidden curriculum can undermine psychological safety in these contexts. Psychological safety stems from a feeling that individuals are comfortable expressing and being themselves, "comfortable sharing concerns and mistakes without fear of embarrassment, shame, ridicule, or retribution" (Torralba et al. 2020).

The hidden curriculum can also erode empathy. In medical practice empathy is described as "detached concern" and viewed as a key element of professionalism. Some studies question how empathy changes during undergraduate training as a result of the subtle influences of the hidden curriculum. The context of the learning environment is vital for fostering empathy. Jeffrey's (2019) exploration of medical school culture revealed several factors which students described as inhibiting their empathy. These factors include a competitive culture where there is pressure to conform and a lack of autonomy. The hierarchy within the medical school contributed to this conforming culture. As consequence of this conforming culture was that students were inclined to keep silent for fear that their lack of medical knowledge would be exposed in their clinical teaching. Others expressed concerns that the conforming culture might inhibit some students from seeking support (Jeffrey 2019).

To understand how the socialization of medical students affects their professional identity formation a study explored how the hidden curriculum influences them during their clinical years. The hidden curriculum influences professional identity formation through three domains: (1) Speeding up – Repetition without reflection ends in a lack of awareness of professional identity formation; (2) Emotional dissonance in the context of negative role modelling; and (3) the conflict between personal and professional life (Silveira et al. 2019).

Further medical education research is needed to address the hidden curriculum. The hidden curriculum may be useful tool for reflection and debate from a critical perspective about issues such as power, patient centeredness, personal resilience, and career pathways in medicine. One solution is by revealing and naming the hidden curriculum, students can be aware of its existence and understand its potential impact. Supporting students to think critically about their experiences and ethical dilemmas may empower them to choose which messages to take on board (Neve and Collett 2018).

Conclusions

The dominant biomedical approach is a deeply entrenched in medical education. Medical school culture is based on a particular form of positivist, scientific logic that embraces rationalism, certainty, and objectification. The culture celebrates competitiveness, heroism, and intellect. A biomedical worldview perpetuates deterministic ways of thinking about sociocultural health disparities as an accepted status quo. Medical schools can, however, advance health equity and educate future health professionals who are responsive to marginalized and vulnerable communities by adopting critical pedagogy and theory (Cavanagh et al. 2019).

Critical theories can help to question underlying assumptions. The application of critical theories to medical education and education research can be a powerful means of changing how medicine is taught and whose voices are heard. The aim should be learning environments where individuals of all races, genders, sexual orientations, and social classes feel recognized, heard, and supported and workplaces that are safe for both practitioners and patients. "Understanding power and privilege has the potential to allow practitioners to connect with their students, humanise their collective practice, and provide better care to their patients" (Sharma 2019).

Traditionally, medical training had little contact with patients. Students rarely had placements outside the hospital or university setting. The scientific content did not include population or social sciences and prioritized laboratory and anatomy dissection sessions instead of consultation skills or clinical simulations.

The global impacts of medical education include: the brain drain of clinicians from under resourced countries and continuing inequalities of access as a consequence of the maldistribution of workforce between rural and urban areas and communities that have high levels of poverty compared to more affluent communities that have better access to health services. Private medical schools are increasing, and economic imperatives are driving the delivery of online learning, while the cost of medical education has increased exponentially. There are many future challenges including: diversity, climate change, integration of the curriculum, interpersonal education, and gaining a better understanding of the hidden curriculum. The underlying core values of medical education are to serve with integrity, compassion, and respect for others and to collaborate for the delivery of quality care. If medicine remains a socially accountable profession, the healthcare needs of underserved populations can be met equitably.

Medical courses that are socially accountable are underpinned by transformative learning theory. They select students from diverse backgrounds, integrate theory and practice, have early exposure to clinical contexts, use a constructivist learning approach that is inclusive, reflective, and responsive to students learning needs. The curriculum is predominantly applied methods such as problem-based and case-based learning so that learners develop clinical knowledge and skills, also preface professionalism, ethics, and leadership; frequent opportunities for experiential simulation education and immerse students in longitudinal integrated clerkships in acute, ambulatory, and community settings.

Medical students and educators are some of the most inspiring, optimistic, and courageous people. Our collective voices can shape the future of medical education towards global equality, and health for those who are most vulnerable.

References

Abelson JS, et al. The climb to break the glass ceiling in surgery: trends in women progressing from medical school to surgical training and academic leadership from 1994 to 2015. Am J Surg. 2016;212(4):566–72.e1.

Ahmed AA, Hwang W-T, Thomas CR Jr, Deville C Jr. International medical graduates in the US physician workforce and graduate medical education: current and historical trends. J Grad Med Educ. 2018;10(2):214–8. https://doi.org/10.4300/JGME-D-17-00580.1.

Anshu, Supe A. Evolution of medical education in India: the impact of colonialism. J Postgrad Med. 2016;62(4):255–9. https://doi.org/10.4103/0022-3859.191011.

Bandura A. *Social learning theory*. Englewood Cliffs, NJ: Prentice Hall. 1977.

Barrows H. An overview of the uses of standardized patients for teaching and evaluating clinical skills. Acad Med. 1993;68(6):443–53. https://doi.org/10.1097/00001888-199306000-00002.

Baugh AD, Vanderbilt AA, Baugh RF. The dynamics of poverty, educational attainment, and the children of the disadvantaged entering medical school. Adv Med Educ Pract. 2019;10:667–76. https://doi.org/10.2147/AMEP.

Bleakley A. Bad faith, medical education, and post-truth. Perspect Med Educ. 2018;7:3. https://doi.org/10.1007/s40037-017-0394-5.

Bleakley A, Brice J, Bligh J. Thinking the post-colonial in medical education. Med Educ. 2008. https://doi.org/10.1111/j.1365-2923.2007.02991.x.

Boelen C, Heck J. Defining and measuring the social accountability of medical schools. Geneva: World Health Organization; 1995. (Unpublished document WHO/HRH/95.7, available on request from Division of Organization and Management of Health Systems, World Health Organization, 1211 Geneva 27, Switzerland).

Boelen C, Woollard R. Social accountability: the extra leap to excellence for educational institutions. Med Teach. 2011;33:614–9.

Boulet J, Bede C, McKinley D, Norcini J. An overview of the world's medical schools. Med Teach. 2007;29(1):20–6.

Boyd VA, Whitehead CR, Thille P, Ginsburg S, Brydges R, Kuper A. Competency-based medical education: the discourse of infallibility. Med Educ. 2018;52(1):45–57.

Bulamba F, Sendagire C, Kintu A, Hewitt-Smith A, Musana F, Lilaonitkul M, Ayebale ET, Law T, Dubowitz G, Kituuka O, Lipnick MS. Feasibility of simulation-based medical education in a low-income country, challenges and solutions from a 3-year pilot program in Uganda. Simul Healthc. 2019;14(2):113–20. https://doi.org/10.1097/SIH.0000000000000345.

Castle M, Fletcher I, Scarpa A, Myers O, Lawrence E. A prospective study of medical student mental health and attitudes of mental illness disclosure. digitalrepository.unm.edu. 2019. https://digitalrepository.unm.edu/hsc_ed_day/39/

Cavanagh A, Vanstone M, Ritz S. Problems of problem-based learning: towards transformative critical pedagogy in medical education. Perspect Med Educ. 2019;8:38. https://doi.org/10.1007/s40037-018-0489-7.

Custers EJ, Ten Cate O. The history of medical education in Europe and the United States, with respect to time and proficiency. Acad Med. 2018;93(3S):S49–54. https://doi.org/10.1097/ACM.0000000000002079.

Davis D. The medical school without walls: reflections on the future of medical education. Med Teach. 2018;40(10):1004–9. https://doi.org/10.1080/0142159X.2018.1507263.

Della Monica M, Mauri R, Scarano F, Lonardo F, Scarano G. The Salernitan School of Medicine: women, men, and children. A syndromological review of the oldest medical school in the western world. Am J Med Genet A. 2013;161A:809–16. https://doi.org/10.1002/ajmg.a.35742.

Duffy TP. The Flexner report-100 years later. Yale J Biol Med. 2011;84:269–76.

Evans DB, Henschen BL, Poncelet AN, et al. Continuity in undergraduate medical education: mission not accomplished. J Gen Intern Med. 2019;34:2254. https://doi.org/10.1007/s11606-019-04949-0.

Farre A, Rapley T. The new old (and old new) medical model: four decades navigating the biomedical and psychosocial understandings of health and illness. Healthcare. 2017;5:88.

Field J. Some current trends in medical education. Bull Med Libr Assoc. 1957;45(1):20–9.

Finkel ML. A call for action: integrating climate change into the medical school curriculum. Perspect Med Educ. 2019;8:265. https://doi.org/10.1007/s40037-019-00541-8.

Frenk J, Chen L, Bhutta ZA, Cohen J, Crisp N, Evans T, Fineberg H, Garcia P, Ke Y, Kelley P, et al. The Lancet Commissions. Health professionals for a new century: transforming education to strengthen health systems in an interdependent world. Lancet. 2010;376:1923–58.

Fulton JF. The history of medical education. BMJ. 1953;2:457.

Giubilini A, Milnes S, Savulescu J. The medical ethics curriculum in medical schools: present and future. J Clin Ethics. 2016;27(2):129–45.

Global Consensus for Social Accountability of Medical Schools. https://healthsocialaccountability.org/. Accessed 19 Oct 2020.

Hafferty FW. Beyond curriculum reform: confronting medicine's hidden curriculum. Acad Med. 1998;73(4):403–7.

Hamdy H, Prasad K, Anderson MB, Scherpbier A, Williams R, Zwierstra R, Cuddihy H. BEME systematic review: predictive values of measurements obtained in medical schools and future performance in medical practice. Med Teach. 2006;28:103–16.

Hani C. Medical education in Southeast Asia. J Med Educ. 1962;37(9):930–7.

Henderson RI, Williams K, Crowshoe LL. Med mini-med school for Aboriginal youth: experiential science outreach to tackle systemic barriers. Med Educ Online. 2015;20:29561.

Hennen B. Demonstrating social accountability in medical education. CMAJ. 1997;156(3):365–7.

Hillen H, Scherpbier A, Wijnen W. History of problem-based learning in medical education. In: Lessons from problem-based learning. Oxford: Oxford University Press; 2010. In 1963, the first simulated patients were introduced in California.

Hoff RG, Frenkel J, Imhof SM, Ten Cate O. Flexibility in postgraduate medical training in the Netherlands. Acad Med. 2018;93(Suppl 1):S32–6. https://doi.org/10.1097/ACM.0000000000002078.

Irby D. Educating physicians for the future: Carnegie's calls for reform. Med Teach. 2011;33:547–50.

Javaid A. The future of medical education: meeting the global standards. Khyber Med Univ J. 2017;9(3):115–6. https://www.researchgate.net/profile/Arshad_Javaid/publication/328463259_THE_FUTURE_OF_MEDICAL_EDUCATION_MEETING_THE_GLOBAL_STANDARDS/links/5bcf50a2a6fdcc204a02196d/THE-FUTURE-OF-MEDICAL-EDUCATION-MEETING-THE-GLOBAL-STANDARDS.pdf. Accessed 16 Jan 2020.

Jeffrey DI. Barriers to empathy: the medical school culture. In: Exploring empathy with medical students. Cham: Palgrave Macmillan; 2019.

Kolb D. Experiential learning. Englewood Cliffs: Prentice-Hall; 1984.

Kötter T. Starting points for resilience promotion in medical education: what keeps future doctors healthy? Aktuelle Urol. 2019;50(2):190–4. https://doi.org/10.1055/a-0834-5954.

Larkins SL, Preston R, Matte MC, Lindemann IC, Samson R, Tandinco FD, Buso D, Ross SJ, Pálsdóttir B, Neusy A-J, on Behalf of the Training for Health Equity Network (THEnet) Measuring social accountability in health professional education. Development and international pilot testing of an evaluation framework. Med Teach. 2013;35(1):32–45.

Larkins S, Johnston K, Hogenbirk JC, Willems S, Elsanousi S, Mammen M, Van Roy K, Iputo J, Cristobal FL, Greenhill J, Labarda C, Neusy A-J. Practice intentions at entry to and exit from medical schools aspiring to social accountability: findings from the Training for Health Equity Network Graduate Outcome Study. BMC Med Educ. 2018;18(1):261. 1472–6920. https://doi.org/10.1186/s12909-018-1360-6.

Latif MZ, Hussain I, Saeed R, Qureshi MA, Maqsood U. Use of smart phones and social media in medical education: trends, advantages, challenges and barriers. Acta Inform Med. 2019;27(2):133–8. https://doi.org/10.5455/aim.2019.27.133-138.

Lave J, Wenger E. Situated learning: legitimate peripheral participation. New York: Cambridge University Press; 1991.

Lawrence C, Mhlaba T, Stewart KA, Moletsane R, Gaede B, Moshabela M. The hidden curricula of medical education: a scoping review. Acad Med. 2018;93(4):648–56. https://doi.org/10.1097/ACM.0000000000002004. Author manuscript; available in PMC 2019 Apr 1.

Le HH. The socioeconomic diversity gap in medical education. Acad Med. 2017;92(8):1071. https://doi.org/10.1097/ACM.0000000000001796.

Lievens F, Peeters H, Schollaert E. Situational judgment tests: a review of recent research. Pers Rev. 2008;37(4):426–41.

Lin HC, Hwang GJ. Research trends of flipped classroom studies for medical courses: a review of journal publications from 2008 to 2017 based on the technology-enhanced learning model. Interact Learn Environ. 2019;27(8):1011–27. https://doi.org/10.1080/10494820.2018.1467462.

Lingard L. What we see and don't see when we look at 'competence': notes on a god term. Adv Health Sci Educ. 2009;14:625. https://doi.org/10.1007/s10459-009-9206-y.

Lovy A, Paskhover B, Trachtman H. Teaching bioethics: the tale of a "soft" science in a hard world. Teach Learn Med. 2010;22(4):319–22. https://doi.org/10.1080/10401334.2010.513196.

Mann KV. Theoretical perspectives in medical education: past experience and future possibilities. Med Educ. 2010. https://doi.org/10.1111/j.1365-923.2010.03757.

Mazotti L, Adams J, Peyser B, Chretien K, Duffy B, Hirsh DA. Diffusion of innovation and longitudinal integrated clerkships: results of the clerkship directors in internal medicine annual survey. Med Teach. 2019;41(3):347–53. https://doi.org/10.1080/0142159X.2018.1472369.

McGaghie WC, Miller GE, Sajid AW, Telder TW. Competency-based curriculum development in medical education – an introduction. Geneva: WHO; 1978. http://whqlibdoc.who.int/php/WHO_PHP_68.pdf

McGaghie WC, Issenberg SB, Petrusa ER, Scalese RJ. A critical review of simulation-based medical education research: 2003–2009. Med Educ. 2010;44:50–63.

McGirr J, Seal A, Barnard A, Cheek C, Garne D, Greenhill J, Kondalsamy-Chennakesavan S, Luscombe GM, May J, McLeod J, O'Sullivan B, Playford D, Wright J. The Australian Rural Clinical School (RCS) program supports rural medical workforce: evidence from a cross-sectional study of 12 RCSs. Rural Remote Health. 2019;19(1):4971–80.

McKivett A, Hudson JN, McDermott D, Paul D. Two-eyed seeing: a useful gaze in Indigenous medical education research. Med Educ. 2020;54:217. https://doi.org/10.1111/medu.14026.

Mian O, Hogenbirk JC, Marsh DC, Prowse O, Cain M, Warry W. Tracking Indigenous applicants through the admissions process of a socially accountable medical school. Acad Med. 2019;94(8):1211–9. https://doi.org/10.1097/ACM.0000000000002636. Can Med Educ J. 2018;9(1):e33–43.

Morgan CJ, Bowmar A, McNaughton S, Flood B. Transformative learning opportunities during interprofessional healthcare practice experiences in higher education: viewed through the lens of a threshold concepts framework. Focus Health Prof Educ. 2019;20(2):41.

Murray RB, Larkins S, Russell H, Prideaux D. Medical schools as agents of change: socially accountable medical education. Med J Aust. 2012;196(10). https://doi-org.ezproxy.flinders.edu.au/10.5694/mja11.11473.

Neve H, Collett T. Empowering students with the hidden curriculum. Clin Teach. 2018;15(6):494–9. https://doi.org/10.1111/tct.12736.

Norman G. Research in clinical reasoning: past history and current trends. Med Educ. 2005;39(4):418–27.

O'Brien BC, Forrest K, Wijnen-Meijer M. A global view of structures and trends in medical education. In: Understanding medical education evidence, theory and practice. Hoboken: Wiley; 2018.

Opalek A, Gordon D. A data model for medical schools and their programs. J Med Regul. 2018;104(1):5–12. https://doi.org/10.30770/2572-1852-104.1.5.

Outcomes for graduates – supplementary guidance for medical schools. 2020. https://www.gmc-uk.org/education/standards-guidance-and-curricula/standards-and-outcomes/outcomes-for-gradu ates/outcomes-for-graduates%2D%2D-supplementary-guidance-for-medical-schools

Owen H. Early use of simulation in medical education. Simul Healthc. 2012;7(2):102–16. https://doi.org/10.1097/SIH.0b013e3182415a91.

Poncelet A, Hirsh D. Longitudinal integrated clerkships: principles, outcomes, practical tools, and future directions. Syracuse: ACE Gegensatz Press; 2016.

Prideaux D. On theory in medical education. 2008. https://doi.org/10.1046/j.1365-2923.2000.00825.

Rees EL, Hawarden AW, Dent G, Hays R, Bates J, Hassell AB. Evidence regarding the utility of multiple mini-interview (MMI) for selection to undergraduate health programs: a BEME systematic review: BEME Guide No. 37. Med Teach. 2016;38(5):443–55. https://doi.org/10.3109/0142159X.2016.1158799.

Reeves S, Perrier L, Goldman J, Freeth D, Zwarenstein M. Interprofessional education: effects on professional practice and healthcare outcomes. Cochrane Database Syst Rev. 2013; (3): Art. No. CD002213. https://doi.org/10.1002/14651858.CD002213.pub.

Rigby PG, Gururaja RP. World medical schools: the sum also rises. JRSM Open. 2017;8(6):2054270417698631. Published 2017 Jun 5. https://doi.org/10.1177/2054270417698631.

Rosen K. The history of medical simulation. J Crit Care. 2008;23(2):157–66. https://doi.org/10.1016/j.jcrc.2007.12.004.

Roth CG, Eldin KW, Padmanabhan V, Friedman EM. Twelve tips for the introduction of emotional intelligence in medical education. Med Teach. 2019;41(7):746–9. https://doi.org/10.1080/0142159X.2018.1481499.

Rourke J. Social accountability in theory and practice. Ann Fam Med. 2006;4(Suppl 1):S45–8. https://doi.org/10.1370/afm.559.

Saraswat M, Lau K, Mazze N, et al. Climate change and global health: training future physicians to act and mitigate. Ottawa: Canadian Federation of Medical Students. 2016. Published online, https://cfms.org/files/position-papers/2016_climate%20change%20and%20gh%20training.pdf

Scanlan GM, Cleland J, Johnston P, et al. What factors are critical to attracting NHS foundation doctors into specialty or core training? A discrete choice experiment. BMJ Open. 2018;8(3): e019911. Published 2018 Mar 12. https://doi.org/10.1136/bmjopen-2017-019911.

Schön D. The reflective practitioner: how professionals think in action. London: Temple Smith; 1983.

Sharma M. Applying feminist theory to medical education. Lancet. 2019;393(10171):493. https://doi.org/10.1016/S0140-6736(18)32595-9.

Shehnaz SI. Privatization of medical education in Asia. Southeast Asian J Med Educ, 2011;5(1). http://seajme.md.chula.ac.th/articleVol5No1/RW2_Syed%20IIyas%20Shehnaz.pdf

Shipman SA, Wendling A, Jones KC, Kovar-Gough I, Orlowski JM, Phillips J. The decline in rural medical students: a growing gap in geographic diversity threatens the rural physician workforce. Health Aff. 2019;38(12):2011. https://doi.org/10.1377/HLTHAFF.2019.00924.

Silveira GL, Campos LKS, Schweller M, Turato ER, Helmich E, Carvalho-Filho MA. "Speed up"! The influences of the hidden curriculum on the professional identity development of medical students. Health Prof Educ. 2019;5(3):198–209. https://doi.org/10.1016/j.hpe.2018.07.003.

Silver J, Ghalib R, Poorman JA, Al-Assi D, Parangi S, Bhargava H, Shillcutt SK. Analysis of gender equity in leadership of physician-focused medical specialty societies, 2008–2017. JAMA Intern Med. 2019;435(3):179–433. https://doi.org/10.1001/jamainternmed.2018.5303.

Skinner H, Bhatti F. Women in surgery. Bull R Coll Surg Engl. 2019;101(Suppl_6):12–4. https://doi.org/10.1308/rcsbull.TB2019.12.

Song P, Jin C, Tang W. New medical education reform in China: towards healthy China 2030. Policy Forum. 2017. https://doi.org/10.5582/bst.2017.01198. In China.

Steven K, Howden S, Mires G, Rowe I, Lafferty N, Arnold A, Strath A. Toward interprofessional learning and education: mapping common outcomes for prequalifying healthcare professional programs in the United Kingdom. Med Teach. 2017;39(7):720–44. https://doi.org/10.1080/0142159X.2017.1309372.

Stoddard HA, Johnson TM II, Brownfield ED. Outcomes, accreditation, interprofessional education, and the Tower of Babel. J Interprof Care. 2019;33(6):805–8. https://doi.org/10.1080/13561820.2019.1593119.

Strasser R, Hogenbirk J, Jacklin K, Maar M, Hudson G, Warry W, Cheu H, Dubé T, Carson D. Community engagement: a central feature of NOSM's socially accountable distributed medical education. Can Med Educ J. 2018;9(1):e33–43.

Tadahiko K. Medical education in Japan. Acad Med. 2006;81(12):1069–75. https://doi.org/10.1097/01.ACM.0000246682.45610.

Taylor TS, Raynard AL, Lingard L. Perseverance, faith and stoicism: a qualitative study of medical student perspectives on managing fatigue. Med Educ. 2019;53(12):1221. https://doi.org/10.1111/medu.13998.

Ten Cate O. Competency-based postgraduate medical education: past, present and future. GMS J Med Educ. 2017;34(5):Doc69. Published 2017 Nov 15. https://doi.org/10.3205/zma001146.

Ten Cate O, Chen HC, Hoff RG, Peters H, Bok H, van der Schaaf M. Curriculum development for the workplace using Entrustable Professional Activities (EPAs): AMEE Guide No. 99. Med Teach. 2015;37(11):983–1002. https://doi.org/10.3109/0142159X.2015.1060308.

Thomas PA, Kern DE, Hughes MT, Chen BY. Curriculum development for medical education: a six-step approach. Baltimore: Johns Hopkins University Press; 2016.

Tomorrow's doctors UK General Medical Council. Tomorrow's doctors: outcomes and standards for undergraduate medical education. London: General Medical Council; 2009.

Torralba KD, Jose D, Byrne J. Psychological safety, the hidden curriculum, and ambiguity in medicine. J Clin Rheumatol. 2020;39:667. https://doi.org/10.1007/s10067-019-04889-4.

Van Schalkwyk SC, Hafler J, Brewer TM, Margolis C, McNamee L, Meyer I, Peluso M, Schmutz A, Spak JM, Davies D, On Behalf of the Bellagio Global Health Education Initiative. Transformative learning as pedagogy for the health professions: a scoping review. Med Educ. 2019. https://doi.org/10.1111/medu.13804.

Vygotsky L. Mind in society: the development of higher psychological processes. Cambridge, MA: Harvard University Press; 1978.

Waheed-Ul-Rahman A, Mills E. Tackling mental health barriers at medical school – insights from fellow medical students. Adv Med Educ Pract. 2019;10:77–8. https://doi.org/10.2147/AMEP.S198993. Macclesfield.

Walker J, DeWitt D, Pallant J, Cunningham C. Rural origin plus a rural clinical school placement is a significant predictor of medical students' intentions to practice rurally: a multi-university study. Rural Remote Health. 2012;12:1908. www.rrh.org.au/journal/article/1908

Wartman SA, Combs CD. Reimagining medical education in the age of AI. AMA J Ethics. 2019;21(2):E146–52. https://doi.org/10.1001/amajethics.2019.146.

Weinstein DF, Thibault GE. Illuminating graduate medical education outcomes in order to improve them. Acad Med. 2018;93:975–8.

Wellbery C, Sheffield P, Timmireddy K, Sarfaty M, Teherani A, Fallar R. It's time for medical schools to introduce climate change into their curricula. Acad Med. 2018;93(12):1774–7. https://doi.org/10.1097/ACM.0000000000002368.

Wenger E. Communities of practice: learning, meaning, and identity. New York: Cambridge University Press; 1998.

Wenghofer E, Klass D, Abrahamowicz M, Dauphinee D, Jacques A, Smee S, Blackmore D, Winslade N, Reidel K, Bartman I, Tamblyn R. Doctor scores on national qualifying examinations predict quality of care in future practice. Med Educ. 2009;43:1166–73.

West C, Graham L, Palmer RT, Miller MF, Thayer EK, Stuber ML, Awdishu L, Umoren RA, Wamsley MA, Nelson EA, Joo PA, Tysinger JW, George P, Carney PA. Implementation of interprofessional education (IPE) in 16 U.S. medical schools: common practices, barriers and facilitators. J Interprof Educ Pract. 2016;4:41–9. https://doi.org/10.1016/j.xjep.2016.05.002.

Whitla DK, Orfield G, Silen W, Teperow C, Howard C, Reede J. Educational benefits of diversity in medical school: a survey of students. Acad Med. 2003;78(5):460–6.

Wilkins KM, et al. Emerging trends in undergraduate medical education: implications for geriatric psychiatry. Am J Geriatr Psychiatry. 2018;26(5):610–3.

Woolley T, Halili SD Jr, Siega-Sur JL, Cristobal FL, Reeve C, Ross SJ, Neusy AJ. Socially accountable medical education strengthens community health services. Med Educ. 2018; 52(4):391–403.

Zendejas B, Wang AT, Brydges R, Hamstra SJ, Cook DA. Cost: the missing outcome in simulation-based medical education research: a systematic review. Surgery. 2013;153(2):160–76.

Surgical Education: Context and Trends

2

David J. Coker

Contents

Where We Have Come From?: A Historical Perspective on Surgical Training in Australia
and New Zealand 30
The Rise of Competency-Based Surgical Training: Moving from Time-Based Training
to Competency-Based Training 31
Curriculum Design in Surgical Education 32
Educational Theory Reflected in Surgical Training Today 34
A New Surgical Training Reality: The Use of Virtual Environments and Simulation 35
The Central Role of Assessment in Surgical Education Today 38
Rethinking Assessment in Surgical Education and Training: Moving Assessment into
the Workplace 39
Moving Beyond Competency to Educating, Training, and Assessing for Performance 42
Conclusion 43
Cross-References 44
References 44

Abstract

This chapter aims to establish for the reader the field of surgical education and
place it within its current context. With respect to context, the author's experience
is in surgical education and training in Australia, which provides some of the
detail for this chapter. It should be stated however that there is significant
contextual similarity between Australia and New Zealand, the United Kingdom,
Canada and the United States.

With regard to trends in surgical practice, the chapter highlights the transition
from traditional apprenticeship models of training to competency-based training.
This fundamental change in the nature of training has led to changes in surgical
education, notably curriculum and assessment design. The advent of new

---

D. J. Coker (✉)
Department of Surgery, Royal Prince Alfred Hospital, Camperdown, NSW, Australia

Discipline of Surgery, University of Sydney, Camperdown, NSW, Australia

© Springer Nature Singapore Pte Ltd. 2023
D. Nestel et al. (eds.), *Clinical Education for the Health Professions*,
https://doi.org/10.1007/978-981-15-3344-0_5

education and training modalities in virtual environments and simulation are discussed, as is their purported role in the training framework.

The chapter concludes by looking beyond the outcome of competence, towards performance which is argued to be the true goal of surgical education and training. Drawing upon expertise theory, notions of routine and adaptive expertise are examined, where again it is argued that education and training should support the development of trainees who demonstrate adaptive expertise. The complexity of the clinical environment has never been greater, and will only continue to become more complex; surgical education and training must produce trainees with the ability to approach novel problems, and develop novel solutions. In this regard, surgical education and training must itself continue to adapt.

Keywords

Surgical Education · Curriculum · Assessment · Competence · Performance · Expertise

Where We Have Come From?: A Historical Perspective on Surgical Training in Australia and New Zealand

To better understand current and future trends in surgical education, an understanding of the past is necessary. For centuries, surgical training throughout the western world was based on an apprenticeship model. Formalized surgical training incorporating both scientific and technical teaching first arose in Germany in the latter half of the nineteenth century (Collins et al. 2007). This integration of basic sciences, with formalized clinical and operative teaching inspired Dr William Halsted to establish the first formalized surgical training program in the English-speaking world at Johns Hopkins Hospital in 1890 (Kerr and O'Leary 1999).

In an Anglocentric manner, surgical training in the United States (US), Canada, the United Kingdom (UK), Australia and New Zealand has been said to reflect a Halstedian model of training for over a century, despite its origins in Germany. The Halstedian model was characterized by a triad of educational principles: knowledge of the basic sciences, research and scholarship, and graduated clinical responsibility for the trainee under the supervision of skilled surgical teachers (Sealy 1999). While knowledge of the basic sciences was a principle of the model, surgical training remained ad hoc and opportunistic, with time in training being central to the delivery of training through exposure to the field of surgery. The centrality of time and exposure to apprenticeship teaching is captured in the oft-quoted surgical aphorism with respect to an operation "see one, do one, teach one."

Innate to the apprenticeship model of training, was the tension between education of the trainee and service provision: the clinical environment inherently dictated the learning environment for the trainee. With the clinical context so drastically changing from that in which Halsted established modern surgical training, the tension between learning opportunities and service delivery reached a point of non-sustainability. A new paradigm of surgical training was required to better align surgical training programs to the outcomes sought at the conclusion of training. In educational scholarship, there was a recognition that:

> In a traditional educational system, the unit of progression is time and it is teacher-centred. In a competency-based training system, the unit of progression is mastery of specific knowledge and skills, and is learner- or participant-centred. (Sullivan 1995)

This recognition filtered through to medical education, and the turn of the twenty-first century saw the establishment of competency-based surgical training.

The Rise of Competency-Based Surgical Training: Moving from Time-Based Training to Competency-Based Training

The Royal Australasian College of Surgeons (RACS) moved to a competency-based training framework in 2003 (Royal Australasian College of Surgeons 2012a), inspired by and adapted from the CanMEDS competency framework established in Canada in 1996 (Frank et al. 1996). It is worth noting that the Accreditation Council for Graduate Medical Education (ACGME) in the US adopted a competency-based framework at around the same time in 1999 (Accreditation Council of Graduate Medical Education 2016). The CanMEDS competency framework comprises 7 competencies, with a central integrating competency of the medical expert, in a "hub and spoke" model.

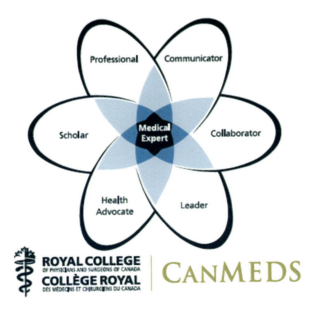

"Copyright © 2015 The Royal College of Physicians and Surgeons of Canada. http://www.royalcollege.ca/rcsite/canmeds/canmeds-framework-e. Reproduced with permission."

The RACS articulated nine competencies, with the addition of judgement – clinical decision-maker and technical expertise to those established in the CanMEDS framework:

1. Medical expertise
2. Judgement – clinical decision making
3. Technical expertise
4. Professionalism and ethics
5. Health advocacy
6. Communication
7. Collaboration and teamwork
8. Management and leadership
9. Scholarship and teaching

The addition of technical expertise in particular reflects the specificity of the RACS competencies to surgical practice, as opposed to the CanMEDS and ACGME six core competencies which apply across the multitude of fields of medical practice. The nine competencies underpin the current Surgical Education and Training (SET) program, introduced just over a decade ago in 2008. The title of the program encapsulates notions of the previous Halstedian apprenticeship model, in recognizing that preparing for a career in surgery requires both theoretical (education) and practical (training) aspects.

Curriculum Design in Surgical Education

The transition to a competency-based training program, and the accompanying focus on education as part of the new SET program, saw all of the surgical specialties in Australia and New Zealand publish explicit curriculum documents. In isolation, each of these curriculum documents are more in keeping with a syllabus, with long lists of learning objectives and the absence of a stated purpose (Grant 2010). The purpose of the SET program, and the accompanying curricula, can be found through the RACS and highlights the primacy of the core competencies in surgical training, where RACS states that the SET program seeks to:

> …ensure that surgical trainees become competent surgeons, who provide safe, comprehensive surgical care of the highest standard to the communities [they] serve. (Royal Australasian College of Surgeons 2019)

Grant (2010) describes four organizational models for curriculum development, all of which may coexist in a given curriculum:

1. Integration
2. Core and options
3. Spiral
4. Modular

In the Australasian context, modular and spiral organization are utilized pragmatically to span the necessary breadth of surgical practice. However, of greatest importance in a curriculum that is instituted while trainees are working in the field, is the use of an integrated model of curriculum design.

The field of surgical practice is necessarily broad, with curriculum documents that often reflect this in terms of their imposing size. The curricula are thus broken into modules, representing discrete, self-contained units, able to studied independently, though there is frequent cross-over of content between modules. A modular structure is important in a non-uniform course of training, allowing learners to study in the order of their choosing reflecting their clinical exposures and experiences.

Curricula documents within Australia and New Zealand surgical specialties reflect the Halstedian principle of graduated clinical responsibilities, though spiral organization (Bruner 1977), with content meant to be revisited throughout the training program with increasing cognitive and practical requirements based on trainees' level of training. In general, the knowledge component of the curriculum, reflecting the competency of medical expertise, is sought early in the training program. As the trainee progresses towards the completion of training there is a shift in focus to judgment and clinical decision-making, representing the application of knowledge to the clinical environment. Technical expertise utilizes the language of Miller's pyramid (Miller 1990), specifically the base ("knows") and the apex ("does") of the pyramid. With increasing experience in training, comes the expectation that trainees will move from a theoretical understanding of technical aspects of surgery, to the practical application of skills.

Vertical integration is central to the delivery of curriculum in surgical training, where trainees are actively engaged in clinical work while also engaged in the process of learning. It is recognized that there is a continuum between full integration at one end, and discipline-based teaching at the other, with surgical training argued to sit far more toward the integrated end of the spectrum (Harden et al. 1984). The curriculum is not completely integrated in that the teaching and learning of the competencies including professionalism, communication, collaboration and teamwork, and management and leadership utilizes a more ad hoc or opportunistic approach outside the formal (explicit) curriculum, as discussed further below.

The structure of curricula across the surgical specialties in Australia and New Zealand, demonstrate the use of well-described organizational models for curriculum design. It is not clear whether this is intentional, or occurs serendipitously. The explicit use of spiral learning, with its recognition that content will be revisited during training with greater levels of sophistication; and the inherent integration of learning the knowledge base of practice within the clinical environment promote deeper learning in the surgical training programs in Australasia.

In introducing the SET program in 2008, RACS stated that each of the nine competencies were vitally and equally important in the achievement of the highest standards of surgical performance (Collins et al. 2007). Contrasting this stated equality of the nine competencies, is the tendency for surgical curricula to focus upon only three of nine competencies: medical expertise, judgement and clinical decision-making, and technical expertise. The other six competencies, what have been termed the "non-technical" skills (Yule et al. 2006), are scarcely referred to, or not at all in the curricula. These competencies are undoubtedly more difficult to encapsulate in terms of objectives, and measurable behaviors within a curriculum, as compared to medical and technical expertise, and judgement and decision-making. What is more, it is posited that supervisors are far less assured in teaching and assessing competencies such as professionalism, communication, leadership and collaboration where they are less able to be directly observed and retrospectively assessed against objective outcomes as the so-called technical skills are.

For the competencies of professionalism, communication, collaboration and teamwork, and leadership and management; their incorporation into the explicit, or formal curriculum, often utilizes "rule-based" approaches to set-down objectives, competencies, and measurable behaviors that seek to define nontechnical behaviors (Coulehan 2005). There is, however. a well-described conflict between the values and rules espoused in the formal curriculum, and the behaviors modelled in the clinical setting, which reflect the hidden curriculum (Snyder 1971; Hafferty and Franks 1994). The role of the hidden curriculum in teaching values and ethical judgment has been previously recognized (Kaufmann and Mann 2010). Teaching and learning nontechnical skills through the hidden curriculum within the clinical context are not in and of itself a problem; however, it does require a consciousness and recognition on the part of supervising surgeons to demonstrate the values and attributes expected of trainees. It is also important that the training experience in its entirety is coherent, where the formal and hidden curriculum are not in conflict so as to fundamentally weaken their implementation.

Educational Theory Reflected in Surgical Training Today

Having looked at the impact of curriculum design on surgical training, it is useful to consider the educational theories that underpin surgical training today. Knowles' principles of adult learning, specifically of andragogy, is central to the delivery of surgical education and training (Knowles 1980). Trainees are expected to take responsibility for their own learning, utilizing the curriculum documents to guide their independent study with little in the way of formalized teaching. The learning process reflects the noncognitive factors identified by Kaufmann and Mann, in their discussion of adult learning principles (Kaufmann and Mann 2010):

1. Pacing
2. Meaningfulness
3. Motivation

The pacing of the learning process is driven by trainees, who are able to meet the learning objectives at a rate appropriate to their needs and the training context in which they find themselves. Balancing this independent pacing is the inherent meaningfulness of curriculum to the clinical environment, and the accompanying motivation to progress in their training.

The traditional apprenticeship approach to surgical education and training remains reflected in the ongoing importance of educational theories of experiential learning, situated learning, and communities of practice. Surgical training is the embodiment of experiential learning, occurring in the practical (clinical) environment, as opposed to the academic context. Trainees inhabit all four phases of Kolb's learning cycle during their training; with progression through symbolically oriented and perceptually oriented learning experiences at the outset of training, culminating in the transition to behaviorally oriented learning experiences towards the completion of training (Kolb 1984). Learner environments reflect levels of supervision, and the progression of trainees toward the ultimate goal of training which is independent practice.

Situated learning and communities of practice see:

> Learners learn how masters walk, talk, and conduct their lives; observe what other learners are doing and what is needed to become part of the community. (Kaufmann and Mann 2010)

Lave and Wenger (2002) would argue that through the course of their training, trainee's immersion in the clinical environment, and their observation of and interaction with consultants and other trainees comprises an essential component of the curriculum. The nontechnical competencies comprising the hidden curriculum, in addition to the technical competencies and particularly the practical components of surgical training, are wellencapsulated by educational theories of situated learning and communities of practice.

A New Surgical Training Reality: The Use of Virtual Environments and Simulation

The move away from the Halstedian apprenticeship model to a competency-based education and training environment has seen a parallel rise in education and training occurring outside the clinical environment through the use of virtual environments and simulation. The increasing complexity of the clinical environment, coupled with factors such as the move to minimally invasive surgery and the competing pressures of service delivery, has led to a re-evaluation of the manner in which surgical trainees are taught and trained. Virtual environments and simulation have been demonstrated as modalities that are capable of addressing the unmet needs in the current training environment.

To understand the increasing interest in, and use of, virtual environments and simulation in surgical training, it is necessary to recognize the significant external factors that influence their implementation. In today's surgical training environment patient safety has rightly taken primacy of place, over and above all other considerations including training opportunities. The traditional surgical aphorism referenced previously of "see one, do one, teach one," is anathema to the primacy of patient safety within today's training environment; where only a trainee with established proficiency in the particular operation should be performing the operation, let alone supervising the operation. An updated surgical training aphorism has been posited as "see one, simulate many deliberately, do one (Stefanidis et al. 2015)." Virtual environments and simulation offer trainees the opportunity to learn in an environment that is completely safe, and free from the inherent risks of the operating theatre. Some have gone so far as to state that the use of simulation-based training is an ethical imperative with respect to patient safety (Ziv et al. 2003).

A further driver for simulation and virtual reality training has been the introduction of safe working hours, and the accompanying reduction in clinical experience and operative exposure of trainees (Kneebone 2011). There can be little argument that the opportunistic training that occurred in the context of the traditional apprenticeship model is not an efficient manner of training, and where time in training is a valuable commodity other means of training to maximize efficiency are needed. Civil posits the hypothetical training of a pilot, who attends the airport each day, and is randomly assigned flight experiences, whereupon after a period of time is regarded as competent in all aspects of flight despite exposure, to highlight the incongruence of surgical education and training under the traditional apprenticeship model (Civil 2009). Virtual environments and simulation offer both improved efficiencies, and the ability to standardize the exposure of trainees.

The key components in successfully establishing virtual environments for training are realism and fidelity. The most successful virtual environments see users suspend belief and accept the environment as real (Evans and Schenarts 2016). Similarly, effective simulation should be realistic, patient-focused, and rooted in the clinical context, embracing complexity as opposed to simplicity and requiring participants to utilize integrated competencies as they would in clinical practice (Kneebone et al. 2007). Neither realism, nor fidelity, are inexpensive when compared at first glance, with traditional training methods occurring in the clinical environment. The comparison is not necessarily that simple; however, with a project analyzing the health economics of the cost of allowing trainees to operate in terms of additional theatre time utilized, finding that the cost of operative training was in the vicinity of US$50,000 per year for one trainee (Bridges and Diamond 1999). Furthermore, a systematic review has found that virtual reality training decreases trainee operative time (Nagendran et al. 2013), thus counterbalancing the cost of virtual reality simulators with likely savings in the utilization of operative time.

The mere availability of virtual environments, and simulation, will not in and of themselves improve training. In order to harness their benefits, they must be integrated within the current training framework. Ideally, a structured and evidence-based virtual reality and simulation curriculum would be implemented in sequence with the current curriculum (Stefanidis et al. 2015). The aviation industry offers an insight into the integration of virtual environments into training, where pilot training utilizes flight simulators at the outset of training to first familiarize apprentice pilots with the cockpit, before progressing through to the simulation of rare emergency situations (McClernon et al. 2011). The transition to actual flight is predicated upon the demonstration of competency in flight simulators using the derived objective measures (Tillou et al. 2016). Virtual environment training in surgery may find its place in a similar phase of training to that of the aviation industry. Indeed, studies into improved operative performance with simulation have demonstrated that it is junior trainees who derive benefit, with senior trainees and consultants seeing no improvement in performance (Loveday et al. 2010).

Virtual environment training aligns with traditional models of skill and expertise development, such as those proposed by Dreyfus and Dreyfus, and Fitts and Posner, which subscribe to the notion that expertise is attained over time and is demonstrated by the ability to practice in an automated fashion in a given domain (Dreyfus and Dreyfus 1986; Fitts and Posner 1967). The empirical evidence for superior performance by experts defined using traditional models of expertise is poor (Ericsson et al. 1993). This has led to the development of new theories of expertise, including Hatano and Inagaki's concept of routine and adaptive expertise, and Ericsson's expert performance approach, which see the attainment of automation as a barrier to expert performance (Ericsson et al. 1993; Hatano and Inagaki 1986).

Central to Ericsson's expert performance approach is the concept of deliberate practice, which comprises four main components (Ericsson et al. 1993):

- Practice with full concentration
- Towards current practice objectives
- Learners receiving or generating immediate feedback
- Training tasks offering opportunities to make repetitions with gradual improvement.

At first instance, virtual environments and simulation would seem well-placed to fulfil the criteria of deliberate practice, though it should be noted that Ericsson would advocate for feedback delivered by a proctor or coach, as opposed to automated feedback generated by a computer (Ericsson 2015). Indeed, for simple psychomotor skills, and even for simplified nontechnical domains, there is certainly a role for virtual environments and simulation to repeatedly practice skills not as easily replicable in the clinical environment, provided learners are motivated to remain in the cognitive and associative phases of learning and actively seek to counteract automaticity with the continual pursuit of improvement.

The question is how far does the transfer of skills honed in virtual environments or simulation extend? An emerging finding in the literature, consistent across the spectrum of simulation from simplistic benchtop models through to high fidelity virtual reality simulators, is that there is a context specificity of learning. Meaning that skills practiced in virtual reality and simulation are poorly generalizable to where the context of the clinical situation diverges from the practiced context (Kirkman 2013). In terms of expertise theory, this context specificity reflects notions of routine, as opposed to adaptive expertise. That is, virtual environments and simulation are adept at achieving efficiency as a primary outcome, though it may fail to develop trainees with the ability to modify their skills to novel problems encountered in the clinical environment, which is the hallmark of adaptive expertise. Employing the language of Ericsson, simulation may promote arrested development, where performance plateaus in an environment without new challenges. Overzealously pursuing deliberate practice of simplified skills divorced and isolated from the complexities of the clinical context may paradoxically prevent trainees from achieving expertise. Kneebone writes that:

> ...simulation's greatest potential is to recreate complexity while protecting patients from harm. [This] complexity lies not only in the technical performance of operations but in the internal development of the clinician. (Kneebone 2011)

Mylopoulos and Farhat have developed the concept of purposeful improvement of practice within the context of adaptive expertise (Mylopoulos and Farhat 2015). Purposeful improvement is central to progressive problem solving where experts continually reinvest cognitive resources gained through routinization into progressively more complex formulations of the problems encountered in their practice (Bereiter and Scardamalia 1993). Virtual environments are fundamentally limited to the scope of their coding in terms of the scenarios faced, though they are and will continue to become more sophisticated with time, they are finite in their scope. The clinical environment though will continue to demand the application of adaptive expertise where novel problems arise, and novel solutions are required. The role of virtual environments may be in the achievement of routine expertise early in training that primes trainees for the development of adaptive expertise within the complex clinical environment. Here they are able to deploy, their freed cognitive space earned in simulation to solve the myriad of nuanced problems that occur in the reality of surgical practice.

The Central Role of Assessment in Surgical Education Today

The relationship between learning and assessment is well established, with the recognition that assessment drives learning (Schuwirth and van der Vleuten 2011a). Indeed, it has been posited that the key purpose of assessment is learning (Norcini and Burch 2007). This contrasts with traditional notions of the purpose of assessment being to distinguish between, and to ensure, the standard of learners (Schuwirth and van der Vleuten 2011a). The tension that exists between these two countervailing viewpoints as to the purpose of assessment manifests in the current era of competency based surgical education, as the difficulty in designing "meaningful assessment[s] of competence" (Lockyer et al. 2017).

The influence of competency-based surgical education is evident in the assessment structure in Australasia, which is primarily concerned with the demonstration of competence by trainees. The means of assessment varies slightly within the SET program for each of the specialties; however, the core elements are:

- Generic and specialty-specific surgical science examinations (written)
- Clinical examination (observed structured clinical examination – OSCE)
- In-training assessment forms and logbooks
- Fellowship examination (written and viva voce)

The primacy of learning objectives in surgical curricula, over and above the teaching and learning experience, is in keeping with a "product model" of education (Stenhouse 1975). It is important to recognize the significant pragmatic benefits of this curriculum structure, and with it the assessment structure, in that it provides clarity and a sense of objectivity for internal stakeholders, and perhaps more importantly external stakeholders where the demonstration of competence is the paramount concern. However, where too great an influence is placed upon learning objectives and the competencies they seek to represent, an environment of superficial learning may result, where trainees seek safe passage through training and examinations, as opposed to a deeper learning and understanding of content.

As discussed previously, the curricula specifically adopt the language of Miller's pyramid, through the use of knows (base of the pyramid) and does (apex of the pyramid), with respect to the learning objectives (Miller 1990). When the assessment structure is appraised using the framework of Miller's pyramid, it can be seen that the focus of the high-stake assessment, specifically the fellowship examination, is generally found toward the base of the pyramid. The question that then arises is whether relatively isolated demonstrations of competence are reliable or valid, particularly when they assume great significance in high stakes assessment? It has been argued that knowledge (knows) and applied knowledge (knows how) may be interesting, but it is the actual performance of trainees (does) that is the desired outcome of training (ten Cate 2006a).

The major assessment of performance, and therefore the apex of Miller's pyramid, in the SET program is the in-training assessments. All of the SET programs utilize in-training assessment, both in a formative and summative capacity. The trainee is assessed against the nine competencies, where the trainee first undertakes a self-assessment, before being assessed by the department led by the term supervisor. The assessment of performance through the in-training assessment is compromised in its effectiveness, by its relative isolation as an assessment of performance.

Rethinking Assessment in Surgical Education and Training: Moving Assessment into the Workplace

In rethinking the assessment structure in surgical training, the question is, how might we more meaningfully assess trainees? If it is accepted that assessment drives learning, then redesigning the assessment structure to better assess trainees would by extension better train trainees. It is suggested that there are two significant conceptual changes that would underpin a redesign of the assessment structure. The first change is a fundamental move from assessment of learning, to assessment for learning within surgical education and training (Martinez and Lipson 1989). The second is the recognition that it is performance, as opposed to competency, that is the most important outcome of training.

To make the transition to assessment for learning, a programmatic assessment approach should be instituted (Schuwirth and van der Vleuten 2011b). A programmatic assessment approach sees:

> ...a variety of informative assessment activities...purposefully selected, combined and arranged in time to constitute a comprehensive programme of assessment that provides a longitudinal flow of information about the [trainee]. (Heeneman et al. 2015)

This flow of information extends to the trainee themselves, where they are required to utilize the information in the form of feedback to employ self-directed learning and thus learn from the assessment process. In a programmatic assessment approach, repeated comprehensive formative assessment and the inherent feedback generated are integral to the flow of information.

In programmatic assessment, "high stakes decisions" would be based upon an aggregate of information to determine progression or promotion (van der Vleuten et al. 2012). This contrasts with the current assessment structure, where the fellowship examination functions as a "gatekeeper," and in essence represents a one-off assessment to determine progression. The quality of this assessment structure when assessed against the criteria outlined by van der Vleuten is questionable (van der Vleuten 1996). A fundamental issue is the underlying validity of the examination, and whether assessing trainees' knowledge domains necessarily extends to assessing their ability to perform the role in the clinical setting. There are also issues of reliability, particularly with regard to the viva voce component of the examination, where a small sampling of cases is presumed to reflect the large breadth of practice a surgeon may encounter. The educational impact of the examination may see trainees aim for superficial breadth of knowledge at the expense of depth of understanding in a bid to overcome the hurdle of the examination. In terms of the other criteria outlined by van der Vleuten (1996), the cost efficiency of this assessment is satisfactory, and perhaps the preeminent criteria with respect to the fellowship examination's retention and role is stakeholder acceptability for both internal and external stakeholders.

Establishing a programmatic assessment approach, and assessment for learning, requires assessment tools that promote a flow of information in the form of feedback. Work-based assessment (WBA) can fill this role in surgical training. At the present time, some but not all of the SET programs utilize WBAs, and where they are utilized it is only early and somewhat sporadically in those training programs, as opposed to an established continual program of WBA as utilized in the United Kingdom context.

Work-based assessment is defined as:

> ...the assessment of working practices based on what trainees actually do in the workplace and predominantly carry out in the workplace itself. (Beard et al. 2009)

WBA reflect assessment, or judgement, based on direct observation in the clinical setting (Norcini 2014). They reflect the apex of Miller's pyramid, in assessing what the trainee actually does in the clinical context. A strength of WBAs is their inherent content and construct validity, where both internal and external stakeholders can readily appreciate the relationship between learning, assessment, and performance.

WBAs fulfil three basic requirements for assessment that facilitates learning (Norcini and Burch 2007):

1. The content of the training program, the competencies expected as outcomes, and the assessment practices are aligned (constructive alignment) (Biggs 1996).
2. Feedback to trainees is an integral part of the assessment process.
3. Assessment events are used to guide learning, and to achieve desired outcomes.

A recent systematic review identified more than 50 WBA tools described in the literature (Barrett et al. 2015). Two of the best studied and most familiar WBAs are the mini-CEX (clinical evaluation exercise) and DOPS (direct observation of procedural skills). The mini-CEX represents that archetypal WBA, where the assessor observes a trainee in a patient encounter. Mini-CEX has demonstrated reliability and validity in outcomes provided there is sufficient sampling (Holmboe et al. 2003); and has been demonstrated to closely correlate with the outcomes of fellowship examinations (Norcini and Burch 2007). DOPS does not have the same depth of evaluation of its validity and reliability, though its inherent similarities with mini-CEX leads to the expectation that it would be similarly reflective of trainee outcomes.

A further WBA that is already utilized by RACS in the sphere of continuing professional development for surgeons and is argued to have scope for introduction into surgical training is multisource feedback (MSF). MSF has been posited to reflect the traditional referral practice of medicine, and the inherent judgment that occurs regarding the performance of an individual (Norcini 2003). It may be seen that MSF is formalizing the ad hoc assessment process that occurred under the apprenticeship model of training, where opinions from a variety of sources within the hospital were sought by supervisors as to the performance of trainees. MSF is distinguished from mini-CEX and DOPS, in that the assessment made relates to longitudinal observation of behavior, as opposed to a discrete encounter. The assessment made in MSF is also unique, in that it has occurred when the trainee has not been conscious of the examination, thus its authenticity is high in its reflection of performance in the clinical environment (Norcini and Talati 2009).

Quality feedback from supervisors is at the heart of WBA, and the accompanying development of a culture of assessment for learning (Bok et al. 2013). The fundamental purpose of feedback is to reduce the discrepancy between current practices and understandings, and desired practices and understandings (Hattie and Timperly 2007). Feedback has been demonstrated to have an overwhelmingly positive effect on clinical performance, where it is effectively delivered (Veloski et al. 2006). Not only does feedback itself improve performance but it has been demonstrated that quality feedback promotes introspection and reflective practice in trainees (Holmboe et al. 2004).

Despite these findings, observational feedback is underutilized in day-to-day clinical practice, where performance is either not directly observed, or more often feedback is not provided to the trainee on performance that is observed. The absence of feedback is of particular concern where the trainee is not meeting the desired level of performance, as underperforming trainees are very unlikely to recognize their own failings in a given domain when tasked with self-assessment (Kruger and Dunning 1999). The most difficult domains for supervisors to deliver effective feedback and achieve remediation on the part of trainees, are the nontechnical domains, particularly professionalism and communication (Torbeck and Canal 2009). This contrasts with the apparent greater level of confidence that supervising surgeons appear to have with respect to recognizing and dealing with deficiencies in technical domains (Sanfey et al. 2013).

A major criticism levelled at WBAs is that they can be reductive, in that they seek to introduce a "tick-box" approach to assessing complex professional behaviors (Crossley 2012). This nihilistic attitude to the use of WBAs has a corrosive effect on their impact in training and has unfortunately been found to be present in some trainers in the United Kingdom where WBA is a compulsory component of the training and assessment structure (Phillips et al. 2015). Poor faculty participation has been identified as the most significant limiting factor in the implementation and success of WBA (Norcini and Burch 2007). Compounding this viewpoint is the placement of assessment in the busy clinical environment, where it must be acknowledged that WBA necessarily impacts upon the time pressures of both trainees and trainers. Faculty development is therefore integral to the success of WBA, as trainers must have an understanding of what they are doing, how they are doing it, and most crucially why it is important (Norcini 2014). The "tick-box" view of WBA ignores the central role of feedback to the assessment process, where regardless of any boxes that are ticked, it is the feedback generated for the trainee that is the most valuable aspect of the assessment process. Regardless of the domain being assessed and the context in which it occurs, feedback is a skill that can be improved with explicit training (Holmboe et al. 2004). Training the trainers should improve the utility of WBA as assessment tools, driving cultural change toward assessment for learning.

Moving Beyond Competency to Educating, Training, and Assessing for Performance

A criticism of competency-based training is that competence is not necessarily a predictor of performance (Rethans et al. 2002); with performance influenced on a moment-to-moment basis by a multitude of internal and external influences (Royal Australasian College of Surgeons 2012b). Grant goes further in advocating that we should abandon notions of competence, as what professionals do is far greater than the sum of parts that can be described in terms of competence (Grant 1999). Within this context, ten Cate has developed the concept of entrustable professional activities (EPAs) as a measure of trainees' actual performance in the clinical environment, where competencies stand alongside EPAs and are inferred from successfully performed professional activities (ten Cate 2005).

EPAs are defined as those professional activities, which together constitute the mass of critical element, which operationally define a profession (ten Cate and

Scheele 2007). EPAs can be seen to formalize the placement of trust by supervisors in trainees, which has always implicitly occurred within the training environment. Entrustment represents the most important outcome of training that being the trainee's readiness to take on professional responsibility and perform the role of the surgeon independently (ten Cate 2006b).

EPAs hold an inherent appeal, in that as with WBAs they represent true constructive alignment, as assessment is made on the basis of the professional activities undertaken. Similar to MSF, the assessment process occurs in a continuous fashion, as opposed to discrete assessment events, adding to their authenticity as trainees are assessed without the consciousness of being assessed, thus representing true performance. They place both learning and assessment firmly within the clinical context, and reflect notions of the traditional apprenticeship model of training where independence is progressively gained as the trust of supervisors is earned. A part of the inherent appeal of EPAs may reflect the fact that it is somewhat of a return to the self-regulation of surgical training and the profession.

The obvious critique of the EPA model of training and assessment is that while it does formalize the notion of trust in the performance of trainees, it constitutes an opaque system, where subjective judgment on the part of trainers form the basis for assessment. This subjectivity is acknowledged by ten Cate, when he writes:

> Supervisors often know who to pick, even if they can't tell exactly why. (ten Cate and Scheele 2007)

It is important to point out that subjectivity does not automatically invalidate or make unreliable an assessment method, where assessors (supervisors) are appropriately trained to make the required judgments of trainees. EPAs place substantial responsibility upon supervisors in terms of their judgment and placement of trust, though as stated above this has always occurred tacitly in surgical training. The degree of subjectivity and the return to internal regulation of surgical training, however, runs counter to expectations of external stakeholders including governing bodies and the public in their ability to scrutinize training in a readily objective fashion. It is worth noting that in the United States, the ACGME has recently introduced the concept of Milestones to all training programs, which are similar in their function to EPAs and provide objective descriptions of performance to facilitate a shared understanding of expected outcomes to both internal and external stakeholders (Accreditation Council of Graduate Medical Education 2016). Furthermore, it needs to be stated that the use of EPAs does not preclude the use of other assessment tools, which can act as objective checks and balances on EPAs.

Conclusion

It is argued that surgical practice has demonstrated the propensity over time to become ever more complex and complicated, and will only continue to do so. Surgery as compared to many other disciplines in medicine is different in its requirement for the consistent and at times concurrent demonstration of technical and nontechnical skills, often simultaneously. Surgical education and training must reflect and adapt to this increasing complexity, which it has already shown the ability to do in moving from an apprenticeship model of training to a competency-based training framework.

Competence, however, is a minimum or benchmark standard. In practice, what is really sought in the clinical context is performance, and perhaps more than that expert performance. With the enshrinement of competencies as the expected standard in surgical training, the questions bear asking as whether we are aiming too low?

The concept of adaptive expertise holds great relevance to surgical practice. Surgery requires the complex integration of multiple competencies both technical and non-technical in all cases encountered on a daily basis. If this is accepted then it is difficult to envisage exactly what would constitute routine practice, albeit there are undoubtedly gradations of complexity. The modern surgeon, more than ever before, must walk steadfastly within the optimal adaptability corridor, balancing the need for efficiency with the need to transition to flexible, innovative, and creative practice when the clinical situation demands this (Schwartz et al. 2005).

Shifting the focus of surgical education and training from the outcome of competency to performance is analogous with a shift from training for routine to adaptive expertise. Mylopoulos and Regher posit that adaptive expertise is not a state of accomplishment, but rather an approach to practice (Mylopoulos and Regehr 2007). Such a statement holds inherent appeal, but poses significant challenges for training. Approaches to practice or mind-sets are difficult to teach and assess, and thus, difficult to standardize, as opposed to competencies which are quite the opposite. Instilling attitudes, habits, and mind-sets in trainees can foreseeably only be achieved within the practical, complex, and compelling environments of the ward, the clinic, and the operating theatre. Thus, despite the many changes in surgical education and training, fostering performance as the outcome of training highlights the continued importance of the Halstedian approach of apprenticeship in surgical training.

Cross-References

▶ Cognitive Neuroscience Foundations of Surgical and Procedural Expertise: Focus on Theory
▶ Entrustable Professional Activities: Focus on Assessment Methods
▶ Focus on Theory: Emotions and Learning

References

Accreditation Council of Graduate Medical Education. The milestones guidebook. Chicago: Accreditation Council for Graduate Medical Education; 2016.

Barrett A, Galvin R, Steinart Y, Scherpbier A, O'Shaughnessy A, Horgan M, Horsley T. A BEME (Best Evidence in Medical Education) systematic review of the use of workplace-based assessment in identifying and remediating poor performance among post-graduate medical trainees. Syst Rev. 2015;4:65–70.

Beard J, Rowley D, Bussey M, Pitts D. Workplace-based assessment: assessing technical skill throughout the continuum of surgical training. ANZ J Surg. 2009;79(3):148–53.

Bereiter C, Scardamalia M. Surpassing ourselves: an inquiry into the nature and implications of expertise. La Salle: Open Court; 1993.

Biggs J. Enhancing teaching through constructive alignment. High Educ. 1996;32:347–64.

Bok HGJ, Teunissen PW, Favier RP, Rietbroek NJ, Theyse LFH, Brommer H, Haarhuis JCM, van Beukelen P, van der Vleuten CPM, Jaarsma DADC. Programmatic assessment of competency-based workplace learning: when theory meets practice. BMC Med Educ. 2013;13:123–31.

Bridges M, Diamond DL. The financial impact of teaching surgical residents in the operating room. Am J Surg. 1999;177(1):28–32.

Bruner J. The process of education. 2nd ed. Cambridge: Harvard University Press; 1977.

Civil ID. Surgical education, training and continuing professional development: crystal ball gazing. ANZ J Surg. 2009;79:214–6.

Collins JP, Gough IR, Civil ID, Stitz RW. A new surgical education and training programme. ANZ J Surg. 2007;77:497–501.

Coulehan J. Today's professionalism: engaging the mind but not the heart. Acad Med. 2005;80(10): 892–8.

Crossley JB. Making sense of work-based assessment: ask the right questions, in the right way, about the right things, of the right people. Med Educ. 2012;46:28–37.

Dreyfus H, Dreyfus S. Mind over machine: the power of human intuition and expertise in the era of the computer. New York: Free Press; 1986.

Ericsson KA. Acquisition and maintenance of medical expertise: a perspective from the expert performance approach with deliberate practice. Acad Med. 2015;90(11):1471–86.

Ericsson KA, Krampe RT, Tesch-Romer C. The role of deliberate practice in the acquisition of performance. Psychol Rev. 1993;100:363–406.

Evans CH, Schenarts KD. Evolving educational techniques in surgical training. Surg Clin North Am. 2016;96(1):71–88.

Fitts PM, Posner MI. Human performance. Belmont: Brooks/Cole; 1967.

Frank J, Jabbour M, Tugwell P, et al. Skills for the new millennium: report for the societal needs working group. Ottawa: Royal College of Physicians and Surgeons of Canada; 1996.

Grant J. The incapacitating effects of competence: a critique. Adv Health Sci Educ Theory Pract. 1999;4:271–7.

Grant J. Principles of curriculum design. In: Swanick T, editor. Understanding medical education: evidence, theory and practice. Oxford: Wiley-Blackwell; 2010. p. 1–15.

Hafferty F, Franks R. The hidden curriculum, ethics teaching, and the structure of medical education. Acad Med. 1994;69:861–71.

Harden RM, Snowden S, Dunn WR. Some educational strategies in curriculum development: the SPICES model. Med Educ. 1984;18:284–97.

Hatano G, Inagaki K. Two courses of expertise. In: Stevenson H, Azuma H, Kakuta K, editors. Child development and education in Japan. New York: W.H. Freeman; 1986.

Hattie J, Timperly H. The power of feedback. Rev Educ Res. 2007;77:81–112.

Heeneman S, Pool AO, Schuwirth LWT, van der Vleuten CPM, Driessen EW. The impact of programmatic assessment on student learning: theory versus practice. Med Educ. 2015;49:487–98.

Holmboe ES, Huot S, Chung J, Norcini JJ, Hawkins RE. Construct validity of the mini-clinical evaluation exercise (mini-CEX). Acad Med. 2003;78(8):826–30.

Holmboe E, Yepes M, Williams F. Feedback and the mini-clinical evaluation exercise. J Gen Intern Med. 2004;19:558–61.

Kaufmann DM, Mann KV. Teaching and learning in medical education: how theory can inform practice. In: Swanick T, editor. Understanding medical education: evidence, theory and practice. Oxford: Wiley-Blackwell; 2010.

Kerr B, O'Leary JP. The training of the surgeon: Dr Halsted's greatest legacy. Am Surg. 1999;65:1101–2.

Kirkman M. Deliberate practice, domain-specific expertise, and implications for surgical education in current climes. J Surg Ed. 2013;70(3):309–17.

Kneebone R. Simulation. In: Fry H, Kneebone R, editors. Surgical education: theorising an emerging domain. London: Springer; 2011.

Kneebone R, Nestel D, Vincent C, Darzi A. Complexity, risk and simulation in learning procedural skills. Med Educ. 2007;41(8):808–14.

Knowles MS. The modern practice of adult education: from pedagogy to andragogy. 2nd ed. New York: Cambridge Books; 1980.

Kolb DA. Experiential learning: experience as the source of learning and development. Englewood Cliffs: Prentice Hall; 1984.

Kruger J, Dunning D. Unskilled and unaware of it: how difficulties in recognising one's own incompetence lead to self-inflated self-assessments. J Pers Soc Psychol. 1999;77(6):1121–34.

Lave J, Wenger E. Legitimate peripheral participation in communities of practice. In: Harrison R, Hanson A, Clarke J, editors. Supporting lifelong learning: perspectives on learning. London: Routledge Farmer; 2002.

Lockyer J, Caraccio C, Chan MK, et al. Core principles of assessment in competency-based medical education. Med Teach. 2017;39(6):609–16.

Loveday BP, Oosthuizen GV, Diener BS, Windsor JA. A randomized trial evaluating a cognitive simulator for laparoscopic appendicectomy. ANZ J Surg. 2010;80(9):588–94.

Martinez ME, Lipson JI. Assessment for learning. Educ Leadersh. 1989;47:73–5.

McClernon CK, McCauley ME, O'Connor PE, Warm JS. Stress training improves performance during a stressful flight. Hum Factors. 2011;53(3):207–18.

Miller GE. The assessment of clinical skills/competence/performance. Acad Med. 1990;65(9):S63–7.

Mylopoulos M, Farhat W. "I can do better": exploring purposeful improvement in daily clinical work. Adv Health Sci Educ Theory Pract. 2015;20:371–83.

Mylopoulos M, Regehr G. Cognitive metaphors of expertise and knowledge: prospects and limitations for medical education. Med Educ. 2007;41:1159–65.

Nagendran M, Gurusamy KS, Aggarwal R, Loizidou M, Davidson BR. Virtual reality training for surgical trainees in laparoscopic surgery. Cochrane Database Syst Rev. 2013;27(8):CD006575.

Norcini J. Peer assessment of competence. Med Educ. 2003;37:539–43.

Norcini J. Workplace assessment. In: Swanwick T, editor. Understanding medical education: evidence, theory and practice. Chischester: Wiley; 2014.

Norcini J, Burch V. Workplace-based assessment as an educational tool: AMEE guide no. 31. Med Teach. 2007;29:855–71.

Norcini J, Talati J. Assessment, surgeon, and society. Int J Surg. 2009;7:313–7.

Phillips AW, Madhaven A, Brookless LR, Macafee DA. Surgical trainers' experience and perspectives on workplace-based assessments. J Surg Educ. 2015;72(5):979–84.

Rethans JJ, Norcini JJ, Baron-Maldonado M, Blackmore D, Jolly BC, LaDuca T, Lew S, Page G, Southgate L. The relationship between competence and performance: implications for assessing practice performance. Med Educ. 2002;36:901–9.

Royal Australasian College of Surgeons. Becoming a competent and proficient surgeon: training standards for the nine RACS competencies. Melbourne: Royal Australasian College of Surgeons; 2012a.

Royal Australasian College of Surgeons. Surgical competence and performance. Melbourne: Royal Australasian College of Surgeons; 2012b.

Royal Australasian College of Surgeons. The SET program. In: Become a surgeon. Royal Australasian College of Surgeons. https://www.surgeons.org/trainees/the-set-program. Accessed 21 July 2019.

Sanfey H, Williams R, Dunnington G. Recognising residents with a deficiency in operative performance as a step closer to effective remediation. J Am Coll Surg. 2013;216(1):114–22.

Schuwirth LWT, van der Vleuten CPM. Conceptualising surgical education and assessment. In: Fry H, Kneebone R, editors. Surgical education: theorising an emerging domain. London: Springer; 2011a.

Schuwirth LWT, van der Vleuten CPM. Programmatic assessment: from assessment of learning to assessment for learning. Med Teach. 2011b;33(6):478–85.

Schwartz DL, Bransford JD, Sears D. Efficiency and innovation transfer. In: Mestre J, editor. Transfer of learning from a modern multidisciplinary perspective. Greenwich: Information Age Publishing; 2005.

Sealy WC. Halsted is dead: time for change in graduate surgical education. Curr Surg. 1999;56: 34–9.

Snyder BR. The hidden curriculum. New York: Knopf; 1971.

Stefanidis D, Sevdalis N, Paige J, Zevin B, Aggarwal R, Grantcharov T, Jones DB. Simulation in surgery: what's needed next? Ann Surg. 2015;261(5):846–53.

Stenhouse L. An introduction to curriculum research and development. London: Heinemann; 1975.

Sullivan RL. The competency-based approach to training: strategy paper no. 1. Baltimore: JHPIEGO Corporation; 1995.

ten Cate O. Entrustability of professional activities and competency-based training. Med Educ. 2005;39:1176–7.

ten Cate O. Trust, competence and the supervisor's role in postgraduate training. BMJ. 2006a;333:748–51.

ten Cate O. Trust, competence, and the supervisor's role in post-graduate training. BMJ. 2006b;333:748–51.

ten Cate O, Scheele F. Competency-based postgraduate training: can we bridge the gap between theory and clinical practice. Acad Med. 2007;82(6):542–7.

Tillou X, Collon S, Martin-Francois S, Doerfler A. Robotic surgery simulator: elements to build a training program. J Surg Educ. 2016;73(5):870–8.

Torbeck L, Canal D. Remediation practices for surgery residents. Am J Surg. 2009;197(3):397–402.

van der Vleuten CPM. The assessment of professional competence: developments, research and practical implications. Adv Health Sci Educ Theory Pract. 1996;1:41–67.

van der Vleuten CPM, Schuwirth LWT, Driessen EW, Dijkstra J, Tegelaar D, Baartman L, van Tartwijk J. A model for programmatic assessment fit for purpose. Med Teach. 2012;34:205–14.

Veloski J, Boex JR, Grasberger MJ, Evans A, Wolfson DB. Systematic review of the literature on assessment, feedback, and physicians' clinical performance: BEME guide no. 7. Med Teach. 2006;28:117–28.

Yule S, Flin R, Paterson-Brown S, Maran N. Non-technical skills for surgeons in the operating room: a review of the literature. Surgery. 2006;139(2):140–9.

Ziv A, Wolpe PR, Small SD, Glick S. Simulation-based medical education: an ethical imperative. Acad Med. 2003;78(8):783–8.

General Practice Education: Context and Trends

3

Susan M. Wearne and James B. Brown

Contents

Introduction	50
The Context of General Practice Training	51
Trends	52
The Need for General Practitioners	52
Changes in General Practices	52
Educational Trends	53
General Practice Specialty Training	53
Educational Philosophies	54
The Structure of General Practice Training	55
Hospital then Community Training	55
General Practice as the Locus of Learning	57
General Practice Training in the Future	57
A Vision of Their Future	58
Early Assessment	58
Learning Based in the Practice	59
Clinical Supervision	59
Graded Introduction to Consulting	59
Educational Resources	60
In-practice Teaching	60
Workshops	60
Programmatic Assessment	61
Summative Assessment	62
Organization	62
Length of Training	63

S. M. Wearne (✉)
Health Workforce Division, Commonwealth Department of Health, Canberra, ACT, Australia

Academic Unit of General Practice, Australian National University, Canberra, ACT, Australia
e-mail: susan.wearne@health.gov.au

J. B. Brown
Eastern Victoria GP Training, Churchill, VIC, Australia

Gippsland Medical School, Monash University , Churchill, VIC, Australia

© Springer Nature Singapore Pte Ltd. 2023
D. Nestel et al. (eds.), *Clinical Education for the Health Professions*,
https://doi.org/10.1007/978-981-15-3344-0_6

Conclusion 63
Cross-References 64
References 64

Abstract

General practitioners (GPs) provision of longitudinal, relationship-based, holistic care to people and communities contributes to cost-effective health systems. Current trends are an increase in complexity of GPs' work as patients age and develop more chronic diseases, and there are increased options for diagnosis and treatment. Practice size has increased as has the number of different health professionals and learners who provide primary care.

Doctors who want to become GPs work in hospital and general practice as GP registrars. These training programs are often based on pragmatics and tradition rather than contemporary educational evidence or theory. Evidence shows that GP registrars learn most by working as GPs in practice under supervision, and there are questions about the relevance of hospital work as a junior doctor, to future work as a GP.

Trends in general practitioner training include early assessment to ensure training builds on strengths and targets educational need; a focus on learning in general practice under supervision, with external education designed complementarily; programmatic work-based assessment and demonstration of learning; and a final assessment process where GPs prove they have developed mastery of their craft.

Keywords

General practice training · General practice supervisors · Learning in practice

Introduction

This chapter considers the context, trends, and future of education in general practice. It is based on the authors' experience as general practitioners (GPs), GP supervisors, and GP academics involved in health and educational policy and in GP educational research.

Susan M. Wearne has worked as a GP, GP supervisor, and academic in England and central Australia. She currently balances her time between a GP clinic and work in health policy for the Australian government, as Senior Medical Adviser in the Health Workforce Division, the Commonwealth Department of Health, Canberra, Australia. The views are expressed are personal and not necessarily those of the Australian government.

James Brown is a GP, GP supervisor, practice owner, and researcher in rural Victoria, Australia. He was awarded an Order of Australia Medal for his work as a medical educator, has been chair of the Australian Directors of Training Committee, and held other leadership roles in GP training. He is currently Director of Education Quality Improvement for Eastern Victoria GP Training.

From 2017 to 2018, Susan joined James, Prof David Snadden, University of British Columbia, Canada, and Dr Catherine Kirby from Eastern Victoria GP Training to research models of GP training in the Netherlands, New Zealand, Ireland, Canada, Australia, and England. This chapter draws on that work which gave perspective on what is important in general practice training, but also what could be done differently. While the research broadened our vision beyond our own experience, it is still a comparatively narrow view. The Besrour Papers (Arya et al. 2017) provide a comprehensive review of general practice training across the globe. We also discuss GPs increasing roles in educating medical students and junior doctors, who have not yet decided on a medical specialty.

The Context of General Practice Training

Health systems with strong primary care are more cost-effective and associated with a more equitable distribution of health in populations, in cross-national and within-national studies (Starfield et al. 2005). GPs' continuity of care (Gray et al. 2003) is associated with reduced hospital admissions (Barker et al. 2017) and increased longevity (Maarsingh et al. 2016). As GPs' roles can vary between countries, we first clarify the definition of general practice that we will use in this chapter, and its North American synonym, family practice.

A general practitioner is usually the first doctor someone sees when they are feeling unwell.

> GPs see it all; the widest variety of conditions and the greatest range of severity in patients of all ages, ethnicities and backgrounds. They are medical detectives, trained to figure out what might be going wrong, how to treat it and who patients should see. (The Royal New Zealand College of General Practitioners 2018)

In rural or isolated areas, GPs often have a broader scope of practice including providing emergency and in-patient hospital services that would usually be the remit of secondary care specialists in urban areas (Robinson et al. 2010; Humphreys et al. 2003; McGrail et al. 2012).

General practice is relationship-based care with GPs developing expertise in people, rather than individual diseases (Stewart 2005). GPs need specific consultation skills (Trumble 2011) and the ability to manage uncertainty (WONCA Europe 2011). Their detective work is holistic as they apply their knowledge of patients' background, biology, sociology, environment, culture, and psychology when diagnosing and managing illnesses (The Royal New Zealand College of General Practitioners 2018). GPs' clinical method creates meaning and links disparate parts of a patient's story into a cohesive narrative that outlines a pragmatic path forward. The European Academy of Teachers in General Practice/Family Medicine agreed features of general practice are shown in Box 1 (European Academy of Teachers in General Practice 2011).

Trends

The Need for General Practitioners

As populations age, more people have an increasing number of complex, chronic medical conditions. Seeing multiple different specialists, each of whom focus on a single element of patient care (or individual organ), becomes inefficient, exhausting, and potentially dangerous (Wallace et al. 2015). Increasingly, generalists are needed who can take a "whole of patient approach" working with patients to identify their priorities and concerns, and juggle their treatment to yield an optimal quality of life (Frenk et al. 2010).

As a result, GPs' work is increasingly complex with consultations covering more issues and more activity per issue: GPs see more presentations of mental illness and chronic disease; manage multi-morbidity (Britt et al. 2008) and polypharmacy (Britt et al. 2010) as well as acute illness; and provide health promotion.

Yet, just while more GPs are needed, in some countries fewer graduates are applying for training. In the UK this is attributed to increasing workloads without commensurate increases in resources, and government initiatives are aimed at addressing this situation (Wass et al. 2016). The United States and Australia face similar challenges, with graduates preferentially choosing non-general practice specialties (American Association for Family Practice 2019; Department of Health 2012).

This makes it essential to encourage doctors into GP training that is high quality, well supported, and focused on developing the skills needed for the role.

Changes in General Practices

It could be argued that some of the challenges facing education in general practice are a result of its own success. Patients are now living long enough to develop chronic disease with different needs because much acute illness can now be treated or prevented with primary care activities such as through immunization.

Since the 1980s there has been an increasing trend to teach medical students and junior doctors in general practice. The success of early teaching initiatives has led to more learners in general practice (Hays et al. 2003). General practice, rather than highly specialized hospitals, has begun to be seen more as the place to learn the generalist skills needed for medical practice (Kidd and Hudson 2007; Kelly et al. 2012). This has turned general practices into major educational environments. Learning outcomes for junior doctors and students were at least equivalent to those achieved in hospitals, with more skills developed in communication, continuity of care, and the benefit of a no-blame culture (Anderson et al. 2015; Henderson

3 General Practice Education: Context and Trends

et al. 2018; Worley et al. 2004). Experience in general practice is advocated not only to increase recruitment to the specialty (Wass et al. 2016) but also to give future hospital doctors better understanding of primary care (Anderson et al. 2015).

Patients have responded positively to learners in general practice (Hudson et al. 2010) and have articulated some benefits, while also identifying how best to involve GP registrars in their care (Bonney et al. 2009). GPs report benefitting from the variety and intellectual challenge of an extended educational role (Weston and Hudson 2014). There are now practices that have learners at all the levels of medical training, and research has shown ways to set up general practices that host multilevel learners comprising medical students, junior doctors, and specialist trainees (Dick et al. 2007, 2019; Stocks et al. 2011; Anderson and Thomson 2009; Morrison et al. 2015; Brown et al. 2015). These increased numbers of learners come from a wider variety of backgrounds as a result of medical migration (Aluttis et al. 2014) and an increased number of postgraduate medical schools.

General practices used to be small, often family-run, organizations. Now single-handed practices are rarer, and many practices are operated from purpose-built premises with multiple doctors, some of whom work part-time. Practice nurses, midwives, health visitors, community pharmacists, and allied health professional increasingly contribute to the delivery of primary care. These larger practices are sometimes run by corporate businesses.

Each additional person learning and working in a practice potentially disrupts the continuity of care that typically occurs in a long-term doctor-patient relationship. So, there is a tension between the extended access and efficiencies of large practices and mutual, personal understanding between a doctor and a patient needed for quality care and professional satisfaction. It has recently been argued that the increased fragmentation of care is directly linked to GP exhaustion and burnout (Zigmond 2019). So, we need to train future GPs to maximize the skills that the primary care team brings to large multiple-doctor practices, without losing GPs' relationships with their patients and their families.

Educational Trends

General Practice Specialty Training

In the UK, and other systems based on the UK model, such as those in Ireland, Australia, and New Zealand, doctors complete one-year hospital internships following graduation from medical school. Internships usually include medical and surgical terms, and in some countries experience in emergency medicine. General registration is granted on completion of internship. This used to be considered sufficient for a career in general practice.

As the discipline of general practice became a specialty in its own right, and the breadth of skills and knowledge needed grew, specific training for general practice was suggested and subsequently required. Dedicated training programs with curricula, training standards, and assessments were established.

In our research of different training programs, we found that differences in programs were based on differences in health care and educational tradition, approaches to educational theory, and how the health system was funded. For example, beginning GP training with hospital-based posts arose from a hospital-based training system with the assumption that hospital practice is good preparation for general practice.

In Australia there is a strong emphasis on GP medical educators (MEs) visiting registrars in practice to observe their consultations and teach. This was introduced because GP supervisors were reluctant to observe their registrars in practice. This reluctance was unsurprising in a fee-for-service system where GPs earn income only when seeing their own patients. Instead, independent GPs were employed as MEs. MEs now play major roles in training in Australia and are perceived as essential to quality training. In the UK, by contrast, the capitation model of general practice funding enabled supervisors to sit in with registrars, and take time out of clinical practice to teach. As a consequence, the UK training programs are run by GPs who have experience as supervisors, and then specialize further in medical education and program management. They too are viewed as essential to quality training.

In the Netherlands the idea of day release educational workshops commenced in the belief that supervisors would need a day off from the intense pressure of teaching registrars. So, day release, where registrars would leave the practice and attend educational workshops, was primarily for releasing the supervisors not the registrars! (Dutch interviewee Eastern Victoria General Practice Training research project 2018 (Brown et al. 2018)).

Knowing the historic rationale for these training activities frees us up to reconsider their role in vocational training into the future. Pragmatism is a major heritage of general practice training and aligns with the discipline itself. Educational theory has also played a significant role over time and will now be discussed.

Educational Philosophies

General practice training mirrors the discipline, and so is primarily about learning how to build trusting relationships, as this anecdote illustrates.

> As a young registrar I asked the GP who ran my training program, when I was going to learn some 'proper medicine', such as how to treat high blood pressure. His riposte was 'the drugs you use to treat high blood pressure will change during your career, but you will always need your communication skills'. He was absolutely right! Now I spend time having similar discussions with young GPs whose focus is on the content and knowledge they think they need. Clearly, that is important too – a GP without any medical knowledge is more friend than physician, but consultation skills remain the foundation of every consultation. (Susan M. Wearne)

The primary approach to teaching general practice has been and continues to be through an apprenticeship relationship. Future GPs start work in general practice, under the supervision of a more experienced and trained educator, their GP supervisor (Wearne et al. 2012).

Educational activities designed to complement work-based learning have been influenced by the educational theories prevalent at the time that the particular activity was instigated. For example, general practice training started in the 1950s in the UK (The King's Fund 2011), which coincided with inquiries that revealed variable standards of care in general practices. At the time, Michael Balint, a psychoanalyst, was prominent with his emphasis on the use of emotion and personal understanding in doctors' work and the therapeutic potential of the doctor-patient relationship (Balint 1957), heavily influenced program development. Consequently, day release workshops were designed around learning communication and consultation skills (Pendleton et al. 2003).

In the Netherlands the initial focus was also on communication skills training and the psychological aspects of practice (Balint 1957). Schon's "reflective practitioner" (Schon 1987) and Kolb's theory of experiential learning (Kolb and Plovnick 1974) influenced their educational approach. Likewise, general practice training in New Zealand emphasized experiential learning as per Kolb (Kolb and Plovnick 1974).

During the 1990s and early 2000s the notion of GP registrars as adult learners was prominent (Brookfield 1986; Knowles 1984). This approach assigned educators the role of facilitating education based on the presumptions that learners were motivated to learn and had valuable experience in general practice to learn from.

In the 2000s the emphasis became the need to prove that training program graduates had met the required competencies of their future profession. Canada was the first country to introduce competency-based training, and the Netherlands followed basing their training on the seven CanMEDs competencies (The College of Family Physicians of Canada 2009). Both countries now use Entrustable Professional Activities (EPAs) to document acquisition of competencies during training (Schultz et al. 2015; Ten Cate 2014).

More recently sociocultural learning theories have been influential highlighting the social basis of learning and the need for GP registrars to learn by doing meaningful work in a community of practice (Lave and Wenger 1991; Wenger 1998; Gamble 2001; Billett 2002).

The Structure of General Practice Training

Hospital then Community Training

In Europe (European Academy of Teachers in General Practice 2011), North America, Australia, and New Zealand, general practice training programs combine experience in hospital post internship with time working under supervision in general practice. The most relevant hospital specialties are considered to be obstetrics and gynecology, pediatrics, mental health, and geriatrics (Royal Australian College of General Practitioners 2013).

In some countries, for example, the UK and Ireland, general practice training schemes arrange the combination of hospital and general practice training deemed necessary. Other countries, such as Australia, expect junior doctors to choose and apply for hospital jobs themselves. Given the breadth of the scope of general practice, it is difficult for trainees to identify which hospital placements are most relevant for general practice training, leading to many working in subspecialties of comparatively limited use for their future career. In Australia, the capacity for junior doctors to select relevant hospital posts has been impacted by a recent increase in the number of junior doctors increasing competition for hospital posts. There are concerns that new GP registrars start their in-practice training with less experience and confidence than their predecessors (West Australia Department of Health 2018).

In Canada there is no internship. Registrars start immediately in general practice and then rotate back into hospital for specific learning, such as in obstetrics or emergency care. In rural areas, these services may be staffed GPs rather than specialists. When the competency-based curriculum was introduced (The College of Family Physicians of Canada 2009; Organek et al. 2012), practicing GPs determined, and now teach, the required competencies taking advice from other specialists at their discretion. GP registrars may combine sessions of community practice with hospital-based care, such as obstetrics, thereby maintaining continuity of care and continuity of learning. Rather than a focus on completing time-based rotations, placements may be modified to ensure registrars acquire necessary competencies. For example, a registrar who needs skills in fracture management may do sessions in the fracture clinic rather than a six-month orthopedics term. Training in Canada also has some "white space": time that GP registrars can use to pursue specific interests or address learning gaps.

Irish training programs also integrate hospital and general practice learning. During hospital terms GP registrars attend half a day per week at GP educational workshops and spend a week in general practice every 6 months, to help them focus their learning and experience on their future career. In some schemes GP MEs run consultation skills training within hospital outpatients. These have generated interest from other specialists in this educational approach.

In Australia recent research has suggested that changes in tertiary hospitals have decreased their suitability to train future GPs (Wearne et al. 2018). The changes include:

- Shorter patient admissions which have reduced the opportunities for junior doctors to observe how illness improves or deteriorates over time (Ash et al. 2012)
- Shorter working hours for junior doctors which has reduced their experience of continuity of care (Detsky and Berwick 2013), reduced their exposure to a varied clinical case-load, episodic education and supervision
- Increasing sub-specialization which means that juniors may experience only a subset of specialist practice (Department of Health 2012)
- Trend to non-urgent chronic disease being managed in general practice, lessening juniors' opportunities to learn these skills in hospital
- Decreasing junior doctor clinical responsibility (Academy of Royal Medical Colleges 2012)
- Twenty-four hour access to pathology and sophisticated diagnostic imaging that is not available in many GP settings including small rural hospitals

These changes, together with a different spectrum on illnesses to general practice, mean that junior doctors in hospitals risk learning illness scripts and methods of management that may not apply to their future work as GPs. Given these concerns with tertiary hospitals as preparation for general practice in Australia, Canadian educators argue that their approach of targeting placements to learning specific skills is preferable (Brown et al. 2018).

General Practice as the Locus of Learning

Although general practice training is principally an apprenticeship model of learning, it has been difficult to find supporting empirical evidence to confirm that registrars do indeed learn from their supervisors and their practices. This gap has recently been addressed with data from a long running study of GP registrars' work.

The **R**egistrars **C**linical **En**counters in **T**raining (ReCEnT) project is an ongoing cohort study of Australian GP registrars' consultations that provides information on registrars' clinical activity, their learning needs. GP registrars record data from 60 consecutive consultations half-way through each 6-month training term (Morgan et al. 2012). They document their case-mix, clinical management, and whether they sought information or assistance from their supervisor or a practice resource, or generated learning goals to be pursued post-consultation. Analysis of this data provides an opportunity to test the effects of off-site and in-practice education.

MEs, from the ReCEnT team, designed off-site educational meetings to teach GP registrars about antibiotic prescribing, de-prescribing in the elderly, and the rational ordering of tests. At the end of the educational sessions GP registrars demonstrated that they knew what to do in applying evidence to written clinical vignettes. They also stated their intentions to change their practice. Despite this knowledge and intent, there was no significant change recorded in their practice (Magin et al. 2016a, b).

Subsequent educational interventions focused on both supervisors and GP registrars. In contrast these sessions did result in changes to GP registrars' practice, which demonstrated how crucial supervisors and their practices are in "teaching" (Magin et al. 2018). Regardless of what GP registrars may know theoretically, if that is not what they see occurring in practice, or are advised to do by their supervisors, then they don't do it. This points to the importance of practice-based learning for general practice training program development.

General Practice Training in the Future

If there was an opportunity to redesign general practice training, what would it look like? In this final section, the best ideas and evidence are collated into a blueprint for the future.

A Vision of Their Future

It is hard to aim for something without a target. Future surgeons know they will perform surgery, and images of emergency physicians fill the media enough for most people to have an idea of what that job might entail. For GPs there are some unhelpful caricatures. "Tears and smears" or "just coughs and colds" misrepresents the significant intellectual challenge of being the diagnostician and manager of the widest scope of practice in medicine. Even harder to show are the relational, business, and creative aspects of practice. Future GPs need accurate and inviting images, and an understanding of good general practice.

Training programs need to explicitly outline their vision of quality general practice. Options include discussions on the definitions and scope of practice, and opportunities for direct observation of different experts in practice to see how their holistic knowledge of patients is used in care (e.g., addressing a patient's family or workplace stresses prior to starting antihypertensive medication). Videos of consultations, reflective essays, or books by GPs and their patients can all help to build understanding. This is particularly important for new GP trainees who undertook their primary training in another country. In a study by Warwick et al., international medical graduates (IMGs) reported that this type of orientation assisted their integration into an unfamiliar health system (Warwick 2014). There are also arguments that this should include messages about social accountability, culturally safe practice, and the need for service in under-served areas (Young et al. 2019).

This vision should capture how GPs interact and work with other health professionals. Time spent with each person working in a practice is invaluable as is time with local pharmacists, community nurses, midwives, and allied health providers.

Early Assessment

Formal assessment of entrants has not been a feature of general practice unlike some other disciplines, such as surgery. There has been an assumption that entrants will come with a similar knowledge and skill base from their basic medical training plus their time in hospitals. A recent recognition that entrants in fact come from a wide variety of prior experience has led to trend for early assessment.

For example, the University of British Columbia in Canada assesses the knowledge and skills of IMGs starting family physician training. General Practice Training Tasmania in Australia conducts a multiple-choice exam and a series of objective structured clinical examinations (OSCEs) for all entrants regardless of previous location of training. Program directors use the results of these tests to direct training to build on individuals' strengths and address their identified gaps.

New Zealand, the Netherlands, Ireland, and Canada conduct knowledge assessments part-way through training.

Learning Based in the Practice

General practice training schemes should be constructed on the premise from both theory and evidence that the primary center of learning general practice is *in* general practice. Training schemes should support in-practice learning, and design workshops and time out of practice to complement in-practice learning. One practical aspect of such support is providing funding so that new recruits to general practice can focus on learning and developing their professional identity, before being required to provide a workforce. This can be a problem in Australia, where the fee for service system requires GP registrars to bill patients in order to cover their own salary (Laurence et al. 2012). Other tensions can exist in countries where GP registrars are salaried, and practices rely on registrars to see large numbers of patients.

A conclusion from our research was that having a GP registrar should be work and cost neutral for the practice and supervisors, such that the extra time in teaching and supervision was balanced by the GP registrar's work or funding. Finding that equilibrium is a challenge for most systems, but it is important to ensure that neither the practice nor the supervisor nor the registrar feels unduly imposed upon by any other.

Clinical Supervision

Effective clinical supervision is required to oversee patient and GP registrar safely, as the latter work and learn in practice. This is explored further in ▶ Chap. 56, "Supervision in General Practice Settings."

Graded Introduction to Consulting

In the apprenticeship model of general practice training, there is a graded introduction to GP registrars having their own list of patients. Initially GP registrars observe experienced GPs, then co-consult and then consult on their own with ready access to their GP supervisor if needed. GP registrars should consult at a pace that meets their educational needs.

Some countries expect GP supervisors to discuss or oversee every patient seen by GP registrars. The Canadian approach is for GP supervisors to write daily field-notes based on their observations of registrar's skills outlining what registrars should continue doing, what to consider and guidance for future learning (Donoff 2009).

In other jurisdictions supervision is "as needed." The problem with this approach is GP registrars' initial "unconscious incompetence" (Ingham et al. 2019). Without being aware of what they don't know, GP registrars are unlikely to know when to ask for help potentially compromising patient safety and registrar learning. For this reason, we advocate for comprehensive oversight of GP registrars when they start in practice to maximize learning from each patient. Over time, as registrars develop expertise, it is reasonable to reduce supervisor input (Kennedy et al. 2005), perhaps to a review of patients, or random case analysis, at the end of each day (Morgan and Ingham 2013).

Educational Resources

If practices are expected to train GPs using up-to-date information and guidelines, it is reasonable for relevant material to be supplied, including (but not limited to) the following:

- Formulary/drug information
- National and local evidence-based guidelines and referral pathways relevant to general practice
- General practice and reference texts
- Information about medico-legal aspects of general practice
- Resource material on relevant legislation – such as on assisted dying, termination of pregnancy, prescribing drugs of addiction
- GPs' role in public health notification of disease
- GPs' role in certification of fitness to work, fitness to drive

In-practice Teaching

In addition to supervision of patient care, GP supervisors run in-practice teaching sessions. Increasingly these are held with multiple level learners (Thomson et al. 2014). This creates efficiency and valuable peer-learning, but must not come at the expense of individual relationships with individual learners, and feedback on their interpersonal skills with patients. It can take skill to create the safe, blame-free educational spaces that GP registrars describe as being so essential to their professional development (Peile et al. 2001). Allowing "just enough" competition between learners at different stages encourages each to do their best. Equally important is a deliberate move away from the historical hallmarks of health professional education of hierarchy, deprecation, and disempowering teaching by humiliation.

Workshops

If the practice is the prime place of learning, what is the role of workshop-based learning outside the practice? The method of teaching should match the learning outcome. There are three broad groups: content; and the skills, behaviors, and attitudes for professional practice.

The considerable content or knowledge needed by future GPs can be learnt via journal articles, textbooks, lectures, or different online media. Information technology delivers content from national and international experts to any learner with a good Internet connection. Podcasts, vodcasts, discussion boards, and quizzes can promote learning between GP registrars across the globe.

Workshops should be used for education that requires interaction with educators and peers. Small groups enable learning enabling peer benchmarking and role modeling. Consultation and communication skills to rehearse relationship-based medical practice are important areas of learning that benefit from this environment.

A summary of the topics suited to teaching in workshops is:

- Consultation skills through the use of role-play, actors, and/or videos
- Rare but important clinical situations that cannot be guaranteed to be seen in practice, e.g., diagnosis and management of ectopic pregnancy, meningitis
- Emergency medicine skills and working in teams
- Gender-sensitive topics such as erectile dysfunction, sexual health, breast lumps
- Ethical and professional practice – such as the GP's role in termination of pregnancy, assisted dying, assessing fitness to drive, and certification for work

Simulation equipment can be useful in teaching some of these topics. For example, simulation models of breast lumps, or prostatic abnormalities, can help GP registrars practice physical examinations in ways that might be too intrusive in clinical practice.

Local program directors should be given freedom to adapt workshops to the local context. This can be learning about injuries related to the local farming industry or the health needs of a refugee population.

Programmatic Assessment

Programmatic assessment is assessment for judging trainee progress both for directing trainee learning and for progress decisions by the training program. GP registrars need to know on what basis progress will be measured and how this will be documented. Historically too many doctors have seemed to advance through training, only to struggle at the final examinations and then require remedial input. Programmatic assessment aims to avoid this situation by providing learners with regular feedback (Schuwirth and Van der Vleuten 2011). A suite of work-based assessments is now used in general practice training, such as case based discussions, direct observation of procedural skills, consultation observations, multisource feedback, and patient satisfaction questionnaires. These assessments help to direct GP registrars' learning, benefit from input from multiple practitioners, and are designed so that remedial intervention can be offered earlier during training.

Judgments of progress can be reassuring for registrars and for program directors, but need to be balanced so that assessment promotes rather than distracts from learning. Repeated and multiple work-based assessments risk a sense of continuous anxiety about assessment. The process of documenting learning, either in hard copy or via an ePortfolio, can have positive effects, particularly if the supervisor also uses the document (Pearson and Heywood 2004). In some countries, GP registrars use portfolios of documented learning for work-based assessments. These are periodically reviewed for evidence of progress in competence and for the training program to decide whether training should continue. However, forcing registrars to complete learning plans can become a "tick and flick" process without much educational impact (Garth et al. 2016).

Summative Assessment

Most GP registrars are required to pass a final assessment to become fully qualified as a GP. There are moves to take assessment as near as possible to the GP registrar's actual practice. This final stage is assessed in New Zealand by a College Fellow visiting the registrar's practice (The Royal New Zealand College of General Practitioners 2016). The College Fellow conducts a multi-modal assessment of the actual practice performance of the doctor to see if their routine work is at the standard expected. Similarly, GP registrars applying to qualify as members of the Royal College of General Practitioners in London have to submit videos of their actual consultations in practice.

The Dutch general practice training program has no final summative assessment but, 6 months into training, video consultations are assessed for communication skills. If a repeat fail occurs 6 months later, GP registrars may be counseled out of training or given another 6-month remediation term. A review of progression assessment is held at the end of the first-year when registrars present a portfolio of their learning in 10 to 12 areas to demonstrate their competence and why they should be allowed to continue training. Similarly, in Canada GP registrars must demonstrate that they have acquired the required competencies; they do also have to successfully pass the College of Family Physician examinations (The College of Family Physicians of Canada n.d.). It is interesting to note the emphasis on the learner proving their competency, rather than the assessor judging their competency.

In Ireland, GP registrars prove their knowledge and competency in an exam, and then develop their performance over the final year, in preparation for transition to independent, unsupervised practice.

Organization

General practice training requires an organization to recruit training practices, place registrars in training sites, coordinate in practice training support, provide out of practice training for registrars and supervisors, assess and monitor registrar progress, and assess and evaluate the performance of the training program. The European Academy of Teachers in General Practice (EURACT) recommends that training

3 General Practice Education: Context and Trends

organizations either be part of or work closely with, universities that run undergraduate general practice placements (Michels et al. 2018). It is usually the professional GP college that sets the training standards, principles, curriculum, and assessments.

Regardless of which organization actually runs training, there is an important role for that organization in ensuring the quality of training both in-practice and out-of-practice. Evaluation activities vary from in-practice feedback to feedback on individual workshops to program evaluation and national surveys of satisfaction with training. Most evaluation programs include visits to practices and direct observation of supervisors and medical educators in action.

Length of Training

In Europe, the length of general practice training ranges from 3 to 6 years. In Canada, there is ongoing discussion about the need to move from two to a third year of general practice training (Buchman 2012). There are currently opportunities to do a third year in specific topics, such as emergency medicine, anesthetics, and care of the elderly. However, there are concerns that graduates with this extra training subsequently prefer working only in their sub-specialty, whereas "generalist" expertise is what is needed. O'Shea 2009 et al demonstrated the benefit of an extra fourth year of training in Ireland which has now become standard. In the UK, there are calls to lengthen training from the current 3 year program (McKinstry et al. 2001; Capewell et al. 2014; de Kare-Silver 2011) and for most of the training to be based in general practice, as hospital experience is seen as having decreasing relevance for general practitioners (O'Dowd 2016).

Conclusion

General practice can provide positive learning environments for students, junior doctors, and specialty trainees (Tate and Ahluwalia 2019). Better understanding of primary care is important for all doctors in the health system, particularly as chronic disease and multi-morbidity require care that transcends the historic divide between community and hospital care. More junior doctors need to be encouraged into general practice training important to address the current trend toward non-GP specialties (Wass et al. 2016).

This chapter has shown how most learning occurs *in* general practice; learning is through relationships and is about relationship based-care. Maintaining high-quality learning in general practice requires deliberate effort and support to GP supervisors and their general practices through specific funding and external organizations. With planning, there is the opportunity to harness educational and technological developments to optimize training within the bounds of the pragmatic and thereby to enhance the capability and competence of future GPs (Tate and Ahluwalia 2019).

> **Box 1 European Academy of Teachers in General Practice**
>
> **The characteristics of the discipline of general practice/family medicine**
> These are that it:
>
> 1. Is normally the point of first medical contact within the healthcare system, providing open and unlimited access to its users, dealing with all health problems regardless of the age, sex, or any other characteristic of the person concerned.
> 2. Makes efficient use of healthcare resources through coordinating care, working with other professionals in the primary care setting, and by managing the interface with other specialties taking an advocacy role for the patient when needed
> 3. Develops a person-centered approach, orientated to the individual, his/her family, and their community
> 4. Promotes patient empowerment
> 5. Has a unique consultation process, which establishes a relationship over time, through effective communication between doctor and patient is responsible for the provision of longitudinal continuity of care as determined by the needs of the patient
> 6. Has a specific decision-making process determined by the prevalence and incidence of illness in the community
> 7. Manages simultaneously both acute and chronic health problems of individual patients
> 8. Manages illness which presents in an undifferentiated way at an early stage in its development, which may require urgent intervention
> 9. Promotes health and well-being both by appropriate and effective intervention
> 10. Has a specific responsibility for the health of the community
> 11. Deals with health problems in their physical, psychological, social, cultural, and existential dimensions

Cross-References

▶ Supervision in General Practice Settings

References

Academy of Royal Medical Colleges. The benefits of consultant-delivered care. 2012.

Aluttis C, Bishaw T, Frank MW. The workforce for health in a globalized context – global shortages and international migration. Glob Health Action. 2014;7(1):23611.

American Association for Family Practice. 2019 Match results for family medicine. 2019. http://aafp.org

Anderson K, Thomson J. Vertical integration – reducing the load on GP teachers. Aust Fam Physician. 2009;38(11):907–10.

Anderson K, Haesler E, Stubbs A, Molinari K. Comparing general practice and hospital rotations. Clin Teach. 2015;12(1):8–13.

Arya N, Gibson C, Ponka D, Haq C, Hansel S, Dahlman B, et al. Family medicine around the world: overview by region: the Besrour Papers: a series on the state of family medicine in the world. Can Fam Physician. 2017;63(6):436–41.

Ash JK, Walters LK, Prideaux DJ, Wilson IG. The context of clinical teaching and learning in Australia. Med J Aust. 2012;196(7):475.

Balint M. The doctor, his patient and the illness. London: Tavistock Publications; 1957.

Barker I, Steventon A, Deeny SR. Association between continuity of care in general practice and hospital admissions for ambulatory care sensitive conditions: cross sectional study of routinely collected, person level data. BMJ. 2017;356:j84.

Billett S. Towards a workplace pedagogy: guidance, participation and engagement. Adult Educ Q. 2002;53(1):27–43.

Bonney A, Phillipson L, Jones SC, Iverson D. Older patients' attitudes to general practice registrars – a qualitative study. Aust Fam Physician. 2009;38(11):927–31.

Britt HC, Harrison CM, Miller GC, Knox SA. Prevalence and patterns of multimorbidity in Australia. Med J Aust. 2008;189(2):72–7.

Britt H, Miller G, Charles J, Henderson J, Bayram C, Pan Y, et al. In: AIHW, editor. General practice activity in Australia 2009–10. Canberra: AIHW;2010.

Brookfield S. Understanding and facilitating adult learning. Milton Keynes: Open University Press; 1986.

Brown J, Morrison T, Bryant M, Kassell L, Nestel D. A framework for developing rural academic general practices: a qualitative case study in rural Victoria. Rural Remote Health. 2015;15(2):3072.

Brown JB, Kirby CN, Wearne SM, Snadden D, Smith M. Final report: review of Australian and International Models of GP vocational education and training. 2018.

Buchman S. It's about time: 3-year FM residency training. Can Fam Physician. 2012;58(9):1045.

Capewell S, Stewart K, Bowie P, Kelly M. Trainees' experiences of a four-year programme for specialty training in general practice. Educ Prim Care. 2014;25(1):18–25.

de Kare-Silver N. Five-year training: a radical rational approach to delivery. Br J Gen Pract. 2011;61(588):464–5.

Department of Health. Section 19AA of the Health Insurance Act 1973: Factsheet: Commonwealth Government of Australia; 2012. http://www.health.gov.au/internet/otd/publishing.nsf/Content/section19AB

Detsky AS, Berwick DM. Teaching physicians to care amid chaos. JAMA. 2013;309(10):987–8.

Dick ML, King DB, Mitchell GK, Kelly GD, Buckley JF, Garside SJ, et al. Vertical integration in teaching and learning (VITAL): an approach to medical education in general practice. [see comment]. Med J Aust. 2007;187(2):133–5.

Dick M-L, Henderson M, Wei Y, King D, Anderson K, Thistlethwaite J. A systematic review of the approaches to multi-level learning in the general practice context, using a realist synthesis approach: BEME Guide No. 55. Med Teach. 2019;41:862–76.

Donoff MG. Field notes. Assisting achievement and documenting competence. Can Fam Physician. 2009;55(12):1260–2.

European Academy of Teachers in General Practice. The characteristics of the discipline of general practice/family medicine. 2011.

Frenk J, Chen L, Bhutta Z, Cohen J, Crisp N, Evans T, et al. Health professionals for a new century: transforming education to strengthen health systems in an interdependent world. Lancet. 2010;376(9756):1923–58.

Gamble J. Modelling the invisible: the pedagogy of craft apprenticeship. Stud Contin Educ. 2001;23(2):185–200.

Garth B, Kirby C, Silberberg P, Brown J. Utility of learning plans in general practice vocational training: a mixed-methods national study of registrar, supervisor, and educator perspectives. BMC Med Educ. 2016;16(1):211.

Gray DP, Evans P, Sweeney K, Lings P, Seamark D, Seamark C, et al. Towards a theory of continuity of care. J R Soc Med. 2003;96:160–6.

Hays R, Sen Gupta T, Veitch C, Chang A, Chapman B, Discher A, et al. Expanding medical education in general practice. Aust Fam Physician. 2003;32:1036–7.

Henderson M, Upham S, King D, Dick M-L, van Driel M. Medical students, early general practice placements and positive supervisor experiences. Educ Prim Care. 2018;29:71–8.

Hudson J, Weston K, Farmer E, Ivers R, Pearson R. Are patients willing participants in the new wave of community-based medical education in regional and rural Australia? Med J Aust. 2010;192:150–3.

Humphreys JS, Jones JA, Jones MP, Mildenhall D, Mara PR, Chater B, et al. The influence of geographical location on the complexity of rural general practice activities. Med J Aust. 2003;179(8):416–20.

Ingham G, Plastow K, Kippen R, White N. Tell me if there is a problem: safety in early general practice training. Educ Prim Care. 2019;30:212–9.

Kelly M, Bennett D, O'Flynn S. General practice: the DREEM attachment? Comparing the educational environment of hospital and general practice placements. Educ Prim Care. 2012;23(1):34–40.

Kennedy TJT, Regehr G, Baker GR, Lingard LA. Progressive independence in clinical training: a tradition worth defending? Acad Med. 2005;80(10 Suppl):S106–11.

Kidd MR, Hudson JN. General practice: a leading provider of medical student education in the 21st century? Med J Aust. 2007;187(2):124–8.

Knowles MS. Andragogy in action: applying modern principles of adult learning. San Francisco: Jossey-Bass; 1984.

Kolb DA, Plovnick MS. Experiential learning theory and adult development. M.I.T. working paper MIT - Massachusetts Institute of Technology, Cambridge, USA. 1974;705–74 .

Laurence C, Docking D, Haydon D, Cheah C. Trainees in the practice – practical issues. Aust Fam Physician. 2012;41(1–2):14–7.

Lave J, Wenger E. Situated learning: legitimate peripheral participation. Cambridge: Cambridge University Press; 1991.

Maarsingh OR, Henry Y, van de Ven PM, Deeg DJ. Continuity of care in primary care and association with survival in older people: a 17-year prospective cohort study. Br J Gen Pract. 2016;66(649):e531–9.

Magin PJ, Morgan S, Tapley A, Davis JS, McArthur L, Henderson KM, et al. Reducing general practice trainees' antibiotic prescribing for respiratory tract infections: an evaluation of a combined face-to-face workshop and online educational intervention. Educ Prim Care. 2016a;27(2):98–105.

Magin PJ, Morgan S, Tapley A, Henderson KM, Holliday EG, Ball J, et al. Changes in early-career family physicians' antibiotic prescribing for upper respiratory tract infection and acute bronchitis: a multicentre longitudinal study. Fam Pract. 2016b;33(4):360–7.

Magin P, Tapley A, Morgan S, Davis JS, McElduff P, Yardley L, et al. Reducing early career general practitioners' antibiotic prescribing for respiratory tract infections: a pragmatic prospective non-randomised controlled trial. Fam Pract. 2018;35(1):53–60.

McGrail MR, Humphreys JS, Joyce CM, Scott A, Kalb G. How do rural GPs' workloads and work activities differ with community size compared with metropolitan practice? Aust J Prim Health. 2012;18(3):228–33.

McKinstry B, Dodd M, Baldwin P. Extending the general practice training year: experience of one model in Scotland. Med Educ. 2001;35(6):596–602.

Michels NRM, Maagaard R, Buchanan J, Scherpbier N. Educational training requirements for general practice/family medicine specialty training: recommendations for trainees, trainers and training institutions. Educ Prim Care. 2018;29(6):322–6.

Morgan S, Ingham G. Random case analysis: a new framework for Australian general practice training. Aust Fam Physician. 2013;42(1):69–73.

Morgan S, Magin PJ, Henderson KM, Goode SM, Scott J, Bowe SJ, et al. Study protocol: the registrar clinical encounters in training (ReCEnT) study. BMC Fam Pract. 2012;13:50.

Morrison J, Clement T, Nestel D, Brown J. Perceptions of ad hoc supervision encounters in general practice training: a qualitative interview-based study. Aust Fam Physician. 2015;44(12):926–32.

O'Dowd A. Significant changes to doctors' training are needed for future-proof workforce, peers are told. BMJ. 2016;355:i6605.

O'Shea EB. What's another year? A qualitative evaluation of extension of general practice training in the West of Ireland. Educ Prim Care. 2009;20(3):159–66.

Organek AJ, Tannenbaum D, Kerr J, Konkin J, Parsons E, Saucier D, et al. Redesigning family medicine residency in Canada: the triple C curriculum. Fam Med. 2012;44(2):90–7.

Pearson DJ, Heywood P. Portfolio use in general practice vocational training: a survey of GP registrars. Med Educ. 2004;38(1):87–95.

Peile E, Easton G, Johnson N. The year in a training practice: what has lasting value? Grounded theoretical categories and dimensions from a pilot study. Med Teach. 2001;23(2):205–11.

Pendleton D, Schofield T, Tate P, Havelock P. The new consultation developing doctor-patient communication. Oxford: Oxford University Press; 2003.

Robinson M, Slaney GM, Jones GI, Robinson JB. GP Proceduralists: 'the hidden heart' of rural and regional health in Australia. Rural Remote Health. 2010;10(3):1402.

Royal Australian College of General Practitioners. RACGP vocational training standards. 2013. http://www.racgp.org.au/education/rtp/vocational-training-standards/

Schon D. Educating the reflective practitioner. San Francisco: Jossey-Bass; 1987.

Schultz K, Griffiths J, Lacasse M. The application of entrustable professional activities to inform competency decisions in a family medicine residency program. Acad Med. 2015;90(7):888–97.

Schuwirth LW, Van der Vleuten CP. Programmatic assessment: from assessment of learning to assessment for learning. Med Teach. 2011;33(6):478–85.

Starfield B, Shi L, Macinko J. Contribution of primary care to health systems and health. Milbank Q. 2005;83(3):457–502.

Stewart M. Reflections on the doctor–patient relationship: from evidence and experience. Br J Gen Pract. 2005;55(519):793–801.

Stocks NP, Frank O, Linn AM, Anderson K, Meertens S. Vertical integration of teaching in Australian general practice–a survey of regional training providers. Med J Aust. 2011;194(11):S75–8.

Tate A, Ahluwalia S. A pedagogy of the particular – towards training capable GPs. Educ Prim Care. 2019;30:198–201.

Ten Cate O. AM last page: what entrustable professional activities add to a competency-based curriculum. Acad Med. 2014;89(4):691.

The College of Family Physicians of Canada. CanMEDs Family Medicine. 2009. http://www.cfpc.ca/uploadedFiles/Education/CanMeds%20FM%20Eng.pdf

The College of Family Physicians of Canada. Certification examination in family medicine. n.d. Accessed 29 Feb 2020. cfpc.ca/FMExam/

The King's Fund. Chapter 2: the evolving role and nature of general practice in England. Inquiry into the quality of general practice in England London. 2011.

The Royal New Zealand College of General Practitioners. Fellowship Regulations effective from 1 December 2016. 2016. https://oldgp16.rnzcgp.org.nz/assets/New-website/Become_a_GP/2017-Fellowship-Regulations-version-1-002.pdf

The Royal New Zealand College of General Practitioners. What is general practice? 2018; 20 January 2018. https://www.rnzcgp.org.nz/RNZCGP/I_m_a_Patient/What_is_general_practice/RNZCGP/Im_a_patient/What_is_general_practice.aspx?hkey=ac794013-53c3-450a-aef3-3958fb26f8fa

Thomson J, Haesler E, Anderson K, Barnard A. What motivates general practitioners to teach. Clin Teach. 2014;11(2):124–30.

Trumble SC. The evolution of general practice training in Australia. Med J Aust. 2011;194(11):S59–62.

Wallace E, Salisbury C, Guthrie B, Lewis C, Fahey T, Smith SM. Managing patients with multimorbidity in primary care. Br Med J. 2015;350:176. https://doi.org/10.1136/bmj.h.176.

Warwick C. How international medical graduates view their learning needs for UK GP training. Educ Prim Care. 2014;25(2):84–90.

Wass V, Gregory S, Patty-Saphon KfHEE. By choice – not by chance Supporting medical students towards future careers in general practice. 2016. https://hee.nhs.uk/sites/default/files/documents/By%20choice%20-%20not%20by%20chance.pdf

Wearne S, Dornan T, Teunissen PW, Skinner T. General practitioners as supervisors in postgraduate clinical education: an integrative review. Med Educ. 2012;46(12):1161–73.

Wearne SM, Magin P, Spike NA. Preparation for general practice vocational training: time for a rethink. Med J Aust. 2018;209:52–4.

Wenger E. Communities of practice; learning, meaning and identity. Cambridge: Cambridge University Press; 1998.

West Australia Department of Health. General practice workforce supply and training. Perth;2018.

Weston KM, Hudson JN. Clinical scholarship among preceptors supervising longitudinal integrated medical clerkships in regional and rural communities of practice. Aust J Rural Health. 2014;22(2):80–5.

WONCA Europe. The European definition of general practice/family medicine. 2011.

Worley PS, Esterman A, Prideaux DJ. Cohort study of examination performance of undergraduate medical students learning in community settings. BMJ. 2004;328:207–9.

Young L, O'Sullivan BG, Peel R, Reeve C. Building general practice training capacity in rural and remote Australia with underserved primary care services: a qualitative investigation. BMC Health Serv Res. 2019;19:338.

Zigmond D. General practice is disintegrating due to its serial reforms. 2019.

Anesthesia Education: Trends and Context

4

S. D. Marshall and M. C. Turner

Contents

Introduction: Challenges of Anesthesia Education	70
Traditional Approaches to Anesthesia Education	72
Selection and Early Vocational Training	73
Assessment During Specialty Training	74
Workplace-Based Assessment	74
Feedback and Planning Sessions	75
Examinations	75
Mandatory Courses	75
Educator Training Programs	75
Communication Training	76
Anesthesia Education in Low Resource Countries	76
In Situ Simulation	77
Quality Improvement and Anesthesia Education	78
Maintenance of Clinical Skills	78
Return to Work Programs	79
Emerging Technologies	79
The Future of Anesthetic Education	80
Practical Skill Acquisition	80
Academic Anesthesia	81
Increased Focus on Wellbeing	81
Social Media	82
Conclusion	82
Cross-References	83
References	83

S. D. Marshall (✉)
Department of Anaesthesia and Perioperative Medicine, Monash University, Melbourne, VIC, Australia
e-mail: stuart.marshall@monash.edu

M. C. Turner
School of Clinical Medicine, The University of Queensland, St Lucia, QLD, Australia

© Springer Nature Singapore Pte Ltd. 2023
D. Nestel et al. (eds.), *Clinical Education for the Health Professions*,
https://doi.org/10.1007/978-981-15-3344-0_8

> **Abstract**
>
> This chapter will outline the unique context of training and maintaining skills in the complex domain of anesthesia as a medical specialty. It will include how clinical skills, communication, decision-making, teamwork, and inter-professional care have traditionally been taught and the challenge of education in this specialty. The chapter will also cover how recent trends in clinical practice have affected the mode of delivery of education including the role of new technologies in delivering these programs. This chapter will focus on the specialty of anesthesia in Australia and New Zealand, with some reference to the practice of anesthesia in the UK.

> **Keywords**
>
> Anesthesia · Education · Continuing education · Clinical skills · Specialist · Pain

Introduction: Challenges of Anesthesia Education

Delivery of education in anesthesia poses a number of unique challenges due to the scope and nature of the work undertaken by the anesthetist and the anesthetic trainee. More than any other specialty, anesthetists must have a firm grasp of the underlying basic sciences – not only those related to earlier pre-clinical training such as anatomy and physiology but also including high school subjects such as physics and chemistry. Unusually, anesthesia is a subject that is not often included in an undergraduate or postgraduate medical school curriculum. When it is included, it is certainly not to the extent of medicine and surgery, and is commonly restricted to less than 3 weeks during the later years of clinical training. Debate about the importance of anesthesia in the undergraduate curriculum has continued for over 30 years (Cooper and Hutton 1995). Nevertheless, pain management is the only subject that appears to be consistently presented to medical students beyond the many that could be taught by anesthetists (Smith et al. 2019).

Anesthesia is therefore a specialty that is predominantly learned following graduation from medical school. Typically, specialized anesthetic training starts after 1 or 2 years of general hospital experience as a junior doctor. As noted, the training includes elements of basic science – some trainees may have not had any exposure to subjects such as physics and chemistry (which are required for the initial professional examinations), while others completed these subjects at a high school level a decade ago, or more recently at an undergraduate university level. This disparity in levels of knowledge at the beginning of a training program can pose a significant challenge to educators and learners alike. Furthermore, the revision of these basic sciences generally occurs at a time when the postgraduate doctor is immersed in a new and often disorientating specialty that has different expectations to previous roles in terms of responsibilities and supervision. The trainee has to learn the basics of the professional role such as consenting patients for anesthesia as well as their clinical role, including how to act in life-threatening emergencies where they have

4 Anesthesia Education: Trends and Context

only a matter of minutes to respond and in circumstances where immediate supervision might not be available. To bridge this education gap, and to minimize the risk to patients, simulation has been enthusiastically taken up by the specialty. Indeed, anesthesia has been at the forefront of simulation training and examination; this will be further explored later in this chapter.

A further challenge to the provision of anesthesia education is the extensive scope of practice of the anesthetist. Training must cover the acute to the chronic: from trauma, hemorrhage, and immediate oxygen delivery problems to the long-term psychosocial difficulties of dealing with persistent pain. These sub-specialized areas have their own additional curriculum within the broader one, but the comprehensive curriculum offered by most physician-delivered anesthesia training is really diverse in range. A specialist anesthetist in a rural or remote area might be involved in managing an intensive care unit, assessing patient fitness for upcoming surgery in a clinic setting in addition to in-hours and after-hours care provision in the operating theatre.

Any training program for anesthesia must be able to deliver effective education across all the contexts of care. This can be difficult in some environments. Traditional medical education has addressed how feedback and coaching can be undertaken in clinic and ward round settings, but the operating theatre environment is not always so conducive to teaching. The room is often noisy with many other professionals within earshot that may make it demanding to provide confidential, honest feedback. The focus is, as it should be, on the safety of the patient at all times. Ensuring vigilance during the maintenance phase of an anesthetic while also concurrently teaching and learning can compromise this focus of both the learner and teacher by dividing their attention between learning and clinical tasks. Teaching encounters may therefore need to be structured differently in this setting.

Indeed, the environment of the teaching itself may be very different in the varied contexts of anesthetic sub-specialization (Carlisle et al. 2016). The role of the anesthetist has evolved from provision of care in the operating theatre environment and has moved into the perioperative medicine space, where anesthetists are entrusted to embrace a holistic approach to patient care by optimizing pre-operative medical conditions via "prehabilitation." With this new role, the anesthetist must learn the unique skills of collaboration and negotiation with other team members and the patient before surgery as well as during surgery. Other non-core specialty rotations such as cardiac perfusion and hyperbaric medicine pose additional challenges.

The final question for the development of anesthesia training is the scale of training required. Anesthetic departments are commonly one of the largest departments, if not the largest department, in most high-income nations' hospitals. Vocational trainees in anesthesia account for about one in ten specialist training positions, and the provision of specialists barely keeps up with demand (O'Dowd 2016). Clearly with cost pressures and an increasing push for safety in anesthesia that has been realized with comprehensive training, the challenges for anesthesia educators are substantial.

Traditional Approaches to Anesthesia Education

Anesthesia, like most medical specialties, has traditionally been taught using the apprenticeship model. Trainees are assigned a mentor, supervisor of training, or teacher for a defined period of time in order to acquire the knowledge and skills to perform as a specialist (JAMA 1924). The mentor also provides the opportunity for role modelling the professional behaviors expected in the job in addition to providing feedback and guidance. In common with other medical specialties, as the role of the profession has become more extensive and more specialized, the trainee rotates among multiple educators, often in different clinical settings. Traditional apprentice/mentor relationships may be difficult to maintain and is unlikely to be appropriate in these situations (Rassie 2017). Training by multiple educators leads to a fragmentation of teaching and a decreased ability to track any trainee deficiencies because a full understanding of an individual's capabilities cannot be held by a single educator (Castanelli et al. 2019). Traditional methods of teaching need to be augmented by methods of effective communication between serial and concurrent educators or via the development of a new model that accounts for the distributed nature of learning.

A defined clinical rotation, for example, in cardiothoracic or pediatric anesthesia, will often be undertaken at a specialist center for those sub-specialties to maximize trainee exposure to these areas. There are further disadvantages to this model of sequential training in different sub-specialties that might not be immediately obvious. At a trainee level, these sub-specialist terms are often in demand, and there is a pressure to get as much out of them as possible. When the broader education system is considered, there may be insufficient workload in some areas for trainees to get enough experience in the time allocated (McIndoe 2012). Furthermore, the concentration of some sub-specialties into a small number of physical locations might result in a lack of access to the experience for some groups of trainees, purely because of their geographical location. An example in Australia, for instance, is trauma anesthesia; some areas have a centralized system with only one or two state trauma centers, limiting the exposure of rural trainees and those outside of these centers to access training in this sub-specialty.

The existence of a rotation-based system for anesthesia training has a more fundamental educational effect; that experience is limited to a defined time period. As we will see later, this can be problematic in moving away from a time-based system of training to a competency-based system. Anesthesia training involves a substantial component of "service delivery" (which may vary between institutions), which is to say that education occurs in conjunction with the provision of work to keep the hospital functioning (Green et al. 2017). As such, education is one part of a trainee's role that also includes after-hours and weekend work in addition to knowledge and skills acquisition from treating patients and traditional book learning. If the after-hours portion of the job is excessive, there may be limited time to access educators, and the effects of fatigue on learning could be significant (McClelland et al. 2017).

Traditional methods of training have included the acquisition of technical skills primarily, or solely, on patients. Clinical skills in anesthesia often have considerable risk of serious complications when starting training. For example, the risk of a trainee with under 3 years of anesthetic experience causing a severe, debilitating headache after an epidural is approximately five times that of a specialist (Haller et al. 2018). Other life-threatening risks are often more difficult to quantify because thankfully they are rare. In some countries, the practice of junior anesthetists undertaking difficult cases without direct supervision has been identified as a risk to patient safety (McIndoe 2012). Guidelines that minimize these out of hours cases, an important component of traditional training, have reduced the volume of emergencies that junior anesthetists are exposed to. In a time-based training program with an after-hours commitment, this has had a substantial effect on experience, necessitating a move away from these traditional teaching models.

Selection and Early Vocational Training

Selection for vocational training has traditionally depended upon interviews and references from colleagues rather than the objective evaluation of personal capabilities and personality traits. Recently however, attention has turned to the use of simulation to select junior doctors to enter specialist anesthesia training (Adams et al. 2009). In a pilot study by Cocciante and colleagues, selection criteria based on communication and non-technical skills were found to have good face validity for selecting the most appropriate candidates (Cocciante et al. 2016). In contrast, personality testing was found to have less support and considered less fair. The likelihood is that simulation testing may soon be routinely used to augment interviews and traditional selection methods such as references and informal observation. The barriers to more widespread use of simulation may be related more to resources and the accessibility of simulation perhaps more than a lack of robust evidence.

Beyond the selection of trainees, there is now a realization that the roles and expected professional attributes of a junior anesthetist are substantially different to their previous role as an "undifferentiated" doctor such as a resident, intern, foundation year doctor, or house officer. Several bodies have attempted to smooth this transition by developing resources to assist junior doctors' progression into the role of a junior anesthetist or intensivist (Joynt et al. 2011). These have traditionally involved a series of skills workshops to develop the required new skills for anesthetic practice such as tracheal intubation, arterial line placement, and central venous catheterization. However, there is a new awareness that other skills, and indeed an orientation to the training program, are required for the new trainee.

The Australian and New Zealand College of Anaesthetists (ANZCA) runs a "Part Zero course," which is a 1-day, face-to-face course, primarily designed for introductory trainees (and occasionally prospective trainees). It is intended to be delivered within the first 2 months of a trainee's commencement of the anesthetic training program. The purpose is to ensure that trainees are equipped with knowledge about the training program and curriculum and are given the opportunity to meet other trainees at the same level. The course is run by the various ANZCA state-based trainee committees and is focused on a centrally developed core curriculum. Part of the content to be delivered is mandatory, but there is autonomy for the regions to adapt some of the program to their local situation. The trainee committees recruit speakers to address trainees on a variety of topics, including the curriculum, workplace-based assessments, and the training portfolio system, as well as on issues such as welfare, professionalism, and performance.

Assessment During Specialty Training

In recent years there has been a shift away from a time-based, apprenticeship approach where trainees spend a minimum amount of time within the overall training scheme, and within that in each sub-specialty. Generally, anesthetic training programs are divided into four discrete training periods – introductory training, when core skills are developed; basic training, with exposure to low complexity cases that facilitate consolidation of these skills and the development of independent practice; advanced training, where more complex patients and sub-specialty cases are managed; and fellowship training, which involves a year or two in an area of interest or sub-specialty training such as pediatric or cardiac anesthesia. There are minimum time requirements for each stage; however trainees may take longer than the specified time to complete each training period, for example, due to examination failure, personal circumstances, and employment conditions precluding the sign off of specialized study units.

In addition, training colleges may specify a minimum pre-determined number of cases or "volume of practice" for each of the specialized study units and for general anesthesia experience. Trainees must log every anesthetic they perform into a logbook or online training portfolio system. By way of example, in Australia and New Zealand, for the specialized study unit of cardiac surgery and interventional cardiology, a trainee must do 20 cardiac surgery and interventional cardiology procedures with a minimum of 11 cases requiring cardiopulmonary bypass and 10 simple cardiological procedures including cardioversion, TOE, or pacemaker checks.

Workplace-Based Assessment

In acknowledgment of the new emphasis on competency-based medical education, there has been a shift toward formative workplace-based assessments (WBAs) (Weller et al. 2017). There are four types currently employed in Australia and New Zealand; direct observation of procedural skills (DOPS), mini clinical evaluation exercises (mini-CEX), case-based discussions (CbDs), and multi-source feedback (MsF) (ANZCA 2018a).

DOPS may be performed on a real patient or in a simulation environment and require assessment of the performance of a particular procedural skill, for example, an anesthetic machine check or a "can't intubate, can't oxygenate" scenario. The

4 Anesthesia Education: Trends and Context

value of DOPS assessment most likely lies in the narrative of what aspects were done well and poorly to guide further supervision, rather than any scoring system.

Feedback and Planning Sessions

Rather than allowing a trainee to struggle and for their performance to drift into failure, in most jurisdictions they are now commonly required to meet with their supervisors of training periodically for a clinical placement review. This often occurs at the beginning of a rotation, so a plan for the subsequent 6 months can be established, and at the end of the rotation so that feedback can be given to the trainee. Each specialized study unit also usually requires an additional meeting with the supervisor at commencement, so that expectations can be conveyed, and at transitions within the training programs. Generally, the aggregated results of the WBAs are reviewed at these points and feedback for improvement given.

Examinations

In the UK and Australasia trainees are required to sit two formal standardized centrally administered summative examinations. Generally, the first examination examines the basic scientific foundations of physiology, pharmacology, and equipment. The second examination is concerned with the safe provision of anesthesia across a range of contexts and sub-specialties.

Mandatory Courses

In Australia and New Zealand there are a number of practical courses that must be completed during anesthetic training. An Advanced Life Support Course (ALS) must be completed during each period of training. The Effective Management of Anaesthetic Crises (EMAC) course must be completed once during training, at any time after the introductory training period and preferably prior to commencement of the provisional fellowship year. Some trainees are also required to complete the Early Management of Severe Trauma (EMST) course, delivered by the Royal Australasian College of Surgeons.

Educator Training Programs

In the last few years there has been a developing interest in the quality of education received by both anesthetists-in-training and specialists. In particular, the skills of the educators have come under some scrutiny, with the realization that well-designed programs with skilled facilitators are more likely to result in higher quality educational outcomes. Illustrative of this are the efforts that have been undertaken by

ANZCA. The "ANZCA Educators program" consists of a 13-module course of study that can be individualized depending on the experience of the educator and their area and scope of educational practice (ANZCA 2019a). The modules are divided into five defined areas, from developing teaching resources through to managing the trainee with difficulties. Similarly a program created by the Royal College of Anaesthetists, "Anaesthetists as Educators," consists of free to access modules tailored for clinicians at different stages of their career, from trainee to senior consultant (RCoA 2019).

Specifically, one of the key skills identified as required by anesthetists with an education role is that of providing feedback to trainees. As a result, ANZCA developed the "Fundamentals of Feedback" training program (ANZCA 2018b). This specifically trains anesthetists to have routine, and occasionally challenging learning conversations with junior staff.

Communication Training

There have recently been advances related to how language can affect patients' perception of pain, discomfort, or risk in anesthetic practice. A branch of psychology termed neurolinguistic programming (NLP) has developed to change how clinicians express these ideas and to improve decision-making and comfort for patients (Cyna et al. 2009). For example, concentrating on the unpleasant sensations rather than the benefit of those sensations can lead to a perception of more pain. An anesthetist that frames contractions of a woman in labor as "another contraction closer to seeing your baby," rather than referring to it directly as "pain" will likely have a patient with less pain as a result (Cyna et al. 2010). Experienced anesthetists are familiar with the effect of a calming tone of voice and neutral language, but these skills are rarely explicitly taught in the clinical setting. Specialized courses on clinical communication are now available for anesthetists, including courses on hypnosis. These courses are increasing in popularity, although are not yet part of mainstream clinical education nor in the training syllabuses.

Discussion of risk and consent is another area of education that is commonly neglected in anesthetic care (Chrimes and Marshall 2018). Often multiple potential options available to the anesthetist can make the explanation of risk of each of these components challenging. For example, in contrast to surgical options, the addition of more invasive monitoring or regional anesthetic techniques might add further procedural risks but with potential overall benefits. Deficits in consent or explanation are often only evident on the rare occasions that an adverse event occurs. Arguably more formal education is needed in this area to address common shortfalls in clinical practice.

Anesthesia Education in Low Resource Countries

The Lancet Commission for Global Surgery in 2015 identified that five billion people in the world do not have access to safe, affordable anesthesia care. It is recognized that anesthetists have an international responsibility to provide quality anesthetic education and capacity building to anesthesia service providers in low-income and middle-income countries in an attempt to improve these conditions (Meara et al. 2015). Courses such as the "Real World Anaesthesia Course" (RWAC) are one example of this (RWAC 2019). The course prepares anesthetists to work in these regions, and also has a small focus on the management of mass casualty critical incidents. Further, participants learn to use draw-over vaporizer techniques in theatre (a technique of general anesthesia no longer practiced in high resource countries) and allows them to participate in lectures, small group discussions, and equipment trouble-shooting sessions. There are also several programs offered to trainees and fellows under the auspices of the Australian Society of Anaesthetists Overseas Development and Education Committee, whose aim is to support and promote anesthesia training in the Pacific and South East Asia.

Another successful and long-running international education initiative, the Essential Pain Management course, is an international program that runs workshops in over 40 countries with the goals of improving pain knowledge and pain management (ANZCA 2019b). Employing a "snowball model" of training that allows early identification of potential instructors, the course is designed to be delivered once to participants then handed over to them to continue to be delivered locally. This is a structure that empowers local health providers and creates a sustainable model that is accepted and culturally embedded within the local setting.

In Situ Simulation

Simulation within operating theatre environments is an increasingly frequent activity, particularly as time within the dedicated simulation center may be limited and the cost of reproducing an operating theatre is restrictive. However, these events are often isolated and confined to a single type of emergency or purpose; sustaining and supporting existing formal education programs and continuing professional development is rarely a focus. For instance, techniques that are learned in a teaching session such as closed loop communication or conflict resolution are rarely reinforced when anesthetists return to the workplace. As a result, behavioral change, clinical practice, and ultimately clinical outcomes might not be affected to the expected degree as the educator intended. Simulation-based programs taking place in dedicated simulation centers and remote from the clinical environment may worsen this reduction in effectiveness. Unless the simulation environment is identical to the clinical setting in terms of equipment, staffing, and processes, the transfer of behaviors is likely to be incomplete.

There has been a trend in simulation education for anesthesia toward in situ simulation within the actual clinical settings that anesthetists work. Clinicians undertaking in situ simulations likely have additional benefits and more complete transfer of clinical skills and behaviors. By performing in their own setting, utilizing their own equipment in the teams they would normally work in, they may identify deficiencies in the environment that can either be corrected or accommodated when actual events occur (Brazil 2017). For example, an anaphylaxis scenario where epinephrine, fluids, and a cognitive aid are immediately to hand will likely lead to an expectation that these will also be rapidly available in an actual emergency (Marshall et al. 2016). However, in the real clinical setting these might not be so readily available and, as a result, implemented late or even not at all. In situ simulation would uncover these deficiencies in the environment and could lead to a change in how equipment and resources are provided that support the education about the early use of epinephrine, fluid, and cognitive aids that have been shown to improve clinical outcomes. This additional safety element to in situ simulation has been observed in other settings, most notably obstetric care where it has been shown to improve neonatal outcomes (Draycott et al. 2006).

Quality Improvement and Anesthesia Education

From one of the most dangerous activities five decades ago, anesthesia is now one of the safest activities undertaken in a hospital environment (Aitkenhead 2005). Applying the principles of safety science and a preoccupation with safety within anesthesia education has no doubt played a key role in this. Morbidity and mortality meetings are an important quality and safety initiative run at a departmental level. Despite the low anesthesia mortality rates, these meetings present excellent opportunity for frank and open discussion about adverse outcomes and near miss events. Both personal and organizational learning occurs at these meetings, often prompting actions that improve overall safety. Furthermore, the open discussion of events creates a culture where further learning about safety is welcomed and expected.

Training programs in anesthesia commonly include a component of quality improvement within them to further grow the culture of safety. The activities within this role include mandatory audits of current practice or research into contentious areas. Rather than pure, or basic science research, these projects are aimed at practical delivery of safe care and reflection on practice.

Maintenance of Clinical Skills

As in other specialties there has been a developing awareness that professional practice requires the clinician to become a "life-long learner" with skills and knowledge constantly evolving with current understanding (Cooper 2017). Variably periods of 3- or 5-year cycles are imposed, during which the clinician must undertake a program of self-directed education. These continuing professional development (CPD) programs are often mandatory for anesthetists to be eligible to maintain registration, or "revalidate" (Roberts 2015).

Some programs have mandatory compliance with specific activities or types of activity. For example, ANZCA's CPD Program is divided into three sections – practice evaluation (patient survey, multi-source feedback, peer review, and clinical audit), knowledge and skills, and emergency responses (airway emergencies, cardiac arrest, anaphylaxis, major hemorrhage, and acute severe behavioral disturbance)

(ANZCA 2014). In the case of the UK's Royal College of Anaesthetists' program, there are no explicitly mandated activities, but independent evaluation and audit may be undertaken to ensure an appropriate breadth of education has been attempted. In addition, some employers mandate courses such as advanced life support or maternity emergency courses are undertaken regularly as a condition of employment (RCOA 2018). These courses are often also accredited toward the CPD programs.

Return to Work Programs

There are a multitude of reasons that flexible work arrangements may be utilized by employers and employees, and it is recognized that return to work following a prolonged period of absence from the workforce can present unique challenges to the anesthetist. With the shift of medical training to a postgraduate qualification, women are entering the workforce later and undertaking anesthetic training during child-bearing years. Extended periods of parental leave may be taken following the birth or adoption of a child. Others have medical or mental health issues requiring a leave of absence, and some doctors find themselves in a care giver role for elderly parents or other family members. The prevalence of these circumstances, and the acknowledgment of the difficulties that returning to work may pose, has led to the development of the Critical care, Resuscitation and Airway Skills in High Fidelity Simulation (CRASH) Course, a return to work course designed to provide practical upskilling and confidence to the anesthetist who has been away from practice for a period of time (Allen 2019). It is predicted that as flexible work arrangements become more accepted by departments, the need for high quality refresher courses aimed at competent anesthetists returning from prolonged periods of leave will be developed.

Emerging Technologies

Anesthesia, perhaps more than most other medical specialties, has become increasingly dependent on technology over the last few years. Techniques that would previously have been thought of as impossible without the use of technology have gradually become commonplace. Examples include the use of ultrasound-guided nerve blocks, depth of anesthesia monitoring, and videolaryngoscopy. Over time the demographics of patients presenting for surgery have become older with more complex comorbidities. Furthermore, surgery is commonly longer and more involved. Nevertheless, the morbidity and mortality associated with anesthesia has decreased in the last few decades (Schnittker and Marshall 2015). There is no doubt that anesthesia has become safer as a result of both new technologies and education. However, this rapid evolution of new technologies poses another problem – that of how we educate both junior and more senior staff about its use.

New techniques are generally reported in journals after (perhaps) trials in animal models and limited evaluation on healthy humans. Dissemination of new skills from this point is not necessarily straightforward. For example, in the case of point of care ultrasound (POCUS), very few practitioners within a department may currently have the skills to perform it competently for nerve blockades or pre-operative gastric assessment of a patient. Even fewer would also be capable of teaching the technique to consultant colleagues or junior staff. These substantially new techniques are generally learned in workshops at conferences or specific specialized courses. However, there are significant resources required to run these workshops in addition to the potential costs of purchasing new equipment. Unless the learning of new techniques is mandated in training programs and continuing professional development programs, there is a risk that these skills become limited to a few isolated pockets of practice. These centers are likely to have one or more clinicians that have a passion for both teaching and the potential of the new technology.

Another risk of introducing new techniques and technology is that they may only be used intermittently by the practitioners. Awake fiber-optic intubation is considered by most anesthetic training programs as a core skill. However, the necessity for most anesthetists to undertake this skill in routine clinical practice is fewer than one instance per year. In this situation it is difficult to truly maintain competency with such infrequent use (Marshall and Chrimes 2016). There are however a subset of anesthetists undertaking regular operating lists where this would be much more frequent, and so the volume and currency of practice needs to be considered when deciding if a new skill is worth pursuing and maintaining. Often the benefits of new technology and skills are not clearly communicated to experienced practitioners, meaning that opportunities to improve care and seek out educational opportunities are commonly missed.

The Future of Anesthetic Education

Practical Skill Acquisition

In comparison to the situation two decades ago, it is now indefensible to put a central venous line into a patient without ultrasound guidance; as a result, there is an increased requirement for trainees to learn ultrasound skills (Scott 2004). As already noted, these skills were often not required when most of the senior clinicians underwent their training, leading to a challenge of how to adequately educate junior staff with emerging technologies. These skills are often not confined to just one application. For example, the use of ultrasound has been extended to point-of-care gastric ultrasound to minimize aspiration risk, bedside echocardiography to diagnose a valvular lesion pre-operatively or the cause of an adverse intraoperative event, and to minimize risk in the use of regional anesthetic techniques. These ultrasound skills will likely become an expected part of every anesthetist's repertoire, and training on simulation models in addition to patients will likely become routine.

Ultrasound training is perhaps one area where Virtual Reality (VR) and Augmented Reality (AR) could be utilized. These simulation techniques involve the trainee interacting with real or simulated equipment and obtaining real-time feedback on their performance. Using AR or VR before interacting with a patient could minimize the risk to performing the procedure on the patient for the first time, by creating good habits and techniques in the handling of equipment (Grottke et al. 2009).

Academic Anesthesia

Increasing competitiveness in the job market in many countries has led to a rise in the acquisition of postgraduate qualifications. Many anesthetic trainees complete qualifications (graduate certificates, graduate diplomas, or masters) in medical education, simulation, perioperative medicine, or public health while they concurrently complete their formal anesthetic qualifications. PhDs are relatively uncommon in the anesthetic space in Australia and the UK, but this seems likely to change in the next few years. Bodies such as the National Institute of Academic Anaesthesia (NIAA) in the UK established in 2008 seem to be key, with one of their stated aims being to "facilitate and support training and continuing professional education in academia" (NIAA 2019). The NIAA supports academic trainees who wish to pursue research by connecting trainees with universities and funding bodies within the UK. Similar approaches in Australia have seen the establishment of state-based trainee-led research networks (Turner and Saric 2019).

Increased Focus on Wellbeing

In recent years there has been a focus on anesthetists, and in particular trainee wellbeing. In a study of 427 Australian anesthetic trainees, 28% were identified as having a K10 score consistent with high or very high distress (Downey et al. 2017). Causes of moderate or severe stress were identified as studying for exams (94.8%), concern about future job prospects (71.3%), critical clinical incidents (69%), and fear of making errors at work (67.1%). The Royal College of Anaesthetists survey conducted in 2017 had similar findings – up to 78% of anesthetists in training had experienced a detrimental impact to their health as a direct result of their employment, with 19% regularly managing self-reported excessive levels of stress associated with their role (RCoA 2017).

At a departmental level, the Long Lives, Healthy Workplaces (LLHW) initiative has been a tripartite response to the issue, led by the Wellbeing of Anaesthetists Special Interest Group that comprises members from ANZCA, the Australian Society of Anaesthetists, and the New Zealand Society of Anaesthetists (Skehan et al. 2018). The LLHW package has been developed in conjunction with Everymind, an institute dedicated to the prevention of mental ill health and suicide. It promotes wellbeing at a departmental level by introducing a toolkit of resources, aimed at primary, secondary, and tertiary prevention of mental ill health, and mental health promotion, which focuses on increasing healthy behaviors.

Social Media

The use of social media platforms is increasing in popularity as a form of knowledge dissemination, and it is likely that this trend will continue. Twitter peer review is a valuable and informal method of post publication peer review. Through social media, readers can ask authors detailed questions about their work that cannot fit into a standard 3000-word journal manuscript. Furthermore, important information such as insights into patient safety issues can be rapidly spread. Recent examples include drawing attention to unsafe fluid warmers (McGuire et al. 2019) and similar ampoules that increase the risk of drug errors (Marshall and Chrimes 2019). Social media can not only start these conversations but lead to lasting and meaningful change for good (Johannsson and Selak 2019).

Examples of Anesthetists and Anesthesiologists with a Strong Social Media Presence

Ed Mariano @EMarianoMD
> Tanya Selak @Gonggasgirl
> Helgi Johannsson @Traumagasdoc
> Laura Duggan @Drlauraduggan
> Tim Cook @Doctimcook
> Stuart Marshall @Hypoxicchicken
> Maryann Turner @MaryannCTurner

Conclusion

Education in anesthesia has undergone a substantial shift in the last two decades. As a specialty, anesthesia has been a pioneer in the modern era of simulation in health education. It now looks to embrace new technologies and ensure more complete translation of these advances into safer care through more responsive curricula and ongoing maintenance of professional skills.

This chapter has canvassed the challenges of anesthesia education, including the different contexts of work, when anesthesia training should commence and the broad scope of modern anesthetic practice including perioperative medicine, critical care, and chronic pain.

Outlining the assessment process, we have reviewed the current flavor of workplace-based assessments, feedback and planning sessions, examinations, and mandatory courses. Medical educators require ongoing teaching, and this concept of lifelong learning has been embraced by anesthetists through educator training programs and communication training. Embracing our responsibility to low- and middle-income country patients, programs have been established to ensure the knowledge and skills required for this type of work are readily available to high-income country anesthetists. In situ simulation is increasingly being employed to improve application of knowledge underpinned by the principles of situated learning. Quality improvement has been a strength of anesthesia and led to its remarkable safety record. Aspects of safety science are now firmly on the anesthesia training curriculum to further progress safety in the face of increasing complexity and patient comorbidities. Maintenance of clinical skills is crucial, and there are a number of opportunities available in this sphere which are underpinned by continuing professional development programs regulated by specialist colleges and professional bodies. The challenges of emerging technologies have been addressed in this chapter, reinforcing the need for continuing education to be orientated to future changes and best clinical practice. Several key areas have been identified where the evolution of medical education has and will be crucial to ensure the workforce is able to adapt to new technologies and techniques. These include the acquisition of practical skills in ultrasound guidance, the future of academic anesthesia, wellbeing, and the increasing use and relevance of social media, including Twitter, in the medical education space.

Cross-References

▶ Developing Health Professional Teams
▶ Embedding a Simulation-Based Education Program in a Teaching Hospital
▶ Learning and Teaching in the Operating Theatre: Expert Commentary from the Nursing Perspective
▶ Simulation for Procedural Skills Teaching and Learning
▶ Well-Being in Health Profession Training

References

Adams D, Sice P, Anderson I, Gale T, Lam H, Langton J, Davies P, Carr A. Validation of simulation for recruitment to training posts in anaesthesia (conference abstract). Anaesthesia. 2009;64:805–6.
Aitkenhead AR. Injuries associated with anaesthesia. A global perspective. Br J Anaesth. 2005;95 (1):95–109.
Allen K. CRASH course – critical care, resuscitation and airway skills in high fidelity simulation. 2019. From https://www.thermh.org.au/health-professionals/continuing-education/anaesthesia-and-pain-management-courses/crash-course
ANZCA. Continuing professional development handbook. Melbourne: ANZCA; 2014.
ANZCA. Anaesthesia training program curriculum v1.8. Melbourne: ANZCA; 2018a.
ANZCA. Fundamentals of feedback course. 2018b. From http://www.anzca.edu.au/resources/learning
ANZCA. ANZCA Educators Program. 2019a. Retrieved 4 Aug 2019, from http://www.anzca.edu.au/training/anzca-educators-program
ANZCA. Essential pain management course. 2019b. From http://fpm.anzca.edu.au/fellows/essential-pain-management
Brazil V. Translational simulation: not "where?" but "why?" A functional view of in situ simulation. Adv Simul. 2017;2(1):20.

Carlisle JB, White SM, Tobin AE. The anaesthetist and peri-operative medicine: migration and evolution. Anaesthesia. 2016;71(S1):1–2.

Castanelli DJ, Weller JM, Chander AR, Molloy EK, Bearman ML. A balancing act: the Supervisor of Training role in anaesthesia education. Anaesth Intensive Care. 2019;47(4):349–56.

Chrimes N, Marshall SD. The illusion of informed consent. Anaesthesia. 2018;73(1):9–14.

Cocciante AG, Nguyen MN, Marane CF, Panayiotou AE, Karahalios A, Beer JA, Johal N, Morris J, Turner S, Hessian EC. Simulation testing for selection of critical care medicine trainees. A pilot feasibility study. Ann Am Thorac Soc. 2016;13(4):529–35.

Cooper AE. The future United Kingdom anaesthetic workforce: training, education, and role boundaries for anaesthetists and others. Br J Anaesth. 2017;119(Suppl 1):i99–i105.

Cooper GM, Hutton P. Anaesthesia and the undergraduate medical curriculum. Br J Anaesth. 1995;74:3–5.

Cyna AM, Andrew MI, Tan SGM. Communication skills for the anaesthetist. Anaesthesia. 2009;64 (6):658–65.

Cyna AM, Andrew MI, Tan SGM, Smith AF. Handbook of communication in anaesthesia and critical care. Oxford, UK: Oxford University Press; 2010.

Downey GB, McDonald JM, Downey RG. Welfare of anaesthesia trainees survey. Anaesth Intensive Care. 2017;45:73–8.

Draycott T, Sibanda T, Owen L, Akande V, Winter C, Reading S. Does training in obstetric emergencies improve neonatal outcome? Br J Obstet Gynaecol. 2006;113:177–82.

Green A, Tatham KC, Yentis SM, Wilson J, Cox M. An analysis of the delivery of anaesthetic training sessions in the United Kingdom. Anaesthesia. 2017;72(11):1327–33.

Grottke O, Ntouba A, Ullrich S, Liao W, Fried E, Prescher A, Deserno TM, Kuhlen T, Rossaint R. Virtual reality-based simulator for training in regional anaesthesia. Br J Anaesth. 2009;103 (4):594–600.

Haller G, Cornet J, Boldi MO, Myers C, Savoldelli G, Kern C. Risk factors for post-dural puncture headache following injury of the dural membrane: a root-cause analysis and nested case-control study. Int J Obstet Anesth. 2018;36:17–27.

JAMA. The spirit of apprenticeship in medicine. JAMA. 1924;83(17):1337–8.

Johannsson H, Selak T. Dissemination of medical publications on social media – is it the new standard? Anaesthesia. 2019;75(2):155–7.

Joynt GM, Zimmerman J, Li TST, Gomersall CD. A systematic review of short courses for nonspecialist education in intensive care. J Crit Care. 2011;26(5):533.e1–e10.

Marshall SD, Chrimes N. Time for a breath of fresh air: rethinking training in airway management. Anaesthesia. 2016;71(11):1259–64.

Marshall SD, Chrimes N. Medication handling: towards practical a human-centred, approach. Anaesthesia. 2019;74:280–4.

Marshall SD, Sanderson P, McIntosh C, Kolawole H. The effect of two cognitive aid designs on team functioning during intra-operative anaphylaxis emergencies: a multi-centre simulation study. Anaesthesia. 2016;71(4):389–404.

McClelland L, Holland J, Lomas JP, Redfern N, Plunkett E. A national survey of the effects of fatigue on trainees in anaesthesia in the UK. Anaesthesia. 2017;72(9):1069–77.

McGuire N, Kelly M, Mustafa E, Hannon J. Fluid warmers, aluminium and what the regulator did. Anaesthesia. 2019;74(11):1354–6.

McIndoe AK. Modern anaesthesia training: is it good enough? Br J Anaesth. 2012;109(1):16–20.

Meara JG, Leather AJM, Hagander L, Alkire BC, Alonso N, Ameh EA, Bickler SW, Conteh L, Dare AJ, Davies J, Mérisier ED, El-Halabi S, Farmer PE, Gawande A, Gillies R, Greenberg SLM, Grimes CE, Gruen RL, Ismail EA, Kamara TB, Lavy C, Lundeg G, Mkandawire NC, Raykar NP, Riesel JN, Rodas E, Rose J, Roy N, Shrime MG, Sullivan R, Verguet S, Watters D, Weiser TG, Wilson IH, Yamey G, Yip W. Global Surgery 2030: evidence and solutions for achieving health, welfare, and economic development. Lancet. 2015;386(9993):569–624.

NIAA. 2019. From https://www.niaa.org.uk/About_Us

O'Dowd A. UK anaesthetist workforce is expanding too slowly, warn experts. BMJ. 2016;353: i3308.

Rassie K. The apprenticeship model of clinical medical education: time for structural change. N Z Med J. 2017;130:66–72.

RCoA. A report on the welfare, morale and experiences of anaesthetists in training: the need to listen. London: RCoA; 2017.

RCoA. Continuing professional development: guidance for doctors in anaesthesia, intensive care and pain medicine. London: RCoA; 2018.

RCoA. Anaesthetists as Educators (AaE) programme. 2019. From https://www.rcoa.ac.uk/anaesthetists-educators-aae

Roberts LJ. Revalidation: implications for Australian anaesthetists. Anaesth Intensive Care. 2015;43:652–61.

RWAC. Real world anaesthesia course. 2019. From http://www.realworldanaesthesia.org

Schnittker R, Marshall SD. Safe anaesthetic care: further improvements require a focus on resilience. Br J Anaesth. 2015;115(5):643–5.

Scott DHT. Editorial II: the king of the blind extends his frontiers. Br J Anaesth. 2004;93(2):175–7.

Skehan J, Hazel G, Tynan R, Fitzpatrick S. Long lives, healthy workplaces. Anaesthetists: improving their mental health and wellbeing. 2018. Retrieved 10 Aug 2019, from https://everymind.org.au/programs/anaesthetists-improving-their-mental-health-and-wellbeing

Smith A, Carey C, Sadler J, Smith H, Stephens R, Frith C. Undergraduate education in anaesthesia, intensive care, pain, and perioperative medicine: the development of a national curriculum framework. Med Teach. 2019;41(3):340–6.

Turner MC, Saric S. Establishing a trainee research network for Queensland anaesthetic registrars: a baseline research engagement survey. Kuala Lumpur: ANZCA ASM; 2019.

Weller JM, Castanelli DJ, Chen Y, Jolly B. Making robust assessments of specialist trainees' workplace performance. Br J Anaesth. 2017;118(2):207–14.

Clinical Education in Nursing: Current Practices and Trends

5

Marilyn H. Oermann and Teresa Shellenbarger

Contents

Introduction	88
Background of Clinical Teaching	88
Outcomes of Clinical Education in Nursing	90
Application of Knowledge and Development of Clinical Judgment	90
Skill Development	90
Professional Identity Formation	91
Cultural Competence	91
Competencies for Quality and Safety in Health Care	92
Models of Clinical Education	92
Traditional Model	93
Partnership or Collaborative Models	94
Preceptorship or Mentoring Model	95
Emerging Clinical Education Models: Collaborative Cluster Model	97
Technology in Clinical Education	98
Clinical Teaching Methods	100
Patient Care Assignment	100
Case-Based Learning	100
Discussions and Clinical Conferences	101
Written Assignments	101
Assessment of Clinical Learning and Performance	102
Conclusion	103
Cross-References	104
References	104

M. H. Oermann (✉)
Duke University School of Nursing, Durham, NC, USA
e-mail: marilyn.oermann@duke.edu

T. Shellenbarger
Department of Nursing and Allied Health Professions, Indiana University of Pennsylvania, Indiana, PA, USA
e-mail: tshell@iup.edu

© Springer Nature Singapore Pte Ltd. 2023
D. Nestel et al. (eds.), *Clinical Education for the Health Professions*,
https://doi.org/10.1007/978-981-15-3344-0_10

Abstract

This chapter examines current practices in clinical nursing education and intended outcomes of clinical experiences for nursing students. The chapter presents models of clinical nursing education, teaching methods used commonly in clinical settings, and technology to support and enhance learning in clinical settings. The chapter concludes with a broad overview of clinical evaluation.

Keywords

Clinical evaluation · Clinical nursing education · Clinical practice outcomes · Clinical teaching · Models of clinical nursing education · Nursing students

Introduction

Clinical practice is an essential component of a nursing curriculum whether preparing for entry into practice as a licensed nurse or for advanced nursing practice. Safe and effective practice requires an extensive knowledge base, the ability to think through complex and often unclear clinical situations and make informed decisions, and a wide range of clinical, technical, and other skills. The clinical learning environment is rapidly changing, and there is recognition of the need to prepare all health care professions students with competencies for improving the safety and quality of care and practicing collaboratively. This chapter describes clinical nursing education and intended outcomes of clinical practice for nursing students, models of clinical nursing education, and common teaching methods. The chapter concludes with a broad overview of clinical evaluation and key concepts.

Background of Clinical Teaching

Nursing is a professional practice-based discipline, distinct from academic disciplines because of the unique practice component. Students learn about nursing and the delivery of care to patients, families, and communities through classroom and clinical learning experiences. Educators guide students and support their learning in the clinical setting as they engage in real-life patient care, practice and refine skills, explore ethical issues, experience nursing roles, process clinical information, and connect theoretical content learned in the classroom to real-life practical situations. In other words, during clinical learning, students have opportunities to apply knowledge and skills in a realistic setting or transfer the knowledge gained in the classroom to the practice setting. Clinical nurse educators guide students to solve clinical problems, develop critical thinking skills, and practice care delivery while serving as a role model demonstrating positive professional work relationships. They also facilitate learner development and socialization as they coach students through the complexities faced in the clinical nursing setting, so the student develops into a competent and safe practitioner prepared to deliver care in the practice setting.

Clinical nurse educators use a variety of teaching-learning approaches that facilitate student learning across diverse settings. Students gain nursing knowledge and skills through simulation and learning laboratories, as well as during engagement in care delivery in health care settings across the delivery spectrum. Educators ensure that students are meeting critical learning outcomes in cognitive, psychomotor, and affective domains so they are prepared to meet the challenges of this practice profession.

Chickering and Gamson (1987), in their classic reference on good practices in undergraduate education, identified seven principles that enhance education. Those practices include: encouraging contact between students and faculty, developing reciprocity and cooperation among students, using active learning techniques, giving prompt feedback, emphasizing time on task, communicating high expectations, and respecting diverse talents and ways of learning. Even though these guidelines provide suggestions for classroom teaching, they can also serve as a guide for good clinical teaching practices in nursing. Additionally, more than just encouraging contact and giving prompt feedback, nursing education research suggests that quality clinical learning experiences require effective interpersonal relationships. Students report that feeling welcome, feeling valued, and having support and supportive relationships are crucial for a clinical learning experience (Dahlke and Hannesson 2016). Through the clinical learning experience, students are exposed to the experiential learning available in the practice setting.

Many of these good teaching practices identified by Chickering and Gamson also align with the National League for Nursing Clinical Nurse Educator Competencies (http://www.nln.org/Certification-for-Nurse-Educators/cnecl/cne-cl-handbook) and the World Health Organization Nurse Educator Core Competencies (https://www.who.int/hrh/nursing_midwifery/nurse_educator050416.pdf). Killingworth (2019), in a review of the literature, identified the following competencies of clinical nurse educators:

- Implement a variety of teaching strategies appropriate for learner needs, desired learning outcomes, content, and context
- Basing teaching strategies in educational theory and evidence-based teaching practices
- Create opportunities for learners to develop critical thinking and clinical reasoning skills
- Promote a culture of safety in the health care environment
- Create a positive and caring learning environment among learners
- Maintain collegial working relationships to promote a positive learning environment
- Show enthusiasm for teaching, learning, and nursing that inspires and motivates students
- Use personal attributes that facilitate learning
- Bridge the gap between theory and practice by connecting clinical learning opportunities to course content
- Foster a safe learning environment that promotes respect and civility

These critical components serve as the foundation for clinical nursing education and help to facilitate student learning in the health care environment.

Outcomes of Clinical Education in Nursing

Clinical practice is an essential component of a nursing curriculum. In practice, students gain new knowledge and master a wide range of clinical, technical, and other skills. In addition to the knowledge and skills to competently care for patients, students also need to develop their ability to think through complex and often ambiguous clinical situations and make informed decisions about actions to take. Experiences with patients provide opportunities for students to develop their clinical judgment skills with guidance and support from the teacher and others in the clinical setting. In most nursing programs, clinical practice time is limited, and as such learning activities should be carefully planned to guide students in meeting specific outcomes and developing essential competencies for practice. The outcomes to be achieved and competencies to be developed through clinical practice provide the framework for student learning and guide the activities in which they engage there.

Application of Knowledge and Development of Clinical Judgment

Clinical practice enables students to apply concepts and knowledge gained in class and through other means of learning in real-life clinical situations and develop their higher-level thinking skills. In clinical practice, students learn to make carefully thought out decisions, guided by the educator or preceptor, that impact patient outcomes (Manetti 2019). Tanner (2006) viewed clinical judgment as the interpretation of a patient's needs or health problems and subsequent decisions about actions to take (or to not act). This judgment process includes four components: (a) noticing (having expectations about the patient and clinical situation based on knowledge of the patient, knowledge gained in courses, and prior experiences); (b) interpreting (interpreting the data and understanding the situation and possible options); (c) responding (deciding on appropriate actions to take); and (d) reflecting (reflecting on the patient's response and modifying interventions based on that response (Tanner 2006). Clinical practice provides essential experience for students to begin to develop their clinical judgment skills and learn to think like a nurse. Lasater et al. (2019) found that this was a developmental process that varied based on learners' individual backgrounds.

Skill Development

In clinical practice, students have an opportunity to build expertise in clinical and procedural skills typically learned earlier in a laboratory or in simulation. The ability to perform skills as a new graduate is critical to transition into practice. Yet studies continue to document that new graduates often lack clinical skills and other entry-level competencies (Missen et al. 2016; Kavanagh and Szweda 2017). To retain skills and build expertise in them, students need deliberate practice: focused, repetitive practice of skills combined with feedback to correct performance errors and guide mastery (Oermann et al. 2015, 2016; Welch and Carter 2018). All too often in nursing programs, students learn to perform skills in a laboratory setting and can demonstrate they know how to perform them, for example, in a skills check-off, but without continued practice, those skills are not retained and gradually decay. Spaced or distributed practice, done over a period of time, improves retention and the ability to transfer a skill to a different context (Soderstrom and Bjork 2015). Clinical experience provides opportunities to practice skills, which not only promotes retention but also enables students to perform skills more quickly and with more confidence.

Professional Identity Formation

In clinical practice, students develop their professional identity as a nurse. This is another outcome of clinical practice. Professional identity is consistent with values of nursing as a profession, such as caring, communication, leadership, and ethics, among others, and is a developmental process through the student's educational program (Hensel 2014; Hensel and Laux 2014). As students care for patients and interact with others in practice, they reflect on these values and what it means to be a nurse. To understand nursing role formation among students, Ostrogorsky et al. (2015) analyzed end-of-term narrative reflections from 34 students over a 15-month program. They identified four major themes: evolving role perception, extending nursing student-patient interaction, engaging with the health care team, and expanding critical thinking. As students progressed through the nursing program, they internalized what it meant to be a nurse, were able to reflect on the meaning of their clinical experiences to their own role development, learned to collaborate as a team member, and became adept at recognizing and managing complications. The researchers also found that regardless of the clinical setting, students' development of their professional identity occurred through authentic clinical experiences. Inherent in this development of a professional identity as a nurse is accepting responsibility for one's own actions and decisions and learning-to-learn.

Cultural Competence

As society becomes more global and multicultural, it is critical for nursing students to learn about different cultures and recognize the impact on culture on care decisions (Carter et al. 2019; de Castro et al. 2019). Students gain this learning in clinical practice as they care for culturally diverse patients and communities. Repo et al. (2017) recommended that to improve cultural competence, nursing students need opportunities to interact with other cultures. These opportunities are available in clinical practice as students care for patients "different from themselves."

Competencies for Quality and Safety in Health Care

The need to improve the quality and safety of care has been well established, and many initiatives have been developed over the years to meet that goal. However, studies still document that patient safety remains a concern in health care settings (Bates and Singh 2018). In clinical practice, nursing students develop competencies essential to providing safe care to patients. They gain knowledge and skills to recognize safety concerns and improve quality of care (including quality improvement); provide patient-centered care (respecting patients' preferences and values, recognizing them as partners in care, and advocating for patients); use research findings and other evidence to guide practice; develop skills in collaboration and teamwork; and use information systems to ensure safe and quality care and for documentation (Altmiller and Armstrong 2017; Horsley et al. 2016; Interprofessional Education Collaborative [IPEC] 2016; Sherwood and Zomorodi 2014). As technologies expand, students will need competencies related to using new technologies such as digital health tools and telehealth, among others (Skiba 2016).

In recent years, there has been recognition globally about the need to improve systems of care to prevent medical errors. One of the initiatives in the United States to meet this goal was the Quality and Safety Education for Nurses (QSEN). The QSEN initiative defined quality and safety competencies for nursing and the knowledge, skills, and attitudes to be developed by students at the prelicensure and graduate levels; many of these competencies are developed in the clinical setting (QSEN 2019). The World Health Organization has developed key resources for improving patient safety, which is one of their global health priorities (https://www.who.int/patientsafety/en/). These resources can be used in the clinical education of nursing and other health professions students.

The World Health Organization and other groups globally have recognized the importance of interprofessional collaboration to patient safety. An important effort to prepare students to work in teams has been the IPEC (2016), which identified core competencies for all health care professions students for collaborative practice (Table 1). Many schools globally have integrated interprofessional simulations and other learning activities for students to learn to work collaboratively; however, students also need experiences in clinical settings such as participating in interprofessional rounds or developing quality improvement initiatives as a team. Table 2 provides a list of the outcomes of clinical practice in nursing programs.

Models of Clinical Education

As health care continues to rapidly change, nurses are faced with increased complexity of care and growth in technology and medical knowledge. Clinical nurse educators need to adequately prepare graduates to confront the ever-changing practice demands they will face. To provide effective and efficient clinical nursing education, various new clinical education models are emerging, and some long-

5 Clinical Education in Nursing: Current Practices and Trends

Table 1 Core competencies for interprofessional collaborative practice: 2016 update

Values/ethics for interprofessional practice: Work with individuals of other professions to maintain a climate of mutual respect and shared values
Roles/responsibilities: Use the knowledge of one's own role and those of other professions to appropriately assess and address the health care needs of patients and to promote and advance the health of populations
Interprofessional communication: Communicate with patients, families, communities, and professionals in health and other fields in a responsive and responsible manner that supports a team approach to the promotion and maintenance of health and the prevention and treatment of disease
Teams and teamwork: Apply relationship-building values and the principles of team dynamics to perform effectively in different team roles to plan, deliver, and evaluate patient/population-centered care and population health programs and policies that are safe, timely, efficient, effective, and equitable

From: Interprofessional Education Collaborative (IPEC) (2016). Copyright, 2016 Interprofessional Education Collaborative[®]. This document may be reproduced, distributed, publicly displayed, and modified provided that attribution is clearly stated on any resulting work, and it is used for noncommercial, scientific, or educational – including professional development – purposes

Table 2 Outcomes of clinical education in nursing

Acquire and integrate knowledge to understand patient conditions and interventions
Apply concepts and knowledge gained in class and through other means of learning to real-life clinical situations
Develop higher-level thinking and clinical judgment skills
Build expertise in clinical, procedural, and other psychomotor skills
Develop professional identity as a nurse
Accept responsibility for own decisions and actions
Provide value- and ethical-based care to culturally and ethnically diverse patients and communities
Develop knowledge, skills, and attitudes for improving the quality and safety of health care
Evaluate and use research and other evidence to guide practice decisions
Communicate effectively with patients, families, other health care providers
Collaborate with other health care professionals in practice settings as team member and leader

Adapted from Oermann et al. (2018), pp 77–78, Oermann and Gaberson (2021), p 256. Reproduced with the permission of Springer Publishing Company, LLC.

established models continue to be used. In the various clinical nursing education models, educators, nursing staff, and students have differing roles and responsibilities. Implementation of these models may be dependent on the students, the clinical agency, and other institutional factors.

Traditional Model

One of the models of clinical nursing education involves a primary educator in a single clinical setting teaching a small group of students ranging in size from approximately 6 to 12. This is a commonly used model of clinical teaching in the

United States and Canada for prelicensure students. In this model, the clinical nurse educator provides support and assists students in delivering patient care usually for one or two clinical days per week for a portion of the day. The clinical educator is responsible for student learning and safe care for the assigned patients as students experience a snapshot of clinical nursing care during this experience. Nursing students learn about clinical practice as they provide total patient care for their assigned patients in parallel with nursing staff. This has been the standard model of clinical nursing education for the past 50 years in the United States (Giddens and Caputi 2020).

Despite this being the oldest and a commonly used model, there is little current description of this model in the literature. When it is described, it is usually part of a comparison with other newer and emerging models. However, given rapid and dramatic changes in health care and higher education, nurse educators and clinical facilities need to examine issues and the problems emerging with the use of this model. For example, it is becoming hard to execute this traditional teaching model with growing competition for clinical sites and with students facing limited continuity of care with patients due to the short length of hospital stays for patients. Nursing programs also face concern about the growing costs of nursing program delivery and limited faculty experience and availability for teaching with this model.

Additionally, during the traditional clinical experience, students may have unproductive time as they wait for the clinical nurse educator's availability to guide their learning and nursing care. At the clinical learning sites, patient census and acuity also impact potential learning opportunities for students in this model of clinical education. These complex and interrelated factors may result in an unpredictable and haphazard approach to learning. Newer models of clinical nursing education are emerging in practice in the literature and offer promising alternatives for clinical nursing education.

Partnership or Collaborative Models

Partnership or collaborative clinical education models between nursing education programs and clinical practice agencies have emerged. The dedicated education unit (DEU) represents the most commonly discussed partnership or collaborative model. DEUs were introduced in the late 1990s in Flinders University in Australia followed by Canada and later the United States, where it has been used for approximately a decade (Dapremont and Lee 2013; George et al. 2017). In this model, the health care facility or unit at a clinical facility develops an exclusive relationship with one nursing program allowing staff nurses to partner with students from that program. DEUs have traditionally been used in acute care setting but more recent literature reports their use in long-term and transitional care settings (Fox 2017; Devereaux Melillo et al. 2014).

In a DEU, students are engaged and immersed with staff nurses who serve as role models for students. Together the student and staff nurse collaboratively participate in the full scope of the nursing role. The students and staff nurses form a partnership or care delivery team while the faculty member serves as a mentor to facilitate the learning. Students benefit from the expertise of the faculty member and the clinical nurse while being exposed to a wide range of clinical experiences. This model also enables students to interact with the interprofessional health care team and gain valuable insight into interprofessional practice.

Early research about this clinical teaching model focused on student, faculty, and staff satisfaction (Rhodes et al. 2012). However, now that DEUs have been used in nursing education for more than a decade, various researchers have conducted studies to assess student learning and outcomes associated with this delivery model. Crawford et al. (2018) conducted a mixed methods study in New Zealand with 42 staff nurses and nurse managers and 24 undergraduate nursing students completing an online survey. They also conducted 6 focus groups with 17 registered staff nurses and 16 undergraduate nursing students. Results suggest that students felt part of the health care team, the DEU structure provided a nurturing and supportive learning environment, and learning partnerships developed. The need for further role clarity for the staff nurses emerged as a challenge of the DEU model.

In another study that moved beyond evaluating satisfaction with DEUs, George et al. (2017) evaluated nursing student self-efficacy in clinical nursing education models. Students working in the studied DEU model demonstrated a statistically significant increase in self-efficacy scores post clinical education compared to students in the traditional clinical education model. This is consistent with the findings of Plemmons et al. (2018), who also found that, of the 272 students in their quasi-experimental study, students participating in the DEU clinical education model had larger statistically significant increases in clinical self-efficacy compared to students in the traditional clinical education model.

Other researchers have also compared DEU teaching models and traditional models and explored specific nursing competencies and professional attributes of nursing students. Rusch et al. (2018) completed a descriptive comparative study of over 300 nursing students in the United States and found that those participating in DEU nursing education scored significantly higher than students participating in traditional nursing education in 26 of 33 competencies and attributes. DEUs offer a supportive and collaborative learning opportunity that may help enhance self-efficacy and clinical competence, thus offering promise as a clinical education model.

Preceptorship or Mentoring Model

Another approach to clinical nursing education involves a preceptorship or mentoring model. This approach draws on apprenticeship theory allowing students to be immersed in learning with an expert. Unlike the DEU model, the preceptorship model does not rely on formal, exclusive partnerships between nursing programs and a clinical unit but are informal, short-term learning opportunities. These experiences may also be known by other names including practicums, preceptorships, clinical coaching model, externship, immersion experiences, and clinical partnerships. Regardless of the name used, these preceptorship models have been used in Canada, the United States, Australia, New Zealand, and the United Kingdom (Lafrance 2018).

The preceptorship or mentoring model involves a clinical immersion experience that is a shorter and intense practicum in a particular clinical setting. Students work closely with staff nurses in a 1:1 or 1:2 ratio in a mentoring or coaching relationship. These experiences are designed to increase student clinical knowledge, skills, and competencies while also promoting role socialization. These concentrated and intensive clinical experiences simulate entry-level professional work. Faculty provide support to the clinical staff preceptors as students refine skills, further develop their clinical judgment, and become socialized to the nursing practice role.

These mentored clinical learning experiences have been discussed in the literature. Fowler, Knowlton, and Putnam (2018) completed a review of the literature of 24 articles from 2005 to 2016 that focused on clinical immersion experiences. They reported that students preferred precepted experiences over a traditional clinical education model. Themes from the review suggest a sense of support and belonging, development of increased self-confidence, an increase in knowledge and skills, the ability to see patient progression, and a feeling of being more prepared for clinical practice. Only three studies examined objective measurements of student performance, and the results were inconclusive, suggesting further research is needed about this clinical teaching approach. In a review by Fowler, Knowlton, and Putnam (2018), immersion experiences were successful in increasing student confidence and nursing skills; however, additional evidence is needed to determine whether these immersion experiences improve graduate readiness for practice.

Other researchers also have discussed these clinical immersion models. A nursing program in the United States reported the use of immersion models to transform clinical teaching across the curriculum. They used five different experiences that enabled students to gain clinical exposure across the care continuum (Shaffer et al. 2018). Although the authors only report their experiences for this single site study, it appears that these models are gaining interest and being adopted by more nursing programs.

Many nursing programs that use this preceptorship or mentoring model provide these clinical experiences near the end of the program of study and use this clinical teaching opportunity to assist students in their transition to practice. Few authors discuss the essential clinical and curriculum foundation needed to ensure a successful learning experience. However, Diefenbeck et al. (2015) discuss the use of three foundational components that are critical to the senior year clinical immersion experience. Students must complete prerequisite field experiences, clinical work experiences, and simulation resource center experiences before engaging in the clinical immersion in their senior year of education. Results from their robust mixed method data collection about the clinical immersion curriculum model suggest that this model is a viable clinical teaching option.

Few authors discuss the best approach for structuring the preceptorship or mentoring model experiences. Kumm, Godfrey, Richards, Hulen, and Ray (2016) sought to determine if there were differences in 8-week and 16-week clinical immersion experiences on students' clinical knowledge, technical skills, critical thinking, communication, professional management of responsibility, and overall performance. They found no statistically significant differences between the groups, suggesting that an 8-week clinical immersion experience may result in appropriate learning outcomes and could offer cost savings for nursing programs. Although research about the preceptorship and mentoring model is limited, this clinical teaching model continues to be used in nursing education.

Emerging Clinical Education Models: Collaborative Cluster Model

As higher education and health care continue to change, clinical nursing education may also be faced with challenges and new clinical education models will appear. One such emerging model is the collaborative cluster model. Maguire, Zambroski, and Cadena (2012) describe a clinical collaborative cluster model for nursing education in which students complete most of their learning experiences in a single health care organization. During each clinical course, students are "matched" with a staff nurse preceptor who provides the clinical education while a clinical faculty offers oversight, makes rounds on the units, and conducts conferencing activities. The specific preceptor working with a student may vary for each course, but the student remains within the same organization throughout the entire nursing program. This model differs from the traditional and preceptorship/mentoring models since it starts at the beginning of the nursing program and does not serve as a single learning experience. This approach to clinical nursing education helps to reduce agency orientation time, allows students to develop strong connections and relationships with staff, and enables students to develop competency with skills and equipment used in the facility. Ultimately, it may serve as a recruitment strategy for the clinical agency, making hiring and orienting new graduates easy. This approach enables graduates to successfully transition to practicing staff nurses: they have had immersed and sustained clinical experiences at the site as a student and are already familiar with the clinical agency.

These findings of the collaborative cluster placement were further supported in a focus group study by Van der Riet, Levett-Jones, and Courtney-Pratt (2018). The authors completed a qualitative study exploring Australian nursing students' perceptions of the collaborative clinical placement model. Six themes were identified from the 14 student participants and included convenience and camaraderie, familiarity and confidence, welcomed and wanted, belongingness and support, employment, and the need for broader clinical experiences. These findings suggest that the collaborative clinical placement model may limit students' stress and improve familiarity with the nursing staff, setting, policies, and clinical environment and thus provide a potential new clinical nursing education model.

In summary, there are four main clinical nursing education models used in nursing programs although many schools use a combination of these models. Table 3 provides a description of each model.

Table 3 Models of clinical nursing education

Model	Description
Traditional	One primary nurse educator in a single clinical setting teaching a small group of nursing students Educator is on site with students
Partnership or collaborative	Academic-practice partnerships between a nursing education program and clinical practice agency (e.g., dedicated education unit) Clinical agency or unit develops an exclusive relationship with one nursing program, with staff nurses providing clinical instruction for students from that program. Faculty guide the staff nurse educators
Preceptorship or mentoring	Based on apprenticeship theory: Students are immersed in learning with an expert (preceptor or mentor) Does not rely on formal, exclusive partnerships between a nursing program and agency but are short-term learning opportunities
Collaborative cluster model	Students complete most of their learning experiences in a single health care agency In each clinical course, students work with a staff nurse preceptor (with faculty guiding the preceptor)

Technology in Clinical Education

Technology has become an integral part of health care, thus representing an area of rapid growth in nursing education. Faculty and students are using technology to support and enhance learning in clinical and classroom settings. Clinical simulation and manikin-based simulation have seen widespread adoption in nursing education during the past 10 years and are commonly used in all clinical areas in nursing programs. Faculty have designed innovative, immersive, experiential simulation approaches using clinical scenarios that portray realistic clinical situations and allow students to have clinical practice opportunities without the risk of patient harm. Simulation also provides standardized learning opportunities in areas that students may not routinely encounter in clinical settings such as high-risk patients or those with uncommon diagnoses. Additionally, these simulated learning experiences allow for active participation within a controlled environment where students can intervene and practice without harm to patients. Nurse educators use a range of task trainers, manikins, simulators, and simulations involving actors portraying patients.

Researchers continue to explore simulation use and gather evidence of its impact on learners, while nurse educators attempt to find the best educational mix of clinical simulation and direct care with patients in clinical facilities. The findings of the national randomized controlled study involving clinical simulation in the United States suggest that up to 50% of traditional clinical practice experiences can be replaced by high-quality simulation and can produce comparable outcomes in prelicensure nursing programs (Hayden et al. 2014). This National Council of State Boards of Nursing simulation study provided educators with empirical support for the claim that high-quality simulation experiences allow students to develop their nursing skills, and the study also provided evidence for continued simulation use in nursing education. The adoption of simulation is now widespread in nursing education, and, given its proliferation, various aspects of simulation-based education are covered in other chapters of this volume.

Three-dimensional (3D) virtual reality simulation represents another innovative technology used in nursing education. Virtual reality simulation has advantages over traditional simulation because of the lower cost, ability to actively engage large numbers of students, convenience, and flexibility in location use. Additionally, virtual simulation offers immersive and problem-based learning and can expose all learners to experiences that may not be available in the clinical setting. Research about virtual simulation suggests that this teaching strategy can enhance students' critical thinking, decision making, clinical reasoning, communication, and skill development (Foronda et al. 2018), thus offering an alternative to other clinical learning experiences.

With the proliferation and access to mobile technology devices such as mobile phones, it is not surprising that the use of this technology is also occurring in clinical nursing education. O'Connor and Andrews (2015), in their literature review of mobile technology use in clinical nursing education, reported that this topic lacks clarity. Many terms such as cell phone, handheld, mobile, tablet PC, and personal digital assistant were found in the literature. This is not surprising as the technology continues to develop, and older devices are replaced with newer devices, applications, and options. This review also suggested that the use of mobile applications has increased student productivity and confidence in their clinical nursing experience. Additionally, students perceive that these devices enhance student clinical learning and knowledge retention.

Mobile technologies may enhance student learning, but there is limited research about their use in clinical nursing education. O'Connor and Andrews (2018) conducted a descriptive cross-sectional study of 200 undergraduate nursing students and reported that just under half used a smartphone application to support clinical learning. When applications were used, students relied on the calculator, drug reference guide, and medical dictionary applications. Although mobile technology can provide efficient data retrieval, interviews with eight undergraduate nursing students in a community practicum revealed unclear expectations for their use of this technology while engaged in this clinical experience (Beauregard et al. 2017). Students reported non-supportive and restrictive cell phone use policies as well as negative views and inconsistent expectations associated with cell phone use in the clinical setting.

Clinical staff and nurse educator experience with technology use, and their lack of acceptance may create missed opportunities for students to access valuable clinical information that could lead to enhance patient care and improved communication. The use of mobile technology can be a powerful aid to clinical teaching and learning; however, connectivity issues, technology literacy, cost, lack of resources, and negative attitudes and stigma may serve as barriers that must be addressed before this technology is widely accepted (O'Connor and Andrews 2015; Beauregard et al. 2017; Mackay et al. 2017). A cultural shift by those in the clinical setting may be necessary before widespread adoption of mobile technology will be embraced as a valuable tool for learning and patient care. Further study demonstrating the benefits of technology integration in clinical nursing education is needed.

Clinical Teaching Methods

In clinical education, regardless of the model used in the school of nursing, the outcomes of clinical practice and competencies to be developed by students guide nurse educators in selecting clinical teaching methods and planning learning activities for students. Competencies are the specific behaviors – knowledge, skills, and attitudes – that students are expected to develop in their clinical practice (Oermann et al. 2018). Educators also consider the level of students in terms of their prior knowledge and experience and characteristics of the clinical setting. Commonly used methods in clinical nursing education are patient care assignment, cases, discussions and conferences, and written assignments.

Patient Care Assignment

Whether an assignment is made by a faculty member from the school of nursing who is also teaching in the clinical setting, or a clinical nurse educator or preceptor, the goal of any patient assignment should be to help students achieve the outcomes described earlier and develop their clinical competencies. All too often students are assigned to provide nursing care to one or a group of patients, but this may not be the best choice for the outcomes or to meet students' individual learning needs. If the goal is collaborative practice, then observation of teams in the clinical setting, with an analysis of team functioning, might be a more appropriate activity than providing complete care to a patient.

To provide more integrated clinical experiences for students, in one school of nursing in the United States, faculty redesigned their clinical practicum to focus on care coordination, transitions of care, primary care, community and population care, advocacy, social justice, person-centered care, and interprofessional collaboration (Shaffer et al. 2018). In each practicum, students have experiences in both acute care and community settings. Clinical educators from both settings work in dyads to teach students across the care continuum.

Case-Based Learning

Other clinical teaching methods include cases, which present scenarios of patients, families, and other clinical situations for students to analyze, propose possible approaches to use, and decide on the best action to take in the situation. Studies support case method for achieving those goals (Li et al. 2019; Thistlethwaite et al. 2012). Cases provide experience in thinking through situations that may be not clear cut. With cases, students can practice identifying possible alternatives, comparing them using research findings and other evidence, thinking through the consequences of different decisions, and deciding on the best decision considering the data provided in the case. Cases and unfolding cases, where the scenario changes as the case unfolds presenting new data for analysis and integration, are effective methods to develop problem solving and clinical judgment skills (Oermann et al. 2018; Hong and Yu 2017). Cases can be used prior to a clinical experience or in postclinical conference. Discussion about cases among peers in the clinical group can challenge students' perspectives and improve their higher-level thinking.

Discussions and Clinical Conferences

Discussions with students, both one-to-one and as a group, need to occur within a supportive learning environment. Discussions about clinical practice provide an opportunity for both the teacher and student to think aloud: verbalizing thoughts about possible decisions in a situation (Burbach et al. 2015). These discussions are for learning – to help students develop their decision-making and clinical judgment skills in a safe environment where they can talk through their reasoning and explore different possibilities with an expert.

Discussions with students as a group are often done as a preconference (prior to beginning a clinical experience) or as a postconference (at its conclusion). Preconferences are important to determine students' learning needs and to identify areas of patient care in which students need further instruction. In postconferences, students have an opportunity to reflect on the care they were provided and their interactions with others in the practice setting. Postconferences also provide a forum for students to discuss ethical issues and situations they encountered or observed in the clinical setting.

While postconferences are typically face-to-face in the clinical setting, they may be held online following the clinical practicum (Hannans 2019). Asynchronous online discussions allow students to reflect on their clinical experiences, interactions with others, and interventions they used. Hannans (2019) used VoiceThread, a Web-based platform for online audio-video discussions to conduct postconferences with her students. With online conferences, students had time to reflect on their clinical experiences, had an equal opportunity to participate in the conference, and learned from peers. In online conferences through careful sequencing of questions by the teacher, students can engage in discussions to develop their critical thinking.

Written Assignments

Written assignments need to be carefully planned to guide students in meeting designated outcomes. All too often in clinical nursing education, students complete the same assignments such as a care plan with each clinical experience and in multiple courses in the nursing program. Instead, assignments should be geared to achieving a particular outcome and should build writing and thinking skills across courses. Through written assignments, students can learn to: (a) locate, analyze, and synthesize evidence and summarize these findings in a paper; (b) analyze concepts and theories and describe how they can be used in patient care or a specific clinical situation; (c) think through problems, potential decisions and actions, and make a judgment about best approaches to use; and (d) communicate ideas in writing, thus developing their writing skills (54). To improve writing skills, students must have feedback on their writing and an opportunity to rewrite sections of a paper (or even the entire paper). As a developmental process, writing skills improve with practice similar to other skills. Ideally, writing assignments for clinical courses should build on one another throughout a course and nursing program. By planning and sequencing assignments across courses, faculty can build students' skills and avoid excessive repetition.

Examples of written assignments for clinical nursing education include:

- Concept map, a graphic arrangement of key concepts related to a patient's care or clinical situation with an explanation of their interrelationships
- Analysis of a clinical situation and alternative approaches that might have been used in the situation with evidence
- Paper that applies concepts, theories, readings, and other literature to a clinical situation
- Nursing care plan
- Analysis of interactions with patients, other health care providers, and with a team
- Analysis of observations in the clinical setting
- Reflective journals providing an opportunity to explore feelings, beliefs, and values; critique clinical experiences and reflect on them; think more deeply about patients and interactions with others; and connect theory to practice (Oermann et al. 2018).

Some of these written assignments can be done in pairs or with small groups of students, rather than as an individual assignment. Group assignments allow students to learn from one another.

Assessment of Clinical Learning and Performance

Through the process of assessment, educators make judgments about students' learning and clinical competencies (Oermann and Gaberson 2021). Typically, this is a cycle of observing performance, providing feedback and additional instruction as needed, and assessing if students are developing the clinical competencies or have achieved them. Assessment of the performance of students cannot be done periodically – it should be an integral part of clinical teaching. Observations of students reveal gaps in learning and performance and suggest areas where more instruction or practice are indicated.

Assessment may be formative (feedback to learners) or summative (at the end of a period of time) (Oermann and Gaberson 2021). Students need to know where their performance is lacking and what to do to improve it. Altmiller (2016) described constructive feedback as providing an unbiased critique of performance, relaying events as they occurred, and correcting errors in a way that reinforces the teacher's intent to guide students' learning and contribute to their success. Since formative assessment provides feedback to improve learning and performance, it should not be graded (Oermann and Gaberson 2021). At the end of a clinical practicum, or some other designated point in time, observations and judgments are synthesized, and educators make a decision (a judgment) if students' performance meets expected competencies. This is a summative assessment and in most programs represents a high-stakes assessment: students are not able to progress in the nursing program without passing the clinical course or achieving selected competencies (Altmiller 2016; Oermann and Gaberson 2021).

The main methods for assessing clinical performance are observing students in practice and rating their performance on a rating tool. Some educators incorporate other assessment methods as part of this process. These include simulations (in which students can assess patients, decide on interventions, and interact with others); simulated patients (individuals trained to consistently portray a patient with a specific diagnosis, or to evoke particular clinical skills that students perform and then can be evaluated); and objective structured clinical examinations (where students rotate through a series of stations in a laboratory and complete various activities and skills, which are then evaluated) (Oermann et al. 2018).

Conclusion

Educators guide students and support their learning in the clinical setting as they engage in real-life patient care, practice and refine their skills, explore ethical issues, experience nursing roles, process clinical information, and connect theoretical content learned in the classroom to real-life practical situations. In most nursing programs, clinical practice time is limited, and learning activities should be carefully planned to guide students in meeting specific outcomes and developing essential competencies for practice. The outcomes to be achieved and competencies to be developed through clinical practice provide the framework for student learning and guide the activities in which they engage there.

Various models have been developed for structuring and delivering clinical education. These include a traditional model with one primary educator in a single clinical setting teaching a small group of students; partnerships or collaborative clinical education models between nursing education programs and clinical practice agencies, e.g., the DEU; preceptorship and mentoring model; and collaborative cluster model. Technology has become an integral part of health care, thus representing an area of rapid growth in clinical nursing education. As well as new technologies, other commonly used methods in clinical nursing education are patient care assignments, cases, discussions and conferences, and written assignments.

The role of the clinical nurse educator is complex. It requires a broad range of teaching skills, expert knowledge relevant to the clinical practice area in which teaching, ability to develop positive relationships with students, and skill in evaluating clinical performance. Evaluation of performance may be formative (feedback to learners) or summative (end of a period of time). Clinical evaluation is an integral part of effective clinical teaching. Regardless of the setting and level of students, clinical nurse educators have a critical role in preparing students with the requisite knowledge and competencies for transition into practice.

Cross-References

► Approaches to Assessment: A Perspective from Education
► Interprofessional Education (IPE): Trends and Context
► Learning and Teaching at the Bedside: Expert Commentary from a Nursing Perspective
► Measuring Performance: Current Practices in Surgical Education
► Nursing Education in Low and Lower-Middle Income Countries: Context and Trends
► Transformative Learning in Clinical Education: Using Theory to Inform Practice

References

Altmiller G. Strategies for providing constructive feedback to students. Nurse Educ. 2016;41:118–9.
Altmiller G, Armstrong G. 2017 National Quality and safety education for nurses faculty survey results. Nurse Educ. 2017;42:S3–7.
Bates DW, Singh H. Two decades since to err is human: an assessment of progress and emerging priorities in patient safety. Health Aff (Millwood). 2018;37:1736–43.
Beauregard P, Arnaert A, Ponzoni N. Nursing students' perceptions of using smartphones in the community practicum: a qualitative study. Nurse Educ Today. 2017;53:1–6.
Burbach B, Barnason S, Thompson SA. Using "think aloud" to capture clinical reasoning during patient simulation. Int J Nurs Educ Scholarsh. 2015;12:1–7. https://doi.org/10.1515/ijnes-2014-0044.
Carter C, Hunt BH, Mukonka PS, Viveash S, Notter J, Toner L. 'I'll never be the same': the impact of an international elective. Br J Nurs. 2019;28:186–92.
Chickering A, Gamson Z. Seven principles for good practice in undergraduate education. AAHE Bull. 1987;39:3–7.
Crawford R, Jasonsmith A, Leuchars D, Naidu A, Pool L, Tosswill L, et al. "Feeling part of a team": a mixed method evaluation of a dedicated education unit pilot programme. Nurse Educ Today. 2018;68:165–71.
Dahlke S, Hannesson T. Clinical faculty management of the challenges of being a guest in clinical settings: an exploratory study. J Nurs Educ. 2016;55:91–5.
Dapremont J, Lee S. Partnering to educate: dedicated education units. Nurse Educ Pract. 2013;13:335–7.
de Castro AB, Dyba N, Cortez ED, Pe Benito GG. Collaborative online international learning to prepare students for multicultural work environments. Nurse Educ. 2019;44:E1–5.
Devereaux Melillo K, Abdallah L, Dodge L, Dowling JS, Prendergast N, Rathbone A, et al. Developing a dedicated education unit in long-term care: a pilot project. Geriatr Nurs. 2014;35:264–71.

Diefenbeck C, Herrman J, Wade G, Hayes E, Voelmeck W, Cowperthwait A, et al. Preparedness for clinical: evaluation of the core elements of the clinical immersion curriculum model. J Prof Nurs. 2015;31:124–32.

Foronda CL, Swoboda SM, Henry MN, Kamau E, Sullivan N, Hudson KW. Student preferences and perceptions of learning from vSIM for Nursing™. Nurse Educ Pract. 2018;33:27–32.

Fowler SM, Knowlton MC, Putnam AW. Reforming the undergraduate nursing clinical curriculum through clinical immersion: a literature review. Nurse Educ Pract. 2018;31:68–76.

Fox J. Creating a dedicated education unit in long-term care. J Gerontol Nurs. 2017;43:23–9.

George LE, Locasto LW, Pyo KA, Cline TW. Effect of the dedicated education unit on nursing student self-efficacy: a quasi-experimental research study. Nurse Educ Pract. 2017;23:48–53.

Giddens JF, Caputi L. Conceptual teaching strategies for clinical education. In: Giddens JF, Caputi LB, Rodgers B, editors. Mastering concept-based teaching. St. Louis: Elsevier; 2020. p. 101–17.

Hannans J. Online clinical post conference: strategies for meaningful discussion using VoiceThread. Nurse Educ. 2019;44:29–33.

Hayden JK, Smiley RA, Alexander M, Kardong-Edgren S, Jeffries PR. The NCSBN national simulation study: a longitudinal, randomized, controlled study replacing clinical hours with simulation in prelicensure nursing education. J Nurs Regul. 2014;5:S3–S40.

Hensel D. Typologies of professional identity among graduating baccalaureate-prepared nurses. J Nurs Scholarsh. 2014;46:125–33.

Hensel D, Laux M. Longitudinal study of stress, self-care, and professional identity among nursing students. Nurse Educ. 2014;39:227–31.

Hong S, Yu P. Comparison of the effectiveness of two styles of case-based learning implemented in lectures for developing nursing students' critical thinking ability: a randomized controlled trial. Int J Nurs Stud. 2017;68:16–24.

Horsley TL, Reed T, Muccino K, Quinones D, Siddall VJ, McCarthy J. Developing a foundation for interprofessional education within nursing and medical curricula. Nurse Educ. 2016;41:234–8.

Interprofessional Education Collaborative. Core competencies for interprofessional collaborative practice: 2016 update. Washington, DC: Interprofessional Education Collaborative; 2016.

Kavanagh JM, Szweda C. A crisis in competency: the strategic and ethical imperative to assessing new graduate nurses' clinical reasoning. Nurs Educ Perspect. 2017;38:57–62.

Killingworth E. Facilitate learning in the health care environment. In: Shellenbarger T, editor. Clinical nurse educator competencies: creating an evidence-based practice for academic clinical nurse educators. Washington, DC: National League for Nursing; 2019. p. 21–37.

Kumm S, Godfrey N, Richards V, Hulen J, Ray K. Senior student nurse proficiency: a comparative study of two clinical immersion models. Nurse Educ Today. 2016;44:146–50.

Lafrance T. Exploring the intrinsic benefits of nursing preceptorship: a personal perspective. Nurse Educ Pract. 2018;33:1–3.

Lasater K, Holloway K, Lapkin S, Kelly M, McGrath B, Nielsen A, et al. Do prelicensure nursing students' backgrounds impact what they notice and interpret about patients? Nurse Educ Today. 2019;78:37–43.

Li S, Ye X, Chen W. Practice and effectiveness of "nursing case-based learning" course on nursing student's critical thinking ability: a comparative study. Nurse Educ Pract. 2019;36:91–6.

Mackay BJ, Anderson J, Harding T. Mobile technology in clinical teaching. Nurse Educ Pract. 2017;22:1–6.

Maguire DJ, Zambroski CH, Cadena SV. Using a clinical collaborative model for nursing education. Nurse Educ. 2012;37:80–5.

Manetti W. Sound clinical judgment in nursing: a concept analysis. Nurs Forum. 2019;54:102–10.

Missen K, McKenna L, Beauchamp A, Larkins JA. Qualified nurses' perceptions of nursing graduates' abilities vary according to specific demographic and clinical characteristics. A descriptive quantitative study. Nurse Educ Today. 2016;45:108–13.

O'Connor S, Andrews T. Mobile technology and its use in clinical nursing education: a literature review. J Nurs Educ. 2015;54:137–44.

O'Connor S, Andrews T. Smartphones and mobile applications (apps) in clinical nursing education: a student perspective. Nurse Educ Today. 2018;69:172–8.

Oermann M, Gaberson K. Evaluation and testing in nursing education. 6th ed. New York: Springer Publishing; 2021.

Oermann MH, Molloy MA, Vaughn J. Use of deliberate practice in teaching in nursing. Nurse Educ Today. 2015;35:535–6.

Oermann MH, Muckler VC, Morgan B. Framework for teaching psychomotor and procedural skills in nursing. J Contin Educ Nurs. 2016;47:278–82.

Oermann M, Shellenbarger T, Gaberson K. Clinical teaching strategies in nursing. 5th ed. New York: Springer Publishing; 2018.

Ostrogorsky TL, Raber AM, McKinley Yoder C, Nielsen AE, Lutz KF, Wros PL. Becoming a nurse: role formation among accelerated baccalaureate students. Nurse Educ. 2015;40:26–30.

Plemmons C, Clark M, Feng D. Comparing student clinical self-efficacy and team process outcomes for a DEU, blended, and traditional clinical setting: a quasi-experimental research study. Nurse Educ Today. 2018;62:107–11.

Quality and Safety Education for Nurses. Website. 2019. Available from: http://qsen.org/

Repo H, Vahlberg T, Salminen L, Papadopoulos I, Leino-Kilpi H. The cultural competence of graduating nursing students. J Transcult Nurs. 2017;28:98–107.

Rhodes ML, Meyers C, Underhill ML. Evaluation outcomes of a dedicated education unit in a baccalaureate nursing program. J Prof Nurs. 2012;28:223–30.

Rusch LM, McCafferty K, Schoening AM, Hercinger M, Manz J. Impact of the dedicated education unit teaching model on the perceived competencies and professional attributes of nursing students. Nurse Educ Pract. 2018;33:90–3.

Shaffer K, Swan BA, Bouchaud M. Designing a new model for clinical education: an innovative approach. Nurse Educ. 2018;43:145–8.

Sherwood G, Zomorodi M. A new mindset for quality and safety: the QSEN competencies redefine nurses' roles in practice. J Nurs Adm. 2014;44:S10–8.

Skiba DJ. Informatics competencies for nurses revisited. Nurs Educ Perspect. 2016;37:365–7.

Soderstrom NC, Bjork RA. Learning versus performance: an integrative review. Perspect Psychol Sci. 2015;10:176–99.

Tanner CA. Thinking like a nurse: a research-based model of clinical judgment in nursing. J Nurs Educ. 2006;45:204–11.

Thistlethwaite JE, Davies D, Ekeocha S, Kidd JM, MacDougall C, Matthews P, et al. The effectiveness of case-based learning in health professional education. A BEME systematic review: BEME Guide No. 23. Med Teach. 2012;34:e421–44.

van der Riet P, Levett-Jones T, Courtney-Pratt H. Nursing students' perceptions of a collaborative clinical placement model: a qualitative descriptive study. Nurse Educ Pract. 2018;30:42–7.

Welch T, Carter M. Deliberate practice and skill acquisition in nursing practice. J Contin Educ Nurs. 2018;49:269–73.

Nursing Education in Low and Lower-Middle Income Countries: Context and Trends

6

Christine Sommers and Carielle Joy Rio

Contents

Introduction	108
International Mobility	110
International Collaboration	112
Distance Learning and Access to Technology	114
National Competency Assessment and Competency Reciprocation Between Countries	115
Cultural Diversity of Students and Faculty Within the Learning Environment	116
Conclusion	117
Cross-References	117
References	117

Abstract

In 2013, the World Health Organization (WHO) estimated there is a need for an additional four (The World Bank Group) million health workers to achieve the Millennium Development Goals (MDGs) (Sousa and Flores 2013). Nurses comprise the largest proportion of health professionals worldwide. Therefore, the quality and quantity of nurses are critical in ensuring the availability and accessibility of safe and effective healthcare. As countries struggle with the crisis on human resources in healthcare, nurses have potential to mitigate the impact of the health workforce shortage (Ng'ang'a and Bryne 2012). Education and training of health professionals, including nurses, is paramount to effectively addressing the shortage in human resources in healthcare (Sousa and Flores 2013). This chapter discusses the current issues related to nursing education in low- and lower-middle-income countries. Background information on low-income countries

---

C. Sommers (✉)
Universitas Pelita Harapan, Jakarta, Indonesia
e-mail: christine.sommers@uph.edu

C. J. Rio
Faculty of Nursing, Universitas Pelita Harapan, Karawaci, Tangerang, Indonesia
e-mail: carielle.rio@uph.edu

© Springer Nature Singapore Pte Ltd. 2023
D. Nestel et al. (eds.), *Clinical Education for the Health Professions*,
https://doi.org/10.1007/978-981-15-3344-0_117

(LIC) and lower-middle-income countries (LMIC) is provided. The key issues of international mobility, international collaboration, distance learning, national competencies, and cultural diversity will be presented.

Keywords

Low-income countries · Lower-middle income countries · Personnel shortages · Faculty qualifications · Health workers crisis · Brain drain · Internationalization · International mobility · Nursing shortage · International council of nurses · Sigma theta tau international · International collaboration · Technology · Partnerships · Massive open online courses · Nursing licensure examinations · Decision-making · Policy development · Cultural diversity · Respect · Cultural and language skill competencies

Introduction

The World Bank updates the system of country classification based on the national income per person or the gross national income (GNI) per capita. The threshold used in classifying countries' income is adjusted over time. In 2018, the World Bank Group defines low-income countries (LIC) as those with a GNI of less than $995 per capita in 2017. Countries with a GNI of $996 to $3,895 per capita in 2017 are classified as lower-middle-income countries (LMIC) (The World Bank Group). According to the 2018 classification by The World Bank Group, 34 (Tjoflåt et al. 2017) countries are classified as LIC and comprise about 10% of the world's population. The majority of LIC are located in Africa, with a few in the Middle East and South Asia (The World Bank Group). There are 47 (Hashimoto and Fujita 2017) countries that are classified as LMIC and comprise about 40% of the world's population. The majority of LMIC are in Africa; Central, South, East and Pacific Asia; and Latin America (The World Bank Group).

Countries classified by the World Bank Group as LIC and LMIC experience scarcity in resources in nursing education and healthcare delivery. The human health resource crisis brought about by personnel shortages and unequitable distribution of health workers, including nurses and nurse educators, is a pressing problem in most LIC. The disparity in healthcare delivery between countries is also reflected in the disparity of the country's nursing education (Dyson 2018). In 2006, WHO (World Health Organization 2006) emphasized that the quantity and quality of health workers is crucial in improving health. The health workforce affects vital components of healthcare delivery such as immunization coverage; primary care; and maternal, infant, and child health. In the recent report of WHO published in 2018, the gaps in maternal, infant, and child health, as well as environmental health, continue as challenges in LIC (World Health Organization 2018).

The quality of education and training that nurses receive has a significant impact on a country's healthcare delivery system. Educational institutions in LIC that train health professionals are confronted with significant limiting factors related to logistics, curricula, human resources, and funding (Cancedda et al. 2015). In some LIC, such as Nigeria where the majority of nurses hold diploma degrees, faculty qualifications limit nursing education and research (Emelonye et al. 2016). In studies in nursing education in the African Sub-Sahara region, researchers have identified that challenges are related to the quantity, quality, and relevance of nursing education. Addressing these challenges in that region would involve reforms in the curriculum, improvement of infrastructures, enhancement of the capability of educators, and strengthening of regulatory frameworks (Bvumbwe and Mtshali 2018).

In 2010, WHO reported that India needs 2.4 million nurses to cover an extremely high nurse-patient ratio of one nurse per 500 patients. It is also projected that by the year 2025, there will be a shortage of ten thousand (10,000) nurses to care for the elderly population in the Caribbean countries (Cohen and Crabtree 2008). The shortage and maldistribution of health workers, including nurses and nurse educators, further aggravates the overwhelming disease burden faced by these countries and other LIC and LMIC (Ng'ang'a and Bryne 2015).

However, it should be noted that the problem of the health workers crisis is not only affecting LIC but also high-income countries. It is projected that in the next 10 (Bvumbwe and Mtshali 2018) years, 40% of nurses in Western countries will retire (Sarfarti 2010). To alleviate the impact of the health workers shortage, high-income countries import health workers from LIC and LMIC (Global Health Workforce Alliance 2013). Thirty-two percent (32%) of Zimbabwe's nurses were employed in the United Kingdom (UK) between 1999 and 2001. The UK is employing nurses from LIC and LMIC such as India, South Africa, and the Philippines (Kingma 2007).

Migration of nurses from LIC contributes to increasing the nursing shortage, resulting in further compromises to the healthcare delivery systems of these countries. The resulting increase in the shortage of nurses creates a heavier workload for the nurses who remain in LIC, thus further strengthening a nurses' desire for migration (Kingma 2007). The problem of the lack of qualified nursing faculty in LIC and LMIC becomes further compounded as some of the more qualified nurses that could teach nursing in those countries migrate to the high-income countries (Global Health Workforce Alliance 2013).

The migration of these qualified nurse educators results in a negative effect on both the quality and quantity of a country's nursing workforce (Sousa and Flores 2013). The impact of the resulting "brain drain" threatens not only the healthcare system but also the education and training of the future generation of nurses in both LIC and LMIC. There are some that consider the "brain drain" as unethical and describe the ethical conflict between the healthcare workers right to migrate and the societal need for them to stay in the source country and care for patients (Kollar and Buyx 2013). They recommend that polices are needed to improve working and living conditions in the source country and polices to prevent migration from LIC and LMIC in the destination countries (Kollar and Buyx 2013).

The WHO Global Code of Practice on the International Recruitment of Health Personnel asserts that ethical international recruitment includes providing information on both the benefits and risks of employment positions for health workers to make informed decisions. The same Code also promotes fair and just recruitment, renumeration, and promotion for migrant health workers. The WHO urges member states importing health workers to provide objective criteria, equal treatment, and legal rights related to employment for both domestically trained and foreign trained health workers (World Health Organization 2010).

International Mobility

The healthcare sector today is experiencing internationalization. This provides opportunities for inter-country movement of health workers and healthcare consumers. International mobilization of health workers, including nurses and nurse educators, is a complex phenomenon that should be viewed from a holistic perspective. Among the reasons why nurses leave their home country are (a) the desire for a better income, (b) improved working conditions, (c) greater opportunities for professional advancement, and (d) in some cases to flee from the political or security instability of their home country (Walani 2015). This international mobility has been identified, along with education and policy regulations, as one theme that helps to describe different factors that has shaped regulatory change in nursing policy worldwide. The trend for nurses to cross borders is increasing due to the major interconnectedness between countries and regions (Stievano et al. 2019).

A major advantage of international mobility is the significant potential in improving nursing education and practice because of the resulting open doors for the exchange of scientific knowledge. At present, nursing students have access to a global perspective of nursing as they gain a broader and more comprehensive understanding of how social, political, economic, and professional issues affect nursing practice (Guksuma et al. 2016). This international mobility in nursing education is viewed as an important step in improving nursing practice and can help to raise the education level of nurses in LIC and LMIC (Stievano et al. 2019). It is believed that increasing mobility in nursing education allows for the improved exchange of nursing knowledge and expertise (Guksuma et al. 2016).

The Association of Southeast Asian Nations (ASEAN) established the ASEAN Economic Community in 2015. Included in the thrust of the ASEAN Economic Community is the mutual recognition of various professions, including nursing, across the ASEAN member countries. Common core competencies were identified to facilitate mutual recognition of professionals in the ASEAN region (Association of Southeast Asian Nations 2017). With this development, modifications in nursing education were made to produce graduates to serve the health needs of their home countries, as well as the wider ASEAN community. The ASEAN Qualifications Reference Framework (Association of Southeast Asian Nations 2014) was developed to assess the qualifications of professionals from ASEAN member countries. The potential of the ASEAN Economic Community framework in improving nurses' competence and mobility is significant. However, there are several challenges that still need to be overcome and include differences in (a) languages spoken and written, (b) national nursing competencies required and expected, (c) national nursing examination requirements, and (d) national nursing regulatory policies and authority boards.

Today, several programs promoting international mobility have been initiated by some countries. For example, in Brazil there is a program that allows undergraduate nursing students to learn from nurse educators in Ireland (Guksuma et al. 2016). Guksuma, Dullius, Godinho, Costa, and Terra (2016) suggest international mobility in nursing education is an essential step in improving both Brazilian and international nursing, and subsequently improving patient care and the health of the populations served.

While it is undeniable that international mobility can positively impact nursing, it is not without disadvantages. Migration causes LIC and LMIC to lose nurse educators and practitioners (Global Health Workforce Alliance 2013). International recruitment of health workers is not a new phenomenon. However, the nursing shortage experienced by developed nations in the recent years has accelerated the migration of nurses from LIC to high-income countries (Dyson 2018). While there may be increase in the number of nursing graduates in LIC, this does not necessarily result in an equal increase in the number of nurses working in the country (Sousa and Flores 2013).

Considering the case of the Philippines, mass production of nurses to meet the demands of developed countries have been observed since the 1950s. There has been a rapid growth in the nursing education sector in the Philippines since the 1980s (Masselink 2009) and the mid-2000s saw the peak in the number of nursing schools. There were approximately 460 nursing schools operating in the Philippines in 2006 (Arends-Kuenning et al. 2015). With the mushrooming of nursing schools came the concern about the decline in the quality of nursing education and decrease in the number of qualified nurse educators (Masselink 2009). Aside from nurses, the economic advantage of working in developed countries has also resulted in a significant number of Filipino physicians to train as nurses. It was reported that 3,500 Filipino physicians were exported as nurses between the years 2000 to 2004 (Brush 2010). This phenomenon has caused an increased burden in the country's healthcare delivery.

It is interesting to note that the role of educational institutions in the migration of nurses is also linked to the fact that migration as a goal for nurses is deeply ingrained in some cultures. Studies have found that many educators support and assist their students in finding employment overseas (Masselink 2009). Researchers that conducted studies in Cape Verde and Fiji found that the prospect of migration is a significant driver for people to pursue higher education (Arends-Kuenning et al. 2015). In general, LIC and LMIC exporting nurses aim to provide global standards for nursing programs, including curriculum and competency standards; therefore, nurse educators are also encouraged to keep pace with these global standards. Ironically, once nurse educators from LIC and LMIC become internationally qualified, they become more desirable for international recruitment by high-income countries (Dyson 2018). There is a persistent trend of highly qualified and advance-degree educated nurses migrating to high-income countries where monetary compensation and working conditions are better. The resulting brain drain of nurses and in the LIC and LMIC further creates negative impact to the quality of patient care and the overall healthcare delivery in those countries (Association of Southeast Asian Nations 2017). It is imperative for a sustainable and collaborative strategy to be established by both the recruiting and the exporting countries.

International Collaboration

International collaboration between high-income and LIC and LMIC has the potential to positively impact nursing education and training and is an opportunity to improve the nursing workforce in those countries (Carr et al. 2016). Through international collaboration, LIC and LMIC have better access to resources that can assist nurses in improving their clinical and service-related skills. This collaboration can also assist in enhancing the research capabilities of the nurses. The impact of international collaboration has the potential to positively impact nursing education and training by improving the competencies of the nursing workforce as well as having the potential to assist in reducing the disease burdens in LIC and LMIC (Ng'ang'a and Bryne 2015).

International collaboration includes initiatives for infrastructure improvement, scholarships for faculty members to pursue advance education, and capacity building activities. An example of an infrastructure improvement is in Bangladesh. In 2010, a healthcare trust developed a partnership with a nursing program at a major university in Scotland to establish a college of nursing in Bangladesh. This international collaboration envisioned providing the training and education of women from an impoverished background in Bangladesh. This collaboration also provided the opportunity to improve the status of nursing as a profession in Bangladesh. Furthermore, the conception and implementation of this college of nursing also addressed the country's human resource needs for healthcare workers. It also championed the view that the education of women is an opportunity to break the cycle of early marriage, pregnancy and poverty in Bangladesh (Grameen Caledonian College of Nursing 2019).

Another example of an international collaboration initiative is the large grant for the development and operation of a simulation laboratory received by a college of nursing in the Philippines from an agency and board in the United States (US). The college of nursing in the Philippines has opened the use of the simulation laboratory to other universities in the Visayas and Mindanao areas in the Philippines, as well as to some countries in the ASEAN region. This simulation facility has provided students with the opportunity to learn evidence-based practices through simulation (Silliman University 2014).

Among the organizations that have played a significant role in facilitating collaboration is the International Council of Nurses (ICN) with its Global Nursing Leadership Institute (GNLI) (International Council of Nurses). The GNLI 2019 program focuses on the nurses' role in the attainment of the United Nation's Sustainable Development Goals. Another collaboration effort to enhance nursing education internationally is the establishment of the Center for Excellence in Nursing Education by Sigma Theta Tau International (Sigma Theta Tau International Honor Society of Nursing 2019). The Center has a variety of programs that are aimed at promoting excellence in nursing education internationally through mentorship, knowledge and skills enhancement, and leadership development.

Another example of an international collaboration focuses on nurse preceptors providing bidirectional education, training, and mentorship with nurses in LIC and LMIC with nurses in other countries (UW Medicine International Nursing Program). The goal of this collaboration is to provide nursing education and training with mutual benefits to both partners and to improve the capacity of the global healthcare community. This is done by providing and training nurse preceptors to work with local nurse champions to create training and education programs based on the results of needs assessment in the LIC and LMIC. Another example of this type of strategy is the bilateral agreement between the USA and the island of St. Vincent which requires the US-based healthcare institutions recruiting nurses from St. Vincent are required to pay the education and training costs for every nurse that is recruited. The reimbursement provided by the recruiting institutions is collected by the St. Vincent government and is reinvested for nursing education and training (Sousa and Flores 2013).

One way to improve the qualifications of nurse educators and at the same time minimize brain drain of nurses in LIC and LMIC is the careful consideration of terms and conditions of international collaboration initiatives. For example, one scholarship program given by the UK government requires the scholarship recipients to serve in their home country for 2 years upon completion of their studies. Failure of a recipient to return to his or her country of origin for at least 2 years is considered a breach of the scholarship conditions (Chevening 2019). A recipient who fails to comply with the required 2 years of service to his or her home country is required to pay back the entire cost of the scholarship. Having clearly defined conditions of the grant or scholarship that emphasizes the dissemination and application of knowledge acquired during the grant/scholarship to the recipient's country of origin contributes to the maximization of the advantages of international collaboration initiatives. LIC and LMIC tend to depend on compulsory service rather than loan repayment as a measure to retain health workers (Sousa and Flores 2013).

The Balik Scientist program of the Department of Science and Technology in the Philippines encourages experts in the different fields of science who are Filipino citizens or of Filipino decent from foreign countries to return to the Philippines on short-term or long-term basis. A public or private institution in need of the scientist's expertise will serve as the host institution. This program allows exchange of knowledge and expertise among Filipinos based in the Philippines and those who have worked overseas (Republic of the Philippines 2017). It is important to note that while countries pursue the highest quality of healthcare for its citizens, health workers have the legal rights to migrate and gain employment in a foreign country (World Health Organization 2010).

International collaborations without thoughtful planning and rigorous implementation can lead to short-term, unsustainable, and donor-driven education initiatives.

To avoid mismatched perceptions, expectations need to be clarified to ensure that gained knowledge and experiences are adapted and contextualized to the local healthcare system (Tjoflåt et al. 2017). Inequalities in healthcare access is one factor to be considered in planning educational and training opportunity for nurses. Empowering aspiring nurses from disadvantaged areas to serve in their area after graduation may improve healthcare access in disadvantages areas (Sousa and Flores 2013). As appropriate for the collaboration, expectations regarding mobility, academic and research policies, quality assurance, degree recognition, sustainability, and funding should be clearly defined (Atherton et al. 2018). The national healthcare needs of LIC and LMIC must be considered alongside the priorities of the collaboration partners in any international collaborative initiative (Cancedda et al. 2015; Ng'ang'a and Bryne 2015).

Another factor to consider when establishing a program of international collaboration for nursing education is clearly articulating a mission, vision, and strategic plan for the collaboration initiative (Kulage et al. 2014). This will involve seeking the perspective of all stakeholders regarding the current strengths present and ensuring that there is alignment with the mission and vision. As relationships are developed for international collaboration, there needs to be cultural awareness, cultural sensitivity, and excellent communication by all involved and in each location. Current strengths can include faculty focused initiatives such as visiting professorships, student-focused initiatives such as service learning, practice-focused initiatives such as working with partners for clinical practice opportunities, and research initiatives such as joint research projects with partners. Ongoing assessment from all stakeholders is required to ensure that the initiatives are aligned with the mission and vision (Kulage et al. 2014).

Distance Learning and Access to Technology

With the opportunities of using technology for the delivery of online learning models, some of the challenges of internationalization can be overcome, as nurses and nursing students can learn from nurse educators and other nurses from different countries, yet still remain in their home country. A challenge to the opportunity of online learning models is that access to the internet varies among and within LIC and LMIC. Internet availability and access can vary from around 15% to 43% in these countries (International Telecommunication Union 2017). Some of the challenges regarding the availability of the Internet are related to the availability and access to high-speed Internet and access to stable electrical power supply (Piletic 2018). In some of these countries, especially in Asia, the increasing availability and accessibility of technology and digital platforms to support online learning models has influenced education (Kiatiwongse and Sciortino 2018). There is an increased drive for online education and learning models, as well as increased availability of technology and access to the Internet (Belawati 2016). This has resulted in more higher education institutions including distance and/or online learning models as part of their strategic plan (Belawati 2016).

The increased availability and accessibility of technology has also enabled unique collaborative partnerships for education in nursing. These partnerships allow for the expertise of nurses and nurse educators in other countries to be shared with nurses and nurse educators in LIC and LMIC. This is important as nurses in these countries, whether they are prepared or not, are charged with meeting an estimated 80% of the healthcare needs of those populations.

For example, responding to needs in Sub-Saharan East Africa, an online nursing curriculum was developed to supplement classroom teaching (Chickering et al. 2018). The online nursing curriculum is now available for use by other nurse educators in low resource countries. The goal of the curriculum is to optimize nursing roles and scope of practice with an emphasis on context, cultural knowledge, and collaborative service; at the same time there is a desire to correct inaccurate public perceptions of nurses and to overcome prohibitive program costs by making the curriculum available as open access (Chickering et al. 2018).

More digital education resources are also becoming available for use in nursing education (Swigart and Liang 2016). Several massive open online courses (MOOCs) and open courseware (OCW) are now available that have content appropriate for nursing. These courses and content are provided through a variety of different providers. The content includes topics on global health, health informatics, clinical terminology, ethics, and nursing care (Swigart and Liang 2016). Most of the content is in the English language with translations and content in other languages becoming increasingly more available.

Increased access to technology and online platforms is enabling nursing programs in LIC and LMIC to explore providing distance learning, online, and hybrid nursing degree programs, as well as continuing education professional development offerings. Careful management and administration of these programs can assist in providing quality nursing education and degrees to a student in their home country (Atherton et al. 2018; Chickering et al. 2018).

National Competency Assessment and Competency Reciprocation Between Countries

The nursing education systems vary widely throughout LIC and LMIC. Even among the countries within the ASEAN compact, there is variation among the standards for nursing licensure examinations and nursing competency qualifications (Efendi et al. 2018). Level and years of education varies among the countries for entry into the nursing workforce. For example, in some countries within the ASEAN compact, it varies from completion of 1 year for a primary or technical nurse on the low end of the spectrum, and completion of 5 years for a professional nurse with a baccalaureate degree in Indonesia on the high end of the spectrum (Efendi et al. 2018). This variation among the nursing education systems and the nursing licensure examinations creates a challenge for migrating between countries and for the comparison between countries (Efendi et al. 2018; Gunawan 2016). The varying regulations and lack of equivalency between nursing education and nursing competencies in the different countries has been a major historical issue and still represents a current challenge (Stievano et al. 2019).

Improving the healthcare in these countries will require that there is ongoing cooperation and dialogue among the nurse educators and administrators to support nursing education and to develop effective health policy (Smith 2014; Koy 2015). As a result of this desire for cooperation and dialogue, it is necessary that nurse leaders in each country have sufficient education to effectively participate in decision-making and policy development for healthcare and nursing education (Smith 2014). In many of these countries, there is a shortage and/or uneven distribution of nurse educators with advanced degrees (Hashimoto and Fujita 2017). This need for education has resulted in a need to provide quality professional development for nurses and increased options for advanced degrees in nursing at the master and doctoral level. Both of these trends, along with the trend for increased access to technology and distance/online learning, will enable more nurse educators to have access to continuing education and to advanced degrees (Hashimoto and Fujita 2017) while staying in their home country or through the opportunity of scholarships to complete advanced degrees in other countries.

Cultural Diversity of Students and Faculty Within the Learning Environment

Among and throughout these countries, there is great cultural diversity of nursing students and nursing educators. There is cultural diversity within the countries itself, as well as migration of nursing students and nurses outside of their home countries, and migration of nursing educators to teach outside of their home countries. Nursing students from culturally diverse backgrounds may have different perspectives on learning (Hsu and Hsieh 2013) and may process information differently (Henze and Zhu 2012). The various cultural values of students will also influence their motivation, their way of thinking, their expectations in groups, and their style of communication (Brown et al. 2013; Coburn and Weismuller 2012; Frambach et al. 2014).

As a result of this diversity, nursing educators need to teach in a culturally congruent manner (Sommers 2014). Teaching in a culturally congruent manner will involve understanding the culture and healthcare system of the country, reciprocating information, being creative and flexible, developing mutual understanding, and fostering mutual grown and development (Conway et al. 2002). Nurse educators must be prepared to teach culturally diverse nursing students using culturally sensitive and inclusive nursing education (Sommers and Bonnel 2020). This will involve using personalized approaches, considering available resources, promoting cultural diversity broadly, and using culturally appropriate active teaching strategies (Sommers and Bonnel 2020).

With the trend for international collaborative partnerships to assist and/or augment professional development and nursing education, it is important that visiting nurses from high income countries recognize and respect local customs and standards when sharing knowledge and providing nursing support (Tjoflåt et al. 2017).

Respecting local customs and sharing knowledge is also important when the professional development and nursing education is provided through online/distance learning methods (Chickering et al. 2018). Mutual respect for others in education will involve engaging others in a manner that respects their cultural integrity, develops a relationship with them, and supports learning by building on their existing knowledge and enthusiasm for learning (Wlodkowski and Ginsberg 2017). Nurses and nurse educators will need to be aware that culture will influence how others learn (Sommers 2018). For nurse educators working outside of their home country, cultural and language skill competencies will also need to be considered and developed (Hashimoto and Fujita 2017).

Conclusion

The trends of international mobility, international collaboration, distance learning and access to technology, national competency assessment and competency reciprocation between countries, and the cultural diversity of students and faculty within the learning environment in LIC and LMIC have the potential to make a difference for nurses, nursing education, patient care delivery, and improved health outcomes in these countries. It is important that the challenges in these trends and their implementation are addressed from a holistic perspective and that the national health needs of LIC and LMIC are the focus of any collaboration and partnership efforts. This will require relationship building, effective communication, clearly defined and mutually established mission and vision, and ongoing evaluation of these efforts by all stakeholders. Careful implementation of international collaboration and international partnerships in addressing the challenges identified in these trends can assist in providing mutual benefits for nurses, nurse educators, and nursing students. These mutual benefits for nurses, nurse educators, and nursing students also have the potential to improve patient care and health outcomes in LIC and LMIC.

Cross-References

▶ Interprofessional Education (IPE): Trends and Context

References

Arends-Kuenning M, Calara A, Go S. International migration opportunities and occupational choice: a case study of Philippine nurses 2002 to 2014. IZA Discussion Paper No. 8881 [Internet]. 2015. Available from: http://ftp.iza.org/dp8881.pdf

Association of Southeast Asian Nations. The ASEAN qualifications reference framework [Internet]. 2014. Available from: https://asean.org/wp-content/uploads/2017/03/ED-02-ASEAN-Qualifica tions-Reference-Framework-January-2016.pdf

Association of Southeast Asian Nations. ASEAN Economic Community [Internet]. 2017. Available from: https://asean.org/wp-content/uploads/2012/05/7c.-May-2017-Factsheet-on-AEC.pdf

Atherton G, Azizan SN, Shuib M, Crosling G. The shape of global higher education: understanding the ASEAN region. 2018;3:1–32. Available from: https://www.britishcouncil.org/sites/default/files/h233_the_shape_of_asean_higher_education_report_final_v2_web_1.pdf

Belawati, T. Open and distance education in Asia. Presentation at the ICDE President Summit, Sydney, Australia. 2016 (November). Retrieved from: https://icde.memberclicks.net/assets/EVENTS/ICDE_Events/PS2016/Presentations/day2-tian-belawati.pdf

Brown AN, Ward-Panckhurst L, Cooper G. Factors affecting learning and teaching for medicines supply management training in Pacific Island Countries – a realist review. Rural Remote Heal [Internet]. 2013;13(2):2327. Available from: http://www.ncbi.nlm.nih.gov/pubmed/23738574

Brush B. The potent lever of toil: nursing development and exportation in the postcolonial Philippines. Am J Public Health. 2010;100(9):1572–81.

Bvumbwe T, Mtshali N. Nursing education challenges and solutions in Sub Saharan Africa: an integrative review. BMC Nurs. 2018;17:3.

Cancedda C, Farmer PE, Kerry V, Nuthulaganti T, Scott KW, Goosby E, et al. Maximizing the impact of training initiatives for health professionals in low-income countries: frameworks, challenges, and best practices. PLoS Med. 2015;12(6):e1001840.

Carr V, Adeyeye O, Marong L, Sarr F. Enhancing nurse leadership capacity in resource-limited countries. Int J Nurs Clin Pract. 2016;3:200.

Chevening. Frequently asked questions: making an application. [Internet]. 2019. Available from: https://www.chevening.org/faq/making-an-application/1577

Chickering MJ, Spies LA, Keating SA, Etcher L. Nurses international's framework for nursing education [Internet]. Nurses International. 2018. Available from: https://nursesinternational.org/nurses-internationals-framework-for-nursing-education-in-low-resource-countries/

Coburn CL, Weismuller PC. Asian motivators for health promotion. J Transcult Nurs [Internet]. 2012;23(2):205–214. Available from: http://www.ncbi.nlm.nih.gov/pubmed/22294332

Cohen DJ, Crabtree BF. Evaluative criteria for qualitative research in health care: controversies and recommendations. Ann Fam Med. 2008;6(4):331–9.

Conway J, Little P, McMillan M. Congruence or conflict? Challenges in implementing problem-based learning across nursing cultures. Int J Nurs Pract [Internet]. 2002;8(5):235–239. Available from: http://www.ncbi.nlm.nih.gov/pubmed/12225349

Dyson S. Critical pedagogy in nursing transformational approaches to nurse education in a globalized world. 1st ed. London: Palgrave Macmillan; 2018.

Efendi F, Nursalam N, Kurniati A, Gunawan J. Nursing qualification and workforce for the Association of Southeast Asian Nations Economic Community. Nurs Forum. 2018;53(2):197–203.

Emelonye A, Aregbesola A, Pitkäaho T, Vehviläinen-Julkunen K. Revisiting nursing research in Nigeria. Int J Med Biomed Res. 2016;5(2):78–85.

Frambach JM, Driessen EW, Beh P, van der Vleuten CP. Quiet or questioning? Students' discussion behaviors in student-centered education across cultures. Stud High Educ [Internet]. 2014; 39(6):1001–21. Available from: https://login.proxy.kumc.edu/login?URL=?url=http://search.proquest.com/docview/1651846279?accountid=28920

Global Health Workforce Alliance. Global health workforce crisis [Internet]. 2013. Available from: https://www.who.int/workforcealliance/media/KeyMessages_3GF.pdf

Grameen Caledonian College of Nursing. About GCCN [Internet]. 2019. Available from: http://gccn.ac.bd/gccn-info/about-gccn/

Guksuma EM, Dullius AA, Godinho MS, Costa MS, Terra FS. International academic mobility in nursing education: an experience report. Rev Bras Enferm. 2016;69:5.

Gunawan J. Diploma nurse: a player or a spectator in ASEAN mutual recognition arrangement? Arch Med Heal Sci. 2016;4(1):157.

Hashimoto M, Fujita N. Toward further professional development of nursing in ASEAN. JOJ Nurs Heal Care. 2017;2(2):555582.

Henze J, Zhu J. Current research on Chinese students studying abroad. Res Comp Int Educ [Internet]. 2012;7(1):90–104. Available from: https://login.proxy.kumc.edu/login?URL=?url=http://search.proquest.com/docview/1140130080?accountid=28920

Hsu LL, Hsieh SI. Development and psychometric evaluation of the competency inventory for nursing students: a learning outcome perspective. Nurse Educ Today [Internet]. 2013;33(5): 492–497. Available from: http://www.ncbi.nlm.nih.gov/pubmed/22727581

International Council of Nurses. Global Nursing Leadership Institute [Internet]. Available from: https://www.icn.ch/sites/default/files/inline-files/GNLIprogrammeoverview_ENG.pdf.

International Telecommunication Union. ICT facts and figures 2017 [Internet]. 2017. Available from: https://www.itu.int/en/ITU-D/Statistics/Documents/facts/ICTFactsFigures2017.pdf.

Kiatiwongse J, Sciortino R. Trans-ASEAN education can play a role in building a regional community. 2018;1–7. Available from: http://theconversation.com/trans-asean-education-can-play-a-role-in-building-a-regional-community-89610

Kingma M. Nurses on the move: a global overview. Health Serv Res. 2007;42(3 Pt 2):1281–98.

Kollar E, Buyx A. Ethics and policy of medical brain drain: a review. Swiss Med Wkly. 2013; 143(October):1–8.

Koy V. Policy recommendations to enhance nursing education and services among ASEAN member countries. Int J Adv Med. 2015;2(September):324–9. https://doi.org/10.18203/2349-3933.ijam20150575

Kulage KM, Hickey KT, Honig JC, Johnson MP, Larson EL. Establishing a program of global initiatives for nursing education. J Nurs Educ. 2014;53(7):371–8.

Masselink LE. Health professions education as a national industry: framing of controversies in nursing education and migration in the Philippines. 2009.

Ng'ang'a N, Bryne MW. Prioritizing professional practice models for nurses in low-income countries. Bull World Health Organ. 2012;90:3–3A.

Ng'ang'a N, Bryne M. Professional practice models for nurses in low-income countries: an integrative review. BMC Nurs. 2015;14:44.

Piletic P. Benefits of using eLearning in developing countries. eLearning Ind [Internet]. 2018;2018:1–7. Available from: https://elearningindustry.com/elearning-in-developing-countries-benefits-using

Republic of the Philippines. Republic Act 11035. Balik Scientist Act 2017 [Internet]. 2017. Available from: https://bspms.dost.gov.ph/home

Sarfarti H. Securing decent pensions for nurses: gaining insights into the issues at stake for an 'atypical' workforce [Internet]. The European Papers on the New Welfare. 2010. Available from: http://eng.newwelfare.org/2010/10/15/securing-decent-pensions-for-nurses-gaining-insights-into-the-issues-at-stake-for-an-'atypical'-workforce/#.XQPHsLwzbic

Sigma Theta Tau International Honor Society of Nursing. Center for excellence in nursing education [Internet]. 2019. Available from: https://www.sigmanursing.org/learn-grow/leadership-new/center-for-excellence-in-nursing-education

Silliman University. Simulation lab supported by $500K ASHA Grant Inaugurated [Internet]. 2014. Available from: https://su.edu.ph/1378-simulation-lab-supported-by-500k-asha-grant-inaugurated/

Smith S. Participation of nurses in health services decision-making and policy development: ensuring evidence-based practice around the globe [Abstracts of Oral Presentations: Evidence Transfer]. Int J Evid Based Healthc. 2014;12:193.

Sommers CL. Considering culture in the use of problem-based learning to improve critical thinking – is it important? Nurse Educ Today [Internet]. 2014;34(7):1109–1111. Available from: https://doi.org/10.1016/j.nedt.2014.03.010.

Sommers CL. Measurement of critical thinking, clinical reasoning, and clinical judgment in culturally diverse nursing students – a literature review. Nurse Educ Pract [Internet]. 2018;30(May):91–100. Available from: https://doi.org/10.1016/j.nepr.2018.04.002

Sommers CL, Bonnel WB. Nurse educators' perspectives on implementing culturally sensitive and inclusive nursing education. J Nurs Educ [Internet]. 2020;59(3):126–132. Available from: http://www.ncbi.nlm.nih.gov/pubmed/32130413

Sousa A, Flores G. Transforming and scaling up health professional education and training [Internet]. World Health Organization 2013. 2013. Available from: https://whoeducation guidelines.org/sites/default/files/uploads/whoeduguidelines_PolicyBrief_Financing.pdf

Stievano A, Caruso R, Pittella F, Shaffer FA, Rocco G, Fairman J. Shaping nursing profession regulation through history – a systematic review. Int Nurs Rev. 2019;66(1):17–29.

Swigart V, Liang Z. Digital resources for nursing education: open courseware and massive open online courses. Int J Nurs Sci [Internet]. 2016;3(3):307–313. Available from: https://doi.org/10.1016/j.ijnss.2016.07.003.

The World Bank Group. Classifying countries by income [Internet]. Available from: http://datatopics.worldbank.org/world-development-indicators/stories/the-classification-of-countries-by-income.html.

The World Bank Group. World Bank country and lending groups [Internet]. Available from: https://datahelpdesk.worldbank.org/knowledgebase/articles/906519-world-bank-country-and-lending-groups.

Tjoflåt I, Melissa TJ, Mduma E, Hansen BS, Søreide E. Mismatched expectations? Experiences of nurses in a low-income country working with visiting nurses from high-income countries. J Clin Nurs. 2017;26(11–12):1535–44.

UW Medicine International Nursing Program. Who we are [Internet]. International Nursing Program. Available from: http://www.internationalnursingprogram.org/who-we-are.

Walani S. Global migration of internationally educated nurses: experiences of employment discrimination. Int J Africa Nurs Sci. 2015;3:65–70.

Wlodkowski RJ, Ginsberg MB. Enhancing adult motivation to learn: a comprehensive guide for teaching all adults. 4th ed. San Francisco: Jossey-Bass; 2017.

World Health Organization. The World Health Report 2006 – working together for health [Internet]. 2006. Available from: https://www.who.int/whr/2006/overview/en/.

World Health Organization. The WHO Global CODE of Practice on the International Recruitment of Health Personnel [Internet]. 2010. Available from: https://www.who.int/hrh/migration/code/code_en.pdf?ua=1

World Health Organization. Increasing the coverage of essential health services [Internet]. 2018. Available from: https://www.who.int/gho/publications/world_health_statistics/2018/EN_WHS2018_Part3.pdf?ua=1

Dr. Sommers has taught for over 25 years in a variety of academic and hospital settings in several countries. Currently, she is the Chief Academic Officer and Executive Dean, Faculty of Nursing at a large university in Southeast Asia. She has published research related to clinical judgment and clinical reasoning, as well as best practices in teaching culturally diverse nursing students. Dr. Rio is a lecturer in the same Faculty of Nursing in Southeast Asia. She has practiced as a nurse in hospital, community, and academic settings in her home country prior to working as a lecturer overseas. With their past and current involvement in different areas of nursing practice in Southeast Asia, the authors have first-hand experiences of the contexts and challenges of nursing education in low- and middle-income countries. Dr. Sommers and Dr. Rio have likewise witnessed the highs and lows of how some lower-middle income countries in Southeast Asia are addressing the gaps in nursing education and healthcare delivery.

Obstetric and Midwifery Education: Context and Trends

7

Arunaz Kumar and Linda Sweet

Contents

Introduction	122
Course Structure	123
Challenges Specific to Obstetric and Midwifery Education	123
Gender Imbalances and Biases	123
Haptic Nature of Learning Skills	124
Hands-On Learning Affordances	125
Preparation for Unpredictable Emergencies	126
Complexity of Clinical Interpretation and Decision-Making Skills	127
Professional Relationships Between Medical and Midwifery Teams	128
New Initiatives to Support Medical and Midwifery Student Learning	129
Learning by Simulation: How Can Simulation Help?	129
Simulation in the Context of Obstetrics and Midwifery Education	130
Interprofessional Education for Medical and Midwifery Staff	130
Readiness for Work: Public or the Private Sector?	131
Conclusion	132
References	132

Abstract

Medical and midwifery healthcare professionals have overlapping working profiles and yet have roles exclusive for each team. This chapter presents an overview of the interface of the two professions and highlights the current topical issues trending in this field. The medical and midwifery workforce both share a joint working space and client-base but their roles can be quite different while caring for the same woman. The challenges of pregnancy and birth complications

---

A. Kumar (✉)
Monash University, Melbourne, VIC, Australia
e-mail: arunaz.kumar@monash.edu

L. Sweet
Deakin University and Western Health Partnership, Melbourne, VIC, Australia
e-mail: l.sweet@deakin.edu.au; linda.sweet@flinders.edu.au

© Springer Nature Singapore Pte Ltd. 2023
D. Nestel et al. (eds.), *Clinical Education for the Health Professions*,
https://doi.org/10.1007/978-981-15-3344-0_11

require a high degree of collaboration and team work from the two professions. This chapter is coauthored by both medical and midwifery educational leads. We are located and knowledgeable from the Australian healthcare system; however, acknowledge many of the issues we raise will resonate with readers from other countries.

Certain characteristics make obstetric medicine and midwifery unique in regard to the skill-sets required. Work-based placements form the cornerstone of clinical learning. Although the curriculum for these respective professions enforces mandatory skills requirement, learners may struggle with presence of scant opportunities to learn from pregnant women. This may be especially due to the intimate nature of maternity care and occurrence of sudden unpredictable emergency pregnancy or birth-related complications. Creative ways of teaching complex skills like haptic procedures, and clinical decision-making in difficult situations, need to be provided. In this chapter, we describe the intrinsic challenges faced by learners of the medical and midwifery professions. We also address these learning issues by describing innovative initiatives to support medical and midwifery student preparation for practice.

> **Keywords**
>
> Undergraduate · Midwife · Obstetrician · Curriculum · Training · Birth · Pregnancy

Introduction

Obstetric medicine and midwifery education have extensive curricula overlap, as both professions relate to care in pregnancy, during labor, and in the postnatal period. Both professions have specialized training pathways, with extensive clinical hands-on and procedural focus. During prevocational training and after completion, obstetricians and midwives need to work together as a team, sometimes in very intense, time-critical settings, to achieve the best pregnancy outcomes for women and their families.

The two professions have significant overlap in working space and in sharing the care for women, and are required to care for women with low- or high-risk pregnancy. However, their roles in healthcare are different. While midwives may be caring for low-risk women independently, doctors and midwives jointly care for women with high-risk pregnancy complications. This professional difference in day-to-day work roles also translates into education and training designed for the individual professions. Curriculum for obstetric trainees is most often centered on complications during pregnancy and childbirth, with scant exposure to low-risk care, while midwifery courses have a significant emphasis on both low-risk and high-risk care. The nature of these courses leads to opportunities for shared learning, with peer interaction between medical and midwifery students and also between practicing midwives and obstetricians on birth units and antenatal clinics. The two groups support learning and clinical work with each other, with the common aim of providing the best possible care to the pregnant woman and her family.

Course Structure

The pathways required to become an obstetrician or a midwife vary, and there is significant international differences, particularly in midwifery. Internationally, to become an obstetrician, qualified doctors are required to undertake postgraduate specialist training. In most countries including Australia, medical students usually receive some education in obstetrics over 6–12 weeks in the final years of their program. Curricula for preregistration medical students are usually designed to equip them with a basic level of core competence in performing examinations and making clinical decisions suited to an intern level. Following 2 or more years in general medical training, qualified doctors may then commence specialist obstetric training. Specialty obstetric training lasts 4–6 years (depending on program and country), with most of that training time spent "on the job" dealing with a variety of clinical complexities. Whereas, midwifery may be studied as an undergraduate or postgraduate program, and may or may not be combined with or subsequent to nursing. There is broad variation in midwifery programs across the world with durations varying from 1–5 years. Regardless of whether an undergraduate or postgraduate course, midwives are able to practice independently following graduation. Midwifery programs are a blend of theory and practice, some with supernumerary workplace learning and some in paid employment models. The goal of midwifery education is to ensure that new graduates are safe to care for women during pregnancy, birth, and the postnatal period, and to consult with and refer to a medical specialist as required.

Challenges Specific to Obstetric and Midwifery Education

With all health professional education programs, there are challenges to be overcome in program design and curricula. Many of these are outlined throughout this book. We focus our discussion on contemporary issues and challenges. These include potential gender bias in learning opportunities, the haptic nature of clinical maternity skills, need for significant hands-on learning opportunities, preparation for unpredictable life-threatening emergencies, the complexity of clinical decision-making, and the professional relationships between medical and midwifery staff.

Gender Imbalances and Biases

Internationally, midwives are predominantly women, while medicine continues to attract similar numbers of men and women. Due to the intimate nature of maternity care, male medical or midwifery students may face gender bias for clinical experiences, especially when it comes to performing intimate examinations (Higham 2006; Alam et al. 2014; Ismail and Kevelighan 2014). Many male students may miss out on learning opportunities and as a result get disillusioned from pursuing these professions (Anfinan et al. 2014). Consequently, there has been a shift in the obstetric workforce with a great number of women than men undertaking specialty training in recent years (Stonehocker et al. 2017). If the decreased preference among male students to consider obstetrics or midwifery as a career path is due to lack of adequate clinical exposure or understanding of the subject (rather than personal choice), alternate measures need to be sought for providing the required training (Dabson et al. 2014; Alam et al. 2014; Siwe et al. 2012). In developed countries, it is uncommon for men to aspire to take up midwifery as a career (Mitra et al. 2018). Male nurses who consider studying midwifery risk feeling singled out and unsupported by families, colleagues, and women (Kantrowitz-Gordon et al. 2014). In Australia, the introduction of graduate entry nursing programs was considered promising to balance the gender ratio of the nursing workforce (McKenna et al. 2016) and therefore increase the potential for Registered Nurse entry into midwifery, but the benefit of this initiative remains to be investigated.

Haptic Nature of Learning Skills

The largely physically intimate nature of obstetric and midwifery practice makes achieving core examination skills complex for both clinical educators and learners. Haptic learning requires an individual's sensitivity to touch, to be combined with the ability to combine partial tactile information about an object into a whole mental image. Clinical skills such as abdominal palpation, assessment of uterine contractions, vaginal examination, speculum examination, and perineal suturing are just some examples that pose challenges for medical and midwifery teaching. These skills are usually taught by a combination of providing theoretical knowledge followed by simulation. Learners often then observe the clinicians perform the procedure in practice, although some of these skills may not be directly visible.

An example is assessing progress of labor, by performing vaginal examination to assess cervix length, dilation, and consistency. These haptic skills, which cannot be visually demonstrated to the learner, are particularly challenging skills to teach and to learn. Learners will often first learn the theoretical steps on how to perform the procedure, why it is necessary, and the physiological and anatomical changes in labor. This is followed by part-task trainer simulation using models to experience the haptic nature of the skill, before progressing to performing intimate examinations on women in clinical practice. However, because of the importance of such assessment to the woman's labor management, this procedure is often done first by the learner, and then by the clinical teacher to verify the assessment result. This requires the woman to consent to two examinations performed in sequence, which is often understandably refused. The ability of the learner to develop such quality assessment skills is reliant on quality simulation models and sufficient authentic experiences in practice. This in turn requires support by the clinicians to seek clinical experiences for the student, and for the student to gain the woman's trust for her to consent to such learning experiences.

A less complex but still haptic skill is assessing the length and strength of uterine contractions. This requires sensitive touch and exposure to a range of uterine activity to develop. In obstetric and midwifery education, there is a range of haptic skills required for practice. Hence, teaching cannot be limited to didactic techniques alone, but requires a significant amount of exposure to both simulated and authentic practice, and a variety of presentations and variations to develop the requisite skills. The simulators used in this context can range from simple plastic or rubber models of the woman's torso (with anatomical landmarks for haptic perception) to highly realistic robotic simulators resembling a real-life woman in labor, responding to verbal and tactile commands. Such equipment is expensive to purchase and maintain.

Hands-On Learning Affordances

Workplace learning is dependent on the duality of what is afforded to the learner and how the learner elects to engage in and learn from the affordance. What constitutes an affordance is not objective or fixed. Affordances are subject to their invitational quality (i.e., welcoming and engaging or restrictive and dismissive) and may bias some learners over others (e.g., females over males). The difficulty in learning clinical skills is accentuated by the sheer numbers of medical and midwifery students with the limited clinical opportunities available to learn from pregnant women. Over the last 10–20 years, there has been an increase in private medical schools and an expansion in capacity of the established medical schools (Lumsden and Symonds 2010), as well as an increase in undergraduate midwifery training opportunities. These changes have resulted in increased numbers of students requiring learning experiences. This has occurred while the birth rate in Australia and across the globe has slowly declined (https://tradingeconomics.com/australia/birth-rate-crude-per-1-000-people-wb-data.html). As described above, not all women who are approached by students will consent to having a student participate in their care, let alone perform assessments or intimate procedures, or allow a student to be present during their labor and birth. To respect the birthing woman's dignity, it is unethical for multiple students to attend a birth solely for the purpose of training, and therefore managing the numbers of learners seeking experiences at any one time may be problematic. This poses challenges for clinical educators trying to ensure a learning culture and seeking to find ways to encourage women to actively participate in the educational needs of medical and midwifery students. It also requires educational institutions to consider the allocation of students to the clinical venues, ensuring the right numbers and skill mix.

With the technological advancements in healthcare, there is an increase in clinicians relying on investigations, like imaging techniques to make clinical assessments. As a result, it has been shown that there has been a noticeable drop in students' confidence in performing clinical examination skills (Pierides et al.

2013). Balancing hands-on learning experiences with the introduction of technologies is an important consideration in medical and midwifery education. In spite of the technology-assisted learning, there are many clinical skills that are unable to be simulated, or that current simulation devices have not been developed or have insufficient realism, hence there remains a reliance on clinical exposure for learning. Some of these skills can be determining fetal lie and presentations, or performing ultrasound examination with the clinical variations that occur in real-life practice. Moreover, in many contexts, technology is not available for clinical practice. It is important, therefore, that students are able to develop core assessment skills with little reliance on technology and build confidence in their abilities.

Preparation for Unpredictable Emergencies

In maternity care, students face the challenge of encountering unexpected clinical emergencies, especially during labor and birth. Most medical and midwifery programs are unable to guarantee sufficient hands-on experiences (e.g., number of births) for learners in diagnosing and managing a clinical emergency, given their unpredictable nature. Two examples may be a cord prolapse, where the baby's umbilical cord can become compressed, or a placental abruption, where the placenta separates from its attachment to the uterus before birth. Both of these situations can make the fetus hypoxic very quickly, with precious few minutes for the healthcare team to deliver the baby as a lifesaving procedure. Such real-life situations cannot be predicted, and therefore, affordances for learning in practice are left to chance. Such emergencies require skills including team working, prioritization, understanding of one's limitations and scope of practice, and escalating care where required (Cornthwaite et al. 2013). The challenge for teaching and learning these skills is not just limited to preregistration programs; it is also a concern for practicing clinicians. Many of these skills can be learnt on the job; however, the added clinical workload and complexity may make the clinical workspace an unsuitable learning environment. After encountering a difficult clinical situation or a procedure, learners may feel stressed (Dabson et al. 2014) or may even experience psychological harm, unless they have had prior exposure to training in a safe environment (Khadivzadeh and Erfanian 2012) where adequate debrief can be provided to deal with stress. Team training courses in obstetric emergencies, such as MOET, ALSO (Advanced Maternal and Reproductive Education Australia), REOT (Medicine ACoRaR), and PRONTO (Walker et al. 2014, 2015), are often restricted to practicing clinicians (Table 1), while a few courses such as PROMPT (Draycott and Crofts 2006; Cass et al. 2011) and ONE-SIm (Kumar et al. 2019) enable undergraduate medical and midwifery students to participate. There remains a challenge on when and how to incorporate emergency training into medical and midwifery career development.

Table 1 Emergency obstetric training for medical and midwifery healthcare professionals

Obstetric simulation training for medical and midwifery healthcare professionals	Brief description
Managing Obstetric Emergencies and Trauma (MOET)	MOET is an advanced course designed by and for obstetricians and anesthetists to improve knowledge and skills for dealing with difficult, serious, and life-threatening conditions in obstetrics.
Rural Emergency Obstetric Training (REOT)	REOT is a course designed for rural doctors and midwives on managing normal birth and birth-related complications.
Programa de Rescate Obstétrico y Neonatal: Tratamiento Óptimo y Oportuno (PRONTO)	PRONTO is a program arising from Mexico on managing maternal and neonatal obstetric emergencies and has been training doctors and nurses in low-middle income settings
Obstetric and Neonatal Emergency Simulation (ONE-Sim)	ONE-Sim is a program for emergency training for obstetric, neonatal medical and midwifery staff, and students.
Practical Obstetric Multi-professional Training (PROMPT)	The PROMPT Maternity Foundation provides a multi-professional training program to improve outcomes for women and their babies. There are various versions for healthcare professionals, prehospital (for paramedics) and for undergraduate students.

Complexity of Clinical Interpretation and Decision-Making Skills

Skills like interpretation of clinical and investigation findings can be difficult as there is no "one" correct or standardized answer to all clinical situations. Interpretation of clinical findings needs to happen in the context of the woman's background history, as with a small change in background risks, decisions about management can be quite variable. An example is of a woman who is a having second pregnancy and now has prolonged labor. If the previous birth was a low-risk normal vaginal birth, her perinatal risks are likely to be low in the current situation. However, if she had a previous caesarean section performed for something like obstructed labor, this situation would be qualified as being high-risk and the woman may require an emergency caesarean section. It is important that medical and midwifery education provide sufficient learning on how best to manage a situation, and that such decisions are based on the woman's history and risk factors, consideration of the resources available, and the desires of the woman herself.

Interpretation of clinical and investigation findings in obstetrics is complex as there is often no standardized answer of what is "normal" versus "abnormal" for the mother and fetus. While pregnancy is a normal physiological phase in a woman's life, and not an illness or a disease, healthcare providers have a unique role in providing medical care and supporting the woman through, what many would call an emotional journey. However, as described in the above section, complications may arise even in women considered to have a low-risk pregnancy. Clinical decision-making may depend on the context of individualized client care. This creates nebulous situations in which it may be difficult to decide a best course of action. An example is cardiotocograph (CTG) findings. The CTG findings need to be interpreted differently depending on whether a woman is in labor, whether there are any underlying complications, and how labor is progressing. Clinical reasoning can be difficult to acquire and may require years of experience; in many cases, this can only be acquired by learning and working immersed in the clinical field.

Professional Relationships Between Medical and Midwifery Teams

Due to overlapping roles in caring for women during pregnancy and birth, obstetricians and midwives usually support each other in their respective clinical roles. When clinical complex situations arise, midwives are expected to make a timely referral to obstetricians, who would then require support from the whole team (including midwifery staff), who all contribute to managing the complex situation. The sharing of roles (which may be similar at times and very different at others) in caring for pregnant/birthing women puts a lot of pressure on medical and midwifery staff to perform together as a team.

As both teams are vested in providing high standard of care (but may have different, educational backgrounds and philosophies), they may occasionally experience professional conflict. Occasionally, disagreement in caring for women may arise due to perception of competition in providing care, a difference of opinion in clinical management, or a hierarchical workplace culture. A workplace conflict possibly due to clinical disconnections is a complex but recurring problem in the healthcare industry and may risk substandard care being provided during birth (Lyndon et al. 2014). The root cause of such disconnect between teams may be the difference in a perceived roadmap to achieve the best clinical outcome; a feeling of being ignored by the dominant team; or a lack of timely action in spite of advice provided, resulting in resignation or disinterest by the team (Lyndon et al. 2014). There may be differences in philosophies of care with a possible increased "medicalization" of birth perceived as being "interventional" by those who espouse women-centered care with minimal intervention in the normal birthing process, compared to those who may consider intervention as a normal practice (Behruzi et al. 2017). Due to these differences in perspectives and practices, some recent interventions with interprofessional education have been introduced for medical and midwifery staff. The intent of these is to learn with and about each other's profession, to develop collaborative practice, and improve teamwork. Improving teamwork requires engaged learners in an interprofessional setting. Learning programs need to address the specific learning needs of the students and also address the learning needs of the team. Some of these educational initiatives that may work for both medical and midwifery students and for their respective teams are described below.

New Initiatives to Support Medical and Midwifery Student Learning

We now shift to educational practices that may address the concerns raised above. In particular, the importance of simulation and the contextual nature of simulation for obstetric and midwifery learning will be addressed, as well as interprofessional education and readiness for varied work contexts.

Learning by Simulation: How Can Simulation Help?

The word "simulate" means to imitate or enact. Simulation is defined by Gaba as "an educational technique that replaces or amplifies real experiences with guided experiences that evoke or replicate substantial aspects of the real world in a fully interactive manner" (Gaba 2007). In the context of healthcare, simulation is a safe educational modality to teach clinical knowledge, facilitate acquisition of skills, and/or develop a change in behavior (Cheng et al. 2015). Simulation can use simple task-trainers (pelvic trainers or birthing models), advanced technology (birth or haptic virtual reality simulators), and/or human input replicating the condition or a situation (with real medical/ midwifery teams). Simulation is an immersive experience, where participants need to be engaged and "buy-into" the simulation for achieving its optimal learning benefits.

In healthcare, artificial clinical situations can be created to mimic the real-world problems for learners of varying degrees of expertise. Simple problems can be created for novices with added levels of complexity for experts. Simulation-based education can provide scaffold learning by breaking learning into independent steps, with components of hands-on learning skills followed by a debrief. Using a customized simulation design, the teaching can be tailored to address the learning needs of the participants.

Simulation can address learning of procedural skills (Nestel et al. 2011), using part-task trainers or modern-day realistic simulators (Scholz et al. 2012), communication and team-working skills (using human patient simulation) or both using a hybrid technique (Siassakos et al. 2010). It can identify and correct system errors by simulating organization processes (Cheng et al. 2015), improve clinical performance by simulating clinical problems, and improve team-based communication skills (Watson et al. 2016) by simulating real-life situations like conflict, breaking bad news, ethical dilemmas, or human error (Azadeh et al. 2016). All of these contribute to improving clinical safety (Cheng et al. 2015), especially when used with increased realism in an in-situ setting (Sørensen et al. 2015).

Simulation in the Context of Obstetrics and Midwifery Education

Simulation can be used to achieve mastery in a procedural skill (McGaghie et al. 2015), where an important or a difficult skill is to be learnt. An example would be vaginal examination in labor, which is an important skill for medical and midwifery students to learn but difficult to teach on women as it can be uncomfortable or even painful (Grynberg et al. 2012). Prior practice on a task trainer can facilitate familiarity with the technique. This will make the teaching of a subsequent examination much easier on either a woman or a simulator (Pugh et al. 2012). Having the opportunity to refine skills in a simulation environment can improve learners' confidence and comfort, and decrease their anxiety (Duffy et al. 2016). Alternatively, simulation can be used for a rarely practiced skill that is difficult for participants to be exposed to in real life. Examples from obstetrics include a rarely required procedural skill, such as the maneuvers needed to deliver shoulders when dystocia occurs, where both time and skill level are crucial (Ennen and Satin 2010); or the treatment of a maternal collapse in cases such as amniotic embolism, where the real occurrence is unpredictable.

Interprofessional Education for Medical and Midwifery Staff

Obstetric and midwifery professionals may work independently or collectively in teams. At times, the care of a woman may be transferred from midwifery to medicine or vice versa. It is important that students learn effective intra- and interprofessional ways of practice. During routine practice, there can be episodes of communication breakdown, which has the risk of development of mistrust within teams or between the members of the two teams. Medical and midwifery students often share the same workspace and patient population. They may support each other's learning by providing peer-learning support. However, due to the difference ways in which the courses are conducted, with faculty independent of each other, students from the two professions frequently may develop bias and differences, which may continue through into their professional lives.

While there seems to be shared and even occasionally blurred boundaries of roles between obstetrics and midwifery (where both midwives and doctors may be providing routine care individually and together as a team), the majority of the medical and midwifery education occurs in silos. Opportunities for combined education for both professions have been introduced but are often limited to clinicians in practice rather than learners at undergraduate level (Kumar et al. 2014, 2017, 2018a). To address this, educational interventions introduced in an interprofessional setting are often tailored to manage complex obstetric emergency situations (which are rare but may occur unannounced even in women with low-risk pregnancies). Opportunities to share learning through nonemergency situations, such as team handover and interdisciplinary team meetings, are only recently being recognized and slowly gaining in popularity. This is primarily due to the mounting evidence of the importance of interprofessional communication to patient safety and the positive benefits of team meetings, case discussions, and handover interactions for team culture.

The interprofessional simulation activities for practicing medical and midwifery staff have been shown to improve medical and midwifery team-based approaches (Crofts et al. 2007; Marshall et al. 2015), leading to improved clinical outcomes (Shoushtarian et al. 2014), and a reduction in maternity claims (Weiner et al. 2016). As discussed earlier in the chapter, the Practical Obstetric Multiprofessional Training (PROMPT) (Promptmaternity. Making child birth safer, together 2018) is one such program that aims to recreate clinical problems either "in-situ" (Sørensen et al. 2015) or in a simulation center, and presents them to participants as realistically as possible. The scenarios are designed specifically for the level of the participants and the facilities available (Draycott et al. 2015). These programs are now becoming a part of routine emergency training for medical and midwifery staff, and are used for credentialing purposes (Kumar et al. 2018b). Many professional education standards now recognize the importance of interprofessional capabilities and now require education providers to incorporate forms of interprofessional learning for collaborative practice in curricula. (Australian Nursing and Midwifery Accreditation Council. Midwife Accreditation Standards 2014). Integrating interprofessional education in undergraduate medical and midwifery education are likely to enhance students' attitudes and future behavior towards interprofessional teams, although this remains to be investigated.

Readiness for Work: Public or the Private Sector?

The post-registration obstetric and midwifery training in the Australian context mostly takes place in public hospital settings. In the final years of educational programs, these health professionals are expected to mimic roles that will be required from an independent practitioner. While medical and midwifery students learn to mirror practices of the senior clinicians they learn from, they may occasionally feel underprepared to practice independently following completion of their education. This is applicable more so in the private practice setting, which the learners may not have been exposed to during their training years. To improve both competence and confidence, post-registration learners may benefit more from an apprenticeship model or by having access to a mentor they can approach, who not only is able to provide advice when the new clinicians face a difficult situation, but is also able to guide them through the day-to-day requirements of practice. This form of intervention may have the potential to assist in taking the novice practitioner gradually towards the expert spectrum, while feeling supported at all stages of learning.

Conclusion

As described above, the common challenges in the learners' journey are difficulty in learning haptic procedures, scant clinical opportunities for learning hands-on skills, and difficulty in managing complex clinical scenarios due to slow gradient of learning clinical reasoning. Learning to work with the other professions can be especially complex in shared work zones, as boundaries of scope of each professional's practice is occasionally blurred and disagreement may occur with regards to clinical management. Besides these issues, a gender bias exists in aspiring practitioners, with relatively low number of male obstetricians and midwives interested to pursue the professions. Initiatives to address the above concerns include simulation based and interprofessional educational programs, along with other interventions that aim to prepare new graduates and clinicians for independent practice. These changing trends in education are aimed towards ensuring competence in procedures and decision-making in new practitioners. In spite of achieving credentialing in independent performance, it is crucial that newly skilled practitioners feel well supported in a team-based structure of interprofessional work communities. Only then, both individuals and teams will work towards the common goal of achieving self-excellence and a shared vision.

References

Advanced Maternal and Reproductive Education Australia. Advanced Life Support in Obstetrics (ALSO) [cited 2019 June 20]. Available from: https://www.amare.org.au/advanced-life-support-in-obstetrics-also/

Alam K, Safdar CA, Munir TA, Ghani Z. Teaching obstetrics and gynaecology to male undergraduate medical students: student's perception. J Ayub Med Coll Abbottabad. 2014;26(4):539–42.

Anfinan N, Alghunaim N, Boker A, Hussain A, Almarstani A, Basalamah H, et al. Obstetric and gynecologic patients' attitudes and perceptions toward medical students in Saudi Arabia. Oman Med J. 2014;29(2):106–9.

Australian Nursing and Midwifery Accreditation Council. Midwife Accreditation Standards. 2014. [cited 2019 20th June]. Available from: http://www.anmac.org.au

Azadeh A, Pourebrahim Ahvazi M, Motevali Haghighii S, Keramati A. Simulation optimization of an emergency department by modeling human errors. Simul Model Pract Theory. 2016;67:117–36.

Behruzi R, Klam S, Dehertog M, Jimenez V, Hatem M. Understanding factors affecting collaboration between midwives and other health care professionals in a birth center and its affiliated Quebec hospital: a case study. BMC Pregnancy Childbirth. 2017;17(1):200.

Cass GKS, Crofts JF, Draycott TJ. The use of simulation to teach clinical skills in obstetrics. Semin Perinatol. 2011;35(2):68–73.

Cheng A, Grant V, Auerbach M. Using simulation to improve patient safety dawn ofa new era. JAMA Pediatr. 2015;169(5):419–20.

Cornthwaite K, Edwards S, Siassakos D. Reducing risk in maternity by optimising teamwork and leadership: an evidence-based approach to save mothers and babies. Best Pract Res Clin Obstet Gynaecol. 2013;27(4):571–81.

Crofts JF, Ellis D, Draycott TJ, Winter C, Hunt LP, Akande VA. Change in knowledge of midwives and obstetricians following obstetric emergency training: a randomised controlled trial of local hospital, simulation centre and teamwork training. BJOG Int J Obstet Gynaecol. 2007;114(12):1534–41.

Dabson AM, Magin PJ, Heading G, Pond D. Medical students' experiences learning intimate physical examination skills: a qualitative study. BMC Med Educ. 2014;14(1):39

Draycott T, Crofts J. Structured team training in obstetrics and its impact on outcome. Fetal Matern Med Rev. 2006;17(3):229–37.

Draycott TJ, Collins KJ, Crofts JF, Siassakos D, Winter C, Weiner CP, et al. Myths and realities of training in obstetric emergencies. Best Pract Res Clin Obstet Gynaecol. 2015;29(8):1067–76.

Duffy JMN, Chequer S, Braddy A, Mylan S, Royuela A, Zamora J, et al. Educational effectiveness of gynaecological teaching associates: a multi-centre randomised controlled trial. BJOG Int J Obstet Gynaecol. 2016;123(6):1005–10.

Ennen CS, Satin AJ. Training and assessment in obstetrics: the role of simulation. Best Pract Res Clin Obstet Gynaecol. 2010;24(6):747–58.

Gaba DM. The future vision of simulation in healthcare. Simul Healthc. 2007;2(2):126–35.

Grynberg M, Thubert T, Guilbaud L, Cordier AG, Nedellec S, Lamazou F, et al. Students' views on the impact of two pedagogical tools for the teaching of breast and pelvic examination techniques (video-clip and training model): a comparative study. Eur J Obstet Gynecol Reprod Biol. 2012;164(2):205–10.

Higham J. Current themes in the teaching of obstetrics and gynaecology in the United Kingdom. Med Teach. 2006;28(6):495–6.

Ismail SIMF, Kevelighan EH. Graduate medical students' perception of obstetrics and gynaecology as a future career specialty. J Obstet Gynaecol. 2014;34(4):341–5.

Kantrowitz-Gordon I, Adriane Ellis S, McFarlane A. Men in midwifery: a National Survey. J Midwifery Womens Health. 2014;59(5):516–22.

Khadivzadeh T, Erfanian F. The effects of simulated patients and simulated gynecologic models on student anxiety in providing IUD services. Simul Healthc. 2012;7(5):282–7.

Kumar A, Gilmour C, Nestel D, Aldridge R, McLelland G, Wallace E. Can we teach core clinical obstetrics and gynaecology skills using low fidelity simulation in an interprofessional setting? Aust N Z J Obstet Gynaecol. 2014;54(6):589–92.

Kumar A, Wallace EM, East C, McClelland G, Hall H, Leech M, et al. Interprofessional simulation-based education for medical and midwifery students: a qualitative study. Clin Simul Nurs. 2017;13(5):217–27.

Kumar A, Kent F, Wallace EM, McLelland G, Bentley D, Koutsoukos A, et al. Interprofessional education and practice guide No. 9: sustaining interprofessional simulation using change management principles. J Interprof Care. 2018a;32(6):771–8.

Kumar A, Sturrock S, Wallace EM, Nestel D, Lucey D, Stoyles S, et al. Evaluation of learning from Practical Obstetric Multi-Professional Training and its impact on patient outcomes in Australia using Kirkpatrick's framework: a mixed methods study. BMJ Open. 2018b;8(2):e017451.

Kumar A, Singh T, Bansal U, Singh J, Davie S, Malhotra A. Mobile obstetric and neonatal simulation based skills training in India. Midwifery. 2019;72:14–22.

Lumsden MA, Symonds IM. New undergraduate curricula in the UK and Australia. Best Pract Res Clin Obstet Gynaecol. 2010;24(6):795–806.

Lyndon A, Zlatnik MG, Maxfield DG, Lewis A, McMillan C, Kennedy HP. Contributions of clinical disconnections and unresolved conflict to failures in intrapartum safety. J Obstet Gynecol Neonatal Nurs. 2014;43(1):2–12.

Marshall NE, Vanderhoeven J, Eden KB, Segel SY, Guise JM. Impact of simulation and team training on postpartum hemorrhage management in non-academic centers. J Matern Fetal Neonatal Med. 2015;28(5):495–9.

McGaghie WC, Barsuk JH, Wayne DB. Mastery learning with deliberate practice in medical education. Acad Med. 2015;90(11):1575.

McKenna L, Vanderheide R, Brooks I. Is graduate entry education a solution to increasing numbers of men in nursing? Nurse Educ Pract. 2016;17:74–7.

Medicine ACoRaR. Rural Emergency Obstetric Training (REOT) [cited 2019 20/6/19]. Available from: https://www.acrrm.org.au/continuing-development/courses/reot

Mitra JML, Phillips KD, Wachs JE. Perceptions of an obstetric clinical rotation by nursing students who are men. MCN Am J Matern Child Nurs. 2018;43(6):330–3.

Nestel D, Groom J, Eikeland-Husebø S, O'Donnell JM. Simulation for learning and teaching procedural skills: the state of the science. Simul Healthc. 2011;6(7 Suppl):S10–S3.

Pierides K, Duggan P, Chur-Hansen A, Gilson A. Medical student self-reported confidence in obstetrics and gynaecology: development of a core clinical competencies document. BMC Med Educ. 2013;13(1):62

Promptmaternity. Making child birth safer, together. 2018. [cited 2019 June 20]. Available from: http://www.promptmaternity.org/what-we-do/training/

Pugh CM, Iannitelli KB, Rooney D, Salud L. Use of mannequin-based simulation to decrease student anxiety prior to interacting with male teaching associates. Teach Learn Med. 2012;24(2):122–7.

Scholz C, Mann C, Kopp V, Kost B, Kainer F, Fischer MR. High-fidelity simulation increases obstetric self-assurance and skills in undergraduate medical students. J Perinat Med. 2012;40(6):607–13.

Shoushtarian M, Barnett M, McMahon F, Ferris J. Impact of introducing Practical Obstetric Multi-Professional Training (PROMPT) into maternity units in Victoria, Australia. BJOG Int J Obstet Gynaecol. 2014;121(13):1710–8.

Siassakos D, Draycott T, O'Brien K, Kenyon C, Bartlett C, Fox R. Exploratory randomized controlled trial of hybrid obstetric simulation training for undergraduate students. Simul Healthc. 2010;5(4):193–8.

Siwe K, Berterö C, Wijma B. Unexpected enlightening of a "female world" male medical students' experiences of learning and performing the first pelvic examination. Sex Reprod Healthc. 2012;3(3):123–7.

Sørensen JL, Navne LE, Martin HM, Ottesen B, Albrecthsen CK, Pedersen BW, et al. Clarifying the learning experiences of healthcare professionals with in situ and off-site simulation-based medical education: a qualitative study. BMJ Open. 2015;5:10.

Stonehocker J, Muruthi J, Rayburn WF. Is there a shortage of obstetrician-gynecologists? Obstet Gynecol Clin N Am. 2017;44(1):121–32.

Walker D, Cohen S, Fritz J, Olvera M, Lamadrid-Figueroa H, Cowan JG, et al. Team training in obstetric and neonatal emergencies using highly realistic simulation in Mexico: impact on process indicators. BMC Pregnancy Childbirth. 2014;14(1):367

Walker DM, Holme F, Zelek ST, Olvera-Garcia M, Montoya-Rodriguez A, Fritz J, et al. A process evaluation of PRONTO simulation training for obstetric and neonatal emergency response teams in Guatemala. BMC Med Educ. 2015;15:117.

Watson BM, Heatley ML, Gallois C, Kruske S. The importance of effective communication in interprofessional practice: perspectives of maternity clinicians. Health Commun. 2016;31(4):400–7.

Weiner CP, Collins L, Bentley S, Dong Y, Satterwhite CL. Multi-professional training for obstetric emergencies in a US hospital over a 7-year interval: an observational study. J Perinatol. 2016;36(1):19–24.

Allied Health Education: Current and Future Trends

8

Michelle Bissett, Neil Tuttle, and Elizabeth Cardell

Contents

Introduction	136
Allied Health Education	136
Definition of Allied Health	136
Context of Allied Health Practice and Education	137
Trends in Allied Health Education	139
Future Trends in Allied Health Education	145
Conclusion	147
Cross-References	148
References	148

Abstract

Allied health is a term used to describe a wide range of health professions which provide care alongside medicine and nursing. This chapter defines allied health before describing key elements of university-delivered allied health education. Key teaching and learning approaches are discussed in addition to the regulatory processes that exist to ensure allied health graduates are competent for practice. The final stages of the chapter explore emerging education and practice trends and how these will shape future allied health education.

M. Bissett (✉)
Discipline of Occupational Therapy, Griffith University, Gold Coast, QLD, Australia
e-mail: m.bissett@griffith.edu.au

N. Tuttle
Discipline of Physiotherapy, Griffith University, Gold Coast, QLD, Australia
e-mail: n.tuttle@griffith.edu.au

E. Cardell
Discipline of Speech Pathology, Griffith University, Gold Coast, Australia
e-mail: e.cardell@griffith.edu.au

© Springer Nature Singapore Pte Ltd. 2023
D. Nestel et al. (eds.), *Clinical Education for the Health Professions*,
https://doi.org/10.1007/978-981-15-3344-0_12

> **Keywords**
>
> Allied health defined · Regulated curriculum · Current and future trends

Introduction

Allied health is a term used to describe a vast range of health professions which provide specialized client care services alongside medicine and nursing. Education programs in allied health professions are typically delivered within universities, and curriculum is highly regulated by university agendas, as well as both national and international profession-specific accreditation standards for education. These standards shape curricula content to ensure that graduates develop competencies that enable them to be registered for practice (as appropriate) and qualified for safe and competent professional practice.

Across the allied health professions, there are some commonalities in the education approaches employed by programs, including the provision of practice education opportunities; engaging students as active learners; and developing expertise in evidence-based practice, cultural competency, and interprofessional practice approaches in healthcare.

This chapter presents current and emerging trends influencing the education of allied health students. Using examples from a range of allied health professions, this chapter explores trends in teaching and learning approaches used to deliver education, and the content typically included in university curricula. In doing so, the chapter illustrates commonalities and variations that exist across the different professions. The latter part of the chapter considers emerging trends in contemporary professional practice and education delivery that will shape the future of allied health education.

Allied Health Education

Definition of Allied Health

Allied health is a broad term used to categorize a range of health professions. The professions classified as allied health vary globally so the definition of this collective group of health professionals can vary, but for the purposes of this chapter, we will consider allied health to include health professionals who require a university degree to qualify and who work outside the professions of medicine, dentistry, and nursing. Numerous professions exist under this broad umbrella including, but are not limited to: audiology, counselling, diversional therapy, exercise physiology, nutrition and dietetics, occupational therapy, orthotics and prosthetics, physiotherapy, podiatry, psychology, radiation therapy, radiography, social work, and speech pathology (Association of Schools of Allied Health Professionals 2018). Originally, allied health professionals were viewed as personnel who provided complementary care to that provided by medical specialists (Schloman 1997) but, in today's healthcare services, allied health professionals are recognized as providing their own core set of expertise that enables them to be autonomous contributors to patient health.

The contribution of allied health to client care is significant, with estimates suggesting that approximately 60% of the healthcare workforce in the United States is classified under the term allied health (Association of Schools of Allied Health Professionals 2018). Within healthcare, allied health professionals work with individuals and communities, across both the lifespan and the healthcare continuum. As an example, physiotherapists are trained to work with children through to older adults, from intensive care units to community-based rehabilitation.

Allied health professionals also contribute to individuals and communities within disability and social care sectors. Examples include speech therapists, who work in early intervention with children in schools, and occupational therapists, who work with refugee and asylum seekers to develop community living skills in their new countries of residence. Regardless of practice context, allied health professionals are required to implement professional expertise merged with expected health constructs, including evidence-based and client-centered practice.

Context of Allied Health Practice and Education

Internationally, allied health professionals are educated in universities (Australian Health Professionals Association 2017; Health and Care Professions Council 2018; Health Professions Council of South Africa 2018) where programs are highly regulated and influenced by profession-specific and university specifications. The level of qualification has changed over time, as allied health professionals have developed increasing autonomy and separation from medicine. Historically, students became qualified through 2-year undergraduate degrees, which progressed to 3 years, then 4 years and, more recently, into postgraduate degrees. This increase in university content is appropriate and parallels the expectations of allied health professionals who, in many countries, now operate as first-contact practitioners without jurisdiction and oversight from the medical and nursing disciplines. It also parallels the increasing expectations in health education to ensure that graduates can implement discipline-specific expertise underpinned by core health competencies, including evidence-based and client-centered practice.

Today, there is still considerable variation between educational requirements in different countries. For example, while some pharmacy programs remain as undergraduate degrees, graduates in the United Kingdom are required to have completed a 4-year master's degree and graduates in North America require an entry-level doctoral degree. There has been an increasing push for postgraduate degrees, particularly in the United States and Canada. In these countries, students typically complete generic undergraduate degrees in health or science with a master's qualification in a particular allied health discipline. Doctoral degrees, which are commonly required in North America, are available for a range of allied health disciplines including audiology, osteopathy, podiatry, and optometry (Seegmiller et al. 2015). These international variations result in the length of tertiary education for students in different professions and different countries ranging from 3 to 7 years.

As many allied health professions require some form of registration, university programs are often required to meet discipline-specific educational standards. National and international professional regulatory bodies stipulate standards for education to ensure that graduates are competent to practice and that patients are safe recipients of healthcare care. University allied health programs undergo processes of accreditation, whereby independent bodies evaluate the educational providers' ability to ensure graduates achieve relevant professional standards. It is customary for programs to demonstrate compliance with university-specific standards, national educational standards, and national and international discipline-specific standards for education and practice. As an example, occupational therapy programs in Australia are required to demonstrate that their students meet:

(i) Graduate outcomes unique to their university (university standards)
(ii) Knowledge and skills against the Australian Qualifications Framework (Australian Qualifications Framework Council 2013) (national educational standards)
(iii) The Occupational Therapy Council of Australia's Accreditation Standards for Entry-Level Occupational Therapy Education Programs (Occupational Therapy Council of Australia 2018) (national profession-specific educational standards)
(iv) Occupational Therapy Board of Australia competency standards (Occupational Therapy Board of Australia 2018) (national profession-specific graduate standards)
(v) Educational standards provided by the World Federation of Occupational Therapists (World Federation of Occupational Therapists 2016) (international profession-specific educational standards).

This example demonstrates the complexity of allied health education and the rigor that exists to ensure graduates are safe and competent to practice.

Concurrent to increasing standards for the education of allied health students, there has also been maturation in the process of teaching these students. Early education of students was *experiential* and embedded within practice settings. In this context, students learnt technical skills relevant to their career through direct contact with care recipients. In the 1980s, as a consequence of increasing regulation, there was a shift in focus, moving away from technical skills training to *classroom-based* education that involved students being more rigorous in their understanding of theories and concepts, and interpretation of research and practice that incorporated research with practical application (Tavakol and Reicherter 2003). Clinical reasoning, the cognitive process of gathering and analyzing data to determine decision-making (Simmons 2010), contributed to this shift and educational programs changed to provide increased theoretical understanding of professional practice. University education, at this time, primarily consisted of didactic teaching approaches where educators provided large quantities of content in lecture-style formats and students were passive receivers of this knowledge. Student learning experiences have been continually monitored by universities. Students express preferences for learning, especially of practical skills, and educators now employ a wide range of educational approaches to provide contemporary allied health education. Despite the increased focus on university-based education, practical opportunities for skill development remained a key component of allied health training.

The acknowledgement of students as active learners has transitioned didactic training to contemporary educational approaches which blend theoretical content with opportunities to practice and translate theory-into-practice. Although the mix of modular university and practice education has long existed, there is now an *integrated* approach which blends knowledge and practice within campus-based learning. In this model, students obtain knowledge and are then provided with a range of practical opportunities to practice skills separate to the experiences provided on traditional fieldwork experiences.

In summary, current allied health education, although unique to each discipline, implements regulated standards and wide-ranging educational approaches to achieve work-ready graduates. This historical development has culminated in several key contemporary approaches and inclusions in allied health education. These trends are now presented.

Trends in Allied Health Education

Professional Practice

Professional practice (also known as fieldwork, work-integrated learning, clinical placement, or practice education) has been a longstanding and important inclusion in allied health education. Through immersion in professional work experiences, students are provided with opportunities to develop competencies required for practice, and required by accreditation bodies, across a range of practice settings. Professional practice addresses the identified theory-into-practice gap, enabling integration of the conceptual/theoretical knowledge obtained on-campus with application with real clients in real professional contexts (Nagarajan and McAllister 2015a). Like other aspects of curriculum design, there is variation between professions in relation to the number of hours required, the timing of the experience within the curriculum, and the range of practice settings that need to be included. Programs typically include multiple professional practice opportunities to match the developmental attainment of proficiency across the degree (Nagarajan and McAllister 2015a). Key learning outcomes are identified for students and they are assessed in a range of ways, including bespoke program-designed measures or nationally applied measures, such as the Competency Based Occupational Standards for Speech Pathologists – Entry Level (Speech Pathology Australia 2017) implemented by Speech Pathology Australia.

Accreditation bodies place a range of stipulations on the provision of professional practice. This includes, but is not limited to:

(i) Who (expertise wise) should supervise students
(ii) How many hours are required to develop competency
(iii) Models of professional practice
(iv) The use of simulation

Some commonalities and variations exist across the professions. Examples include:

Supervision of Students In Australia, students in several professions including speech pathology and physiotherapy must be supervised by an educator from their profession, but discipline specific supervision is not essential for rehabilitation counselling students (McAllister and Nagarajan 2015).

Hours of Professional Practice The British Dietetic Association (British Dietetic Association 2017) requires students to complete a minimum of 1000 hours of professional practice, compared to 360 hours specified by Exercise and Sports Science Australia for exercise physiology students (Exercise and Sports Science Australia 2019). The Occupational Therapy Council of Australia (Occupational Therapy Council of Australia 2018) expects practice across the life span and healthcare continuum, and the Australian Physiotherapy Council requires placement hours to be allocated to prescribed areas of practice (such as musculoskeletal and cardiorespiratory physiotherapy) without specifying the number of hours required (Australian Physiotherapy Council 2006).

Models of Professional Practice Historically, clinical education of allied health professionals used apprenticeship-style models with 1:1 supervision by supervisors. Over time, evidence has emerged to support the effectiveness of ratios of from 2:1 to 4:1 (Lekkas et al. 2007), and peer/pair models, which often combine supervisor expertise and feedback with peer feedback. Student-as-educator models (Lekkas et al. 2007) are increasingly being used, in part due to challenges in sourcing sufficient supervisors and placements. This model transfers the student experience from being solely learner to also educator. Role-emerging opportunities, where students engage with training sites in which their profession does not have an existing role (Lekkas et al. 2007; Rodger et al. 2008), are also increasing.

International Classification of Functioning, Disability and Health (ICF)

The World Health Organization's International Classification of Functioning, Disability and Health (ICF) (World Health Organization 2001) provides a logical foundation for allied health education, as it offers consideration of health and illness from a cellular level, through to body systems and onto the individual and community-living perspective. The framework presents an international approach to understanding functioning and disability through a shared language and conceptualization (World Health Organization 2001). The ICF provides a multifaceted framework for coding and understanding information related to health including diagnosis and the personal and environmental influences on disease. The ICF acknowledges that a person's functioning and disability result from the interplay between their health condition, intrinsic features of the individual, and a broad range of environmental and contextual factors (Bickenbach 2008). The framework is useful in the allied health context as disciplines are able to identify where and how their profession is conceptualized internationally and enables students to understand the contributions of their own disciplines and make comparisons to the contributions made by other disciplines (Snyman et al. 2016). It provides students with a structure for describing and understanding illness, health determinants, and health outcomes (Snyman et al. 2016), and educationally can provide a framework for clinical reasoning (Darrah et al. 2006). As the framework can be contextualized with broad health concepts including ethics and human rights, a key strength in education is that the ICF can provide a basis for shared education across student allied health professionals. The articulated complexity of health makes clear the importance of a range of health professionals to contribute to client care and brings together notions of interprofessional (e.g., multidisciplinary and interdisciplinary) healthcare which are key conceptualizations of allied health service provision. Educationally, the ICF is a sound foundation for interprofessional education.

Interprofessional Education

Interprofessional education (IPE), the provision of educational experiences to students from a range of different health disciplines (Olson and Bialocerkowski 2014; Boshoff et al. 2019), is defined as at least two distinct disciplines sharing learning experiences which enable them to learn "from, with and about each other" (Hammer and Vasset 2019). IPE is now commonplace within university curricula and mandated in several countries and disciplines. In education, IPE typically involves the use of case-based or simulated learning experiences where small groups of health professions students work together to develop knowledge and skills relevant to specific target clients. In doing so, they develop knowledge and skills about their own discipline and that of other health professionals. Sessions may be synchronous or asynchronous, online, and be completed at one point in time or develop over several classes or weeks (Olson and Bialocerkowski 2014). Studies demonstrate that IPE in allied health education is effective (Olson and Bialocerkowski 2014) and that students undergo a positive learning experience (Reddington et al. 2018) through which they can develop knowledge and skills required for collaborative professional practice (Reeves et al. 2010). As the development and implementation of IPE activities has increased within health education, there are now documented and common competencies that have been established for needs of all health profession students. These include knowledge relating to the practice of other allied health professions and skills in developing patient goals in collaboration with other health professionals (O'Keefe et al. 2017). Research evidence now illustrates the value of IPE activities to graduate development and practice. Consequently, many professions are now required to include IPE into university curriculum (Gray et al. 2015; Zorek and Raehl 2013; Long et al. 2014).

Professional practice education provides a further opportunity for students to obtain IPE experiences. There is an assumption that interprofessional learning during study may translate into interprofessional graduate practice (Rodger et al. 2008). A recent systematic review (Boshoff et al. 2019) identified over 25 studies that described the provision of an IPE student professional practice, most commonly with students from occupational therapy, physiotherapy, pharmacy, social work, and speech pathology. Included studies described students completing interprofessional assessment, goal setting, intervention planning, and intervention implementation. Positive outcomes were identified from both allied health students and the recipients of their therapy.

Cultural Competency and Safety

In acknowledgment of the health inequities that exist for indigenous peoples, ethnic minorities, and other population groups globally, there has been increasing interest in implementing health curricula that addresses these gaps. Content specifically addressing culture and cultural influences on health is a common requirement of accreditation bodies to ensure that allied health graduates have the knowledge and skills to provide effective healthcare to clients from a range of cultural backgrounds. This content focuses primarily on cultural competence and culturally safe practice.

Cultural competence relates to developing knowledge and skills and attitudes whereby learners understand their own culture in interactions with others (Kurtz et al. 2018; Williamson and Harrison 2010). Cultural safety, an extension of cultural competence, requires health professionals to reflect on the power imbalances that potentially exist between the healthcare professional and patient and attempt to create healthcare interactions that are safe from the patient perspective (National Aboriginal and Torres Strait Island Health Worker Association 2016; Laverty et al. 2017). These important knowledge, skills, and attitudes, and their aligned cultural principles, are now considered as essential graduate competencies in certain allied health programs in some countries. For example, The Physiotherapy Board of New Zealand dictates that cultural competence is essential for safe and effective practice, and outlines knowledge, skills, and attitudes relevant for all areas of physiotherapy practice (Physiotherapy Board of New Zealand 2016). A review by Kurtz et al. (2018) identified that cultural safety education was provided through a range of educational experiences ranging from didactic classroom-based activities to cultural immersion practice education. The authors highlighted the importance of collaborative partnerships with indigenous people, supported by university policy, as being imperative to successful and sustainable outcomes for students.

Another trend in allied health education relates to internationalization as part of the university curriculum. This is based on the assumption that international experiences prepare students to be global citizens and to be able to work in diverse cultural contexts (Useh 2011). These strategies are typically incorporated through either "Internationalisation of Curriculum" or "Internationalisation at Home" approaches (Nagarajan and McAllister 2015b). In the internationalization of curriculum approach, students are provided with opportunities for student mobility grants where they can study aspects of their degree in an alternate cultural context. In Australia, the Federal government provides the "New Colombo Plan" (Australian Government Department of Foreign Affairs and Trade 2019), which aims to increase

Australian student knowledge of the Indo-Pacific area through short- and long-term study, internships, practice education, and research opportunities. With government support, universities offer these grants to support students' exposure to such international opportunities. In the "Internationalisation at Home" approach, students obtain an understanding of international and global perspectives of health integrated into on-campus curricula. Examples of such approaches include case studies using clients from different cultural backgrounds, consideration of healthcare in low-resource environmental contexts, and practice education with unique cultural groups within the country of education (Nagarajan and McAllister 2015b). Again, this trend is of increasing interest to accreditation and registration bodies because of its importance in the development of the cultural competence of graduates.

Simulation

Simulation has been defined as "...an array of structured activities that represent actual or potential situations in education and practice" (Lopreiato et al. 2016, p. 32) and has always been a part of the education of allied health professionals. Simulation-based education is now an accepted and approved method of teaching and learning that is being adopted by health educators (Ryall et al. 2016) for health students. From the very beginning of allied health education, students were engaged in simulation-based learning when they practiced techniques on each other to develop procedural skills. The trends in simulation since then have mirrored the trends described in previous sections in relation to allied health education. Although peer practice and role play still form an important component of procedural learning, the changes in simulation-based learning correspond with the change in the focus of education from procedural ability to active learning related to processes and clinical reasoning. Gradually simulation progressed through more structured role play to now include a range of formalized, highly sophisticated structures with clearly defined learning objectives (Tuttle and Grant 2019).

Simulation-based learning includes a wide range of structures, technologies, and environments that have become more used and accepted as an educational approach in the past two decades. Common features of simulation-based learning environments are that they can offer a range of real-life scenarios and experiences for students without the safety or ethical concerns that can occur when students are working with real patients (Ryall et al. 2016; O'Shea et al. 2019; Bridge 2016). The modalities of simulation include: (i) physical task trainers, (ii) academics or actors portraying patients in patient-centered scenarios, (iii) a range of computer-based approaches, and (iv) hybrid forms that combine different types of simulation (Tuttle 2018). While task trainers are, at least initially, used to develop procedural skills, the other forms of simulation are able to align with the development of higher-level skills such as clinical reasoning and problem-solving. Computer-based approaches range from simple exposition of scenarios with linear progressions and the "choose your own adventure" options that are possible through adaptive learning environments, to gamification and fully immersive virtual or augmented reality. In all of these cases, control of the simulation by educators enables the simulation to be graded in complexity for students across the years of their degree. Students can enhance their confidence, resilience, and hands-on experience by experiencing simulated real-life scenarios in clinical situations without direct contact with real patients (Ryall et al. 2016; O'Shea et al. 2019).

As well as the modalities and learning objectives of simulation changing over time, so too has its place in curricula. Initially simulation was primarily used for either learning or assessing procedural skills on campus. For example, the assessment of procedural skills might involve a fellow student playing the role of patient. In particular, patient-centered, digital, or hybrid simulations have moved the use of simulation to later in the curricula, where students are learning and practicing higher-level skills. The increasing number of students across allied health professions has driven the need to find creative means of increasing capacity. In response, simulation is used in several professions to replace clinical placement hours or to make placements more effective by better preparing students for clinical placements (Tuttle and Horan 2019).

Within allied health, replacement of all or part of clinical placement time by simulated clinical placement hours has been shown to not be inferior to traditional placements in disciplines including physiotherapy (Watson et al. 2012) and occupational therapy (Imms et al. 2018). As a result, simulation has been acknowledged as an appropriate model for replacing some clinical placement hours by a range of governing bodies, including the Health and Care Professions Council in the United Kingdom, and the Australian Health Practitioner Regulation Agency. Although there are some innovative examples of simulation using technology, including virtual and augmented reality in radiology (Gunn et al. 2018), pharmacy, and physiotherapy (Tuttle 2018), the use of these digitally enhanced tools is in its infancy.

Consumer and Patient Involvement in Allied Health Education

Consumer engagement has long been a fundamental component of allied health education, primarily through professional practice experiences. Today, consumers in health education in on-campus learning activities is supported by health policy and accrediting bodies as a strategy to develop graduate expertise in providing client-centered approaches to therapy. The approaches range from consumers sharing "lived experiences" of health and illness (patient educators), through to being partners in curriculum design, teaching, assessment, and evaluation (consumer academics) (Towle et al. 2010). There is documented evidence that consumer involvement can enable students to develop clinical skills, change attitudes towards disability, and develop empathy (Perry et al. 2013). Furthermore, there is evidence that consumers can facilitate assessment of students without negatively impacting student engagement nor performance (Logan et al. 2018).

Mental health curriculums appear to lead the way in consumer involvement and a growing body of evidence is emerging to understand experiences of health students, educators, and consumers in the educational experiences. In summary, student views have been mixed, with some students perceiving consumer involvement as worthwhile, while other students have raised concerns about whether consumers can provide representative (rather than individual) views of the consumer experience (Happell et al. 2014). "Consumer academics," people with lived experiences who are being increasingly employed by universities in academic roles, are being trained in educational design to support their involvement in teaching and learning (Hanson and Mitchell 2001). As the health sector moves towards greater consumer participation and decision-making in their healthcare, allied health training programs will need to take this into account.

Future Trends in Allied Health Education

The twenty-first century has seen new frontiers emerge in allied health education to create work-ready graduates. Interprofessional learning and learning through simulation have quickly become business-as-usual curricular activities, and there has been a surge in digitally enabled learning through online offerings of programs, courses, and interactive learning activities. Indeed, many universities now incorporate their "digital campus" in their promotional activities and metrics. Into the 2020s and beyond, allied health education will become increasingly responsive to health sector and workforce needs. Disruptive forces such as e-health to support healthcare practice and new educational foci will be key drivers for new knowledge and skills in allied health education, along with new professional perspectives.

E-Health

Telepractice

Telepractice utilizes telecommunication technology as a medium to provide healthcare services. As examples, telephone or videoconferencing facilities are now used to link health professionals to clients, caregiver, and other professionals responsible for delivering care to the client. Through these mediums, therapists can complete assessment, intervention, consultation, and/or supervision (Speech Pathology Australia 2014). Across many allied health professions (e.g., physiotherapy, psychology, speech pathology), much evidence now supports equivalent individual and group therapy outcomes from telepractice compared to face-to-face delivery, as well as telepractice's value in specialist clinical consultation and remote supervision of students (Australia et al. 2015). Telepractice improves the reach of services through overcoming geographical constraints to access and overcoming time constraints through more flexible service options for consumers. Hence, the future workforce will need the knowledge and technological capabilities for delivering the best quality evidence-based care, and all allied health training programs will need to include such education.

Digital Capabilities

The new world of learning will see a greater emphasis on building digital capabilities. For allied health students, the digitization of electronic medical records contrasts with paper-based records and will require a new practical skill set on recording. In addition, routine patient and service management will require allied health professionals to have well-developed data analytic skills to enable them to access big data to use, interpret, and make predictions that will translate into efficiencies in workflow and information access, enhance patient care and quality of life, and optimize healthcare costs. A strong commitment to creating a digitally capable health workforce for the future can be seen in Australia through a 7-year $55 million government-funded *Digital Health Cooperative Research Centre* (2018–2024). In the university sector, graduate certificates and diplomas in health data and analytics have begun to appear. With electronic record management systems now "live" in many work facilities, training digital capabilities will become an imperative and core domain in allied health education.

Business, Marketing, and Entrepreneurship Skills

Global workforce trends have changed markedly over the last decade for allied health graduates. Increasingly, graduates are starting their working lives in the private sector rather than in the public or non-for-profit (NFP) sectors which, historically, have been the main employers. This trend largely is a result of the imbalance between the slower rate of growth of public and NFP jobs relative to annually increasing numbers of allied health students emerging from more university training programs. Although most new graduates move into established private workplaces where they are well supported and mentored, a baseline level of business, marketing, and entrepreneurship acumen is nonetheless required. It must be noted that, specifically, for the private practice market, some national allied health regulatory authorities recommend a certain number of years of experience before working as a sole private practitioner (e.g., Speech Pathology Australia). In preparing graduates for working in the private sector, many allied health university programs have capstone seminars with topics targeting this area. The inclusion of business, marketing, and entrepreneurial skills have not been a core unit in allied health education but are likely inclusions in coming years.

Microcredentials

A microcredential is "a certification of assessed learning that is additional, alternate, complementary to or a formal component of a formal qualification" (Oliver 2019). In essence, they are mini-qualifications that extend and assess a person's knowledge, skills, and/or experience in a particular content area (Oliver 2019). As the name suggests, microcredentials are smaller than traditional diploma or degree qualifications. However, the intent is that these "nanodegrees" can be stacked together to provide full or partial credit towards designated courses or qualifications. Already gaining traction, microcredentials are now offered through traditional education providers, industry, and private providers across Europe, the United Kingdom, North America, Australia, and Asia. For example, a 2019 review reported that in the United States, there were between 500,000 and 750,000 microcredential programs, and in Australia, 36 out of 42 Australian universities were either offering or developing microcredentials in some form, primarily as standalone *Massive Open Online Courses* (MOOCs) or bundled online units (Oliver 2019).

Microcredentials can perform an important role for upskilling the workforce including supporting professional development, lifelong learning, and lifewide learning perspectives; further, they offer flexibility and (often) affordability for the learner. However, for professional preparation programs in universities, micro-credentials are a potential disruptive force against the traditional notions of how allied health education is structured and delivered. It is feasible that allied health courses can be developed with embedded microcredential units. If these units have a dual professional development application for learners in the workforce to update and validate new knowledge and skills, this represents a win for all. However, attention will be needed to ensure that embedding microcredentials into allied health coursework creates additional and tangible value to university students beyond merely being a novel way to deliver courses. Certainly, in the aforementioned areas such as e-health and business and marketing, microcredentials may be an excellent starting point for weaving these through allied health curricula, or as stackable units in an elective subject.

The Multiskilled Allied Health Professional

The arrival of digital and automation technologies will change the workforce, and by 2030, up to 14% of the global workforce may need to change occupational categories (Manyika et al. 2017). Allied health has distinct professions with distinct identities and scope of practice. However, in response to a global growing need for allied health services in the community, a broadening of scope of practice in the future is a real possibility. Australia has successfully tested these waters through the 2013 Allied Health Rural Generalist Pathway (Services for Australian Rural and Remote Allied Health 2012). This strategy aimed to improve health outcomes in rural and remote areas through upskilling allied health professionals with additional capabilities from disciplines other than their own, to enable multidisciplinary care in rural healthcare teams where the presence of multiple allied health disciplines was not possible.

To meet the predicted growing demand for allied health services, universities may need to consider developing training programs for a new type of allied health worker. This professional could graduate with core skills that overarch several professions (e.g., physiotherapy, occupational therapy, speech pathology, audiology, exercise physiology, nutrition, and dietetics). This new multiskilled allied health professional would serve as a conduit between the "pure" allied health professional that exists in the United Kingdom, Europe, Asia-Pacific, and North America and the allied health assistant, to provide public education, basic screening and diagnostic programs, and deliver essential interventions. Although currently a controversial proposition, and much work would be required by universities and regulatory authorities to determine the shape and scope of this new profession, it is difficult to argue that such a profession will not be required to meet the diverse and burgeoning needs of healthcare in the future.

Conclusion

In summary, education in allied health has moved from a simple, directly experiential, predominantly apprenticeship model in the early stages of many professions to a sophisticated, diverse, and multifaceted aspect of university-based health professional education. The nature of clinical education has not just responded to new evidence and workforce trends in allied health professions but have often foreshadowed or even fostered new directions in clinical practice.

Although there has been an increased specialization in allied health and a corresponding increase in the number of allied health professions, current trends include disruptive models of care and education which, paradoxically, may foster greater specialization in disciplines and practitioners as well as more generalist practitioners. Moving into the future, there are a number of potential disruptors including blurring or even dissolution of professional boundaries, inter- and/or cross-disciplinary supervision during clinical placements, an increase in virtual and augmented realities, new e-health frontiers, and changes in the structure of higher education which make the future of allied health education both exciting and uncertain.

Cross-References

▶ Competencies of Health Professions Educators of the Future
▶ Future of Health Professions Education Curricula
▶ Practice Education in Occupational Therapy: Current Trends and Practices
▶ Simulation as Clinical Replacement: Contemporary Approaches in Healthcare Professional Education
▶ Simulation for Clinical Skills in Healthcare Education
▶ Supporting the Development of Patient-Centred Communication Skills

References

Association of Schools of Allied Health Professionals. What is allied health? 2018. Available from: http://www.asahp.org/what-is

Australia SP, Burns C, Hill A, Baldac S, Cook M, Erickson S, et al. Telepractice in speech pathology position statement. Melbourne: Speech Pathology Association of Australia Inc; 2015.

Australian Government Department of Foreign Affairs and Trade. New Colombo Plan. 2019.

Australian Health Professionals Association. Allied health accreditation. 2017.

Australian Physiotherapy Council. Australian standards for physiotherapy. 2006. Available from: https://www.nwivisas.com/media/521998/Australian-Standards-for-Physiotherapy.pdf

Australian Qualifications Framework Council. Australian qualifications framework. 2nd ed. 2013. Available from: https://www.aqf.edu.au/sites/aqf/files/aqf-2nd-edition-january-2013.pdf

Bickenbach JE. ICF and the allied health professions. Adv Physiother. 2008;10(3):108–9.

Boshoff K, Murray C, Worley A, Berndt A. Interprofessional education placements in allied health: a scoping review. Scand J Occup Ther. 2019;early online view:1–18.

Bridge P. Radiotherapy educational research: a decade of innovation. J Radiother Pract. 2016;15(1):5–14.

British Dietetic Association. Practice education. 2017. Available from: https://www.bda.uk.com/training/practice/home

Darrah J, Loomis J, Manns P, Norton B, May L. Role of conceptual models in a physical therapy curriculum: application of an integrated model of theory, research, and clinical practice. Physiother Theory Pract. 2006;22(5):239–50.

Exercise & Sports Science Australia. 2019. Available from: https://www.essa.org.au/Public/EDUCATION_PROVIDERS/Practicum.aspx

Gray JM, Coker-Bolt P, Gupta J, Hisson A, Harmann KD. Importance of interprofessional education in occupational therapy curricula. Am J Occup Ther. 2015;69(suppl 3):1–14.

Gunn T, Jones L, Bridge P, Rowntree P, Nissen L. The use of virtual reality simulation to improve technical skill in the undergraduate medical imaging student. Interact Learn Environ. 2018;26(5):613–20.

Hammer H, Vasset F. Interprofessional learning in the simulation laboratory: nursing and pharmacy students' experiences. J Res Interprof Pract Educ. 2019;9(1):1–14.

Hanson B, Mitchell DP. Involving mental health service users in the classroom: a course of preparation. Nurse Educ Pract. 2001;1(3):120–6.

Happell B, Byrne L, McAllister M, Lampshire D, Roper C, Gaskin CJ, et al. Consumer involvement in the tertiary-level education of mental health professionals: a systematic review. Int J Ment Health Nurs. 2014;23(1):3–16.

Health & Care Professions Council. Standards for education and training. 2018. Available from: https://www.hcpc-uk.org/standards/standards-relevant-to-education-and-training/set/

Health Professions Council of South Africa. Overview. 2018. Available from: https://www.hpcsa.co.za/Registrations

Imms C, Froude E, Chu EMY, Sheppard L, Darzins S, Guinea S, et al. Simulated versus traditional occupational therapy placements: a randomised controlled trial. Aust Occup Ther J. 2018;65(6):556–64.

Kurtz DLM, Janke R, Vinek J, Wells T, Hutchinson P, Froste A. Health sciences cultural safety education in Australia, Canada, New Zealand, and the United States: a literature review. Int J Med Educ. 2018;9:271–85.

Laverty M, McDermott DR, Calma T. Embedding cultural safety in Australia's main health care standards. Med J Aust. 2017;207(1):15–6.

Lekkas P, Larsen T, Kumar S, Grimmer K, Nyland L, Chipchase L, et al. No model of clinical education for physiotherapy students is superior to another: a systematic review. Aust J Physiother. 2007;53(1):19–28.

Logan A, Yule E, Taylor M, Imms C. Mental health consumer participation in undergraduate occupational therapy student assessment: no negative impact. Aust Occup Ther J. 2018;65(6):494–502.

Long S, Schwarz BW, Conner-Kerr T, Cada EA, Hogan R. Priorities, strategies, and accountability measures in interprofessional education. J Allied Health. 2014;43(3):37E–44E.

Lopreiato JO, Downing D, Gammon W, Lioce L, Sittner B, Slot V, et al. Healthcare simulation dictionary. 2016. Available from: https://www.ssih.org/Dictionary

Manyika J, Lund S, Chui M, Bughin J, Woetzel J, Batra P, et al. Jobs lost, jobs gained: Workforce transitions in a time of automation. McKinsey Global Institute. 2017. https://www.mckinsey.com/~/media/McKinsey/Industries/Public%20and%20Social%20Sector/Our%20Insights/What%20the%20future%20of%20work%20will%20mean%20for%20jobs%20skills%20and%20wages/MGI-Jobs-Lost-Jobs-Gained-Report-December-6-2017.pdf

McAllister L, Nagarajan SV. Accreditation requirements in allied health education: strengths, weaknesses and missed opportunities. J Teach Learn Graduate Employability. 2015;6(1):2–24.

Nagarajan SV, McAllister L. Integration of practice experiences into the allied health curriculum: curriculum and pedagogic considerations before, during and after work-integrated learning experiences. Asia-Pacific J Cooperat Educ. 2015a;16(4):279–90.

Nagarajan S, McAllister L. Internationalisation of curriculum at home: imperatives, opportunities and challenges for allied health education. J Teach Learn Graduate Employability. 2015b;6(1):88.

National Aboriginal and Torres Strait Island Health Worker Association. Cultural safety framework. 2016. Available from: https://www.natsihwa.org.au/cultural-safety-framework

O'Keefe M, Henderson A, Chick R. Defining a set of common interprofessional learning competencies for health profession students. Med Teach. 2017;39(5):463–8.

O'Shea M-C, Palermo C, Rogers GD, Williams LT. Simulation-based learning experiences in dietetics programs: a systematic review. J Nutr Educ Behav. 2019;early view.

Occupational Therapy Board of Australia. Australian occupational therapy competency standards. 2018. Available from: http://www.occupationaltherapyboard.gov.au/Codes-Guidelines/Competencies.aspx

Occupational Therapy Council of Australia. Accreditation standards for Australian entry-level occupational therapy education programs. 2018. Available from: https://www.otcouncil.com.au/wp-content/uploads/OTC-Accred-Stds-Dec2018-effective-Jan2020.pdf

Oliver B. Making micro-credentials work for learners, employers and providers. Melbourne: Deakin University; 2019.

Olson R, Bialocerkowski A. Interprofessional education in allied health: a systematic review. Med Educ. 2014;48(3):236–46.

Perry J, Watkins M, Gilbert A, Rawlinson J. A systematic review of the evidence on service user involvement in interpersonal skills training of mental health students. J Psychiatr Ment Health Nurs. 2013;20(6):525–40.

Physiotherapy Board of New Zealand. Standard: culutral competence. 2016. Available from: https://www.physioboard.org.nz/sites/default/files/CulturalCompetenceMay2016.pdf

Reddington AR, Egli AJ, Schmuck HM. Interprofessional education perceptions of dental assisting and radiologic technology students following a live patient experience. J Dent Educ. 2018;82(5):462–8.

Reeves S, Goldman J, Burton A, Sawatzky-Girling B. Synthesis of systematic review evidence of interprofessional education. J Allied Health. 2010;39(3):198–203.

Rodger S, Webb G, Devitt L, Gilbert J, Wrightson P, McMeeken J. Clinical education and practice placements in the allied health professions: an international perspective. J Allied Health. 2008;37(1):53–62.

Ryall T, Judd BK, Gordon CJ. Simulation-based assessments in health professional education: a systematic review. J Multidiscip Healthc. 2016;9:69–82.

Schloman BF. Mapping the literature of allied health: project overview. Bull Med Libr Assoc. 1997;85(3):271–7.

Seegmiller JG, Nasypany A, Kahanov L, Seegmiller JA, Baker R. Trends in doctoral education among healthcare professions: an integrative research review. Athl Train Educ J. 2015;10(1):47–56.

Services for Australian Rural and Remote Allied Health. The allied health rural generalist pathway. 2012. Available from: https://sarrah.org.au/ahrgp

Simmons B. Clinical reasoning: concept analysis. J Adv Nurs. 2010;66(5):1151–8.

Snyman S, van Zyl M, Müller J, Geldenhuys M. International classification of functioning, disability and health: catalyst for interprofessional education and collaborative practice. In: Forman D, Jones M, Thistlethwaite J, editors. Leading research and evaluation in interprofessional education and collaborative practice. London: Palgrave Macmillan; 2016. p. 285–328.

Speech Pathology Australia. Telepractice in speech pathology – position statement. 2014. Available from: https://www.speechpathologyaustralia.org.au/SPAweb/Members/Position_Statements/spaweb/Members/Position_Statements/Position_Statements.aspx?hkey=dedc1a49-75de-474a-8bcb-bfbd2ac078b7

Speech Pathology Australia. Competency-based occupational standards for speech pathologists – entry level. 2017. Available from: https://www.speechpathologyaustralia.org.au/SPAweb/SPAweb/Resources_for_Speech_Pathologists/CBOS/CBOS.aspx

Tavakol K, Reicherter PEA. The role of problem-based learning in the enhancement of allied health education. J Allied Health. 2003;32(2):110–5.

Towle A, Bainbridge L, Godolphin W, Katz A, Kline C, Lown B, et al. Active patient involvement in the education of health professionals. Med Educ. 2010;44(1):64–74.

Tuttle N. The use of an online adaptive learning platform as an adjunct to live simulated clinical encounters. In: Sing I, Raghuvanshi K, editors. Emerging technologies and work-integrated learning experiences in allied health education. Hershey, IGI Global; 2018. p. 93–105.

Tuttle N, Grant G. Varieties of simulation experience. 2019;Forthcoming 2019.

8 Allied Health Education: Current and Future Trends

Tuttle N, Horan S. Replacing content teaching with an intensive just-in-time simulation-based learning activity improves physiotherapy student performance on clinical placements. 2019; forthcoming 2019.

Useh U. Internationalisation of higher education: inclusion of socio-cultural skills in a physiotherapy programme. J Hum Ecol. 2011;36(1):1–7.

Watson K, Wright A, Morris N, McMeeken J, Rivett D, Blackstock F, et al. Can simulation replace part of clinical time? Two parallel randomised controlled trials. Med Educ. 2012;46(7):657–67.

Williamson M, Harrison L. Providing culturally appropriate care: a literature review. Int J Nurs Stud. 2010;47(6):761–9.

World Federation of Occupational Therapists. Minimum standards for the education of occupational therapists (revised). Forrestfield: Author; 2016.

World Health Organization. ICF: international classification of functioning, disability and health. Geneva: World Health Organization; 2001.

Zorek J, Raehl C. Interprofessional education accreditation standards in the USA: a comparative analysis. J Interprof Care. 2013;27(2):123–30.

Dental Education: Context and Trends

9

Flora A. Smyth Zahra and Sang E. Park

Contents

Introduction	154
The Societal and Regulatory Contexts	155
The Patient Context	156
The Learner Context	157
Trends in Delivery of Dental Education Toward a More Holistic Approach for Both Patients and Learners	159
Conclusion	163
Cross-References	163
References	163

Abstract

Educating the current generation of dental students to deliver optimal care is particularly challenging at a time when the rate of both technological and societal changes is particularly rapid and the future role of the clinician is less predictable than with previous cohorts. This chapter considers trends in the delivery of dental education that support a more holistic approach to both patient care and learning given the present societal and regulatory contexts. Considering that the practice of dentistry is arguably one of the most stressful of all the health professions, the current high rates of student mental ill health and the link between burnout and reduced patient care, dental curricula should include self-care and wellness. There must also be more emphasis on the sociocultural determinants of health, critical appraisal skills, and educating for advocacy against global oral health

---

F. A. Smyth Zahra (✉)
Faculty of Dentistry, Oral & Craniofacial Sciences, King's College London, London, UK
e-mail: flora.smyth_zahra@kcl.ac.uk

S. E. Park
Office of Dental Education, Harvard School of Dental Medicine, Boston, MA, USA
e-mail: sang_park@hsdm.harvard.edu

© Springer Nature Singapore Pte Ltd. 2023
D. Nestel et al. (eds.), *Clinical Education for the Health Professions*,
https://doi.org/10.1007/978-981-15-3344-0_14

inequalities. To date, the focus on knowledge and technical skills has neglected the vital role of personal and professional identity formation, given that the education of dentists follows a transformational professional development model. The authors advocate active learning through case-based collaborative methods, authentic assessment, and a humanistic learning environment with dialogue and reflection. Emancipatory pedagogy with curricular content that looks beyond the bioscientific to the humanities nurtures students' personal and professional identity formation through transformational learning and provides them with more strategies for lifetime learning and the complexity of professional practice.

Keywords

Ambiguity · Humanistic · Holistic · Sociocultural · Complexity · Advocacy · Emancipatory pedagogy · Reflexivity · Flourishing

Introduction

Healthcare delivery in the twenty-first century is a Gordian knot of complexity. Educating the current generation of students for their practicing lifetimes, inspiring their commitment to continuing professional development at a time of rapid and accelerating pace of change both within the biomedical sciences and more generally society as a whole while simultaneously instilling within them delivery of compassionate care, is just as challenging for dental educators as any others within the health professions. Oral health is intrinsically linked to systemic health and impacts both self-esteem and quality of life. It has a significant socio-behavioral dimension, ensuring patient compliance is fundamental to achieving good treatment outcomes. It is also illustrative of a major twenty-first-century inequality in access to care, particularly among disadvantaged communities, minority ethnic groups, and the homeless, which has contributed to growing health disparities.

Many of the generation, born between 1996 and 2010, have been described as exhibiting attitudinal changes compared to previous groups: having high expectations and high esteem, yet at the same time often exhibiting low levels of perseverance, low attention span, and low tolerance of ambiguity, while also being reticent to ask for help (Twenge and Campbell 2009). Disenchantment and burnout among medical and dental students are prevalent, with high levels of stress and cynicism reported in dental schools (Apelian et al. 2014). Directly related is evidence of declining levels of patient empathy as students progress through their clinical courses (Brazeau et al. 2010), which impacts on patient safety (Gerada 2017). Doctors, dentists, and veterinarians have consistently higher rates of suicide than other professional groups (Roberts et al. 2013).

At the heart of dental education is the close triangular relationship between the operating student, their clinical supervisor who is both a facilitator and role model, and each individual patient. This follows the "context-specific" transformative model of professional development (Kennedy 2005) where the learner, encouraged in "discourse and critical reflection," (Mezirow 1990) constructs his/her own knowledge and in doing so gains increased professional autonomy.

Both the delivery of healthcare and the education of healthcare professionals have been described as inherently sociocultural (Napier et al. 2014). Some medical educators have argued that developing student humanistic skills through the role modeling of caring practice and "serious engagement with the medical humanities" is "key to fostering their professionalism" (Cohen 2007). Despite the trend in both US and UK medical schools to incorporate aspects of the humanities into their curricula, it is only in the last few years that this has been pioneered in dentistry (Smyth 2018). As models of dental education have shifted from apprenticeship to competency-based and as we prepare our students for a future we cannot fully predict, much more should be done beyond a focus on knowledge and technical skills. We must support student professional identity formation and personal development; nurture their cultural awareness, reflection, advocacy, and critical thinking skills with more emphasis on the complexities and ambiguities of clinical practice, global oral health disparities, sustainability, and difficult judgment calls; and employ different epistemologies to enable them to address the sociocultural aspects of patient care.

The Societal and Regulatory Contexts

Oral diseases are largely preventable, the causes are well known, and the progression of the two most common diseases, dental caries and periodontal disease, may be controlled by relatively inexpensive simple measures. Oral and oropharyngeal cancers, however, both potentially fatal, continue to increase in some population groups with oral cancer being the sixth most common cancer in the world (Warnakulasuriya 2009). While there has been improved oral health and increasingly high demand for cosmetic procedures among the more affluent in many countries, other community groups globally exhibit high levels of disease with associated physical pain, loss of function, and lowered self-esteem. There are particular concerns regarding the vulnerable, children living in poverty, the homeless, and the elderly, many of whom are living with complex comorbidities. Inequalities in access to oral healthcare and changing disease patterns have led to a review of the distribution and roles of the UK dental workforce (Health Education 2018). Others have claimed that there is overspecialization within the profession and that dentistry has become disassociated from medicine (Cohen et al. 2017). As the era of the general dental surgeon, draining acute dental abscesses and extracting teeth, evolves to the management of more chronic conditions and supporting patient behavior change, there have been calls for the mouth to be "put back in the body" and for interdisciplinary teams of dentists, therapists, and hygienists working alongside their medical and nursing colleagues in primary care settings to deliver integrated care with more emphasis on disease prevention rather than mechanical intervention (Health Education 2018; Cohen et al. 2017).

As dental educators, accountable to the regulatory and accreditation bodies entrusted by the public to produce a safe competent workforce, we have a fundamental obligation to create "healthcare professionals that match what societies need" (Aretz 2011). Therefore, set against the current complex backdrop of rapid and ongoing rates of change in global health, the pressure for healthcare providers to improve access and quality of care, yet simultaneously be more cost-effective and responsive to the needs of their local communities, means "transformation must also occur in the educational systems" (Lucey et al. 2018). Acknowledging that "change is here," the American Dental Education Association Commission on Change and Innovation in Dental Education highlighted five external influences already impacting and shaping the delivery of healthcare globally: "technology, education, demographics, healthcare, and environment" (Palatta et al. 2017). Ensuring dental programs that produce "future-ready" graduates for their practicing lifetimes in an era of constant change, the Commission stated that, "Person-centered health care will become the dominant model in health systems" and "Graduates will be educated in a transformative learning environment" (Palatta et al. 2017). The Association for Dental Education in Europe (ADEE), advocating best practice within the European dental curriculum, emphasized the need for learning that ensures "student preparedness," for an interprofessional, collaborative team working in society, that keeps the patient and safety paramount (Field et al. 2017). Health Education England's review of dental education and training infrastructure highlighted the need for more leadership and management teaching within the undergraduate curriculum, and for the wider workforce to adopt a "proportionate universalism" approach to reducing inequalities and inequities, ensuring that the individuals within interprofessional and multidisciplinary teams have appropriate skill levels to deliver "on prevention priorities in a range of settings and are targeted at vulnerable or high-risk groups" (Health Education 2018).

The Patient Context

The move away from mainly acute, interventionist dental treatment to one of managing often chronic conditions and foregrounding, the sociocultural determinants of health, prevention, the patient, and their individual context all necessitate a transition from a purely biomedical model of clinical practice. With this change in disease pattern and presentation, dentistry has been criticized in being slow to change from a "paternalist, reductionist model of healthcare" based on Cartesian positivism (Apelian et al. 2014). Person-centered care is based on philosophies of holism and has been defined as a model that levels the hierarchies between clinician and patient, treating the whole person within his/her own individual context, "putting people and their families at the center of decisions and seeing them as experts, working alongside professionals to get the best outcome" (Walji et al. 2017). Since 2015, this principle of shared decision-making, evidence-based, but in partnership with values, has become the basis of consent to all medical treatment and is the legal underpinning of person-centered care. Effective communication with empathy and compassion, cultural humility, advocacy skills, and multi-perspective thinking has therefore become much more important in this clinical context, with knowledge from the humanities and behavioral and social sciences vital to deliver a twenty-first-century model of care.

Dental education has therefore evolved in recent years to reflect these many changes in patient care. A new focus in person-centered assessment has shifted predoctoral clinical learning from a student requirement-driven educational model to a person-centered and patient-driven care model. An example of this initiative is the case completion curriculum (Park et al. 2011; Park and Howell 2015a), which requires completion of assigned patient cases. The traditional clinical procedure-centered system required that dental students satisfy procedural requirements for each discipline-specific guideline as part of their assessment for competence and criteria for graduation. This teaching model inadvertently promoted student- and faculty-driven patient care rather than person-centered care. With the new assessment model, analysis of retrospective data and the student perspective surveys conducted (Park and Howell 2015a) indicate that the case completion clinical curriculum, in which the comprehensive management of the patient is the priority, encouraged student providers to perform quality patient care and to learn the importance of patient management. This change in clinical education can improve the quality of comprehensive care delivered to patients by student providers and commit to the comprehensive person-centered care model.

The Learner Context

Many of our students, on entering university, crave "belongingness," (Thomas 2012) fear judgment and failure, and are risk-averse and unable to tolerate ambiguity. This period of significant personal change has been described as one of "high risk, a quantum leap of multiple complex transitions" (Health Education England 2019). Mental ill health for this generation of university students born between 1996 and 2010 who have grown up with wide access to social media, smartphones, and the Internet has increased in recent years, with rates of anxiety, depression, and burnout higher still among medical and dental students (Health Education England 2019; Elani et al. 2014).

UK dental practice, compared to colleagues in general medical and veterinary practice, other professions, and other countries, is known to be a highly stressful profession with the top stressors being fear of litigation and increased regulation together with increased negligence claims from patients (Toon et al. 2019). Unsuccessfully managed chronic workplace stress may result in occupational burnout syndrome, which manifests as "energy depletion or exhaustion; (distancing) or feelings of negativism or cynicism related to one's job; and reduced professional efficacy" (World Health Organisation 2019). Therefore, perhaps understandably, levels of self-reported distress and burnout are "alarmingly high" with many UK dentists feeling "persecuted" and undervalued by the public and the media (Toon et al. 2019). Since professional identity and job satisfaction are so closely related to sense of self-worth and emotional well-being, morale among teams "where nobody wants to see you" is low, with many UK dentists feeling lonely or isolated, practicing defensive dentistry, and attempting to minimize possibility of error amid a culture of blame and public distrust (Hayer and Wassif 2019). Since low morale of healthcare teams directly affects patient care (RCP 2015), there are calls to "rehumanize" the dental team, improve psychological well-being in the face of the mental and emotional challenges dentists face, and improve the leadership and systems they work within (Hayer and Wassif 2019).

Dental programs are recognized as a challenging combination of academic and professional learning, with many students finding the course stressful (Colley et al. 2018). Dental education follows a context-specific transformational model of professional development (Kennedy 2005; Smyth Zahra 2018). Within the dental learning environment, it has been reported that students are "entrenched" and their "fear of being humiliated and failing surpasses their desire to learn" (Bedos et al. 2018a).

Educationalists argue that transformative learning, crucial to personal and professional development and axiomatic of a higher education, requires the learner to take risks and challenge previously held assumptions (Mezirow 2006; Wenger 1998). Paradoxically, the perspective change that transforms the peripheral newcomer to a confident participant within the university community and the dental profession after graduation necessitates the learner to engage his/her vulnerabilities in order first "to belong" and then to progress in "becoming" professional (Wenger 1998). Some feel that a largely biomedical curriculum, didactically taught, with emphasis and assessment of knowledge acquisition, is not conducive to students perceiving any value in allowing themselves to be vulnerable, opening up and engaging with patients in a person-centered context (Bedos et al. 2018a). There is a feeling that as educators, we should be doing more to support our students in their learning and preparing them for the stress of practice (Colley et al. 2018). This may prove to be the most challenging role yet that we have as dental educators, with a student cohort reporting more mental health issues than previous. This same student cohort is simultaneously risk-averse and therefore at a disadvantage for the transformational learning necessary for their own personal and professional development; intolerant of ambiguity in unpredictable rapidly changing times; and on graduation entering a working environment at extreme risk of burnout.

An educational model that engages the learners to take an active part in their own learning may have an important role in developing reflective dental practitioners invested in continuous lifelong learning. Various educational pedagogies that promote active learning have been utilized in healthcare education in recent years, including the flipped classroom, which emphasizes a learner-centered teaching where the learner rather than the teacher is the focus (Barr and Tagg 1995). The new vision for dental education builds on interactive approaches to scholarship that foster active learning and critical thinking. This pedagogy presents a shift from surface, fragmented learning to integrated, coherent, case-based, and deep learning; from passively conveying course content to encouraging interactive reasoning; from the standard lecture model to the flipped classroom model; from the rigidity of large classrooms and small-group problem-based learning tutorials to experimentation with different interactive group sizes and principles of team-based learning; and to a better balance between an interactive learning environment, on the one hand, and higher expectations and student accountability for their own learning on the other. A learning sequence comprising self-study, team study, group learning, and reflection is the foundation of the new teaching approach. The role of instructors is changed from deliverer of content to coach, mentor, and guide during educationally purposeful interactive classroom activities which encourage collaboration and nurture self-directed learners keen to carry on learning throughout their professional lives (Park and Howell 2015b).

Trends in Delivery of Dental Education Toward a More Holistic Approach for Both Patients and Learners

Rapid advances in biomaterials science, nanotechnologies, informatics, and tissue engineering continue to drive change in clinical dental practice. Research into genetics, cell biology, and biomarkers have enabled the development of personalized risk assessment tools for caries and periodontal diseases, with the advent of salivary diagnostic markers linking the mouth and therefore the role of the dentist to systemic health and interprofessional collaboration across healthcare teams (Iacopino 2007). Given the complexity of healthcare provision in the current climate, there have been concerns that "Professional education has not kept pace with these challenges, largely because of fragmented, outdated, and static curricula that produce ill-equipped graduates" (Frenk et al. 2010). In an effort to produce clinicians who are better equipped to deal with the reality of clinical practice and have a deeper understanding of both their own local contexts and the wider societal needs, dental undergraduate education has been moving away from a consultant-led, discipline-specific, didactic model of teaching. The traditional emphasis on technical expertise, transmission of knowledge, lecture attendance, and assessment-driven learning was criticized for being "stagnant [and] overcrowded" (Iacopino 2007), producing graduates with inadequate critical thinking abilities, unable to problem-solve or appraise the latest clinical research for the benefit of their patients, and ill-prepared to embrace a professional lifetime of continual learning.

Recent years have therefore seen the move, informed by patient and societal needs in common with medical education, toward a more flexible, integrated, competency-based curriculum over 4–5 years, often with hygienists and therapists trained alongside over 2 years. Supervised by their clinical teachers, dental students, unlike their medical peers, work in interdisciplinary teams from a very early stage in their education, often carrying out irreversible procedures and managing their own patients' pain and anxiety. The teaching is typically small group. Much of the learning within the culture of this community of practice is informal by nature, often with unintended "hidden curriculum" learning outcomes. The twenty-first-century curriculum, redesigned from teacher-led and process-driven to outcome- and competency-based; from knowledge acquisition to knowledge application; and from summative assessment of facts to a more authentic assessment of performance necessitating ongoing individualized formative feedback, has placed the focus firmly on the learner. This approach in turn is now enabling better delivery of person-centered care in the university environment.

Mirroring the centrality of the patient in shared decision-making about their own care, competency-based dental education sees the student as a partner in their education. Six broad competencies, critical thinking, professionalism, communication and interpersonal skills, health promotion, practice management, and informatics and patient care, are proscribed in the USA (Palatta et al. 2017). In Europe, four domains have been specified to produce a "safe beginner," professionalism, safe and effective clinical practice, patient-centered care, and dentistry in society, with suggested methods of teaching, learning, and assessment mapped across the four domains (Field et al. 2017).

The shift in focus from teacher to learner has drawn attention to the learning environment. An ideal dental education should promote a holistic student development supported by humanistic pedagogy that "inculcates respect, tolerance, understanding, and concern for others" (Commission on Dental Accreditation 2016) and "critical thinking, lifelong learning, scientific discovery and integration of knowledge" (Haden et al. 2006). Values-based medicine has emerged as a "complementary partner component" to evidence-based medicine in clinical decision-making (Piele 2013). Likewise, humanistic pedagogy is relational and values-driven, nurtured by faculty role modeling "mentoring, advising and small group interaction" (Commission on Dental Accreditation 2016). Fundamental to a contemporary dental education, one that nurtures students, supports clinical decision-making, and aims to deliver person-centered care, is that students are enabled to learn to how to think critically for themselves, exhibit cultural humility (Tervalon and Murray-Garcia 1998), ask the right questions, and have the necessary flexibility to carry on learning and self-critiquing throughout their lifetimes. Person-centered education has its roots in humanistic psychology, the centrality of phenomenology (Heidegger 1962), sense of free will or personal agency, the belief that personal growth is a basic human motive, (Maslow 1946) and that to support this "self-actualization" the learning environment should be authentic, accepting, and empathic (Rogers 1983). It follows that "students who are respected, learn to respect their patients, both present and future, as living human beings, as individuals with a diversity of backgrounds, life experiences, and values" (Haden et al. 2006), and in this way humanistic educational practices underpin development of dentists who practice holistic patient care.

Some challenges to competency-based, humanistic dental education and delivery of holistic patient care still exist, however. There are reports from some students of "belittlement," a hidden curriculum of; faculty exhibiting poor role modeling; and students copying their teachers "entrenched in a biomedical model in which they reduce people to organs and diseases" (Bedos et al. 2018a). Others have noticed a tension that dentistry involves both "complex human behaviours that demand an interpretive holistic approach and complex biological mechanisms that require a deductive, reductionist approach" (Apelian et al. 2014).

Patient care should be practiced using a systemic approach and should provide patient treatment that meets the standard of care for the dental profession by integrating research evidence with patient needs and values. Therefore, curriculum development involves a critical evaluation of the literature and application of evidence-based practice. Specifically, dental education uses evidence in evaluating treatment options, selection of clinical procedures, and material selections for optimum treatment outcomes for patients. Integration and application of evidence-based dentistry (EBD) occur at various levels through school committees, discipline and departmental meetings in support of patient care, and clinical practice to determine treatment modalities, dental materials, and devices, evaluating them using literature to support the applicability of these modalities into clinical practice. The ability to critically appraise and assess the appropriateness of material and device selection as well as to understand when there is sufficient evidence to support adopting new technology is a critical skill the dental educators seek to impart in students.

Given the prevalence of oral health inequalities globally and amid the calls to place much more emphasis on educating to address the social determinants of health, clinical dentistry has been "slow to join this movement[...] reform undergraduate and postgraduate curricula[...] and 'develop competency frameworks' [addressing] 'social dentistry'" (Bedos et al. 2018b). Much more should be done to nurture students' cultural awareness, reflection, advocacy, and critical thinking skills, with more emphasis placed on the complexities and ambiguities of clinical practice, oral health inequities, service learning, difficult judgment calls, and employing different epistemologies to enable the students to address the sociocultural aspects of patient care. The domination of bioscientific curriculum content has been directly challenged on the basis that many aspects of clinician roles are "socio-culturally based and thus not supported by scientific knowledge" (Kuper et al. 2017). Identification of interrelated themes derived from Canada's list of physician competencies includes "epistemology, social justice, power, culture, ambiguity, contextualization, differences, and self-awareness" which underline the fact that clinical teaching needs to look beyond the confines of the biosciences to the humanities and social sciences.

There is a paucity of literature in dental education regarding personal development and professional identity formation, the link between student well-being and patient care, and the need to "embed resilience" and management of stress in the dental quote to curriculum (Colley et al. 2018). The exclusion of self-care and wellness from most dental curricula is arguably an educational dereliction of duty of care, given the harsh reality of clinical dental practice and the increase in mental health disorders of current student cohorts. There are weaknesses too and further development needed with the present competency-based frameworks. The more complex aspects of competence "knowledge, professional and ethical attributes, (reflective practice) [may] be overlooked" (Chuenjitwongsa et al. 2018). If these are not assessed alongside attributes of humanistic care such as empathy, cultural humility, and compassion just because they are complex, then these too may be perceived as unimportant.

There have been calls for dental educators to encourage "critical consciousness" and address implicit bias through transformative learning approaches and dialogue (Bedos et al. 2018b). One US dental school has called for "rethinking" of knowledge in dental education, drawing on critical social theory arguing that emancipatory knowledge including reflexivity and self-knowledge nurtures the skills required for lifelong learning, ethical decision-making, and addressing oral health inequalities (Whipp et al. 2000). This learning model, with the incorporation of the flipped classroom educational methodology and case-based collaborative learning (CBCL) methods, has reshaped predoctoral dental education (Krupat et al. 2016).

The CBCL method incorporated into the flipped classroom reinforces team-based discussion and promotes self-directed learning. In the new educational format, students receive pre-learning resources prior to class sessions in order to process basic information. Pre-assessment for in-class discussion is determined before class, and class time is devoted to case discussion to reinforce deeper learning and applied knowledge exercises. The case-based collaborative learning format in the classroom continues to support team-based discussion and problem-solving with strong emphasis on student-driven learning and student-centered teaching. This pedagogical model promotes problem-solving and critical thinking as students engage in active learning and develop their communication skills. The educational methodology emphasizes student accountability for their own learning in order to contribute to team discussions and participate in the class. These pedagogical models also encourage students to learn from each other through increased peer-to-peer interactions in a collaborative learning environment.

Emancipatory pedagogy emerged from the fundamental belief that education is always political and should play a role in creating a just and democratic society (Freire 1970). It is, therefore, a more radical approach to providing a humanistic education, focussing on social inequity, critical thinking, reflection, and discussion in an atmosphere of mutual respect between student and facilitator and critical consciousness, the ability to "intervene in reality in order to change it" (Freire 1970) to foster deep understanding and promote transformation.

If the nature of clinical care is about anything, it is about people, societies, clinicians, and patients. The disciplines of the humanities by definition are concerned with human nature, society, and culture. The needs of any society change over time, but the fundamental characteristics of human nature remain the same. The humanities, through comparative and critical approaches, provide reliable learning resources to develop critical thinking and interrogative and advocacy skills.

As early as 1980, one US educator had argued that without any background in philosophy, history, and culture, there was a risk of creating dentists who would be "technicians unable to make creative judgments" (Neidle 1980).The American Dental Association 20 years later advised schools to "include cultural and linguistic concepts in dental curricula – principles of self-awareness, respect for diversity, and sensitivity in communication" (Haden et al. 2006).

The work piloted and subsequently embedded in a UK dental curriculum has shown for the first time how humanities approaches support humanistic pedagogy, personal and professional identity formation (Smyth Zahra 2018). Exposure to humanities epistemologies frees the students to make meaning (Kennedy 2005) and incorporate "a commitment to self -evaluation and self- critique that is synonymous with cultural humility" (Tervalon and Murray- Garcia 1998). This holistic approach to both the learner and patient (Haden et al. 2006) raises the level of the students' critical thinking as evidenced by their written reflections. They gain self-awareness in the process, and further, as they start to consider the impact of the sociocultural environment on patients, they develop a consideration of "other-awareness" through transformative, emancipatory learning (Kuper et al. 2017; Bourdieu 1980).

Conclusion

Dental education should include active learning methods, authentic assessment, a person-centered care model, and a humanistic learning environment. Development of cultural humility and critical thinking skills are also essential, with growth in self-awareness relative to others necessary for self-care, countering confirmation biases, acquiring integrity and wisdom in the process. By learning to reflect beyond the critical to a higher emancipatory level, students start to develop the necessary "epistemological curiosity" (Freire 1970) to carry on discovering for themselves what the professional practice of dentistry entails and what lifetime learning really means. Students cannot learn all they need to know about person-centered care, the sociocultural environment, advocacy for inequity, and addressing inequalities in access to care from the biosciences alone. Therefore, from an early stage, throughout their learning, it is recommended that they should also engage with the humanities which offer contexts and ways of thinking that can inform aspects of clinical care, personal development, and professional identity formation.

Cross-References

▶ Arts and Humanities in Health Professional Education
▶ Dental Education: A Brief History
▶ Developing Professional Identity in Health Professional Students
▶ Transformative Learning in Clinical Education: Using Theory to Inform Practice

References

Apelian N, Vergnes JN, Bedos C. Humanizing clinical dentistry through a person- centred model. Int J Whole Pers Care. 2014;1(2):31–37

Aretz H. Some thoughts about creating healthcare professionals that match what societies need. Med Teach. 2011;33(8):608–13. https://doi.org/10.3109/0142159X.2011.590389.

Barr R, Tagg J. From teaching to learning – a new paradigm for undergraduate education. Change. 1995;27(6):13–25.

Bedos C, Apelian N, Vergnes J-N. Commentary on "An officer of the 10th Battalion, Cameronians (Scottish Rifles) leads the way out of a sap and is being followed by the party". Acad Med. 2018a;93:1802–3. https://doi.org/10.1097/01.ACM.0000549821.79641.12.

Bedos C, Apelian N, Vergnes J-N. Time to develop social dentistry. JDR Clin Trans Res. 2018b;3(1):109–10. https://doi.org/10.1177/2380084417738001.

Bourdieu P. The logic of practice. Stanford: Stanford University Press; 1980.

Brazeau C, Schroeder R, Rovi S, Boyd L. Relationships between medical student burnout, empathy, and professionalism climate. Acad Med. 2010;85(10):s33–6. https://doi.org/10.1097/ACM.0b013e3181ed4c47.

Chuenjitwongsa S, Oliver R, Bullock A. Competence, competency-based education, and undergraduate dental education: a discussion paper. Eur J Dent Educ. 2018;22:1–8.

Cohen J. Viewpoint: linking professionalism to humanism: what it means, why it matters. Acad Med. 2007;82(11):1029–32.

Cohen L, Dahlen G, Escobar A, Fejerskov O, Johnson N, Manji F. Dentistry in crisis: time to change. La Cascada Declaration. Aust Dent J. 2017;62(3):258–60. https://doi.org/10.1111/adj.12546.

Colley J, Harris M, Hellyer P, Radford D. Teaching stress management in undergraduate dental education: are we doing enough? Br Dent J. 2018;224:405–7.

Commission on Dental Accreditation. In: Accreditation standards for dental education programmes. 2016. http://www.ada.org/~/media/CODA/Files/predoc.ashx. Accessed 19 July 2019.

Elani H, Allison P, Kumar R, Mancini L, Lambrou A, Bedos C. A systematic review of stress in dental students. J Dent Educ. 2014;78:226–42.

Field J, Cowpe A, Walmsley D. The graduating European dentist: a new undergraduate curriculum framework. Eur J Dent Educ. 2017;21(Suppl. 1):2–10. https://doi.org/10.1111/eje.12307.

Freire P. Pedagogy of the oppressed. Harmondsworth: Penguin; 1970.

Frenk J, Chen L, Bhutta Z, Cohen J, Crisp N, Evans T, et al. Health professionals for a new century: transforming education to strengthen health systems in an interdependent world. Lancet. 2010;376(9756):1923. https://doi.org/10.1016/S0140-6736(10)61854-5.

Gerada C. Why has medicine become such a miserable profession? In: thebmjopinionblogsbmj.com [online]. 2017. http://blogs.bmj.com/. Accessed 19 July 2019.

Haden N, Andrieu S, Chadwick D, Chmar J, Cole J, George M, et al. The dental education environment. J Dent Educ. 2006;70(12):1265–70.

Hayer N, Wassif H. A lonely business: reflections on the wellbeing and morale of dental teams. Br Dent J. 2019;226(8):559–61. https://doi.org/10.1038/s41415-019-0205-y.

Health Education England. Advancing dental care education and training review: final report. 2018. https://www.hee.nhs.uk/sites/default/files/documents/advancing_dental_care_final.pdf. Accessed 19 July 2019.

Health Education England. NHS staff and learners' mental wellbeing commission. London: NHS England; 2019. https://www.hee.nhs.uk/sites/default/files/documents/NHS%20%28HEE%29%20-%20Mental%20Wellbeing%20Commission%20Report.pdf. Accessed 19 July 2019.

Heidegger M. Being and time (trans: Macquerrie J, Robinson E). New York: Harper and Row; 1962.

Iacopino A. The influence of "new science" on dental education: current concepts, trends, and models for the future. J Dent Educ. 2007;71(4):450–62.

Kennedy A. Models of continuing professional development: a framework for analysis. J In-service Educ. 2005;31(2):235–250

Krupat E, Richards J, Sullivan A, Fleenor T, Schwartzstein RM. Assessing the effectiveness of case-based collaborative learning via randomized controlled trial. Acad Med. 2016;91(5):723–9. https://doi.org/10.1097/ACM.0000000000001004.

Kuper A, Veinot P, Leavitt J, Levitt S, Li A, Goquen J, et al. Epistemology, culture, justice and power: non-bioscientific knowledge for medical training. Med Educ. 2017;51(2):158–73.

Lucey C, Thibault T, ten Cate O. Competency-based, time -variable education in the health professions: crossroads. Acad Med. 2018;93(3):s1–5.

Maslow A. Problem-centering vs. means-centering in science. Philos Sci. 1946;13:326–31.

Mezirow J. Fostering critical reflection in adulthood. San Francisco: Jossey-Bass; 1990.

Mezirow J. An overview of transformative learning. In: Sutherland P, Crowther J, editors. Lifelong learning: concepts and contexts. New York: Routledge; 2006.

Napier A, Ancarno C, Butler B, Calabrese J, Chater A, Chatterjee H, et al. The Lancet Commissions. Culture and health. Lancet. 2014;384(9954):1607–39.

Neidle E. Dentistry-ethics-the humanities: a three-unit bridge. J Dent Educ. 1980;44(12):693–6.

Palatta A, Kassebaum D, Gadbury-Amyot C, Karimbux N, Licari F, Nadershahi N, et al. Change is here: ADEA CCI 2.0 – a learning community for the advancement of dental education. J Dent Educ. 2017;81(6):640–8. https://doi.org/10.21815/JDE.016.040.

Park S, Howell T. Implementation of a patient-centered approach to clinical dental education: a five-year reflection. J Dent Educ. 2015a;79(5):523–9.

Park S, Howell T. Implementation of a flipped classroom educational model in a predoctoral dental course. J Dent Educ. 2015b;79(5):563–70.

Park S, Timothe P, Nalliah R, Karimbux N, Howell T. A case completion curriculum for clinical dental education: replacing numerical requirements with patient-based comprehensive care. J Dent Educ. 2011;75(11):1411–6.

Piele E. Evidence based medicine and values based medicine: partners in clinical education as well as in clinical practice. BMC Med. 2013;11:40.

RCP. Work and wellbeing in the NHS: why staff health matters to patient care. 2015. https://www.rcplondon.ac.uk/file/2025/download?token=XX7kKnq1. Accessed 19 July 2019.

Roberts S, Jaremin B, Lloyd K. High risk occupations for suicide. Psychol Med. 2013;43(6):1231–40.

Rogers C. Freedom to learn for the 80s. New York: Merrill Wright; 1983.

Smyth ZF. Clinical humanities; informal, transformative learning opportunities, where knowledge gained from humanities epistemologies is translated back into clinical practice, supporting the development of professional autonomy in undergraduate dental students. MedEdPublish. 2018. https://doi.org/10.15694/mep.2018.0000163.2

Tervalon M, Murray-Garcia J. Cultural humility versus cultural competence: a critical distinction in defining physician training outcomes in multicultural education. J Health Care Poor Underserved. 1998;9(2):117–22.

Thomas L. Building student engagement and belonging in higher education at a time of change: final report from the what works? Student retention and success programme. Higher Education Academy, Action on Access, HEFCE and Paul Hamlyn Foundation, York; 2012.

Toon M, Collin V, Whitehead P, Reynolds L. An analysis of stress and burnout in UK general dental practitioners: subdimensions and causes. Br Dent J. 2019;226:125–30.

Twenge J, Campbell W. The narcissism epidemic: living in the age of entitlement. New York: Free Press; 2009.

Walji M, Karimbux N, Speilman A. Person-centered care: opportunities and challenges for academic dental institutions and programs. J Dent Educ. 2017;81(11):1265–72.

Warnakulasuriya S. Global epidemiology of oral and oropharyngeal cancer. Oral Oncol. 2009;45(4–5):309–16. https://doi.org/10.1016/j.oraloncology.2008.06.002.

Wenger E. Communities of practice: learning, meaning, and identity. New York: Cambridge University Press; 1998.

Whipp J, Ferguson D, Wells L, Iacopino A. Rethinking knowledge and pedagogy in dental education. J Dent Educ. 2000;64(12):860–6.

World Health Organisation. In: Burn-out an "occupational phenomenon": international classification of diseases. 2019. https://www.who.int/mental_health/evidence/burn-out/en/. Accessed 19 July 2019.

Interprofessional Education (IPE): Trends and Context

10

Lyn Gum and Jenn Salfi

Contents

Introduction	168
Background: Context	168
Effective Interprofessional Education: Guiding Principles	169
Competencies and Frameworks	170
Challenges in IPE	171
Challenges in Evaluation	172
Challenges in Delivery of IPE/Pedagogy	173
Theories to Underpin IPE	174
Facilitator Skills	174
IPE Settings	175
Future Trends	175
Conclusion	177
Cross-References	177
References	177

Abstract

Effective interprofessional practice is imperative in the delivery of safe, ethical, quality care in today's complex and ever-changing health-care system. The ability to communicate and function effectively in teams, in addition to an ongoing commitment to provide client-centered care, has been declared essential in collaborative relationships. Interprofessional education (IPE) has the potential to develop these competencies, to foster a mutual respect among health and social care providers, ultimately serving as the foundation for a collaborative workforce that is better prepared to respond to the challenges

---

L. Gum (✉)
College of Nursing and Health Sciences, Flinders University, Adelaide, SA, Australia
e-mail: lyn.gum@flinders.edu.au

J. Salfi
Nursing, Brock University, St. Catharines, ON, Canada
e-mail: jsalfi@brocku.ca

© Crown 2023
D. Nestel et al. (eds.), *Clinical Education for the Health Professions*,
https://doi.org/10.1007/978-981-15-3344-0_15

and complexities of the current health-care environment (World Health Organization, Framework for action on IPE & collaborative practice. WHO, Geneva, 2010). This chapter provides a brief overview of IPE, before providing details about its current context and trends as we look to the future to prepare a collaborative workforce that has learned how to work in an interprofessional team and is competent and confident to do so.

Keywords

Interprofessional education · Interprofessional collaborative practice · Competencies · Interprofessional learning · Theory · Interprofessional practice

Introduction

Interprofessional education (IPE) occurs when students of "two or more professions learn with, from, and about each other to improve collaboration and the quality of care" (Centre for the Advancement of Interprofessional Education [CAIPE] 2002, p. 6). CAIPE, a UK-based charity established in 1987, is an international voice for IPE and collaborative practice. IPE encompasses learning in both academic and clinical settings and aims to develop the required knowledge, skills, and attitudes required for interprofessional collaboration. Interprofessional collaboration (or interprofessional collaborative practice) occurs when individuals from different professional backgrounds work together with patients, families, carers, and communities to deliver the highest quality of care, ultimately strengthening health systems and improving overall health outcomes (WHO 2010). After nearly 60 years of research and enquiry, the World Health Organization (2010) and its multiple partners acknowledge there is sufficient evidence to support the relationship between effective interprofessional education and successful interprofessional collaborative practice.

Background: Context

Interprofessional education is not a new concept and can be described in the literature as taking on many different shapes and forms. IPE has been successfully delivered via case-based discussions and simulation-based learning, online learning, incorporated into anatomy dissection learning environments, as well as into work-based clinical environments, where students experience cultural contexts and workplace demands working alongside other professionals. However, there is still some debate around when to introduce IPE, with some educators arguing against the introduction of IPE at the undergraduate level. Some believe that most students at this level have not acquired a sense of their own professional characteristics or sufficient practical experience to be able to experience the full benefits of IPE and that premature introduction of IPE could have negative repercussions because it might interfere with the establishment of a distinct professional identity (Michalec et al. 2017).

Conversely, research has also revealed advantages associated with integrating IPE within undergraduate curricula – specifically in innovative and interactive interprofessional environments (Fernandes et al. 2015; Hammick et al. 2007; Solomon and Salfi 2011). By embedding IPE within the content and the process of an entire undergraduate, pre-licensure curriculum, there is a recontextualization of the traditional uni-professional knowledge, into a knowledge of one's unique and valuable professional role within an interprofessional practice. As students progress throughout their professional curriculum, they are afforded the opportunity to accumulate essential knowledge, skills, attitudes, and confidence necessary to be an effective member of a health-care team upon graduation (Salfi et al. 2012).

An overview of the current context and research literature on IPE supports that interprofessional education is beneficial both before and after registration or licensure as a professional. Exposing pre-licensure students to IPE helps to cultivate mutual trust and respect for other professionals' knowledge and skill set, confronts misconceptions and stereotypes, and dispels prejudice and rivalry between professional groups (CAIPE 2017), while engaging in IPE post-licensure (as a practicing professional) aims to maintain and sustain interprofessional competencies and positive collaborative attitudes gained in effective pre-licensure IPE experiences. Exposure to the hierarchy and stereotypes that still exist in clinical practice is realities that have been identified to have a negative impact on a student's interprofessional attitude, creating conflict between how one wishes to practice and what results in a fast-paced clinical world (Schutt 2016). Research has revealed that even after several years, graduates greatly appreciated and were still able to recall what they had learned from participating in effective pre-licensure IPE experiences; however, it's also been revealed that exposure to the reality of the clinical environment over time has the potential to erode some of the positive collaborative attitudes and behaviors gained from these effective IPE experiences (Zheng et al. 2018), hence making the case for IPE to be offered both before and after gaining professional license.

Effective Interprofessional Education: Guiding Principles

The timing of the delivery of IPE is just as critical as the content and process of interprofessional education. CAIPE (2017) has identified several key principles to assist in the development of effective IPE. A few key principles that should always be considered when designing and implementing IPE experiences include (a) the opportunity to learn about one's own scope of practice, as well as that of other professionals; (b) opportunities should be grounded in mutual respect, honoring the distinctive experiences and expertise that each participant brings to the team from their respective backgrounds; and (c) providing the opportunity for students to develop and refine essential competencies required for collaboration (CAIPE 2017).

Another key principle of effective IPE is that it should not be viewed in isolation but rather as a continuum over a pre-licensure curriculum, and continuously revisited and reinforced as the student develops as a professional. This continuum should be planned with intentional and shifting goals for each level of the learner and should use a variety of pedagogical methodologies (Salfi et al. 2012; Grice et al. 2018).

Embedded within these key principles of effective IPE are several competencies (knowledge, skills, and behaviors) that are required for interprofessional collaborative practice which, although similar, may vary slightly across academic institutions and countries. IPE competency frameworks aim to provide a common lens through which a variety of professionals can understand, implement, and assess team-based practices.

Competencies and Frameworks

Across the globe, there exist several frameworks outlining key competencies required for effective interprofessional collaboration. These competencies serve to guide interprofessional education learning experiences and assessments, as well as inform optimal clinical performance and quality of care. For the purposes of brevity, we will outline only a few of these frameworks in this chapter.

On an international level, the WHO (2010) established its commitment to IPE with its publication of the *Framework for Action on Interprofessional Education and Collaborative Practice*. This framework outlines six key interprofessional learning domains required for collaborative practice: teamwork, roles and responsibilities, communication, learning and critical reflection, relationships with the patient, and ethical practice (which involves understanding the stereotypical views of other health workers held by self and others). Similar to these six learning domains are the six core competencies outlined in the Canadian Interprofessional Competency Framework (Canadian Interprofessional Health Collaborative (CIHC) (2010), which include team functioning, role clarity, communication, collaborative leadership, conflict resolution, and patient/client/family/community-centered care.

One year later, two more IPE competency frameworks emerged, with similar competencies identified. The Australian Interprofessional Capability Framework (Curtin University 2011) identified communication, role clarification, team function, conflict resolution, and reflection as the five capabilities required for a collaborative practice-ready workforce. A few years later, the Interprofessional Education Collaborative (IPEC) expert panel in the United States listed roles and responsibilities, interprofessional communication, teamwork/team-based care, and values and ethics as their four key competencies required for collaboration (updated in 2016).

To help guide the development of IPE at the curriculum level, a number of frameworks have also been proposed. A notable framework includes the University of British Columbia (UBC) framework: the UBC model of IPE. This model conceptualizes IPE in three stages of learning that students progress through during their interprofessional training: exposure, immersion, and mastery (Charles et al. 2010). Exposure-level IPE strategies are primarily knowledge based and enhance awareness of the scopes of practice of all health and social care professions within a team (Charles et al. 2010). Some examples of IPE strategies that are exposure level might include interviewing and shadowing other professionals, as well as observing multidisciplinary panel discussions.

Immersion-level IPE strategies require higher levels of interaction between professional groups. Individuals are required to communicate and collaborate, and participate in shared decion-making and problem-solving (Charles et al. 2010). Some examples of immersion-level IPE strategies include communication skills labs (Solomon and Salfi 2011) and gross anatomy dissection courses (Fernandes et al. 2015).

Mastery-level IPE strategies are the most complex, as individuals integrate their interprofessional knowledge and skills in an ongoing team environment (Charles et al. 2010). These IPE strategies are of long-term duration, and there is an ongoing opportunity to be actively engaged in a team. Mastery-level strategies are better suited for practicing professionals, as opposed to undergraduate level students in health professional programs.

Miller's (1990) pyramid is another well-known framework referred to widely, which outlines the logical sequence of levels of competence (knows, knows how, shows how, does) in that levels of competence are much like steps – the underlying level is the building block for the next level. Salfi et al. (2012) developed an IPE framework incorporating key concepts from both Miller and Charles et al. (2010) that was specifically designed to educate and prepare a large number of students (2000+), across multiple academic sites, for effective collaborative practice.

In order to develop competencies that were context-specific, one Australian university partnered with a primary health service to produce an interprofessional capability framework (Gum et al. 2013). Unique to the framework is bridging the theory gap between education and practice, its design inclusive of the broad skills and aptitudes required for interprofessional collaborative practice and can be adapted to all levels of learning (i.e., entry to practice) (Gum et al. 2013). While the development of the interprofessional capability framework resulted from a collaborative process between the university and the health sector, all agreed that for the model to be successful, it requires ongoing support and leadership (Gum et al. 2013).

Unfortunately, very little research exists detailing and evaluating the incorporation of the abovementioned interprofessional competencies across the span of an entire health-care curriculum. Although interprofessional competency frameworks serve as a guide for educators in planning how they can best prepare their students for collaborative practice, several barriers and challenges exist in the planning, implementation, sustainability, and evaluation of IPE. The final half of the chapter will provide a brief overview of some of these challenges, as well as the resulting trends in the field of IPE.

Challenges in IPE

While the aim of IPE seems relatively simple, that is, the concept that by learning with, from, and about each other, students and health professionals will be more collaborative together in the workplace, demonstrating evidence of its effectiveness is complex. As with most research, the more robust the evidence, the more difficult it becomes, for example, to show how IPE can ultimately achieve a change for the better in regard to patient outcomes is more difficult than demonstrating the impact on the learner/s. As IPE is becoming more formally enacted worldwide, leaders need to know how IPE, more specifically, impacts patients, populations, and organizations (Institute of Medicine (IOM) 2015).

Challenges in Evaluation

A frequently-utilized model for measuring IPE outcomes is Kirkpatrick's educational outcomes model, introduced and extended by Barr et al. (2005). This model has been modified for use by Yardley and Dornan (2012) as a grading standard when evaluating evidence (see Table 1).

Measurement and outcomes in relation to Levels 1–2 above are predominant in the literature and indicate IPE is generally well received, but lacks quality evidence (Reeves et al. 2017). Cochrane reviews and systematic reviews have attempted to gather more robust evidence in relation to the latter levels (3–4) which require evidence of change. In a Cochrane review, Zwarenstein et al. (2009) explored interventions designed to change interprofessional collaboration and found it hard to draw generalizable inferences, suggesting that more rigorous studies and qualitative methods were needed. Following this, Reeves et al. (2013) updated their previous review, and due to the small number of studies and heterogeneity of interventions and outcome measures, were unable to draw generalizable inferences about the effectiveness of IPE. Reeves et al. (2013, p. 5) defined IPE *interventions* as occurring:

Table 1 With permission of Yardley and Dornan (2012) ©

Impact of intervention studied
Code the level of impact being studied in the item and summarize any results of the intervention at the appropriate level. Include both predetermined and unintended outcomes.
Kirkpatrick Hierarchy
Level 1 Participation: covers learners' views on the learning experience, its organization, presentation, content, teaching methods, and aspects of the instructional organization, materials, and quality of instruction.
Level 2a Modification of attitudes / perceptions: outcomes relate to changes in the reciprocal attitudes or perceptions between participant groups toward the intervention / simulation.
Level 2b Modification of knowledge / skills: for knowledge, this relates to the acquisition of concepts, procedures, and principles; for skills, this relates to the acquisition of thinking / problem-solving, psychomotor, and social skills.
Level 3 Behavioral change: documents the transfer of learning to the workplace or willingness of learners to apply new knowledge and skills.
Level 4a Change in organizational practice: wider changes in the organization or delivery of care, attributable to an educational program
Level 4b Benefits to patient / clients: any improvement in the health and well-being of patients / clients as a direct result of an educational program

> When members of more than one health or social care (or both) profession learn interactively together, for the explicit purpose of improving interprofessional collaboration or the health/well being (or both) of patients/clients. Interactive learning requires active learner participation, and active exchange between learners from different professions.

In order to allow sound conclusions about IPE effectiveness, Reeves et al. (2013) suggested that studies must compare IPE interventions to profession-specific interventions, examine the processes of IPE using high levels of evidence, and undertake cost-benefit analyses.

Thistlethwaite et al. (2015) proposed that a more effective way to evaluate IPE is to find out what type of educational interventions work, in what context, and to what degree. This focus suggests an alternative evaluation framework from the traditional outcomes-based approach which often seeks generalizable conclusions, to a realism view where there may be multiple interpretations of the results (Thistlethwaite et al. 2015).

Among the plethora of systematic and scoping reviews, Reeves and colleagues updated their previous best evidence medical education (BEME) review (Hammick et al. 2007), publishing a further BEME review in 2016 on the effects of IPE (Reeves et al. 2016). In order to understand the contextual factors and educational processes, they re-employed the 3P (presage-process-product) model (Biggs 1993). The presage factors are described as the sociopolitical context for education, including those within it, such as the teachers and learners (Reeves et al. 2016). The process factors include how the teaching and learning were undertaken; and the product factors were the outcomes from the learning or educational experience (Reeves et al. 2016).

Presage, that is the IPE context, was found to be of significance in relation to IPE success (Reeves et al. 2016). Timetabling and space issues continue to make implementation difficult. Therefore, support is required from organizations, local IPE leaders, and managers to help with making IPE viable. Reeves et al. (2013) also found that for learners, prior experiences, age, professional background, and gender affected their attitudes toward IPE. While they found that high-quality facilitation was necessary for effective interprofessional learning, there was limited evidence available in relation to the characteristics of an effective IPE facilitator (Reeves et al. 2013). This is explored in the next section.

Challenges in Delivery of IPE/Pedagogy

Interprofessional education can be taught in a variety of ways. Having determined the importance of key competencies to guide learning and assessment, firstly there is a need to focus on the appropriate environment, such as how and where *learning with others* will occur (McCarthy and DiGiovanni 2017). For example, can the IPE transition beyond the classroom, and how will it be assessed? Whether students are experiencing IPE in the clinical or classroom setting, it will be necessary to determine how students will be able to not only learn *with each other*, but also how they will learn *from* and *about* each other.

Theories to Underpin IPE

While there is no one single theory to guide IPE, learning theories will need to be considered to optimize curricula development and learning outcomes. In order for interprofessional learning to take place, the teacher will need to plan *how* the learning is going to be facilitated. Use of educational theory will ensure the learning is authentic and places emphasis on the process (interaction between students) rather than just the content to be learned. Consequently, the complexity of IPE usually requires teaching methods to be guided by more than one theory. For example, social learning theories support the social dimensions of interprofessional learning, and complexity theory will focus on how each individual contributes to interprofessional care (Hean et al. 2018). Perspectives and approaches to IPE theories have been widely reported (Barr 2013; Barr et al. 2005; Bluteau and Jackson 2009; Carpenter and Dickinson 2008; Clark 2006; Colyer 2008) including scoping and systematic reviews (Hean et al. 2018; Reeves et al. 2007; Suter et al. 2013).

Hean et al. (2018) reviewed the theories used in the literature for interprofessional learning from 1988 to 2015, finding that reflective learning, identity formation, and contact hypothesis were widely used, and reporting on many others such as constructivist and social constructionist theories. Theories such as contact hypothesis and adult learning theory contribute to learning and curricula content as well as the training of the facilitators who will be accountable for the safe learning environment (Hean et al. 2018). Communities of practice theory are an ideal approach to interprofessional education learning as it is viewed as being situated in a certain context, where its members can socially interact and contribute to the team (Sargeant 2009; Wenger et al. 2002).

The advantage of using socio-material theory for teaching pre-licensure health professional students is that learning occurs through dynamic and relational processes and fits well with the aims of IPE (McMurtry et al. 2016; Oates 2016). Drawing upon theories such as complexity theory, cultural-historical activity theory and actor-network theory inform on how to focus on social interactions and relationships rather than on individual acquisition of knowledge (McMurtry et al. 2016).

Theoretical awareness is vitally important to ensure IPL is focused on those processes which are grounded in context and experience rather than pre-determined outcomes. It is highly recommended to become familiar with the features of group and system-level theories as they provide effective frameworks for addressing the multiple components and sometimes unpredictable nature of IPE.

Facilitator Skills

The settings where interprofessional education opportunities may be undertaken by students vary widely; however, the skill of the facilitator must also be considered. For example, both faculty academics and local educators in practice settings are responsible for effective interprofessional learning between students. O'Carroll et al. (2018) demonstrated there are practical and logistical issues with organizing and

10 Interprofessional Education (IPE): Trends and Context

implementing interprofessional learning in a practice setting, as well as misconceptions about IPE as an educational process by educators. Also described as teacher characteristics or a presage factor, the quality of facilitation has been found to be critical to the success of IPE (Reeves et al. 2016). Importantly, IPE educators must provide a non-threatening environment where different behaviors and attitudes are well managed. One of the purposes of IPE is to reduce the power imbalance across professions (Collin et al. 2010) by finding common ground. IPE facilitators may need to challenge assumptions (Phelan et al. 2006) and should allow students to explore the differences between professions.

IPE Settings

Interprofessional practice settings are the most obvious for students to access interprofessional learning experiences. These experiences can vary in terms of being able to integrate with or observe collaborative practice; however, placing more value on IPE and quality educators in practice settings has the potential to provide many innovative opportunities for students (O'Carroll et al. 2018). Notwithstanding, there are many barriers to overcome including consideration for the alignment of the higher education and community organizations in implementing IPE, and how it is to be sustainable (Bennett et al. 2010). Innovative programs have emerged, such as the Interprofessional Health Mentors program at the University of British Columbia elective patient-as-teacher initiative where a patient mentor is an integral part of interprofessional student group meetings (Towle et al. 2014). Student-run clinics are proving successful, as they can serve as a sustainable source of primary care. One exemplar is a free clinic run by the Yale University, United States, where students are exposed to the provision of community health care while experiencing working in a health-care team (Scott and Swartz 2015). Meanwhile, peer-led IPE simulation was found to be an effective way to not only gain respect for other professions' roles and responsibilities but to be able to gain leadership and management skills (Lairamore et al. 2019). Additionally, student leadership, where student groups form steering committees and have input into the design and delivery of IPE for their peers, is a powerful approach to providing long-term sustainability, by promoting interest among their peers, academics, and the general public (Hoffman et al. 2008).

Future Trends

This chapter has discussed the current context and challenges associated with the delivery and evaluation of IPE and will conclude with considerations for future interprofessional education, with respect for how both academia and practice settings can bridge together, to further enable IPE.

We cannot train students to be interprofessional practitioners if the teams they interact with are not working collaboratively together. IPE has a role to play globally, to overcome increasing health challenges such as diabetes, non-communicable diseases, cancers, cardiovascular disease, dementia, and mental health issues (Sunguya et al. 2014; Thistlethwaite et al. 2019). This is because IPE can potentially lead to interprofessional collaboration, reducing the burden of health care on one profession by sharing it among all health workers (WHO 2010). Currently developing countries who want to roll out IPE are learning from developed countries due to increased collaborations (Sunguya et al. 2014). In a systematic review, Sunguya et al. (2014) summarized the many challenges to IPE implementation for both *developing* and *developed* countries including curriculum, leadership, resources, stereotypes/attitudes, student variety, teaching, enthusiasm, and accreditation. Health systems will need to be organized in a way to be responsive to change, such as addressing the requirements for the development of interprofessional collaboration (Thistlethwaite et al. 2019). Continuing professional development is currently profession-driven and can compete with organizational priorities, and therefore approaches are needed where there is consideration for how different professions might undertake joint professional development (Gum et al. 2019).

The field of "health professions education" has emerged this century as part of the reform recommended to address the gaps in health care failing to provide quality care (Greiner and Knebel 2003). Emphasis following reports such as *To Err is Human* (Donaldson et al. 2000) on having a better prepared health professional workforce has been responsible for a whole new industry in health professions education. Notwithstanding, there is now a plethora of journals, conferences, and academic appointments which span all disciplines and professions in health care. This is exciting for IPE, as the vision for health system reform has led to interprofessional education and collaborative practice being more of value and recognized across all professions.

Value-based health care is one example of how to organize health care for the benefit of the patient. Not only is there a respect for patients but also for all of the different professions involved in their care (Thistlethwaite 2012). Globally, value-based health care is on the rise and could be considered as a way to support and further develop interprofessional collaborative practice. Collaborative team-based models of care are needed to develop effective interprofessional working relationships and enable quality health outcomes. In the university setting, a collaborative learning culture will assist to integrate IPE into curriculum. By definition, this would entail all faculty contributing through interactions, forming relationships, and being able to learn and develop knowledge together. Therefore, building interprofessional academic communities of practice could be one strategy to contribute to the culture change and be widened to include clinicians external to the university (Gum and Schoo 2014). Universities should also consider how they can utilize their simulation laboratories to provide not only training for students but for faculty and clinicians (Andrews 2017). Simulation-based IPE is an effective strategy for promoting collaborative, interprofessional teamwork and effective communication (Decker et al. 2015). This way, relationships can be strengthened, paving the way for a more collaborative curriculum.

With the objective to increase global networking and sharing of ideas for interprofessional development, a confederation named Interprofessional.Global (Global Confederation for Interprofessional Education and Collaborative Practice, https://interprofessional.global/the-confederation/), formerly the World Coordinating Committee, is a way of becoming more involved in interprofessional education and collaborative practice. Networking is an important strategy to widely disseminate research, resources, and tools for effective IPE.

Conclusion

Interprofessional education maintains a focus on the development of health and social care professionals in order to provide effective interprofessional collaborative practice. This chapter has provided a brief overview of interprofessional education and its current context and challenges, as we continue to learn and evaluate how best to prepare a collaborative workforce that is able to respond to the challenges and complexities of the current health-care environment.

Cross-References

▶ Communities of Practice and Medical Education
▶ Developing Health Professional Teams
▶ Developing Patient Safety Through Education
▶ Learning and Teaching in Clinical Settings: Expert Commentary from an Interprofessional Perspective
▶ Learning with and from Peers in Clinical Education
▶ Simulation for Clinical Skills in Healthcare Education
▶ Supporting the Development of Patient-Centred Communication Skills

References

Andrews EA. The future of interprofessional education and practice for dentists and dental education. J Dent Educ. 2017;81(8):186–92. https://doi.org/10.21815/JDE.017.026.

Barr H. Toward a theoretical framework for interprofessional education. J Interprof Care. 2013;27 (1):4–9.

Barr H, Koppel I, Reeves S, Hammick M, Freeth D. Effective interprofessional education: argument, assumption and evidence. Carlton: Blackwell Publishing; 2005.

Bennett P, Gum L, Lindemann I, Lawn S, McAllister S, Richards J, ... Ward H. Faculty perceptions of interprofessional education. Nurse Educ Today. 2010;31(6):571–76.

Biggs JB. From theory to practice: a cognitive systems approach. High Educ Res Dev. 1993;12(1): 73–85.

Bluteau P, Jackson A. Interprofessional education: unpacking the early challenges. In: Bluteau P, Jackson A, editors. Interprofessional education: making it happen. Hampshire: Palgrave Macmillan; 2009.

Canadian Interprofessional Health Collaborative (CIHC). A national interprofessional competency framework. Vancouver: CIHC; 2010.

Carpenter J, Dickinson H, editors. Interprofessional education and training. Bristol: The Policy Press; 2008.

Centre for the Advancement of Interprofessional Education (CAIPE). Interprofessional education – today, yesterday and tomorrow (Barr, H). Higher education academy, learning & teaching support network for health sciences & practice. Occasional Paper 1. 2002. https://www.caipe.org/resources/caipe-publications. Accessed 14 July 2019.

Centre for the Advancement of Interprofessional Education (CAIPE). Interprofessional education guidelines. 2017. https://www.caipe.org/resources/publications/caipe-publications/caipe-2017-interprofessional-education-guidelines-barr-h-ford-j-gray-r-helme-m-hutchings-m-low-h-machin-reeves-s. Accessed 14 July 2019.

Charles G, Bainbridge L, Gilbert J. The University of British Colombia model of interprofessional education. J Interprof Care. 2010;24:9–18.

Clark P. What would a theory of interprofessional education look like? Some suggestions for developing a theoretical framework for teamwork training. J Interprof Care. 2006;20(6):577–89.

Collin K, Paloniemi S, Mecklin JP. Promoting inter-professional teamwork and learning: the case of a surgical operating theatre. J Educ Work. 2010;23(1):43–63. https://doi.org/10.1080/13639080903495160.

Colyer H. Embedding interprofessional learning in pre-registration education in health and social care: evidence of cultural lag. Learn Health Soc Care. 2008;7(3):126–33.

Curtin University. Interprofessional capability framework. Faculty of Health Sciences. 2011. https://healthsciences.curtin.edu.au/wpcontent/uploads/sites/6/2017/11/interprofessional_A5_broch_1-29072015.pdf. Accessed 10 July 2019.

Decker SI, Anderson M, Boese T, Epps C, McCarthy J, Motola I, ... Scolaro K. Standards of best practice: simulation standard VIII: simulation-enhanced interprofessional education (Sim-IPE). Clin Simul Nurs. 2015;11(6):293–97. https://doi.org/10.1016/j.ecns.2015.03.010.

Kohn LT, Corrigan JM, Donaldson MS, editors. To err is human: building a safer health system, vol. 6: Washington (DC): National Academies Press; 2000.

Fernandes A, Palombella A, Salfi J, Wainman B. Dissecting through barriers: a mixed-methods study on the effect of interprofessional education in a dissection course with health care professional students. Anat Sci Educ. 2015;8:305–16.

Greiner AC, Knebel E. Health professions education: a bridge to quality. Washington: National Academies Press; 2003.

Grice G, Thomason A, Meny L, Pinelli N, Martello J, Zorek J. Intentional interprofessional experiential education. Am J Pharm Educ. 2018;82:6502.

Gum LF, Schoo AM. Building an Interprofessional Academic Community around Health Professional Educators. Paper presented at the Australian and New Zealand Health Professional Education, Brisbane; 2014.

Gum L, Lloyd A, Lawn S, Richards J, Lindemann I, Sweet L, et al. Developing an interprofessional capability framework for teaching healthcare students in a primary healthcare setting. J Interprof Care. 2013;27:454–60. https://doi.org/10.3109/13561820.2013.807777.

Gum LF, Sweet L, Greenhill J, Prideaux D. Exploring interprofessional education and collaborative practice in Australian rural health services. J Interprof Care. 2019:1–11. https://doi.org/10.1080/13561820.2019.1645648.

Hammick M, Freeth D, Koppel I, Reeves S, Barr H. A best evidence systematic review of interprofessional education (BEME guide no. 9). Med Teach. 2007;29(8):735–51.

Hean S, Green C, Anderson E, Morris D, John C, Pitt R, O'Halloran C. The contribution of theory to the design, delivery, and evaluation of interprofessional curricula: BEME guide no. 49. Med Teach. 2018;40(6):542–58. https://doi.org/10.1080/0142159X.2018.1432851.

Hoffman S, Rosenfield D, Gilbert J, Oandasan I. Student leadership in interprofessional education: benefits, challenges and implications for educators, researchers and policymakers. Med Educ. 2008;42:654–61.

Institute of Medicine (IOM). Measuring the impact of interprofessional education on collaborative practice and patient outcomes. Washington, DC: National Academies Press; 2015.

Interprofessional Education Collaborative (IPEC). Core competencies for interprofessional collaborative practice: 2016 (update). 2016. https://nebula.wsimg.com/2f68a39520b03336b410 38c370497473?AccessKeyId=DC06780E69ED19E2B3A5&disposition=0&allo worigin=1. Accessed 23 July 2019.

Lairamore C, Reed CC, Damon Z, Rowe V, Baker J, Griffith K, VanHoose L. A peer-led Interprofessional simulation experience improves perceptions of teamwork. Clin Simul Nurs. 2019;34:22–9. https://doi.org/10.1016/j.ecns.2019.05.005.

McCarthy JW, DiGiovanni JJ. The interprofessional education environment: places and pedagogies. Paper presented at the Seminars in speech and language; 2017.

McMurtry A, Rohse S, Kilgour KN. Socio-material perspectives on interprofessional team and collaborative learning. Med Educ. 2016;50:169–80. https://doi.org/10.1111/medu.12833.

Michalec B, Giordano C, Pugh B, Arenson C, Speakman E. Health professions students' perceptions of their IPE program. Potential barriers to student engagement with IPE goals. J Allied Health. 2017;46:10–20.

Miller G. The assessment of clinical skills/competence/performance. Acad Med. 1990;65:S63–7.

O'Carroll V, McSwiggan L, Campbell M. Practice educators' attitudes and perspectives of interprofessional collaboration and interprofessional practice learning for students: a mixed-methods case study. J Interprof Care. 2018:1–10. https://doi.org/10.1080/13561820.2018. 1551865.

Oates M. Socio-material theory: an alternate view of interprofessional team learning. Med Educ. 2016;50:160–2.

Phelan AM, Barlow CA, Iversen S. Occasioning learning in the workplace: the case of interprofessional peer collaboration. J Interprof Care. 2006;20(4):415–24. https://doi.org/10. 1080/13561820600845387.

Reeves S, Suter E, Goldman J, Martimianakis T, Chatalalsingh C, Dematteo D. A scoping review to identify organizational and education theories relevant for interprofessional practice and education. Calgary Health Region & QUIPPED – Queen's University Inter-Professional Patient-Centred Education Direction. 2007. http://meds.queensu.ca.proxy1.lib.umanitoba.ca/quipped/assets/ScopingReview_IP_Theories_Dec07.pdf. March 2011.

Reeves S, Perrier L, Goldman J, Freeth D, Zwarenstein M. Interprofessional education: effects on professional practice and healthcare outcomes (update). Cochrane Database Syst Rev. 2013;3: CD002213. https://doi.org/10.1002/14651858.CD002213.pub3.

Reeves S, Fletcher S, Barr H, Birch I, Boet S, Davies N, ... Kitto S. A BEME systematic review of the effects of interprofessional education: BEME guide no. 39. Med Teach. 2016;38(7):656–68. https://doi.org/10.3109/0142159X.2016.1173663.

Reeves S, Palaganas J, Zierler B. An updated synthesis of review evidence of interprofessional education. J Allied Health. 2017;46(1):56–61.

Salfi J, Solomon P, Allen D, Mohaupt J, Patterson C. Overcoming all obstacles: a framework for embedding interprofessional education (IPE) into a large, multi-site BScN program. J Nurs Educ. 2012;51:106–10.

Sargeant J. Theories to aid understanding and implementation of interprofessional education. J Contin Educ Health. 2009;29(3):178–84.

Schutt H. An investigation of the relationship between interprofessional education, interprofessional attitudes, and interprofessional practice. Unpublished doctoral dissertation, University of East Anglia, Norwich; 2016.

Scott EA, Swartz MK. Interprofessional student experiences on the HAVEN free clinic leadership board. J Interprof Care. 2015;29(1):68–70. https://doi.org/10.3109/13561820.2014.934339.

Solomon P, Salfi J. Evaluation of an interprofessional education communication skills initiative. Educ Health. 2011;11:616.

Sunguya B, Hinthong W, Jimba M, Yasuoka J. Interprofessional education for whom? – challenges and lessons learned from its implementation in developed countries and their application to developing countries: a systematic review. PLoS One. 2014;9(5):e96724. https://doi.org/10.1371/journal.pone.0096724.

Suter E, Goldman J, Martimianakis T, Chatalalsingh C, DeMatteo DJ, Reeves S. The use of systems and organizational theories in the interprofessional field: findings from a scoping review. J Interprof Care. 2013;27(1):57–64.

Thistlethwaite J. Values-based interprofessional collaborative practice: working together in health care. New York: Cambridge University Press; 2012.

Thistlethwaite J, Kumar K, Moran M, Saunders R, Carr S. An exploratory review of pre-qualification interprofessional education evaluations. J Interprof Care. 2015;29(4):292–7. https://doi.org/10.3109/13561820.2014.985292.

Thistlethwaite JE, Dunston R, Yassine T. The times are changing: workforce planning, new health-care models and the need for interprofessional education in Australia. J Interprof Care. 2019;33(4):361–8. https://doi.org/10.1080/13561820.2019.1612333.

Towle A, Brown H, Hofley C, Kerston RP, Lyons H, Walsh C. The expert patient as teacher: an interprofessional health mentors programme. Clin Teach. 2014;11(4):301–6. https://doi.org/10.1111/tct.12222.

Wenger E, McDermott RA, Snyder W. Cultivating communities of practice. Boston: Harvard Business School Press; 2002.

World Health Organization (WHO). Framework for action on IPE & collaborative practice. Geneva: WHO; 2010.

Yardley S, Dornan T. Kirkpatrick's levels and education 'evidence'. Med Educ. 2012;46:97–106. https://doi.org/10.1111/j.1365-2923.2011.04076.x.

Zheng YH, Palombella A, Salfi J, Wainman B. Dissecting through barriers: a follow-up study on the long-term effects of interprofessional education in a dissection course with healthcare professional students. Anat Sci Educ. 2018;12:52–60.

Zwarenstein M, Goldman J, Reeves S. Interprofessional collaboration: effects of practice-based interventions on professional practice and healthcare outcomes. Cochrane Database Syst Rev. 2009; 3(3):CD000072: pp. 1–24.

Global Surgery and Its Trends and Context: The Case of Timor-Leste

11

Sean Stevens

Contents

Introduction 182
Global Surgery and Timor-Leste 182
    Global Surgery 182
    Timor-Leste 190
Conclusion 198
Cross-References 198
References 198

> **Abstract**
>
> This chapter introduces the topical and burgeoning field of global surgery, a global health priority requiring an educational solution. Global surgery is defined and the path from "neglected step-child of global health" to global health priority is described. The key role of the clinical education of health professionals in improving global access to safe, effective, timely, and affordable surgical care is examined. Theories to guide the development of surgical education and training programs in low- and middle-income countries (LMIC) are critically reviewed through the analysis of practical examples. The challenges of surgical education and training in LMICs will be explored through the case study of Timor-Leste, a low-income country in Southeast Asia that was decimated by war after gaining independence in 2001.

> **Keywords**
>
> Global surgery · Surgical workforce · Surgical education · Surgical training · Low- middle-income countries · Timor-Leste

---

S. Stevens (✉)
Department of Surgery, Austin Health, University of Melbourne, Melbourne, VIC, Australia
e-mail: sean.stevens@austin.org.au

© Springer Nature Singapore Pte Ltd. 2023
D. Nestel et al. (eds.), *Clinical Education for the Health Professions*,
https://doi.org/10.1007/978-981-15-3344-0_124

Introduction

Global surgery has been defined as "an area of study and practice focussed on improving health outcomes for those who need surgical care, with a special emphasis on underserved populations" (Meara et al. 2015a).

Global surgery has only recently established itself on the global health agenda. Indeed, "global surgery" is a relatively new concept. Traditionally, the global health community focused on infectious diseases such human immunodeficiency virus (HIV), malaria, and tuberculosis (TB). Interventions to address these diseases – immunization programs, for example – tend to have been vertically integrated in health systems. This comes with the benefit of reduced costs and complexity but does not strengthen the overall health system (Meara et al. 2015a).

In contrast, "surgery" has generally not been conceptualized as a "disease" and thus not considered alongside prominent infectious diseases for the global health communities' attention. However, as a treatment modality, surgery "address(es) the breadth of human disease – infections, non-communicable, maternal, child, geriatric and trauma-related disease and injuries" (Meara and Raykar 2016). Thought of in this way, a significant proportion of the global burden of disease is attributable to conditions that are treated by surgery; an estimated one-third all deaths are due to disease requiring surgical care (Meara et al. 2015a). This is more than HIV, TB, and malaria combined (Meara et al. 2015a). Further, the burden of surgical disease is unequally distributed toward poorer countries; globally 90% of deaths from injuries occur in LMICs and 99% of maternal deaths occur in low-income countries (Peden et al. 2002; Debas et al. 2006).

Improving surgical care requires horizontally integrated interventions, specifically targeted toward strengthening health systems. Such approaches are inevitably complex and expensive. This contributed to the historical perception of surgery by the global health community as a luxury of high-income countries. For decades, this perception consigned surgery to being "the neglected step-child of global public health" (Farmer and Kim 2008).

Global Surgery and Timor-Leste

Global Surgery

Against these perceptions and despite the complexity and expense, there is evidence that interventions to improve access to surgical care can be highly cost-effective (Mock et al. 2015). A standard measure of the cost-effectiveness of interventions is the number of disability adjusted life years (DALYs) averted by the intervention. Examples of cost-effective surgical interventions include cleft lip repair (US$10–110 per DALY averted), inguinal hernia repair (US$10–100 per DALY averted), cataract surgery (approximately US$50 per DALY averted), and emergency caesarean section (US$15–380 per DALY averted) (Mock et al. 2015). These compare favorably with widely practiced global health interventions such as oral rehydration solution (more than US$1000 per DALY averted) and antiretroviral therapy for HIV (approximately US$900 per DALY averted) (Mock et al. 2015). Moreover, cost-effectiveness has been shown to be greatest in Africa and South East Asia, regions with the greatest burden of surgical disease (Laxminarayan and Ashford 2008). This led the authors of the Disease Control Priorities Project to conclude that surgical care "...can be highly cost-effective – even on par with widely accepted preventive health care such as child immunisations" (Laxminarayan and Ashford 2008).

The combined revelation of the high global burden of diseases treatable with surgical care and the cost-effectiveness of surgical interventions led to a major investigation into global surgery: the "Lancet Commission on Global Surgery" (Meara et al. 2015a). This seminal publication is the most comprehensive analysis on the topic of global surgery. The report estimated that 5 billion people lack access to timely, safe, and affordable surgical care. Review of surgical interventions in LMICs showed that "investing in surgical services in LMICs is affordable, saves lives and promotes economic growth" (Meara et al. 2015a). The report concludes that surgery should be viewed as an "indivisible, indispensable part of health care" and therefore integral to achieving universal health coverage (Meara et al. 2015a). Achieving universal coverage of essential surgery in LMIC is estimated to avert 1.5 million deaths and 77 million DALYs annually (Meara et al. 2015a).

The findings of the Lancet Commission thrust surgery into prominence on the global health stage. Subsequently, at the 2015 World Health Assembly, the resolution to "Strengthen Emergency and Essential Surgical Care and Anaesthesia as a part of Universal Health Coverage" was passed (WHA 2015).

With surgery now a priority on the global health agenda, attention turned toward upscaling surgical capacity in LMICs to achieve universal health coverage of surgical care. This involves a multidisciplinary and multisectorial response, interrelatedly involving infrastructure development, procurement of equipment and supplies as well as raising and sustaining human resources. Alongside new strategies, traditional strategies such as private nonprofit hospitals, surgical missions from high-income countries, and task shifting to lesser trained health workers may continue to contribute toward upscaling surgical capacity (Pollock et al. 2011).

A key component of any strategy aimed at long-term sustainable upscaling of surgical capacity is the training and retaining of local surgeons (Meara et al. 2015a). Placed within a text on clinical education in the health professions, this chapter will focus on global surgery in the context of developing surgical training programs in LMICs.

Surgical Workforce in LMICs: Shortages and Maldistribution

Globally, there is a surgical workforce shortage. An estimated 72% of the world's population lives in countries with a surgical workforce shortage (Meara et al. 2015a). Compounding the issue of surgical workforce shortages is the maldistribution of the existing surgical workforce both globally and nationally. Shortages are greatest in LMICs and in rural areas. In LMICs, there is a shortage of approximately one million surgical, anesthetic, and obstetric (SAO) providers (Campbell et al. 2013). Within

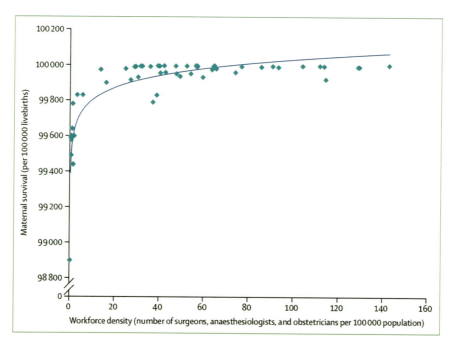

Fig. 1 Relationship between surgical workforce density and maternal survival rates for 50 countries. (From Meara et al. 2015b. Reproduced with permission)

countries, the surgical workforce is concentrated in urban areas leading to rural scarcity (Spiegel et al. 2011).

Surgical workforce shortages are harmful; surgical workforce density has been shown to correlate with specific health outcomes. As shown in Fig. 1, a ratio of less than 20 surgeons, anesthetists, and obstetricians (SAO) per 100,000 people is associated with increased rates of maternal death (Meara et al. 2015a). Above 40 SAO per 100,000 people, the benefit in reducing maternal death was minimal. This has led to the ratio of SAO per unit of population being promoted as a metric for measuring the adequacy of surgical workforce density, with a recommended target of 20–40 SAO per 100,000 people (Meara et al. 2015a).

Surgical Training in LMICs

Rickard et al. conducted a systematic review of postgraduate surgical training in LMICs (Rickard 2016). This review analyzed postgraduate surgical training programs in 34 LMICs representing Latin America and Caribbean, sub-Saharan Africa, Middle East and North Africa, Europe and Central Asia, East Asia, and Pacific and South Asia. Some LMICs have well-established surgical training programs, in the case of South Africa since as early as 1944. In contrast, other LMICs in same geographic region, such as Malawi and Rwanda, have commenced local surgical training programs as recently as 2005. Financial support for trainees is primarily from the government sometimes with additional private sponsorship. When government sponsorship is provided, a period of return of service post-training is sometimes required. The majority of surgical training programs award trainees a Master in Medicine degree, which generally requires submission of a thesis or dissertation. The syllabus of the surgical training programs in LMICs was generally "broad-based with the goal of having trainees work in rural or district hospitals" (Rickard 2016). While there was significant heterogeneity between curricula, most postgraduate surgical training programs in LMICs follow a similar structure; "after secondary school, most trainees complete 6 years of undergraduate training, 1 year of internship, and 4–5 years of postgraduate training" (Rickard 2016).

Challenges of Surgical Training in LMICs

Key challenges facing the development of surgical training programs in LMICs are discussed in the following section.

Local Versus Overseas Surgical Training

In many LMICs, a lack of in-country training opportunities has meant that surgical specialization has necessitated overseas training. While this arrangement may provide trainees with high-quality training not available locally, there are disadvantages for LMICs. Firstly, doctors-in-training are removed from the local health system, which is already likely to be experiencing a medical workforce shortage (Gruen 2006). Secondly, curricula may reflect Western rather than local needs (Gruen 2006). Thirdly, the exposure of doctors from LMICs to work and lifestyle in high-income countries may be a contributory factor toward the phenomenon of "brain drain" (Mullan 2005). In contrast, locally conducted surgical training provides continuity of the local surgical workforce and increases doctor retention in LMICs (Cameron et al. 2010). Locally conducted surgical training also provides contextualization of training to local needs and resource availability (Mutabdzic et al. 2013). For example, typhoid perforation of the small bowel and abdominal tuberculosis are common presentations in some LMICs but are rare in most high-income countries (Qureshi et al. 2011).

Institutions

To develop surgical training programs in LMICs, a strong and cohesive network of institutions working collaboratively is required. Governments have responsibility for providing funding, developing policy, and ensuring regulation. State or national institutions overseeing registration, certification, and continuing professional development are important for ensuring high individual standards of performance. Other national or regional institutions may accredit and regulate training providers, such as the role of the College of Surgeons in East, Central, and South Africa (COSECSA) to ensure surgical training programs provide a high standard of education. Universities or colleges provide the academic underpinning of a surgical training program and are usually responsible for administration. Teaching hospitals are the interface between academia and surgical practice and are responsible for the provision of surgical training. Additionally, an accredited local medical school is an important precursor to a locally populated surgical training program. Lastly, strong institutions alone are not enough; institutions need to work collaboratively to efficiently progress the development of a surgical training program (Qureshi et al. 2011).

Educational Faculty

A successful surgical training program requires a motivated, competent, and supported educational faculty to develop, administer, and deliver the program (Ezeome et al. 2009). Yet, in some LMICs there is no local experience with postgraduate training and very limited faculty resources (Cameron et al. 2010). Hampering the development of educational faculties has been the globally pervasive attitude that qualification as a medical specialist confers the ability to educate effectively (OFlynn et al. 2017). However, surgeons are generally not being trained to be educators (OFlynn et al. 2017).

Numerous strategies have successfully been employed to drive faculty development in LMICs. The Royal College of Surgeons in Ireland collaborated with COSECSA to develop Train the Trainer programs for surgical trainers. These courses have now been conducted in all 14 COSECSA countries. Following completion of the course, surgeons are recognized as COSECSA accredited trainers. Surgeons can complete further training to become master trainers and be accredited to deliver the COSECSA Train the Train courses (OFlynn et al. 2017). Online strategies have also been shown to be effective. In a comparison between online educational curricula designed for US surgeons with curricula designed for sub-Saharan African surgeons, both cohorts of African surgeons found the curricula beneficial (Goldstein et al. 2014).

In addition to faculty development, strategies to overcome faculty limitations are being sought. Sharing faculty teaching sessions between institutions by teleconferencing or the mail out of DVD recordings has proved successful in sub-Saharan Africa (Hadley and Mars 2011). Other innovative solutions include bypassing the need for faculty and utilizing online educational tools that can provide learners with feedback on task performance (Bunogerane et al. 2018).

Surgical Training Program Development

To inform surgical training program development, an understanding of the existing surgical capacity is required. The "situational analysis" tool developed by the Global Initiative for Emergency and Essential Surgical Care is the most widely used method for assessing surgical capacity, having been used in at least 54 LMICs (WHO 2018). The survey tool evaluates a country's health facilities, human resources, equipment, supplies, and the surgical interventions performed.

Sierra Leone was one of the first countries to use the situational analysis tool to create a snapshot of the entire country's surgical capacity. The country had ten fully trained surgeons to service a population of 5.3 million, with only one surgeon being under 50 years of age (Kingham et al. 2009). These findings demonstrated obvious need for urgent renewal of the already drastically inadequate surgical workforce.

Also employing the situational analysis tool, Rwanda found that 80% of surgery was performed in the 41 district hospitals while 80% of surgeons worked in the three referral hospitals (Petroze et al. 2012). Following this finding, the Rwandan Ministry of Health established the objective of having a trained surgeon in each of the 41 district hospitals by 2018 and tripled the intake of surgical trainees (Rickard et al. 2015).

Such assessments of surgical capacity may also reveal unexpected opportunities. A study in Sierra Leone surprisingly showed that most surgical procedures – and almost all orthopedic procedures – in the country were performed in private hospitals (Bolkan et al. 2015). Thus, the Sierra Leonean private sector was identified as an untapped potential for surgical training that could be incorporated into future national surgical training plans.

Mutabdzic et al. presented a model for developing a contextually appropriate surgical training program in a LMIC based on their experience in Botswana (Mutabdzic et al. 2013). The model consists of three key components. The first is an analysis of the procedures being performed within the country to identify the required operative proficiency of local surgeons, such as by using the situational analysis tool. The second was to select a simple preexisting framework on which to base a written curriculum. In the Batswana case, the Surgical Council of Resident Education curriculum for USA general surgery trainees was used. The final element was to utilize expert local opinion to adapt the template curriculum to suit local needs.

Using a preexisting framework on which to base a curriculum is convenient but needs to be done with caution. A comparison of Rwandan and USA general surgery trainee logbooks showed that while total operative caseload was similar, the types of cases were very different (Rickard et al. 2015). USA trainees performed high numbers endoscopy, laparoscopy, and pancreatic surgery compared to Rwandan trainees. In contrast, Rwandan trainees obtained experience in urology, neurosurgery, and orthopedics which was uncommon for USA trainees. This operative mix was considered more appropriate training for the Rwandan general surgeon who may be required to be the single surgeon in a district hospital (Rickard et al. 2015).

Equipment and Infrastructure

Predictably, reliable access to safe and effective equipment and infrastructure is a challenge in many LMICs. As well as limiting service delivery, there is a subsequent impact on surgical training opportunities.

A survey of sub-Saharan neurosurgical trainees and trainers found that 71% of respondents identified lack of equipment as the number one barrier to neurosurgical training at their institution (Sader et al. 2017). In Egypt, surgical trainees are based in underresourced public facilities. Yet an estimated 80% of the general pediatric surgical workload is performed in the better resourced private health care sector, representing a lost learning opportunity for trainees (Elhalaby et al. 2012).

Innovative solutions to equipment and infrastructure problems exist. Equipment limitations have been successfully addressed through the utilization of low-cost simulation, such as the locally assembled laparoscopic box trainers for US$30 in place of expensive laparoscopic trainers (Andreatta et al. 2014). In South Africa, the difficulty of conducting surgical training in a poorly resourced public hospital was overcome through the establishment of an academic private hospital owned and run by the University of the Witwatersrand and accredited for surgical training (Degiannis et al. 2009).

Relationships Between High- and Low-Income Countries

While high-income countries (HICs) have much to offer LMICs – funding, resources, workers, and expertise – there is also a risk of harm.

Historically, HICs' involvement in surgical care in LMICs focused on service delivery – rather than education and training – and predominantly involved short-term surgical trips. Such trips typically involved visiting surgeons from HICs arriving in LMICs and performing a large volume of clinical work in a short space of time before departing. While often contributing to a reduction in elective surgery waiting times and providing people with treatment closer to their local community, issues with the traditional model of short-term surgical trips are well documented (Butler 2016).

Short-term trips – particularly if infrequent – provide limited opportunity for the development of strong relationships between visiting and host surgeons or familiarity with the local environment. This may be associated with a lack of necessary planning to identify local needs for the visiting surgical team to address. There may be a lack of awareness regarding local culture, customs, and practices resulting in visiting teams inadvertently causing offence to their hosts. Unfamiliarity with local patterns of disease may lead to patient harm due incorrect diagnoses and treatments while inexperience with resource limitations may lead to excessive resource consumption. Additionally, there may be poor coordination with other visiting teams and local government reducing the overall impact of the trip on local health care provision. Finally, aftercare is an issue as, when visiting surgeons leave, local surgeons are left with the responsibility of coordinating postoperative care which may be beyond the expertise or capacity of local services to provide (Butler 2016; DeGennaro Jr et al. 2012).

At a population level, poorly integrated short-term surgical trips have little impact on the performance of the overall health system. As the trips do not build local capacity to provide surgical services, an unmet need for surgery persists. The reliance on short-term trips to meet this need is unsustainable and creates dependency on international help. Additionally, while short-term trips *may* provide an opportunity for education and training, the focus of such trips is typically service provision and local trainees may actually be denied learning opportunities, particularly if visiting surgeons come with their own perioperative support team (Asgary and Junck 2013; Wolfberg 2006).

There is a long history of faith-based organizations (FBO) contributing to surgical care and training in LMICs. This has been particularly significant in Africa where an estimated 30–70% of all health infrastructure is owned or operated by FBOs (Butler 2016). An advantage of FBOs is their permanency which overcomes many of the issues with short-term surgical trips. Some FBOs have significantly contributed to local surgical training. The Pan-Africa Academy of Christian Surgeons has established six surgical training programs spread across Kenya, Ethiopia, Gabon, and Cameroon based on US curricula in collaboration with Loma Linda University in California (Pollock et al. 2011). These programs vary from 2 to 5 years in duration and receive various levels of accreditation with COSECSA from Member to Fellow status (Pollock et al. 2011). Like short-term surgical trips, FBOs are also associated with issues of sustainability and local self-sufficiency in delivering both surgical care and training (Butler 2016).

With short-term surgical trips and FBO, LMICs are perceived as "recipients" and HICs as "donors," with the implication of an unbalanced power relationship. The trend in recent years has been toward new models of engagement whereby HICs and LMICs collaborate as equal "partners." The nature of the partnership between HICs and LMICs is heterogenous. The partnership may occur at the level of individuals, institutions, or governments. The work involved may include deployment of HIC surgeons to LMIC to perform clinical, educational, or administrative tasks. Through partnerships between HIC and LMIC collaborators, short-term surgical trips have been remodeled. By improving integration with local existing service provision and incorporating educational objectives, short-term surgical trips can contribute to augmenting health system performance while also promoting sustainability (Butler 2016).

Partnering with HICs has been demonstrated to be a particularly effective method for LMICs to develop educational faculties for surgical training programs (Mutabdzic et al. 2013). Guyana sought to create the country's first postgraduate surgical training program but lacked faculty resources and local expertise with postgraduate training. A partnership was formed with the Canadian Association of General Surgeons to address this deficit and the program has successfully graduated at least 14 locally trained surgeons (Cameron et al. 2010). Similarly, Malawi developed a five-year surgical training program in partnership with the University of North Carolina in the USA and University of Haukeland in Norway that has been accredited by COSECSA (Qureshi et al. 2011).

One of the longest running partnerships regarding surgical training program development is between Australia and Papua New Guinea (PNG) (Gruen 2006; Kevau and Watters 2006). In 1975, a surgical training program was commenced in PNG with significant Australian involvement. After 30 years, this program was locally taught and administered with minimal external support. A key lesson from this program was the need for international partners to make long-term commitments and that the nature of these relationship be carefully considered. The PNG surgical program deliberately avoided seeking accreditation from the Royal Australasian College of Surgeons (RACS). This encouraged local ownership and contextualization of the program to PNG. Additionally, only specialist training relevant to PNG, but not available in-country, was provided externally. This program design has contributed to 97% of locally trained PNG nationals continuing to practice in-country (Watters et al. 2019). As surgical capacity expanded, the nature of the relationship changed. Initially, expatriates performed the bulk of the surgical work, this evolved into expatriates teaching local doctors to perform surgery and finally into expatriates playing a mentoring and supervisory role in the local delivery of the surgical training program (Gruen 2006; Kevau and Watters 2006).

Although partnerships seem a preferable model for HIC engagement with LMICs, the risk of inadvertent harm remains. For example, as surgical programs tend to be modeled on the curriculum of partner HIC there is the potential for lack of local contextualization (Mutabdzic et al. 2013). Similarly, there are issues with sustainability if the local program is dependent upon HIC involvement for ongoing survival of their surgical training program (Mutabdzic et al. 2013). Additionally, there are also potential social, cultural, and political consequences. When Western institutions export their medical curricula to LMICs, packaged up with the curricula are Western values, attitudes, and culture which are then imposed on LMICs of non-Western culture (Bleakley et al. 2011). This process has been criticized as "colonialism via the back door," a creeping form of "neo-colonialism in a post-colonial era" (Bleakley et al. 2011). Numerous surgical societies have recently published guidelines for the conduct of culturally aware, safe, and effective partnerships with recommendations from HIC and LMIC perspectives (Butler et al. 2018). A common theme among these recommendations is that whatever the nature of the engagement between the HIC and LMIC, promoting education and training should be of high priority (Butler 2016).

Timor-Leste

Background of Timor-Leste

Timor-Leste is a country with a population of 1.2 million people situated on the eastern part of the Timor Island, which is located to the north of Australia separated by the Timor Sea (CIA 2018) (Fig. 2).

Previously known as East Timor, Timor-Leste was under colonial occupation from Portugal for 400 years. Days after withdrawal of the Portuguese in 1975, Timor-Leste came under military occupation from Indonesia. Following 24 years of resistance, an UN-supervised referendum was held in 1999 whereby a majority of Timorese people voted for Timor-Leste to establish independence from Indonesia (CIA 2018). This result triggered a violent response from anti-independence Timorese militias which devastated the nation: 75% of the Timor-Leste population became displaced and the majority of public and private infrastructure was destroyed (CIA 2018). Disruption was particularly significant in the health sector due to the additional insult of mass emigration of doctors (who were mostly of Indonesian nationality) (WHO 2000). A World Health Organization situation report from 2000 counted 25 Timorese doctors remaining in the region and only one doctor with specialist training (WHO 2000). These events culminated in the collapse of the health system in Timor-Leste (WHO 2000).

The international community, through both government and nongovernment organizations, has supported Timor-Leste's recovery and development. The development of the health system has been described as occurring in three overlapping phases, each characterized by the varying involvement of Timorese in the delivery of medical and surgical care (Guest et al. 2017a). During the first phase (2001–2004), specialist services were largely delivered by expatriate health practitioners in the

11 Global Surgery and Its Trends and Context: The Case of Timor-Leste

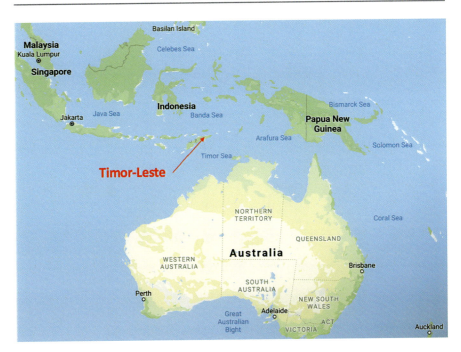

Fig. 2 Timor-Leste and surrounding countries. (Adapted from Google Maps 20.11.2019)

relative absence of local specialist practitioners. The second phase (2005–2010) saw an increased ability for Timor-Leste to provide primary care and international support to allow Timorese doctors to pursue overseas specialist training. Additionally, the transition from the first to second phase saw expatriate specialists increasingly working alongside Timorese doctors in training and mentoring roles (RACS 2013). This transition is well demonstrated by a retrospective audit of three 1-year periods which showed a significant increase in the number of surgical procedures conducted under the supervision of expatriate surgeons and involving a Timorese doctor: from 10% in 2001 to 51% in 2006 to 77% by 2010 (Guest et al. 2017a). The third phase (since 2011) has seen the return of overseas trained Timorese specialists to provide clinical care and occupy leadership positions within their health service (Guest et al. 2017a). This has freed up expatriates from service provision and enabled the creation of a local faculty for delivering education and training programs. Thus, a key feature of the third phase has been the introduction of formal postgraduate medical training in Timor-Leste.

Surgical Care in Timor-Leste

Over the past two decades, Timor-Leste has made tremendous advances in the capacity to deliver surgical care. However, numerous shortfalls are still evident.

Timor-Leste, with 0.9 SAO per 100,000 people, has one of the lowest-density surgical workforces in the world (Guest et al. 2017b), well below the recommended target of 20–40 SAO per 100,000 people (Meara et al. 2015a). In contrast, nearby Australia has one of the highest-density surgical workforces in the world with 63.9 SAO per 100,000 people (Guest et al. 2017b). Low surgical workforce density is associated with poor performance in other metrics used to measure surgical care delivery: timely access to surgery and surgical volume.

Timely access to surgery is defined as the "proportion of the population that can access, within 2 h, a facility that can do caesarean delivery, laparotomy, and treatment of open fracture" (Meara et al. 2015a). These procedures are designated as "Bellwether procedures" because the ability to perform these procedures implies the skills and resources to perform a broad range of emergency and essential surgical procedures. The Lancet Commission in Global Surgery recommended 80% of a countries' population should be able to access these Bellwether procedures within 2 h (Meara et al. 2015a).

In Timor-Leste, three hospitals perform the Bellwether procedures and are accessible by 50% of the population within 2 h (Guest et al. 2017b). This coverage could be improved to 80% if two of the existing district hospitals gained the ability to perform Bellwether procedures (Guest et al. 2017b). In contrast, there are 112 hospitals in Australia performing Bellwether procedures and they are accessible to 98.85% of the population within 2 h (Guest et al. 2017b).

The Lancet Commission in Global Surgery also recommended a target of 5,000 operations per 100,000 people annually as this surgical volume is estimated to represent surgical need. Timor-Leste is well below this target, performing 433 operations per 100,000 people annually (Guest et al. 2017b). In comparison, Australia performs 10,156 operations per 100,000 people annually (Guest et al. 2017b).

Increasing the surgical workforce density is clearly necessary for increasing access to surgery and surgical volume in Timor-Leste. For Timor-Leste to achieve the minimum target of 20 SAO per 100,000 people the surgical workforce in Timor-Leste will need to be upscaled significantly – from 12–260 SAO. Thus, Timor-Leste faces a major challenge to raise and sustain their surgical workforce (Timor-Leste. 2011).

Surgical Education and Training in Timor-Leste

The initial pathway for Timorese doctors to obtain specialist training was via government or international scholarships to train overseas. This was associated with numerous issues. Firstly, overseas training meant removing a doctor from the already underserviced local medical workforce that needs their services (Gruen 2006). Secondly, the overseas destination needed to be suitable in terms of language, culture, educational standard, disease patterns, and resource utilization and this proved difficult to achieve. Several of the initial trainees sent for overseas specialty training were unsuccessful in completing their studies for a variety of the abovementioned reasons (Guest et al. 2017a).

Postgraduate Diploma in Surgery

The Timor-Leste Government declared the strategic goal of becoming self-sufficient in the provision of specialist surgical and medical services by 2030 and do so through "in-country" training (Timor-Leste. 2011). Thus, an 18-month postgraduate diploma (PGD) was introduced in a variety of specialty areas: surgery, anesthesia, obstetrics, pediatrics, and internal medicine. The expectation was that graduates from this program would then be better prepared to undertake overseas specialist surgical training. Longer term, the plan was to develop the diploma into a master's program and achieve self-sufficiency in the local training of specialists.

The PGD was a joint enterprise between RACS, the Ministry of Health, and the national university (Universidade Nacional de Timor Lorosa'e) (RACS 2015). The PGD is delivered through the national university with trainees based at the national teaching hospital (Hospital Nacional Guido Valadares). RACS has been involved in developing the curriculum, contributing to teaching and providing follow-up mentoring and supervision to ensure the quality of the diplomas (AusAID 2012).

The first PGD cohort commenced in 2012 and nine Timorese doctors graduated in 2013 including three in surgery (DFAT 2014). The surgical graduates possess the skills to manage simple bone fractures, treat complex wounds, and identify critically ill patients in regional settings who require higher levels of care (RACS 2015).

Development of a surgical training program was first considered by RACS upon becoming involved in Timor-Leste 2001. Thus, 12 years of continuous involvement underpinned the graduation of the first PGD surgical graduates (RACS 2015). This is an important insight into the reality of developing a surgical training program in a postconflict low-income country that despite relative government stability and significant long-term international support almost a generation was required to establish a basic level surgical training program.

Another insight regarding health system development from the case study of Timor-Leste is the potential for unexpected events that can lead to changing priorities. Cuba has played a major role in strengthening the Timor-Leste health system, specifically by repopulating the medical workforce. In 2010, Cuba sent 230 Cuban doctors to Timor-Leste (Asante 2014). Furthermore, Cuba has subsequently trained (in Cuba) approximately 1000 Timorese doctors (RACS 2015). Thus, by 2013, a major priority for the Ministry of Health became the successful integration of the newly graduated Cuban-trained Timorese doctors into the Timor-Leste health system. RACS was requested to suspend the PGD programs and focus on this new task of assimilating the Cuban-trained doctors instead (Guest et al. 2017a). Jointly, RACS, the Ministry for Health, and the national university created and began conducting a two-year internship program called the Family Medicine Program (FMP) for the Cuban-trained Timorese doctors (DFAT 2014).

Despite the two-year disruption, the introduction of the FMP has also served to benefit the PGD programs. A major challenge with the PGD programs had been trainee selection due to both a lack of suitable applicants and a rigorous selection process. Now, the FMP betters prepares applicants to enter the PGD programs and the summative assessment at the conclusion of the first and second year of FMP provides an objective tool for discriminating the best applicants (Stevens 2018). Table 1 summarizes the time course of the PGD in Surgery in Timor-Leste and the number of trainees in each cohort.

Table 1 Timeline of postgraduate diploma (PGD) in surgery in Timor-Leste

Date	Stage of PGD in Surgery	Number of trainees
Feb 2012 to July 2013	PGD in Surgery cohort 1	3
June 2014 to June 2015	Embargo on PGD in Surgery, Family Medicine Program (FMP) commenced	–
July 2015 to Jan 2017	PGD in Surgery cohort 2	4
July 2017 to 2018	PGD in Surgery cohort 3	6
2019–2020	PGD in Surgery cohort 4	3

Challenges in Surgical Education and Training in Timor-Leste

The remainder of this chapter will discuss various challenges encountered in developing and delivering a surgical education program in Timor-Leste. These include surgeons as educators, selection of trainees, language barriers, career pathways, and equipment and infrastructure.

A qualitative study (Stevens 2018) explored the challenges of conducting a surgical education and training program in Timor-Leste (Stevens 2018). Semistructured interviews with trainees, surgeons, and administrators engaged in the Timorese training program were undertaken. Data was analyzed using iterative thematic analysis and the identified challenges were organized into the following key themes.

Surgeons as Educators

Timorese surgeons have powerful motivation to train junior doctors:

> "I train you [surgical trainees] because you are the future. I am a citizen of this country. One day, I will come to the hospital and become a patient, and I will want to be treated properly. That's why I need to train you." (Stevens 2018)

However, such motivation may wane when surgeons are busy, their income is spread widely, and training is not remunerated.

> "Passion alone cannot fulfil everything that you need. [A doctor may need to provide for their] children, parents and extended family. You know from the $610 per month that a doctor gets in Timor, it goes everywhere. It does not stay in the house." (Stevens 2018)

Even if surgeons are motivated, they may lack knowledge, skills, and experience in being a trainer. As such, the delivery of "train the trainer" courses have been well received in Timor-Leste.

> "We need more people that have experience [in] teaching. I don't have that. The way I train [surgical trainees], the way I teach them is just [to] follow [the way] I've been trained and [taught]." (Stevens 2018)

Language Barriers

Language in surgical training is a complex and unique challenge in Timor-Leste. Timorese speak their local language, Tetum, and an Indonesian language, Bahasa.

Having previously been a Portuguese colony, most people also speak Portuguese. The current MBBS program is taught by Cubans – either in Cuba or Timor-Leste – in Spanish. To prepare, medical students undertake training in Spanish before commencing their medical studies. Additionally, English proficiency also needs to be acquired as textbooks, postgraduate programs, and clinical ward rounds in Timor-Leste are conducted in English.

Teaching is conducted in English for several reasons. As there are consultants from Cuba, China, Australia, and other countries working in Timor-Leste, a common language for communicating in the hospital is required, which has emerged to be English. Additionally, training in English prepares graduates of the PGD in Surgery program to undertake further specialization training in the region (e.g., Fiji or Papua New Guinea) which is also usually conducted in English.

Consequently, trainees' proficiency with English impacts on their educational capabilities.

> "If they don't understand, or really struggle with English, then...it is a major constraint...English is the major constraint to learning, in my view." (Stevens 2018)

In response to this challenge, trainees are provided with English education during the FMP.

> "Before [the trainees] enter a [postgraduate] diploma program, RACS provide a very good English class." (Stevens 2018)

This initiative has been reported to have had a significant impact on the trainees' ability to perform well during postgraduate training.

> "So, it's a year of English that makes the difference with the FMP. That makes a difference more than the year of medicine." (Stevens 2018)

Career Pathways

The pathway for a Timorese doctor to become a surgeon has significantly evolved since the introduction of the PGD in Surgery in 2012 (Table 2). The trend has been toward a more structured – albeit incomplete – pathway. Prior to 2012, a Timorese doctor would initially need to complete their medical qualification, work as a general practitioner, and hope for a government scholarship to fund overseas surgical specialty training. Now, a Timorese doctor would likely have completed the FMP and PGD in Surgery prior to overseas surgical specialty training.

However, scholarships to undertake overseas surgical specialty training are difficult to obtain. Previously, RACS had provided scholarships for trainees to undertake surgical specialty training abroad. Access to these scholarships had previously seemed reliable.

> "Previously was really clear; if you had good attitude, good preparation, you will go [overseas for surgical specialty training]." (Stevens 2018)

Table 2 Career pathways for a Timorese to become a qualified surgeon across different time periods and cohorts of the Postgraduate Diploma (PGD) in Surgery. (Bachelor Medicine Bachelor Surgery (MBBS), General practitioner (GP), Family Medicine Program (FMP))

Year	Pre-2012	2012	2015-
PGD in Surgery cohort	Pre-PGD	Cohort 1	Cohorts 2+
Level of education	MBBS	MBBS	MBBS
	GP (variable)	GP (variable)	+/− GP (variable)
	Overseas surgical specialization training (4 years)	PGD in Surgery (18 months)	FMP (12 months)
	Qualified surgeon	Overseas surgical specialization training (4 years)	PGD in Surgery (18 months)
		Qualified surgeon	Overseas surgical specialization training (4 years)
			Qualified surgeon

This clarity regarding career pathways after completion of the PGD in Surgery had a motivating effect on trainees.

> We, [the PGD in Surgery trainees], thought this [scholarship] was going to continue. We were really enthusiastic. We thought our future was brighter than what we're seeing now, so we worked hard (Stevens 2018).

However, since the introduction of the postgraduate diplomas, RACS has ceased funding scholarships for overseas specialization training. Trainees cannot afford to self-fund specialization training and therefore they are dependent on receiving government scholarships. Such scholarships have not been reliably rewarded to graduates of the PGD in Surgery program. These doctors continue to work in Timor-Leste as general doctors but cannot do further specialization training. This uncertainty regarding career pathways is a cause of angst among trainees and has impacted on trainee motivation.

> "The trainees have seen the results of [those who] graduated from the diploma and think, "I'm not going anywhere!". So, no motivation." (Stevens 2018)

In-country specialization training is established for pediatrics. A key challenge to developing a full specialization program in surgery within Timor-Leste is equipment and infrastructure limitations.

Equipment and Infrastructure

As may be expected in a low-income country such as Timor-Leste, equipment and infrastructure challenges restrict not only surgical care but also educational opportunities.

Extensive limitations exist for basic and essential surgical equipment in Timor-Leste:

"Almost weekly we run out of stock of medication, instruments, theatre gowns etc etc." (Stevens 2018)

Consequently, there is a reduction in the provision of local surgical care:

"Sometimes theatre is cancelled because of surgical reasons. . .like patient has comorbidities that have not been sorted out. . .but most of the cancellations are due to unnecessary things like no gowns, no water, no medications." (Stevens 2018)

Similarly, there are significant limitations in infrastructure, particularly in regard to diagnostic facilities such as radiology and pathology. The outcome is patients are sent overseas for their surgical care.

"Only cytology is here. So, for those cases that need to be worked up histologically we will send through to Indonesia for their diagnostic and staging and operation." (Stevens 2018)

Of note, it is more often equipment and infrastructure limitations rather than lack of surgical expertise that lead to patients being referred overseas for treatment.

"All general surgeons can perform mastectomy here but because there is no histology here we send [patients] overseas." (Stevens 2018)

Equipment and infrastructure limitations have a detrimental effect on surgeon morale and maintenance of competency with subsequent complications for surgical education and training in Timor-Leste.

"At the moment it is very tiring. We have not enough resource to do things. . .The conditions make the doctors become frustrated and lose their enthusiasm." (Stevens 2018)

Sending patients overseas for treatment comes at both a financial and educational cost:

"[Regarding] the referral [of patients overseas], we. . .not only lose financial[ly] but we also lose the opportunity to train and to show to the [trainee] how we are dealing with the cases." (Stevens 2018)

The educational cost of equipment and infrastructure limitations is the impediment to developing a full surgical specialization program in Timor-Leste.

"Looking at the present situation, it is impractical and actually it will be laughable." (Stevens 2018)

Conclusion

Most of the global population lack access to safe, timely, and affordable surgical care leading to excess morbidity and mortality. Addressing this inequity is a global health priority and the clinical education of health professionals is at the heart of the solution. Experienced faculty delivering locally contextualized surgical training programs in well-resourced settings offer the greatest prospect of sustainably upscaling the global surgical workforce and delivery of surgical care, especially in LMICs. This requires investment in health system strengthening, alignment between government and training institutions, and carefully negotiated partnerships between LMICs and HICs. In LMICs especially, there needs to be investment in developing faculties of surgical educators capable of conducting surgical training programs. Individually, health professionals in HIC engaging with LMICs should see their role as transitioning from providing surgical services to supporting surgical education and training program initiatives. A coordinated global approach to surgical education and training at macro-, meso-, and microlevels is essential to achieving universal access to safe, timely, and affordable surgical care.

Cross-References

▶ Future of Health Professions Education Curricula
▶ Learning and Teaching in the Operating Room: A Surgical Perspective
▶ Nursing Education in Low and Lower-Middle Income Countries: Context and Trends
▶ Surgical Education: Context and Trends
▶ Surgical Training: Impact of Decentralization and Guidelines for Improvement

References

Andreatta P, Perosky J, Klotz J, Gamble C, Ankobea F, Danso K, et al. Pilot study outcomes from a resource-limited setting for a low-cost training program for laparoscopic surgical skills. Int J Gynaecol Obstet. 2014;125(2):186–8.

Asante A. Retaining doctors in rural Timor-Leste: a critical appraisal of the opportunities and challenges. Bull World Health Organ [Internet]. 2014;92:[277–82 pp.].

Asgary R, Junck E. New trends of short-term humanitarian medical volunteerism: professional and ethical considerations. J Med Ethics. 2013;39(10):625–31.

AusAID. Training young doctors in East Timor. Canberra: Australian Agency for International Development; 2012.

Bleakley A, Bligh J, Browne J. In: Hamstra S, editor. Medical education for the future: identity, power and location. New York: Springer; 2011.

Bolkan HA, Von Schreeb J, Samai MM, Bash-Taqi DA, Kamara TB, Salvesen O, et al. Met and unmet needs for surgery in Sierra Leone: a comprehensive, retrospective, countrywide survey from all health care facilities performing operations in 2012. Surgery. 2015;157(6):992–1001.

Bunogerane GJ, Taylor K, Lin Y, Costas-Chavarri A. Using touch surgery to improve surgical education in Low- and middle-income settings: a randomized control trial. J Surg Educ. 2018;75(1):231–7.

Butler MW. Developing pediatric surgery in low- and middle-income countries: an evaluation of contemporary education and care delivery models. Semin Pediatr Surg. 2016;25(1):43–50.

Butler M, Drum E, Evans FM, Fitzgerald T, Fraser J, Holterman AX, et al. Guidelines and checklists for short-term missions in global pediatric surgery: recommendations from the American Academy of Pediatrics Delivery of Surgical Care Global Health Subcommittee, American Pediatric Surgical Association Global Pediatric Surgery Committee, Society for Pediatric Anesthesia Committee on International Education and Service, and American Pediatric Surgical Nurses Association, Inc. Global Health Special Interest Group. J Pediatr Surg. 2018;53(4):828–36.

Cameron BH, Rambaran M, Sharma DP, Taylor RH. International surgery: the development of postgraduate surgical training in Guyana. Can J Surg. 2010;53(1):11–6.

Campbell J, Dussault G, Buchan J. A universal truth: no health without a workforce. Recife: World Health Organisation; 2013.

CIA. World FactBook: Central Intelligence Agency; 2018. Available from: https://www.cia.gov/library/publications/the-world-factbook/geos/tt.html

Debas HGR, McCord C, et al. Disease control priorities in developing countries. 2nd ed. New York: Oxford Press; 2006.

DeGennaro VA Jr, DeGennaro VA, Kochhar A, Nathan N, Low C, Avashia YJ, et al. Accelerating surgical training and reducing the burden of surgical disease in Haiti before and after the earthquake. J Craniofac Surg. 2012;23(7 Suppl 1):2028–32.

Degiannis E, Oettle GJ, Smith MD, Veller MG. Surgical education in South Africa. World J Surg. 2009;33(2):170–3.

DFAT. Aid program performance report 2013–14 Timor-Leste. Canberra: Department of Foreign Affairs and Trade; 2014.

Elhalaby EA, Uba FA, Borgstein ES, Rode H, Millar AJ. Training and practice of pediatric surgery in Africa: past, present, and future. Semin Pediatr Surg. 2012;21(2):103–10.

Ezeome ER, Ekenze SO, Ugwumba F, Nwajiobi CE, Coker O. Surgical training in resource-limited countries: moving from the body to the bench – experiences from the basic surgical skills workshop in Enugu, Nigeria. Trop Doct. 2009;39(2):93–7.

Farmer PE, Kim JY. Surgery and Global Health: a view from beyond the OR. World J Surg. 2008;32(4):533–6.

Goldstein SD, Papandria D, Linden A, Azzie G, Borgstein E, Calland JF, et al. A pilot comparison of standardized online surgical curricula for use in low- and middle-income countries. JAMA Surg. 2014;149(4):341–6.

Gruen RL. Template for surgical training in resource-poor countries. ANZ J Surg. 2006;76(10):871–2.

Guest GD, Scott DF, Xavier JP, Martins N, Vreede E, Chennal A, et al. Surgical capacity building in Timor-Leste: a review of the first 15 years of the Royal Australasian College of surgeons-led Australian aid programme. ANZ J Surg. 2017a;87(6):436–40.

Guest GD, McLeod E, Perry WRG, Tangi V, Pedro J, Ponifasio P, et al. Collecting data for global surgical indicators: a collaborative approach in the Pacific region. BMJ Glob Health. 2017b;2(4):e000376.

Hadley GP, Mars M. e-Education in paediatric surgery: a role for recorded seminars in areas of low bandwidth in sub-Saharan Africa. Pediatr Surg Int. 2011;27(4):407–10.

Kevau I, Watters DA. Specialist surgical training in Papua New Guinea: the outcomes after 10 years. ANZ J Surg. 2006;76(10):937–41.

Kingham TP, Kamara TB, Cherian MN, Gosselin RA, Simkins M, Meissner C, et al. Quantifying surgical capacity in Sierra Leone: a guide for improving surgical care. Arch Surg. 2009;144(2):122–7. discussion 8.

Laxminarayan R, Ashford L. Using evidence about "best buys" to advance Global Health. Disease Control Priorities Project; 2008.

Meara J, Raykar N. The sustainable development goals and surgery: is a 'moon shot' the answer? Los Angeles Times. 2016 Mar 8, 2016; Sect. World and Nation.

Meara JG, Leather AJM, Hagander L, Alkire BC, Alonso N, Ameh EA, et al. Global surgery 2030: evidence and solutions for achieving health, welfare, and economic development. Lancet. 2015a;386(9993):569–624.

Meara JG, Leather AJ, Hagander L, Alkire BC, Alonso N, Ameh EA, et al. Global surgery 2030: evidence and solutions for achieving health, welfare, and economic development. Surgery. 2015b;158(1):3–6.

Mock CN, Donkor P, Gawande A, Jamison DT, Kruk ME, Debas HT. Essential surgery: key messages of this volume. In: Debas HT, Donkor P, Gawande A, Jamison DT, Kruk ME, Mock CN, editors. Essential surgery: disease control priorities, vol. 1. 3rd ed. Washington, DC; 2015.

Mullan F. The metrics of the physician brain drain. N Engl J Med. 2005;353(17):1810–8.

Mutabdzic D, Bedada AG, Bakanisi B, Motsumi J, Azzie G. Designing a contextually appropriate surgical training program in low-resource settings: the Botswana experience. World J Surg. 2013;37(7):1486–91.

OFlynn D, OFlynn E, Deneke A, Yohannan P, da Costa AA, OBoyle C, et al. Training surgeons as medical educators in Africa. J Surg Educ. 2017;74(3):539–42.

Peden M, McGee K, Krug E. Injury: a leading cause of the global burden of disease, 2000. Geneva: World Health Organisation; 2002.

Petroze RT, Nzayisenga A, Rusanganwa V, Ntakiyiruta G, Calland JF. Comprehensive national analysis of emergency and essential surgical capacity in Rwanda. Br J Surg. 2012;99(3):436–43.

Pollock JD, Love TP, Steffes BC, Thompson DC, Mellinger J, Haisch C. Is it possible to train surgeons for rural Africa? A report of a successful international program. World J Surg. 2011;35(3):493–9.

Qureshi JS, Samuel J, Lee C, Cairns B, Shores C, Charles AG. Surgery and global public health: the UNC-Malawi surgical initiative as a model for sustainable collaboration. World J Surg. 2011;35(1):17–21.

RACS. Consultation on Australia's relationship with Timor-Leste. Melbourne: Royal Australian College of Surgeons; 2013.

RACS. Building health in Timor-Leste. Surg News. 2015:26–7.

Rickard J. Systematic review of postgraduate surgical education in Low- and middle-income countries. World J Surg. 2016;40(6):1324–35.

Rickard JL, Ntakiyiruta G, Chu KM. Identifying gaps in the surgical training curriculum in Rwanda through evaluation of operative activity at a teaching hospital. J Surg Educ. 2015;72(4):e73–81.

Sader E, Yee P, Hodaie M. Barriers to neurosurgical training in sub-Saharan Africa: the need for a phased approach to global surgery efforts to improve neurosurgical care. World Neurosurg. 2017;98:397–402.

Spiegel DA, Choo S, Cherian M, Orgoi S, Kehrer B, Price RR, et al. Quantifying surgical and anesthetic availability at primary health facilities in Mongolia. World J Surg. 2011;35(2):272–9.

Stevens S. Exploring surgical education & training in Timor-Leste: what are the challenges and how are they interrelated? University of Melbourne; 2018.

Timor-Leste. Timor-Leste strategic development plan 2011–2030. Dili; 2011.

Watters DA, McCaig E, Nagra S, Kevau I. Surgical training programmes in the South Pacific, Papua New Guinea and Timor Leste. Br J Surg. 2019;106(2):e53–61.

WHA. Strengthening emergency and essential surgical care and anaesthesia as a component of universal health coverage. Geneva: World Health Assembly; 2015.

WHO. East Timorese health sector situation report. World Health Organisation; 2000.

WHO. Emergency and essential surgical care: World Health Organisation; 2018. Available from: http://www.who.int/surgery/globalinitiative/en/

Wolfberg AJ. Volunteering overseas – lessons from surgical brigades. N Engl J Med. 2006;354(5):443–5.

Surgical Training: Impact of Decentralization and Guidelines for Improvement

12

Christine M. Cuthbertson

Contents

Introduction 202
    Hybrid Distant and Direct Surgical Training 203
    The Challenges of Providing Surgical Education at a Distance 203
    Skills Teaching in Distance Education 204
    Educational Techniques That Support the Surgical Training Program 204
    The Impact of Decentralized Training on Assessment 208
    Other Challenges of Distance Education 209
    Opportunities in Blending Distance and Face-to-Face Education 211
Conclusion 213
Cross-References 213
References 213

Abstract

Future surgeons must develop operative and other skills such as decision-making, operative planning and self-awareness, in addition to traditional medical skills and knowledge. In larger, well-resourced hospital situations, this training can be provided easily. However, smaller hospitals may struggle to provide suitable breadth.

Increasingly, distance education is used to supplement training in smaller hospitals. Education may be coordinated by a central faculty, with the cohort in geographically distributed hospitals, or the cohort may be taught almost entirely by distance syllabus in some circumstances. This creates a spoke and hub educational structure, which has specific limitations and challenges. A combination of central regulation or credentialing faculty with peripheral workplace resident or registrar working placements is a common pattern in surgical training and education. The central hub may only manage assessment and standards, or it

---

C. M. Cuthbertson (✉)
Monash Rural Health, Bendigo, Monash University, North Bendigo, VIC, Australia
e-mail: Christine.Cuthbertson@monash.edu

© Springer Nature Singapore Pte Ltd. 2023
D. Nestel et al. (eds.), *Clinical Education for the Health Professions*,
https://doi.org/10.1007/978-981-15-3344-0_132

may provide formalized education to the whole cohort. The various hospitals (or spokes) are responsible for direct workplace teaching, including technical and nontechnical patient management skills. A curriculum designed to take advantage of this pattern will improve quality, and potentially, trainee outcomes.

This system is effectively a hybrid of direct workplace education and distance education. True distance education, where the educator and the student are geographically separated, is less common in surgical education, but can be used in remote, rural, and low resource settings. In this chapter, I will focus primarily on distance education, but in sympathy with a hybrid approach.

For the purpose of clarity, the term "surgical trainee" will be used to refer to all junior doctors progressing towards a career in surgery. Depending on the educational system, these might be residents or registrars or medical officers. Likewise "surgical training" is the education program that is used to develop these doctors and usually combines teaching of technical skills, base knowledge, and non-clinical skills.

Keywords

Surgical education · Surgical training · Postgraduate education · Distance education · E-learning · Residency teaching · Residency training

Introduction

Single site surgical training is limited to larger hospitals, where there are sufficient clinical jobs to support a dedicated education program. Training programs that use clinical positions across multiple hospitals are also common. Many countries have an uneven distribution of the medical workforce between rural centers and bigger cities (McCusker 2004; Bruening and Maddern 2009; Mercier et al. 2019). Countries that have a rural/metropolitan workforce disparity are increasing training times in regional settings to improve retention, which increases this geographic distribution (Bruening and Maddern 2009; Mercier et al. 2019; Wearne et al. 2015). Where trainees are located in different towns or suburbs, distance or hybrid education design is useful to provide accessible education. Naturally, these types of educational programs can also be used for provision of training over larger distances, such as in lower resource settings (Nartker et al. 2010; Battat et al. 2016; Geissbuhler et al. 2007), or even restricted access to face-to-face training due to pandemics (Tuma et al. 2021; Nicholas et al. 2021; Al-Balas et al. 2020).

It is clearly more complex to design an education program that provides equal opportunities to all participants, regardless of their physical location. Smaller centers have less administrative support and a smaller academic faculty (Battat et al. 2016). Educators also have to be available to all groups in some form, which usually leads to a larger workforce, with less formal training in education. Smaller sites will also have limits in the clinical skills of available teaching staff (McCusker 2004; Bruening and Maddern 2009). In addition to this, clinical teaching staff may be part time or volunteers (Collins et al. 2007; Sandhu 2018). Faculty are increasingly expected to teach in domains and structures different from what they experienced, which is perhaps reflected in an increasing number of faculty taking postgraduate education (Morris and Swanwick 2018).

Hybrid Distant and Direct Surgical Training

One solution adopted to resolve these tensions is a hybrid model, combining both distant and face-to-face education. Medical and surgical education can be imagined as two streams: applied or patient facing and non-applied or nontechnical education. Applied training occurs in all clinical settings and is usually embedded in a hospital placement. It might include applied anatomy ("What is that structure?"), technical skills training ("Retract more with your left hand"), and nontechnical teaching ("How would you explain risk management to this patient?"). This education is grounded in the clinical experience and fits well into workplace teaching, provided by clinical hospital supervisors.

Many training programs also use non-applied or pure education programs like lectures, tutorials, online modules, or simulation sessions. As these are not directly linked to a hospital setting, they can be administered independent of their workplace. Options for this include intensive "boot-camps" (Yeh et al. 2017) distance or online learning modules (Jayakumar et al. 2015; Wu et al. 2009), self-education (Artino and Jones 2013; Kassab et al. 2011; McGann et al. 2021), or rolling face-to-face education in different locations. This centralized portion can be scheduled to allow a full-time independent educator, while allowing those with less time or experience to focus on workplace training (Anthony and Muralidharan 2019).

The Challenges of Providing Surgical Education at a Distance

Traditional strategies in surgical training have emphasized self-directed learning guided by a published curriculum. Formal teaching might consist of lectures, or online content, such as modules, or even podcasts or simulations (Collins et al. 2007). Attendance at centralized short skills courses has also been used (Yeh et al. 2017). However, surgical training is not limited to synchronous teaching, and embracing newer flexible technologies may facilitate better educational outcomes (Booth et al. 2009).

Distance learning has restrictions that should be recognized in order to create an optimum environment. Distance students may be prone to isolation and their progress may be more difficult to track (Harwood et al. 2018). This can be alleviated with video conferencing and other community-building techniques (Locatis et al. 2010). Providing teaching material to multiple sites can be complex and may lead to reliance on online content over physical or other material (Williams et al. 2021; Berndt et al. 2017). However, some skills are difficult to teach in pure distance mode and require innovative approaches (Williams et al. 2021; Wright et al. 2012).

There are also limitations based specifically on using distance learning as a component of a bigger program, which can cause conflicts between face-to-face responsibilities and distance responsibilities (O'Grady et al. 2010).

Distance education has advantages over conventional education. Students or trainees are able to plan their own time flexibly, to adapt to their working environment (Harwood et al. 2018). Students with special needs can adapt the program to be easier to access. Travel is reduced, which improves overall safety for those learning in addition to full-time working obligation. Reduced use of face-to-face teaching also means educators' have more time to spend on areas requiring more flexibility, like well-being, student progress, and extension programs (McQueen et al. 2021a, b).

Some techniques, such as asynchronous learning (de Jong et al. 2013; Burnette et al. 2009) and online one-many content or MOOC teaching (Pickering and Swinnerton 2017) can be specifically used to overcome some limitations of distance learning.

Skills Teaching in Distance Education

Skills and technical teaching in true distance mode is very challenging. Ultimately, clinical exposure is required to learn clinical skills well (Hernandez et al. 2018), although simulation can be used to facilitate learning and competency assessment. Multiple solutions exist to facilitate skills teaching, including boot camp-style centralized teaching (Yeh et al. 2017; Kassam et al. 2021; Wang et al. 2020), crowdsourced feedback (Dai et al. 2017), and self-directed teaching (Nayar et al. 2020). The design of this support will differ according to program resources.

Simulation is a useful addition to ward and theatre-based teaching, but it can be difficult to provide in a peripheral setting, particularly where the experience of the trainees is variable. As simulation can be experienced away from the clinical setting, this may be provided by the central hub in teaching camps or training weekends (Yeh et al. 2017) (expanded in later sections). This approach is financially and education-ally viable, as the facilities can be set up or rented for brief periods and provided to each cohort in a group. This allows trainees to work at an appropriate skill level.

Telemonitoring of procedures can also be used to improve training. This involves the mentoring or supervision of a distant operation, leveraging video and audio linkup. Technical skill development and telementoring have been shown to be suitable for advanced and infrequent surgery, particularly in video-assisted surgery (Snyderman et al. 2016). This also promotes the development of distant faculty over a longer time.

Educational Techniques That Support the Surgical Training Program

Technology Enhanced Learning

Technology enhanced learning (TEL) is the most obvious innovation to facilitate distance education (Ellaway 2018). Many distance education courses use blended learning, incorporating both face-to-face (online or real life) and digital content. Electronic resources are more scalable, adapt to different educational styles, and allow asynchronous access of material (Ellaway 2018; Masters and Ellaway 2008). Technology can be used as support only, or as pure content, without any educator or mediator present (Ellaway 2018). Online videos have been shown to enhance learning of practical skills (Hamm et al. 2013). Technological tools can also facilitate peer-to-peer interactions and social support, and even class discussions that might be impossible if limited to traditional formats (Ellaway 2018). Technology can also increase student engagement in education by flattening the relationship between tutors and students (Masters and Ellaway 2008). Furthermore, as discussion is more malleable, the students can shift the focus, facilitating a student-centered experience.

Limitations to Digital Solutions

It is important to note that technical limitations may limit online access, and these are more common in regional or rural centers and smaller hospitals. Internet-based tools are limited by available internet speed, and some online tools may even be limited by the slowest user (Nartker et al. 2010; Ellaway 2018). This can be ameliorated by allowing students to download particularly large files offline, or overnight, but can still limit video use (Masters and Ellaway 2008). Students may only be able to access the internet through a hospital provider, which may have security limitations and firewalls (Masters and Ellaway 2008). The burden of software purchase may also fall to the trainee, increasing the cost of training (Masters and Ellaway 2008).

Design of digital approaches is also important to usability. Poor design may simply broadcast information to students without following up outcomes or input (Locatis et al. 2010). As workplace e-learners are often well-versed in technology, a poorly designed user experience can amplify frustrations (Booth et al. 2009).

Technological solutions also are prone to other risks of distance education. There may be an imbalance between on-site and distance participants in a hybrid program (Locatis et al. 2010). A key risk in this area is managing the trainee's time obligations with their clinical workplace and educational obligations. Online teaching can contribute to this burden (Locatis et al. 2010).

Maintaining Connection Online

Technology can also foster collaboration and community with a geographically dispersed cohort (Locatis et al. 2010; Jones-Bonofiglio et al. 2018). Noninteractive online tuition is associated with lower student satisfaction and poorer educational outcomes (Nartker et al. 2010; Booth et al. 2009; Locatis et al. 2010; Jones-Bonofiglio et al. 2018). Blended courses, where students have met facilitators and other members of the cohort in person, foster authenticity and a feeling of safety (Booth et al. 2009; Locatis et al. 2010). Interaction with a teacher or moderator is a key factor in maintaining progress in online teaching (Jordan et al. 2013).

Flipped classroom approaches can maximize the value of face-to-face time, by having the students cover the coursework in a self-directed way, before having a face-to-face or online discussion (Jones-Bonofiglio et al. 2018). With this pattern, the teacher can adapt to issues in class time, rather than teach core material.

Boot Camps and Intensive Face-to-Face Teaching

Short centralized intensive classes or boot camps can be used to facilitate distance education (Yeh et al. 2017). These intensives can be structured as short workshops over 2 or 3 days, which may risk overscheduling if provided on weekends or days off. Blocks of 1–2 weeks are an effective alternative, as they provide space to focus on learning and study. Boot camps can cover non-patient facing skills like judgment and communication (Collins et al. 2007; Hernandez et al. 2018), as well as simulation opportunities (Sandhu 2018). In addition, subject experts or specialized staff like actors can be scheduled (Anthony and Muralidharan 2019).

There are numerous advantages of this approach, including planned access to expensive or bulky equipment or labs and improved flexibility. A boot camp program can be changed every time, in contrast to online or distance teaching modules that usually are less agile. External courses in relevant areas like leadership, ethics, team management, or research skills can also be integrated into the program, which reduces faculty burden, while providing expert tuition (Sandhu 2018).

Self-Directed Learning

Self-directed learning has always been a cornerstone of surgical education, typically with little moderation except by published curriculum. This approach works well with a geographically distributed student group, as long as they have equal access to required resources. Learner control has been shown to be a key value point in existing distance education programs (Booth et al. 2009), and the program should leverage this opportunity to allow the trainee to direct their own program to some degree, but maintain teacher interaction where possible (Jordan et al. 2013).

Effective design can make self-directed learning very flexible. Self-directed simulation programs in technical skills can be effective, if they are administered over time, and incorporate self-assessment tools (Wright et al. 2012). Group assignments can be successful even if participants are not colocated (Booth et al. 2009).

Resource availability may be an issue. For example, assignments may require resources that have different availability in different settings. In addition to internet speed mentioned above, some settings might have less complex patients, less specialized support staff, or supervising surgeons, which may limit the complexity of work. Resources that can be accessed asynchronously promote flexible self-directed learning (Jordan et al. 2013).

Resource availability can be included in program design. Self-directed learning can be based around various resources – traditional physical textbooks, online repositories, podcasts, social media, or other portable education techniques. Traditional paper-based texts are expensive to maintain and a burden to smaller hospital libraries, but distributed paper materials are typically a lower cost alternative (Nartker et al. 2010). Institutional online journal subscriptions and health coalition sites, like UpToDate, can also be helpful.

New Media in Surgical Education

New media such as social media and portable education tools can also be used to support education (Sterling et al. 2017). It is not time restricted and it is user moderated, so provides personalized content (Hamm et al. 2013). Microblogging services, such as twitter, can actually be used to moderate the available material, via discussion with experts, and the ethical and practical comments that act as footnotes to the linked material. Educational material can be accessed on longer form sites, such as wikis, blogs, and microblogs, or streaming video sites (Hamm et al. 2013; Sterling et al. 2017). Blogs have been used to support journal clubs and other ongoing education programs (Sterling et al. 2017). A single topic can be viewed in many different formats, which allows the student to tailor their own learning experience according to preference (Glick and Yamout 2012).

Podcasts can allow moderated asynchronous content, such as discussion of papers (Sterling et al. 2017) and lecture content (Samuels et al. 2020; White et al. 2011; Sandars 2009). Dedicated academic podcasts can improve outcomes over traditional didactic education and unsegmented podcasts (Abate 2013). These types of media can also be used effectively for exam revision (Shantikumar 2009). Additionally, many podcasting platforms are accessible publicly, augmenting the teaching material that a single site can provide (White et al. 2011).

Microblogging platforms such as Twitter are increasingly used for education support. Information provided via these platforms is difficult to review, making it more unreliable than moderated material (Brady et al. 2017; Vukušić Rukavina et al. 2021). However, social media platforms are excellent at providing peer support and community, often using hashtags (Ovaere et al. 2018), backchannel discussion and highlighting new research and information (Sterling et al. 2017). If students understand the limitations of crowdsourced information, microblogging platforms can be a useful adjunct.

Peer-Led Education

With a geographically dispersed cohort and a part-time volunteer faculty (Anthony and Muralidharan 2019), peer-led education is a useful tool (Rees et al. 2016).

The creation of learning communities can facilitate this. In this model, a group of learners is intentionally created with an assigned faculty member (Hernandez et al. 2018). This model allows a forum-based discussion. It also allows emotional support, longitudinal cohort development, and forms the basis for individualized learning plans. Facilitation of community is important (Booth et al. 2009) and can be effectively provided within peer education (MacMillan et al. 2016). Online and distance programs could consider a student-only discussion forum (Booth et al. 2009). An alternative strategy might be to facilitate social media interaction between students, with dedicated groups or hashtags.

Facilitating Asynchronous Education

One of the key challenges in surgical education is finding the balance between service provision and education. Trainees are often studying in addition to long paid working hours and on call schedules, including weekend commitment (O'Grady et al. 2010). Provision of education should not limit clinical exposure in the workplace, so flexible and asynchronous access is vital (Booth et al. 2009).

Technology can facilitate geographically dispersed and asynchronous education modalities, allowing education where it was previously too difficult (Jones-Bonofiglio et al. 2018; Eggermont et al. 2013). An example is an online lecture or webinar which is able to be accessed later by a trainee who was on call, who then can still participate in the ongoing discussion (Vo et al. 2019). In fact, social media is a boon to health informatics, as it is by nature not time restricted, and can have inherent opportunities for clarification by expert moderators' comments (Hamm et al. 2013). Blogs, microblogs, and vodcasts provide greater access to groups of experienced clinicians at any time of the day (Glick and Yamout 2012).

However, purely asynchronous delivery reduces interaction between faculty and students, which can impair educational outcomes and satisfaction (Englander and Carraccio 2018). A danger of asynchronous curriculum development is expansion of time obligation, as one is no longer limited to 24-hour clock. Many trainees work a full-time job (O'Grady et al. 2010) and may not have protected training time. Defeating the limitations of time, scheduling can also lead to challenges to the concepts of "working hours" and "non-working hours" (Masters and Ellaway 2008), and create a situation where trainees essentially have no personal or recovery time. Reviews have demonstrated that educational programs with greater flexibility of administration, with built in "Catch-up" time, are much more accessible for students, as they allow for individual differences in sick leave, conferences, and busy work time (Booth et al. 2009).

Ideally, a blend of synchronous and asynchronous techniques is likely to lead to the best outcomes for students and educators (Jones-Bonofiglio et al. 2018).

The Impact of Decentralized Training on Assessment

As we move away from exit assessment and toward longitudinal and programmatic assessment, the faculty workload and impact increases (Morris and Swanwick 2018). It also becomes more difficult to manage a decentralized cohort (Sandhu 2018; Udemans et al. 2018). Assessment is easier if there is an increased focus on workplace low-stakes assessment, although significant faculty training is required (Schut et al. 2021). A focus on entrustable professional activities make assessment more accessible and consistent with inexperienced faculty (Ten Cate et al. 2017).

Automatic assessment can be used, although digital identity verification becomes more important (Masters and Ellaway 2008), particularly when assessment is based on asynchronous participation. Online systems with automatic assessment have some limits assessing clinically relevant tasks. Crowdsourced, nonexpert can be used to assess and give feedback on recorded tasks, which might be useful for formative and lower stakes assessment (Dai et al. 2017).

Higher stakes exams are demanding from an administrative point of view and are more commonly held as a massed cohort in a central location (Torre et al. 2021). This approach will also be required for assessments requiring specialized staff or equipment. However, online and virtual assessment techniques have developed through the experience of social restrictions due to pandemic (Hauer et al. 2021; Graffeo et al. 2020). These innovations may be useful in post-pandemic education but are unlikely to completely replace face-to-face assessment. While online tests are easy to administer, this mode of assessment limits the types of assessment that can be provided. Online testing also favors those more familiar with its use (Ellaway 2018).

Other Challenges of Distance Education

Reduced Community

Distance education communities can suffer from lack of community (Locatis et al. 2010; Bernard et al. 2004). The use of synchronous online teaching such as webinars can create an adequate sense of presence to counteract this feeling (Locatis et al. 2010). Social media of various types can also foster community, as can online student discussion groups (Ovaere et al. 2018). Many distance course designs consider assessment and parity, but community and isolation are also important. Solutions will vary according to group size and balance of distance and in person education, and may include private online forums or chat rooms, for both faculty and students.

Difficulty with Monitoring Longitudinal Progress

Trainees at risk may also be overlooked, as they are not seen in the context of their cohort. Lack of engagement may mask genuine issues with content, and this is difficult to detect, particularly when trainees have serial appointments at different hospitals, which hide patterns of behavior. Supervisors also do not trust official portfolios (Schut et al. 2021; Castanelli et al. 2020). This effect is mitigated by longitudinal assessment using different modalities, and particularly with longitudinal mentor or supervisor involvement (Torre et al. 2021; Bok et al. 2018).

Digital Privacy

A further risk of increasing online education is the online permanence of classroom or discussion room transcripts. There is a potential risk that a person's career can be read from medical school forward. For example, there is a potential confidentiality burden when the historical classroom conversations of the future head of department are discoverable (Ellaway 2018). Online privacy and security measures might include closed classrooms, digital destruction of discussions, and other measures (Thoma et al. 2020).

Faculty Support and Development

Dedicated faculty training for distance curriculum is important, as traditional teaching skills are not directly transferable (Nartker et al. 2010). This is particularly difficult in surgical training, as one workplace faculty member may interact with a single trainee, where another might have responsibility for many. Achievement of education standards in each area relies, in part, on a preexisting education culture in the department (Sandhu 2018), as well as focused faculty development and support. Peripheral faculty (in clinical workplaces) are primarily responsible for clinical and technical teaching, as well as trainee well-being, and future career advice (Anthony and Muralidharan 2019). Educators might be involved in curriculum development and centralized assessment. In both instances, formal faculty development is recommended (Gunderman 2011).

Unfortunately, the development of peripheral faculty has the same challenges as distance education of trainees (Morris and Swanwick 2018). In addition, education responsibilities may be part time or casual and often are not remunerated.

Training of the peripheral faculty might focus applied skills including surgical skills development, feedback, coaching, reflection, and other skills that support clinical learning. Flexible options for educator training are required in order to not increase the burden on volunteers. Incorporating education development activities into regular continuing medical education gives surgeons development opportunities (Morris and Swanwick 2018). Telemonitoring and mentoring of faculty can also be used to facilitate faculty development (Williams et al. 2021; Snyderman et al. 2016; Augestad et al. 2013). This reduces the travel burden for faculty and improves outcomes and can be adapted to the specific limitations of the hospital location.

Education-Centered Workplace

One of the challenges of surgical training is the conflict between education and service provision. Workplace learning may also be undervalued, because it has less focus than formal education (Morris 2018); however, workplace learning is vital because it allows contextualization of knowledge (Wilkinson 2017). When training programs are planned with intention, they can be designed as educational centered workplaces. This can be matched by improved patient outcomes (Hernandez et al. 2018). An example would be a pediatric residency program set up with "teaching units" with restricted patient-doctor ratios, married to "service units" to manage the remainder of community need. Due to the increased patient, family, and community involvement in each health care admission, the patients on the teaching unit had better outcomes and lower readmission rates (Hernandez et al. 2018). Another approach is to remove tasks with both low clinical and educational impact from registrar responsibilities, increasing the quality of the working time (Hernandez et al. 2018). This workplace design can facilitate both workplace learning and assessment.

Workplace assessment and teaching needs to adapt to different competencies, and it needs to adapt to reflect feedback and assessment (Wilkinson 2017). This is an ideal place to implement the cycle of learning. Effective intervention offers just-in-time information with effective briefing, well-supervised practice, and timely feedback (Wilkinson 2017). The workplace is an ideal place to teach team-training and team science, as well as interdisciplinary work (Sandhu 2018). This casual, apprenticeship-style workplace learning can be augmented by the nomination of a workplace mentor, guest speakers, real case studies, and problem-based scenarios (Booth et al. 2009).

Opportunities in Blending Distance and Face-to-Face Education

If we embrace the diversity of the surgical training cohort, including their time pressures and geographic decentralization, we can provide quality distance education. This is facilitated by a blended or dual curriculum with a central "theoretical and simulation" faculty and a peripheral workplace focusing on applied surgical education. This can combine online and face-to-face contact to effectively to maximum advantage. The main risks of the distance component are disengagement and irrelevance of content. The risks of peripheral workplace education relate to lack of consistency and disconnection with the cohort – the trainee who becomes "lost in the system."

With this in mind, the roles of the workplace and central educational hub are different (see Table 1). The central hub can more easily focus on longitudinal development, exam preparation, nonclinical skills, simulation, and nontechnical skills. The peripheral workplace might focus on personalized supervision and feedback, coaching, applied development of technical and nontechnical clinical skills, and professional identity development. Both should work in concert to ensure there is balance between service and education requirements to reduce trainee burnout.

Suggestions for Improving Distance Education Programs

Distance education programs can be designed to combine distance modules with face-to-face learning in an effective way. Student-centered clinical sites can also be developed to maximize the value of workplace education (Hernandez et al. 2018). However, as demonstrated during pandemic-associated restrictions, many standard surgical education programs can be adapted to distance paradigms (Tuma et al. 2021; Al-Balas et al. 2020; Hauer et al. 2021; Schmitz et al. 2021).

In development of a distance or hybrid program, the following issues should be considered:

1. **Longitudinal continuity to monitor progression and safety**. This might be provided by a stable workplace or by central educational hub.
2. **Student support and community**. Distance education has reduced community within the training level or cohort, but this can be deliberately improved with online forums and discussions or central boot camp or training opportunities.
3. **Opportunities for training in surgical skills**, including both workplace training and simulation training opportunities.
4. **Assessment design**. Assessments can be administered in different environments. A longitudinal portfolio is particularly useful if trainees move through different sites and progression needs to be monitored.
5. **Digital security and safety**, as many distance courses are administered online.
6. **Faculty support**, tailored to the needs of faculty who might have different responsibilities, particularly in hybrid program design.

Table 1 Hub and spoke model of surgical education

	Peripheral or workplace environment	Central environment or hub
Typical relationship with trainees	Single multiple rotations of discrete time period (usually months)	Whole cohort oversight from acceptance into surgical training to assessment and qualification.
Clinical exposure	Each rotation exposes trainee to a single clinical unit which may be specialized, with experts in that clinical field. There is exposure to clinical cases and situational learning	None. Simulation, and technology enhanced modes only
Typical faculty skills	Expert in one clinical field. May have much less training in education, but is usually familiar with mentoring a trainee through clinical experiences	Can employ experienced and qualified surgical educators to manage the program. Experts can be employed for short courses.
Typical faculty restraints	Often part time or casual, and may not be directly remunerated for education	Can be dedicated educators. May have limited face-to-face exposure to trainees. Depending on expertise may not be registered surgeons
Typical education style	Teaching on the run. May have limited formal nonclinical training time Inconsistent training across rotations, both in exposure and faculty skill	Formal education within the limits of distance constraints, either by providing the distance curriculum or central skills camps or courses This may involve online lecture, webinar, asynchronous online courses, reading lists, and short face-to-face courses and assessments
Educational strengths	Skills teaching Trainee development over rotation Mentoring and professional identity formation	Focus on breadth of curriculum Can leverage expert tutors in specialty or uncommon areas
Resources	Variable resources depending on the clinical communities served. Physical resources in libraries, simulation equipment, and infrastructure may be limited	May be better funded, with better facilities or equipment
Assessment strengths	Short clinical assessments Assessment of professional skills Competence assessment (in field of expertise)	Assessment for the whole cohort, such as high-stakes exams or high-stakes committees. Monitoring of longitudinal progress including logbooks and trainees at risk of poor progressing Benchmarking and credentialing
Limitations	Small trainee group More limited resources (physical library, simulation equipment, etc.)	Likely to be at a distance from some or most of the cohort
Typical cohort	One or few trainees in one location, or varying educational level	Care for the entire cohort both cross-sectionally and longitudinally

Conclusion

Surgical trainees are at risk of isolation, and workforces are distributed geographically in many states and countries. This may be exacerbated by natural disasters or health crises. In many centers, there has been rapid adoption of distance education programs. By reflecting on what is known about distance and flexible education, educational outcomes of surgical training might be improved into the future. Curriculum design should allow space for trainees to work and recreate while maintaining longitudinal progress and standards. Faculty development should focus at least partly on inspiring more student-centered approaches, by discussion of different successful rotation and hospital administrative design. The use of a deliberate approach will allow development of more flexible surgical training into the future.

Cross-References

▶ Screen-Based Learning
▶ Technology Considerations in Health Professions and Clinical Education

References

Abate KS. The effect of podcast lectures on nursing students' knowledge retention and application. Nurs Educ Perspect. 2013;34(3):182–5.

Al-Balas M, Al-Balas HI, Jaber HM, Obeidat K, Al-Balas H, Aborajooh EA, et al. Distance learning in clinical medical education amid COVID-19 pandemic in Jordan: current situation, challenges, and perspectives. BMC Med Educ. 2020;20(1):341.

Anthony A, Muralidharan V. The contemporary context of surgical education. In: Nestel D, Dalrymple K, Paige JT, Aggarwal R, editors. Advancing surgical education: theory, evidence and practice [Internet]. Singapore: Springer; 2019. p. 17–31. https://doi.org/10.1007/978-981-13-3128-2_3.

Artino AR, Jones KD. AM last page: self-regulated learning – a dynamic, cyclical perspective. Acad Med. 2013;88(7):1048.

Augestad KM, Bellika JG, Budrionis A, Chomutare T, Lindsetmo R-O, Patel H, et al. Surgical telementoring in knowledge translation – clinical outcomes and educational benefits: a comprehensive review. Surg Innov. 2013;20(3):273–81.

Battat R, Jhonson M, Wiseblatt L, Renard C, Habib L, Normil M, et al. The Haiti medical education project: development and analysis of a competency based continuing medical education course in Haiti through distance learning. BMC Med Educ. 2016;16(1):275, s12909-016-0795-x.

Bernard RM, Abrami PC, Lou Y, Borokhovski E, Wade A, Wozney L, et al. How does distance education compare with classroom instruction? A meta-analysis of the empirical literature. Rev Educ Res. 2004;74(3):379–439.

Berndt A, Murray CM, Kennedy K, Stanley MJ, Gilbert-Hunt S. Effectiveness of distance learning strategies for continuing professional development (CPD) for rural allied health practitioners: a systematic review. BMC Med Educ. 2017;17(1):117.

Bok HGJ, de Jong LH, O'Neill T, Maxey C, Hecker KG. Validity evidence for programmatic assessment in competency-based education. Perspect Med Educ. 2018;7(6):362–72.

Booth A, Carroll C, Papaioannou D, Sutton A, Wong R. Applying findings from a systematic review of workplace-based e-learning: implications for health information professionals. Health Info Libr J. 2009;26(1):4–21.

Brady J, Kelly M, Stein S. The trump effect: with no peer review, how do we know what to really believe on social media? Clin Colon Rectal Surg. 2017;30(04):270–6.

Bruening MH, Maddern GJ. Rural surgery: the Australian experience. Surg Clin North Am. 2009;89(6):1325–33.

Burnette K, Ramundo M, Stevenson M, Beeson MS. Evaluation of a web-based asynchronous pediatric emergency medicine learning tool for residents and medical students: EVALUATION OF A WEB-BASED ASYNCHRONOUS PEM LEARNING TOOL. Acad Emerg Med. 2009;16:S46–50.

Castanelli DJ, Weller JM, Molloy E, Bearman M. Shadow systems in assessment: how supervisors make progress decisions in practice. Adv Health Sci Educ. 2020;25(1):131–47.

Collins JP, Gough IR, Civil ID, Stitz RW. A new surgical education and training programme. ANZ J Surg. 2007;77(7):497–501.

Dai JC, Lendvay TS, Sorensen MD. Crowdsourcing in surgical skills acquisition: a developing technology in surgical education. J Grad Med Educ. 2017;9(6):697–705.

de Jong N, Verstegen DML, Tan FES, O'Connor SJ. A comparison of classroom and online asynchronous problem-based learning for students undertaking statistics training as part of a Public Health Masters degree. Adv Health Sci Educ. 2013;18(2):245–64.

Eggermont S, Bloemendaal PM, van Baalen JM. E-learning any time any place anywhere on mobile devices. Perspect Med Educ. 2013;2(2):95–8.

Ellaway RH. Technology-enhanced learning. In: Swanwick T, Forrest K, O'Brien BC, editors. Understanding medical education [Internet]. Chichester: Wiley; 2018. [cited 2021 Jun 1]. p. 139–49. https://doi.org/10.1002/9781119373780.ch10.

Englander R, Carraccio C. A lack of continuity in education, training, and practice violates the 'Do No Harm' principle. Acad Med J Assoc Am Med Coll. 2018;93(3S Competency-Based, Time-Variable Education in the Health Professions):S12–6.

Geissbuhler A, Bagayoko CO, Ly O. The RAFT network: 5 years of distance continuing medical education and tele-consultations over the Internet in French-speaking Africa. Int J Med Inform. 2007;76(5–6):351–6.

Glick PL, Yamout SZ. Social media for surgeons: understand it, embrace it, and leverage it for our profession and our patient. Surgery. 2012;152(5):941–2.

Graffeo CS, Elder BD, Van Gompel JJ, Daniels DJ. Digitally decentralised mock oral board examination for neurological surgery trainees. Med Educ. 2020;54(9):854–5.

Gunderman RB. Education matters. In: Achieving excellence in medical education [Internet]. London: Springer; 2011. [cited 2021 Jun 1]. p. 1–16. https://doi.org/10.1007/978-0-85729-307-7_1.

Hamm MP, Chisholm A, Shulhan J, Milne A, Scott SD, Klassen TP, et al. Social media use by health care professionals and trainees: a scoping review. Acad Med. 2013;88(9):1376–83.

Harwood KJ, McDonald PL, Butler JT, Drago D, Schlumpf KS. Comparing student outcomes in traditional vs intensive, online graduate programs in health professional education. BMC Med Educ. 2018;18(1):240.

Hauer KE, Lockspeiser TM, Chen HC. The COVID-19 pandemic as an imperative to advance medical student assessment: three areas for change. Acad Med J Assoc Am Med Coll. 2021;96 (2):182–5.

Hernandez RG, Hopkins A, Dudas RA. The evolution of graduate medical education over the past decade: building a new pediatric residency program in an era of innovation. Med Teach. 2018;40(6):615–21.

Jayakumar N, Brunckhorst O, Dasgupta P, Khan MS, Ahmed K. e-Learning in surgical education: a systematic review. J Surg Educ. 2015;72(6):1145–57.

Jones-Bonofiglio KD, Willett T, Ng S. An evaluation of flipped e-learning experiences. Med Teach. 2018;40(9):953–61.

Jordan J, Jalali A, Clarke S, Dyne P, Spector T, Coates W. Asynchronous vs didactic education: it's too early to throw in the towel on tradition. BMC Med Educ. 2013;13(1):105.

Kassab E, Tun JK, Arora S, King D, Ahmed K, Miskovic D, et al. 'Blowing up the barriers' in surgical training: exploring and validating the concept of distributed simulation. Ann Surg. 2011;254(6):1059–65.

Kassam A-F, Singer KE, Winer LK, Browne D, Sussman JJ, Goodman MD, et al. Acquisition and retention of surgical skills taught during intern surgical boot camp. Am J Surg. 2021;221(5):987–92.

Locatis C, Berner ES, Hammack G, Smith S, Maisiak R, Ackerman M. An exploratory study of co-location as a factor in synchronous, collaborative medical informatics distance education. BMC Res Notes. 2010;3(1):30.

MacMillan TE, Rawal S, Cram P, Liu J. A journal club for peer mentorship: helping to navigate the transition to independent practice. Perspect Med Educ. 2016;5(5):312–5.

Masters K, Ellaway R. e-Learning in medical education guide 32 Part 2: technology, management and design. Med Teach. 2008;30(5):474–89.

McCusker BJ. Training our future rural medical workforce. Med J Aust. 2004;180(12):651–2.

McGann KC, Melnyk R, Saba P, Joseph J, Glocker RJ, Ghazi A. Implementation of an E-learning academic elective for hands-on basic surgical skills to supplement medical school surgical education. J Surg Educ. 2021;78(4):1164–74.

McQueen S, Mobilio MH, Moulton C. Fractured in surgery: understanding stress as a holistic and subjective surgeon experience. Am J Surg. 2021a;221(4):793–8.

McQueen SA, Hammond Mobilio M, Moulton C. Pulling our lens backwards to move forward: an integrated approach to physician distress. Med Humanit. 2021b;medhum-2020-012100.

Mercier PJ, Skube SJ, Leonard SL, McElroy AN, Goettl TG, Najarian MM, et al. Creating a rural surgery track and a review of rural surgery training programs. J Surg Educ. 2019;76(2):459–68.

Morris C. Work-based learning. In: Swanwick T, Forrest K, O'Brien BC, editors. Understanding medical education [Internet]. Chichester: Wiley; 2018. [cited 2021 Jun 1]. p. 163–77. https://doi.org/10.1002/9781119373780.ch12.

Morris C, Swanwick T. From the workshop to the workplace: relocating faculty development in postgraduate medical education. Med Teach. 2018;40(6):622–6.

Nartker AJ, Stevens L, Shumays A, Kalowela M, Kisimbo D, Potter K. Increasing health worker capacity through distance learning: a comprehensive review of programmes in Tanzania. Hum Resour Health. 2010;8(1):30.

Nayar SK, Musto L, Baruah G, Fernandes R, Bharathan R. Self-assessment of surgical skills: a systematic review. J Surg Educ. 2020;77(2):348–61.

Nicholas C, Hatchell A, Webb C, Temple-Oberle C. COVID-19 and the impact on surgical fellows: uniquely vulnerable learners. J Surg Educ. 2021;78(2):375–8.

O'Grady G, Loveday B, Harper S, Adams B, Civil ID, Peters M. Working hours and roster structures of surgical trainees in Australia and New Zealand: working hours of Australasian trainees. ANZ J Surg. 2010;80(12):890–5.

Ovaere S, Zimmerman DDE, Brady RR. Social media in surgical training: opportunities and risks. J Surg Educ. 2018;75(6):1423–9.

Pickering JD, Swinnerton BJ. An anatomy massive open online course as a continuing professional development tool for healthcare professionals. Med Sci Educ. 2017;27(2):243–52.

Rees EL, Quinn PJ, Davies B, Fotheringham V. How does peer teaching compare to faculty teaching? A systematic review and meta-analysis. Med Teach. 2016;38(8):829–37.

Samuels JM, Halpern AL, Carmichael H, Christian NT, Travis CEM, Jaiswal K, et al. This surgical life – an exploration of surgical department podcasting. J Surg Educ. 2020;77(5):1257–65.

Sandars J. Twelve tips for using podcasts in medical education. Med Teach. 2009;31(5):387–9.

Sandhu D. Postgraduate medical education – challenges and innovative solutions. Med Teach. 2018;40(6):607–9.

Schmitz SM, Schipper S, Lemos M, Alizai PH, Kokott E, Brozat JF, et al. Development of a tailor-made surgical online learning platform, ensuring surgical education in times of the COVID19 pandemic. BMC Surg. 2021;21(1):196.

Schut S, Maggio LA, Heeneman S, van Tartwijk J, van der Vleuten C, Driessen E. Where the rubber meets the road – an integrative review of programmatic assessment in health care professions education. Perspect Med Educ. 2021;10(1):6–13.

Shantikumar S. From lecture theatre to portable media: students' perceptions of an enhanced podcast for revision. Med Teach. 2009;31(6):535–8.

Snyderman CH, Gardner PA, Lanisnik B, Ravnik J. Surgical telementoring: a new model for surgical training: surgical telementoring. Laryngoscope. 2016;126(6):1334–8.

Sterling M, Leung P, Wright D, Bishop TF. The use of social media in graduate medical education: a systematic review. Acad Med. 2017;92(7):1043–56.

Ten Cate O, Tobin S, Stokes M. Bringing competencies closer to day-to-day clinical work through entrustable professional activities. Med J Aust. 2017;206(1):14–6.

Thoma B, Warm E, Hamstra SJ, Cavalcanti R, Pusic M, Shaw T, et al. Next steps in the implementation of learning analytics in medical education: consensus from an international cohort of medical educators. J Grad Med Educ. 2020;12(3):303–11.

Torre D, Rice NE, Ryan A, Bok H, Dawson LJ, Bierer B, et al. Ottawa 2020 consensus statements for programmatic assessment – 2. Implementation and practice. Med Teach. 2021;1–12

Tuma F, Kamel MK, Shebrain S, Ghanem M, Blebea J. Alternatives surgical training approaches during COVID-19 pandemic. Ann Med Surg. 2021;62:253–7.

Udemans R, Stokes M-L, Rigby L, Khanna P, Christiansen J. Educational renewal of physician training in Australia and New Zealand: multiple educational innovations in a complex environment. Med Teach. 2018;40(6):627–32.

Vo T, Ledbetter C, Zuckerman M. Video delivery of toxicology educational content versus textbook for asynchronous learning, using acetaminophen overdose as a topic. Clin Toxicol. 2019;57(10): 842–6.

Vukušić Rukavina T, Viskić J, Machala Poplašen L, Relić D, Marelić M, Jokic D, et al. Dangers and benefits of social media on E-Professionalism of health care professionals: scoping review. J Med Internet Res. 2021;23(11):e25770.

Wang W, Ma H, Ren H, Wang Z, Mao L, He N. The impact of surgical boot camp and subsequent repetitive practice on the surgical skills and confidence of residents. World J Surg. 2020;44(11): 3607–15.

Wearne SM, Dornan T, Teunissen PW, Skinner T. Supervisor continuity or co-location: which matters in residency education? Findings from a qualitative study of remote supervisor Family Physicians in Australia and Canada. Acad Med. 2015;90(4):525–31.

White JS, Sharma N, Boora P. Surgery 101: evaluating the use of podcasting in a general surgery clerkship. Med Teach. 2011;33(11):941–3.

Wilkinson TJ. Kolb, integration and the messiness of workplace learning. Perspect Med Educ. 2017;6(3):144–5.

Williams TP, Klimberg V, Perez A. Tele-education assisted mentorship in surgery (TEAMS). J Surg Oncol. 2021;124(2):250–4.

Wright AS, McKenzie J, Tsigonis A, Jensen AR, Figueredo EJ, Kim S, et al. A structured self-directed basic skills curriculum results in improved technical performance in the absence of expert faculty teaching. Surgery. 2012;151(6):808–14.

Wu BJ, Dietz PA, Bordley J, Borgstrom DC. A Novel, web-based application for assessing and enhancing practice-based learning in surgery residency. J Surg Educ. 2009;66(1):3–7.

Yeh DH, Fung K, Malekzadeh S. Boot camps: preparing for residency. Otolaryngol Clin North Am. 2017;50(5):1003–13.

Mental Health Education: Contemporary Context and Future Directions

13

Christopher Kowalski and Chris Attoe

Contents

Introduction	218
Contemporary Context	219
Clinical	219
Educational	220
The Need for Change	222
Future Directions	223
Adopting the Right Approach	223
Getting the Design Right	228
Conclusion	242
Key Learning Points	243
Cross-References	243
References	243

Abstract

This chapter aims to orient the reader to contemporary context in mental health education while outlining current developments and new theoretical directions for the field.

Fragmented healthcare systems and the interrelatedness of mental and physical ill health necessitate integrated and collaborative ways of working in mental healthcare. At the same time, a lack of trained mental health professionals means that other health professionals will need to become competent in the assessment and management of mental health difficulties if population mental health is to improve.

C. Kowalski (✉)
Oxford Health NHS Foundation Trust, Oxford, UK
e-mail: chris.kowalski@nhs.net

C. Attoe
Maudsley Learning, South London and Maudsley NHS Foundation Trust, London, UK
e-mail: chris.attoe@kcl.ac.uk

© Springer Nature Singapore Pte Ltd. 2023
D. Nestel et al. (eds.), *Clinical Education for the Health Professions*,
https://doi.org/10.1007/978-981-15-3344-0_123

Given this, it is important to develop educational interventions that prepare healthcare professionals of all specialties to deliver mental healthcare. Here, novel ways of thinking about the pedagogy of mental health education are required. This includes reviewing the requisite learning outcomes and the pedagogical mechanisms required to achieve them. Innovative educational methods – including interprofessional education, co-production, and technology-enhanced learning – will be important in ensuring that future workforces are adequately prepared for working with those with mental health needs.

Keywords

Mental health education · Psychiatry · Psychotherapy · Interprofessional education · Technology-enhanced learning · Co-production · Humanism

Introduction

Although mental health education is an expanding field, our understanding of how best to educate health professionals for mental healthcare is still somewhat limited.

Given the increasing burden of mental health difficulties globally, it is clear that efforts to improve population mental health will need to be supported by high-quality educational initiatives. As such, our theoretical knowledge of how to achieve the varied learning outcomes required to ensure effective mental healthcare requires improvement.

Practically speaking, mental health education must support both the prevention and treatment of mental ill-health as well as the promotion of good mental well-being. To do so, it must seek to shift individual attitudes toward roles and responsibilities in these activities particularly where such attitudes prevent collaborative and holistic approaches to care.

While mental health professionals must lead efforts to improve population mental health, for this effort to be truly successful, *all* healthcare professionals will need to engage with the mental health needs of their service users. This imperative is borne out in the evidence on the interrelatedness of mental health and physical health and the impact that unmet need in either has on overall morbidity (Attoe et al. 2018; Lake and Turner 2017).

Furthermore, given the pervasive impact of mental ill health in all settings – be this social, occupational, or educational – promoting good mental health will need to become a collective responsibility of all of society rather than the sole responsibility of healthcare professionals (Longley et al. 2001).

As such, mental health education should not be delivered solely in the healthcare arena going forward, but in other institutions – both privately and publicly owned – as well. Only then can mental health difficulties be supported in a truly holistic way.

In this chapter, the clinical and educational contexts in which mental health education takes place will be discussed. In addition, new theoretical directions and potential instructional design elements will be considered. In particular, the need for alternative learning outcomes around altering healthcare professionals' disposition toward, and approach to, the delivery of mental healthcare will be discussed as will the pedagogical mechanisms that might be leveraged to achieve such outcomes. The specific educational methods through which such mechanisms might be actioned – including interprofessional education (IPE), co-production, and technology-enhanced learning (TEL) – will also be examined. Finally, past, present, and future uses of these methods in mental health education are outlined and their implications considered.

Despite focusing primarily on health professions education, some implications for mental health education outside of healthcare are also outlined.

Contemporary Context

Clinical

Globally, the prevalence of mental health difficulties appears to be increasing (Whiteford et al. 2013). The impact of this on individuals' social and occupational functioning, as well as their physical health, is keenly felt in healthcare, the workplace, education, the judicial system, and, most importantly, individuals' personal lives.

Given the societal and financial implications of poor mental health, not to mention its impact on quality of life, promoting good well-being appears to be an increasing priority on many government agendas (World Health Organization 2013; Eaton et al. 2011). In some countries, this has resulted in increased funding for mental health services (Liese et al. 2019). However, there is still a major discrepancy between funding in mental healthcare as compared to physical health specialties (Shah and Beinecke 2009). In addition, the chronic underfunding and under-resourcing of mental healthcare historically means that professionals are playing catch up in relation to improving the prevention and treatment of mental ill health (Patel et al. 2018).

Unsurprisingly, given this underfunding, healthcare systems globally are struggling to meet the mental health needs of an ever-expanding population. This is exacerbated by fragmented models of care that prevent effective collaboration across organizations (World Health Organization 2005).

Mental healthcare is particularly reflective of the problems of fragmented healthcare systems due to the pervasiveness of mental ill health, and its accompanying impact on morbidity, across all healthcare settings. In line with this, there is increasing recognition of the importance of addressing the overlap of mental and physical ill health in the manifestation of illness (Attoe et al. 2018). That is to say, physical health problems cannot be viewed in isolation from the mental health effects that they have and vice versa. This necessitates integrated models of care as well as effective interprofessional working. Similarly, individuals' mental health needs require support across the entire care continuum from primary to specialist care and from community to hospital settings.

Healthcare policy makers are beginning to develop strategies for creating systems that can meet healthcare needs in an efficient and effective manner. Where such transformative solutions are being devised, there needs to be similar thought given to transforming educational approaches so that healthcare professionals are prepared for the demands of working in these new systems. This requires a close examination of current educational paradigms and methods and the development of new practices that are commensurate with future working models.

An additional obstacle that governments are facing here is the fact that, globally, the number of psychiatrists and other mental health professionals does not match current demand (Saxena et al. 2007). Given the difficulties in recruiting to mental health posts, healthcare systems are having to rely more heavily on healthcare professionals from other specialties when managing mental health difficulties.

However, the relative impoverishment seen in mental healthcare funding is replicated in education settings, meaning that healthcare professionals may, at the time of qualification, have had limited exposure to mental health issues as well as inadequate education in caring for those with mental health needs (Happell 2010).

Thus, mental health education must adapt to take into account professionals whose specialist training may not have incorporated significant components related to mental healthcare. This leads to an additional educational conundrum in that such professionals may not feel that it is their role to engage in mental healthcare alongside their usual clinical work and yet will be called upon to do so.

Additionally, only a small proportion of those with mental health difficulties are actually seen in specialist healthcare contexts. Many individuals suffer from poor mental well-being to a degree that does not require specialist input but which, nevertheless, requires recognition and support. There is an additional imperative going forward, therefore, of enabling those working in schools and higher education institutions, workplaces, and places of worship, among others, to recognize and address mental health difficulties confidently and competently.

Educational

Pedagogically speaking, mental health education has followed the same trends seen in health professions education more broadly (albeit often lagging behind in adopting new innovations in the field, e.g., simulation). Educational methods and settings are generally similar to those of other specialties – although there is, inevitably, less focus on procedural skills given the nature of mental healthcare.

Most mental health education makes the same distinction between types of learners – e.g., undergraduate, postgraduate, and continuing professional development – with initiatives tending to focus on one professional group rather than being delivered interprofessionally. This means that the current frameworks within which mental health educational programs are developed are often not best suited to the delivery of complex multidisciplinary and cross-agency initiatives.

In line with education for other specialties, mental health education has tended to adhere to a biomedical model of "illness" – reflecting the dominant discourse in mental healthcare itself historically. However, this has been increasingly replaced by psychological and biopsychosocial models of mental disorder which, in turn, has affected the emphasis of educational activities (e.g., focusing more on psychotherapeutic skills rather than on eliciting psychopathology) (Kinderman 2005; Pilgrim 2002).

With regard to learning outcomes, emphasis is often placed on the attainment of competencies for practice – mirroring the dominant competency-based paradigms adopted in health professions education generally. Some differentiating features that have emerged, however, are an increased emphasis on reflection as central to professional development (Horton-Deutsch et al. 2012); a specific focus on supervision as integral to training and continuing practice (Severinsson 1995); and the importance of a solid foundation of communication and relational skills (e.g., therapeutic engagement, empathy, and compassion) (Ditton-Phare et al. 2017). At the same time, there appears to have been an increased focus on engaging service users in education – in line with the trend for increased co-production in mental healthcare service delivery (Clark 2015).

The importance of psychotherapeutic practice in improving service user outcomes in mental health has led to a specifically unique area of educational practice in mental health – namely, the development of initiatives for teaching psychotherapeutic techniques. Importantly, teaching in this area typically eschews a competency-based focus, instead focusing on the qualities of clinician-service user interaction and on clinician approach when experimenting with specific therapeutic techniques.

While communication skills training is common in health professions education, the teaching of psychotherapeutic skills goes further in focusing more deeply on the dynamic – that is, the unconscious processes at work – and relational aspects of mental healthcare practice. Techniques that have been employed in teaching these skills include the following: role-play, review of actual taped sessions, and simulated patients. Indeed, teaching in this area has often been keen to adopt the technological advances seen in health professions education generally (Ravitz and Silver 2004).

With regard to educational research, psychotherapeutic theory, in particular, highlights the complex areas of thought that researchers need to grapple with if they are to generate the knowledge needed for educators to adequately understand how best to deliver mental health education.

Unfortunately, academic thought into the specific pedagogical nuances of the field has generally been lacking. In particular, analysis of the mechanisms by which learning outcomes related to mental healthcare might be achieved has been poor. This may reflect a lack of interest in the academic community as well as a deficit in academic funding for educational research in mental health (in line with the general underfunding of clinical services).

The Need for Change

The current clinical and educational context in which mental health education is delivered highlights the challenges that need to be surmounted in order to develop educational programs that result in meaningful differences to population mental health. In particular, the clinical and organizational reality of healthcare delivery must be reflected more in educational initiatives (Frenk et al. 2010).

To do this, alternative conceptualizations of the aims of educational practice will be required. In particular, educators must continually ask themselves: "Given the current landscape, what learning outcomes do we need to aim for in order to achieve meaningful clinical outcomes?"

Since mental healthcare will be delivered in an increasingly integrated and collaborative fashion, specific learning outcomes around interprofessional collaboration and joint-working will be required.

To achieve these effectively, educational initiatives will need to both confer skills for this way of working *and*, given the inevitable reliance on non-mental health professionals for mental healthcare, alter individuals' orientation toward working with mental health difficulties. Such an approach will inevitably support clinicians from a variety of disciplines and professional backgrounds to engage meaningfully, and to work collaboratively, with service users. At the same time, in order to remove further barriers to care, educators must come up with ways to directly address the issue of clinician stigma toward those with mental illness (and, additionally, toward those who work in mental healthcare) (Henderson et al. 2012; Rao et al. 2009).

Mental ill health is fundamentally shaped by interpersonal and societal influences, resulting in complex and varied expressions of illness even where individuals are ostensibly suffering from the same disorder. Where mental health education has evolved to incorporate alternatives to a purely biomedical model of illness, it must seek to directly engage with this complexity more deeply. It can do this by incorporating the various theoretical paradigms applied to understanding mental disorder – biomedical, cultural, sociological, and psychological – and by seeking to develop educational interventions that aid learners to synthesize these views into a more holistic whole.

At the same time, there is an imperative, in line with person-centered models of care, to move away from the concept of educating for assessing and treating "illness" or "disorder" toward focusing on strength-based approaches, preventative practice, and early intervention. This will require a significant shift in the majority of existing approaches to developing educational interventions.

In order to achieve this, greater involvement of service users is required. While educators are beginning to involve service users more, things must go further such that service users are incorporated into every aspect of education for mental healthcare as standard. In this way, it might be possible to truly transform healthcare delivery in a meaningful way for those suffering with mental health difficulties.

If we agree that mental healthcare should be a universal responsibility of all of society, then a significant societal shift in attitudes toward mental illness is required. Again, this will require educators to deliver initiatives to alter negative, or inhibitory, attitudes while at the same time skilling up larger communities of non-clinical individuals in order that they might better understand mental ill health and promote good mental well-being.

Finally, we live in an ever-changing age where technological advances directly shape how learners consume and process material. While TEL offers increased access to education, as well as vast potential scalability, in mental health education, the incorporation of such techniques risks failing to prepare learners for the inherently human and dynamic aspects of mental healthcare.

Clinically speaking, therapeutic success is often fundamentally rooted in what a service user and clinician co-create together by virtue of being present with one another. This cannot easily be replicated by technological means. That said, and given the increasing trend toward remote learning and working generally, mental health educators will have to adapt their practice to embrace TEL and find ways within it to preserve the teaching of those qualities of mental healthcare that are grounded in the interpersonal.

Future Directions

Before considering the specifics of the educational methods that can be employed to address some of the imperatives above, it is important to review the overarching approach that educators should adopt when considering mental health education for the future.

While incorporating the subsequent approaches and methods would be preferable, the realities of the local context in which education is delivered will necessarily impose some parameters on any proposed interventions. What follows should, therefore, be considered a template rather than a mandate.

Adopting the Right Approach

In health professions education, consideration of educational paradigms is often overlooked in favor of analyzing techniques and modes of delivery. Similarly, pedagogical theory, and understanding the mechanisms of learning, often comes second to establishing the efficacy of educational interventions.

Given this, and the fact that mental health educational research has been underprivileged historically, educators are faced with a double deficit in pedagogical theory for mental health education. This makes developing new theoretical approaches to this activity problematic as there is a scarcity of evidence to go on.

A starting point from which to outline a new way of thinking about mental health education is to define the types of learning outcomes required. This provides an accessible and learner-centered means of articulating what educators should be seeking to achieve (Maher 2004). Next, consideration of the models and mechanisms of learning that can be leveraged to achieve these outcomes is needed. Finally, an overarching paradigm, or philosophy, about mental health education generally is necessary in order to anchor future learning activities.

This section considers new conceptualizations of learning outcomes and explores relevant models of learning. In addition, the paradigm of humanism is considered as a possible overarching tenet for mental health education.

Learning Outcomes and Pedagogical Paradigms

Learning outcomes in mental health education have most often focused on the acquisition of knowledge and skills for mental healthcare. These outcomes have usually been derived from competency frameworks or from higher learning institutions' curricula (which themselves often focus on competencies) (Delaney et al. 2011).

If we consider that future mental health education must prepare clinicians for working in complex healthcare systems, while at the same time altering the attitudes of some professional groups in relation to their perceived roles and responsibilities in caring for those with mental health needs, then it quickly becomes apparent that competencies frameworks are not sufficiently nuanced to capture the types of learning outcomes that future mental health education needs to be aiming for.

Merely constructing objectives from such frameworks neglects the importance of altering individuals' mindsets so that they privilege working with mental health needs. Additionally, the need to impact on the interpersonal aspects of mental healthcare delivery is overlooked.

Going forward, learning outcomes cannot be constructed solely around gaining skills and competences. Rather they should focus on outcomes that promote certain *ways* of working or, indeed, being. This necessitates a broader, and more complex, conception of learning outcomes.

One approach here is to differentiate between outcomes that focus on *acquisition* (e.g., skills; knowledge) from those that emphasize *participation* (e.g., identity; membership; disposition toward) (Sfard 1998). This allows us to begin to articulate those outcomes that are important for ensuring that healthcare professionals *actually* adopt new ways of working with those with mental health needs – whether this be performing interprofessional collaboration more effectively or simply engaging with the mental health needs of their service users more.

Here we are dealing with the complex task of effecting a fundamental shift in individuals' relationship to their work as well as in their organizing principles and values. Interestingly, ideas from the practice of mental healthcare itself may be useful here since much psychotherapeutic treatment seeks to effect lasting intrapsychic and interpersonal change in a similar manner (Bateman et al. 2010).

In order to achieve this task, mental health education would benefit from taking a more person-centered and holistic approach to learners. This recognizes that complex outcomes of this nature oblige us to focus on promoting individuals' awareness of both their own positions in relation to mental healthcare and of the internal barriers which may be preventing them from altering their ways of working.

Here a humanistic view of education is required. This proposes that, for education to be successful in a profound and meaningful way, it must incorporate the feelings and cognitions of the individual into the learning event. Humanism requires educators to develop interventions that "cultivate deeper sensory and emotional experiences" (Ringness 1975) while also seeking to facilitate "students' self-actualisation and fulfilment of their full potential" (DeCarvalho 1991). A humanistic paradigm has the added benefit in mental health education in that it "fits," philosophically speaking, with the ethos of mental healthcare itself.

In addition to promoting better self-awareness and internal change, humanistic approaches might be employed to improve empathy toward oneself and others (Marcus 1999). This may be important for addressing stigma toward those with mental health difficulties – a potential barrier to effective working with this demographic – and for improving interprofessional working.

Compounding the issue of stigma is the fact that mental health education has generally applied a disease-centered model to individuals' difficulties. This belies some of the more recent developments in treatment where a shift in focus to recovery and strengths-based approaches to care has taken place (Schrank and Slade 2007). By taking this pathology-focused approach, educators may be detracting from the improvements that can be possible in mental healthcare and unwittingly reinforcing stigmatizing attitudes.

In order to move away from focusing on *problems* to building on *strengths,* a re-evaluation of the discourse that existing learning outcomes play into is required. Rather than developing outcomes focused on "disorder," a more hopeful and positive discourse – one rooted in strength-based narratives – could be developed. In this way, it may be possible to influence professionals' attitudes toward mental health difficulties further and impact even more positively on their practice.

In line with this idea is the imperative to train clinicians to practice more holistically when managing mental health difficulties (Naylor et al. 2017). This will require learning outcomes related to higher-order learning – e.g., metacognition and synthesis (Paris and Winograd 1990). Such outcomes should not only support clinicians to incorporate numerous theoretical paradigms for understanding mental health difficulties into their treatment planning, but they should also help practitioners to engage with service users' physical health; ensure a person-centered focus while operating within the logistical limitations of modern healthcare systems; maintain cultural sensitivity; and maintain awareness of the social determinants of health throughout treatment planning.

All this is not to say that educators should ignore more routine *acquisition* type outcomes – that is, ensuring professionals acquire the necessary clinical skills for mental healthcare. Certainly, this will be needed in areas where there is little experience of, or familiarity with, mental health difficulties. However, in order for this learning to be meaningful, we need to move further in our educational aspirations toward outcomes that are related to sophisticated performance of these skills and that are focused on influencing participation in mental healthcare generally. This must include, in particular, interprofessional collaboration between individuals, teams, and agencies. An approach that recognizes that higher-order learning of this kind does not always have to follow the initial attainment of acquisition type outcomes is required. This would allow for a more comprehensive and integrated approach to preparing learners for the complexity of mental healthcare practice.

If we are to teach such nuanced and complex skills well, then clinical experts will require a solid foundation in teaching skills and pedagogical theory in order that they might better develop and facilitate training to elicit these outcomes. This will involve better understanding the means by which lasting intrapsychic and interpersonal change can be achieved in learners.

Box 1 outlines some examples of potential future learning outcomes that educators may wish to aim for in mental health education.

> **Box 1 Examples of Potential Future Learning Outcomes**
> For learners to:
>
> - Develop a disposition towards working with individuals' mental health difficulties.
> - Attain skills in working with strength-based models of mental healthcare.
> - Synthesise different conceptual models of mental health difficulties in order to achieve a holistic understanding of treatment needs.
> - Acquire greater empathy and understanding towards those suffering from mental ill health.
> - Engage in cross-speciality and cross-agency interprofessional working processes.
> - Develop a feeling of membership to a community that privileges interprofessional working.

Models of Learning

In order to achieve the types of learning outcomes above, consideration must be given to the learning models that may facilitate the complex changes required. A number of models may be relevant to the task. These share a commonality in that they focus on psychological processes around identity and experience rather than the accumulation of knowledge or skills.

Experiential Learning

Experiential learning is well-embedded in health professions education – most notably in the field of simulation (Zigmont et al. 2011). In mental health education, there is a general trend toward experiential teaching methods with the recognition that, given adequate reflection, concrete experiences have the capacity to facilitate lasting internal change. By providing learners with the opportunity to directly engage in alternative ways of being, experiential learning can facilitate changes in individuals' orientation toward certain activities (Fenwick 2001).

One of the most powerful means by which experiential learning achieves its effect, at least from a psychological point of view, is through the stimulation of strong emotional reactions (Finch et al. 2015; Zeivots 2016). In part, this might be mitigated through emotionally charged events being better embedded in memory (Christianson 2014).

Affective Learning

The learning achieved through emotional events can be termed "affective learning." This form of learning views the learner in their entirety – both intellect and feelings – and considers the processing of emotions as both therapeutic and enabling. As such, it fits well with a humanistic approach to education.

Affective learning is felt to promote "greater appreciation for differences, tolerance of ambiguity, and feelings of courage, self-trust and inner strength" (Neumann 1997). Such outcomes may be instrumental in eliciting the internal change that is required in promoting outcomes around participation – e.g., disposition toward and feelings of membership – as well as in tackling stigma.

Transformative Learning

Transformative learning involves a "psycho-cultural process of constructing and appropriating new or revised interpretations of the meaning of one's experience" (Taylor 2000). As such, it may be key in promoting learning outcomes related to individuals' values and beliefs.

Transformative learning privileges critical reflection. This reflection occurs in relation to the recognition, acknowledgment, and processing of emotions. Personal change occurs through the combination of activating emotional processes; exploring feelings; reflecting upon these; and promoting self-examination and self-understanding (Mezirow 1991). As such, transformative learning often co-exists with affective learning.

Psychodynamic Theories of Learning

Within mental healthcare itself, there is a recognition of the importance of addressing dysfunctional interpersonal processes; promoting intrapsychic change; enhancing self-realization; and promoting self-actualization – that is "the desire to become...everything that one is capable of becoming" (Maslow 1943). These ideas are not too dissimilar to the type of change required to achieve participation-based learning outcomes.

Psychodynamic theories of learning help us to understand, and subsequently navigate, the internal barriers that may be encountered in seeking to alter individuals' mindsets toward an activity or, indeed, group of people. By supporting learners to recognize the unconscious experiences that may be triggered for them in the delivery of mental healthcare, educators may be more successful at facilitating lasting personal change (Karagiannopoulou 2011).

Social Theories of Learning

Given the importance of interprofessional collaboration in mental healthcare in the future, consideration around social theories of learning – that is, theories that directly engage with the group dynamics involved in educating individuals – is required. Theories, such as social identity theory (Tajfel and Turner 1986), self-categorization theory (Turner 1999), and social cohesion, might all be leveraged to influence clinicians' relationship to joint-working. This might be achieved by promoting identification with other professionals, by fostering affective bonds, and through interventions that lead learners to collectively categorize themselves as interprofessional collaborators.

Activity Theory

Social theories of learning highlight that, for mental health education to be successful, educational activities must speak to the social and contextual relationships that exist in real life between learners. Activity theory is one means of incorporating this complexity (Engeström 2001). Instructional activities that replicate how social organization and artifacts mediate social action may embed learning more effectively due to learners ascribing more meaning to the thought processes triggered and tasks undertaken as part of these activities. This would again be important for altering individuals' attitudes toward their roles and responsibilities in mental healthcare.

Getting the Design Right

Having outlined some of the theoretical considerations for mental health education in the future, three instructional design concepts that will be key in operationalizing the learning theories above are now presented. These concepts will be crucial in ensuring that the development of educational initiatives fits the context in which mental healthcare is delivered in future. They are the following:

- Interprofessional education (IPE)
- Co-production
- Technology-enhanced learning (TEL)

Each of these areas is, of course, pertinent to health professions education more widely, but their application in mental health education specifically needs consideration.

The following discussions aim to guide the reader in their consideration of these concepts for their own needs in the hope that they might integrate these ideas into their current practice.

Interprofessional Education

Given the increasing complexity of mental healthcare systems in the future, IPE will be an imperative going forward. In particular, educational initiatives will need to adapt to include non-healthcare partners – e.g., education, private sector companies, and voluntary sector organizations – in order to ensure that appropriately skilled support is in place to promote good population mental health.

Conceptually, various types of IPE will be required – including initiatives that: improve multidisciplinary working in mental health teams; address treatment barriers at the mental-physical interface; improve joint-working between primary and secondary care; and improve co-working between healthcare and non-healthcare organizations.

There have been some excellent examples of the use of IPE for these aims (Box 2). Two of these examples in particular have sought to increase the complexity of IPE by ensuring that cross-specialty and cross-agency approaches are used. This should be the default going forward with educators continually striving to improve the sophistication and ambition of their IPE projects.

Box 2 Case Studies of Interprofessional Mental Health Education

(i) *Multidisciplinary*

Lavelle et al. (2017) developed an in-situ, interprofessional simulation course around managing medical emergencies in mental health settings in London, UK. In-patient ward teams were trained together around a variety of scenarios in half-day sessions over 8 weeks. Participants reported improved confidence and knowledge for managing medical emergencies along with improved communication, self-reflection, and team-working. Critical incident reporting increased post-intervention reflecting better recognition of potential near-misses.

(ii) *Cross-speciality*

Fernando et al. (2017) developed an interprofessional simulation course for mental health and physical health specialists in general hospitals and primary care in London, UK. Scenarios focused on assessment and management of service users with both physical and mental health needs. Participants reported increased knowledge and confidence in, as well as improved attitudes for, this work. Various non-technical skills were privileged in qualitative feedback including: teamwork, reflection, communication and leadership.

(iii) *Cross-agency*

Woodside-Jiron et al. (2019) developed a trauma-informed, resiliency-based, interprofessional graduate course for child welfare, mental health, and education students in the US. This aimed to improve trauma-informed collaborative practice for working with children and families in historically siloed components of service provision. The intervention comprised of creating an "academy" which delivered hybrid graduate courses, both face-to-face and online. Findings demonstrated improved trauma-specific knowledge and skills; increased professional self-efficacy; and improved interprofessional collaborative relationships and knowledge of systems outside of one's own.

Adapting IPE interventions to include those from a diverse range of professional backgrounds increases both the richness and sophistication of learning by ensuring that there is a diversity of views taken into account when exploring the complexities of mental healthcare (Priest et al. 2008). Such interventions might also allow educators to speak directly to the sociological and dynamic aspects of interprofessional working – that is, to unpack the interpersonal and systemic factors that either facilitate or impede care.

By taking an interprofessional approach, mental health educators can adapt individuals' professional development so that they can come to more easily complement each other's roles, thereby improving overall clinical care (Illingworth and Chelvanayagam 2007). In addition, by designing IPE in such a way as to operationalize affective, transformative, and social models of learning, educators might be more effective at altering mindsets toward the importance of interprofessional working in mental healthcare.

Finally, IPE can be used to address stigma toward those suffering from, and working with, mental health difficulties by allowing learners to critically reflect on their own values and beliefs in relation to others.

Developing IPE initiatives does not come without challenges. In particular, educators will need to navigate the following:

- *Negative attitudes toward IPE and mental illness* – while impacting on the value professionals attribute to working interprofessionally is an aim of IPE itself, before such events can take place a baseline level of enthusiasm toward IPE is required. This is particularly important in key management personnel who will be in the position to authorize the resources required for developing and delivering IPE and to ensure learners are released from their work responsibilities to attend. Support of this kind may be lacking in non-mental healthcare settings due to stigmatized attitudes toward mental illness along with negative beliefs about IPE itself. For the latter, these include a lack of perceived value; fear of having too high a workload; and a lack of respect for other health professionals (Lawlis et al. 2014).

- *Organizational systems that are not structured to support interprofessional working* – there is an inherent problem with educating individuals to work interprofessionally when current healthcare systems do not promote this way of working. Organizational boundaries make the development and delivery of IPE logistically, and financially, difficult while, in mental healthcare specifically, the following issues with collaborative working across systems have been identified: a lack of models for collaboration; different professional cultures and methods; lack of shared channels of communication; and differences in management, financing, and legislation (Kristensen et al. 2019).

  However, it is only through ensuring that future healthcare professionals privilege interprofessional ways of working that we can hope to guarantee mental healthcare systems that are designed in such a way as to support effective collaboration.

- *Development of robust pedagogical rationales* – given the above difficulties, educators must be confident that their IPE initiatives are truly worth the time and effort. This means ensuring clear pedagogical frameworks for how to achieve desired interprofessional learning outcomes along with robust evidence for IPE's efficacy in mental health education. Given the general lack of evidence for this to date, there is a somewhat circular aspect here in that more IPE initiatives are required in order to provide the pedagogical justification for their existence. As such, all mental health IPE initiatives should aim for high-quality evaluations that demonstrate that they make a difference to service user care and experience. This, in turn, requires educators to have both pedagogical know-how *and* access to financial, and human, resources.

Co-production

Co-production, that is, where professionals and service users share power in the planning and delivery of services, has long been privileged in mental healthcare (Clark 2015; Lewis 2014; Needham 2008; Rose et al. 2002). The inclusion of those with lived experience is vital in understanding how services can better meet the needs of those they serve. In particular, this approach recognizes the importance of empowerment, autonomy, and self-efficacy in recovery from mental ill health such that the concept is mutually beneficial for both healthcare provider and service user.

Despite this precedent, co-production in mental health education is taking longer to embed. Where historically service users have often been engaged for the purposes of demonstration – e.g., of different psychopathology – they have not often had direct input into the development of educational interventions themselves.

Here a distinction between true co-production and routine service user involvement is beneficial, with the former necessitating an in-depth collaborative process from conception through to delivery and even evaluation.

Various models and frameworks for co-production exist along with evidence for its efficacy and guidelines for its implementation (Attoe et al. 2017; National Survivor User Network 2015; Slay and Stephens 2013). Generally, successful approaches to co-production in mental health can best be explained by outlining their guiding principles (Cahn 2000; Minghella and Linsky 2018). These include the following:

- People as assets
- Building existing capabilities
- Reciprocity and mutuality
- Engaging peer networks
- Blurring roles and valuing diversity
- Facilitating collaborative change

These principles emphasize the strengths-based approach that contemporary mental healthcare has begun to privilege. Similarly, they align well with the holistic ethos of a humanistic educational paradigm.

Various types of co-produced initiatives exist in mental health education (Box 3).

Box 3 Case Studies of Co-production in Mental Health Education

(i) *Undergraduate education*

The COMMUNE project (Horgan et al. 2018) delivered co-produced mental health education for undergraduate nursing students. As part of this multi-centre project, focus groups with nursing academics and experts by experience were used to determine key themes to guide co-produced educational practice. The opportunity to encourage consideration of the whole person and their strengths, beyond their diagnosis, and to promote reflection and self-awareness of personal values by staff, were highlighted as important outcomes.

(ii) *Interprofessional education*

Davies et al. (2014) developed a national awareness training programme on Personality Disorder for an interprofessional audience of clinicians in the northwest of England. Development of the programme involved co-production and co-delivery at scale, with experts by experience involved throughout. Evaluations demonstrated improvements in understanding, capability and efficacy along with reduced negative emotional reactions. Qualitative themes highlighted the training's effectiveness along with key considerations for delivering co-produced programmes.

(iii) *Continuing professional development*

Recovery Colleges - institutes which aim to provide co-produced, co-delivered education for service users, carers and staff - have been developed around the world (Perkins et al. 2018). Training courses aim to promote improved mental health and sustained recovery from mental illness by fostering collaborative approaches to meeting health needs. Recovery Colleges exemplify good practice in co-produced health education by ensuring that service users are involved in an equal and reciprocal partnership with professionals.

Certain areas of mental health education have engaged more significantly with co-production – notably in the teaching of intellectual disability. Here, co-produced education has been used to meet a variety of higher-order learning outcomes (Attoe et al. 2017; Billon et al. 2016; Hall and Hollins 1996; Grech et al. 2012; Thacker et al. 2007; Thomas et al. 2014). Such initiatives have often incorporated voluntary and community sector partners in order to develop sustainable working relationships and to integrate co-produced training into their routine educational programs. This has involved the appropriate compensation of service users for their time on terms that suit them and that are sensitive to their welfare needs (Minghella and Linsky 2018).

Co-produced educational initiatives are generally facilitated by: the presence of an infrastructure that enables service user involvement; agreed ways of working; support for those with lived experience to access and contribute to the co-production process (e.g., reasonable adjustments); and collaboration with community groups and networks.

Crucially, co-production in education, as in clinical service delivery, may be an important means by which mental health professionals can contribute to service users' recovery and ensure maintenance of their well-being (Fairlie 2015). At the same time, engaging service users in education might support the fostering of positive discourses around mental health and eschew the dominant historical focus on "illness" and "disease." Similarly, co-production embodies the moral imperative for adopting a person-centered approach to mental healthcare and so may be important in dispelling stigmatized attitudes toward those suffering from mental health difficulties (Horgan et al. 2018).

To drive engagement in co-production in the future, strong educational leadership will be important. This will require the fostering of an openness and willingness to work and educate in this way as well as the development of infrastructures that facilitate service user involvement. Existing initiatives that support co-production in clinical service delivery may provide a good organizational starting point for maximizing service user inclusion in education (Minghella and Linsky 2018).

At the same time, the barriers to educators engaging with co-production will need to be navigated. These can include uncertainty or unfamiliarity with the approach; practical concerns around cost, time, and welfare implications; an inhibitory working culture; fear of conflict; and organizational pressures (Colham et al. 2016; Minghella and Linsky 2018).

Going forward, continued work of this kind will better socialize educators, learners, and organizations to co-production. This can be advanced further with training to ensure healthcare professionals know how to operationalize co-production appropriately (Owen et al. 2004). Here, educators must be able to openly reflect on which service users come to be involved in co-production and consider how to ensure that certain lived experiences are not neglected in favor of those that are "easier" to represent or that are more forthcoming during recruitment.

As we develop our understanding of this area further, the nuances and complexities of co-production in mental health education will need exploration. In particular, a coherent narrative of the principles of co-production and their relation to pedagogical theory is required. Here, educators must consciously align their approach to co-production with the aforementioned learning outcomes and models so that initiatives can meet the complex educational needs of future healthcare professionals.

Technology-Enhanced Learning

The current technological age creates enormous possibilities for health professions education. As in other specialties, mental health education has begun to explore new technological modalities of teaching.

The reach that TEL interventions can have is particularly important when considering the need to skill up vast groups of healthcare professionals for mental healthcare. Similarly, if suitable, interventions might easily be disseminated to other organizations so that non-healthcare professionals might learn more about how to support those with mental health difficulties.

Given the technological era we live in, there is an additional imperative to develop a digitally literate mental health workforce for the future (Topol 2019). Having professionals engage with TEL will, in itself, be an important means of achieving this.

However, the application of TEL technologies brings with it unique quandaries. In particular, is the use of virtual technologies an appropriate and ethical way of teaching for mental healthcare practice?

Here, various developments in TEL are presented along with future considerations for such technology. It is important to note that there is considerable variation in the nomenclature of TEL methods in the literature – with the terms "virtual" and "simulation" particularly being attributed to a wide variety of interventions. Attempts have been made to differentiate them as best possible in the separate sections below. Here interventions are discussed in order of increasing technological complexity.

Video-Based Interventions

Video-based teaching has been much employed in mental health education. Its main uses have been:

- To enhance learners' exposure to diagnostic assessment and psychopathology (e.g., Sturgeon 1979; Miller and Tupin 1972; Garralda 1989)
- To provide feedback and evaluation on interviewing and psychotherapeutic technique (e.g., Bailey et al. 1977; Abbass 2004; Gorrindo et al. 2011)
- To stimulate discussion of theoretical issues (e.g., Parkin and Dogra 2000)
- To develop clinical reasoning and decision-making skills (e.g., Pantziaras et al. 2015)
- To evaluate the interpersonal and introspective factors at play during an interview (Roeske 1979)

The types of videos used range from tapes of real clinical sessions to videos of human simulated patients (SPs) to commercial movie clips.

Over time, video-based interventions have moved from classroom teaching to online with the development of branching, interactive scenarios that incorporate video footage (Ekblad et al. 2013; Gorrindo et al. 2013; Lamont and Brunero 2013; Sunnqvist et al. 2016; Pantziaras et al. 2015).

Interactive patient scenarios of this kind will sit alongside other online options for learners in the future. While the latter interventions may generate more excitement due to their novelty, the ability of videos to demonstrate the dynamic aspects of mental healthcare, along with real-life presentations of psychopathology, mean that they will continue to be an integral component of teaching for many.

However, given advances in film-making, and the expectations that this may engender in learners, the sophistication and quality of educational videos will almost certainly have to improve if we are to maintain learner engagement. This may involve more considered thought around camera angles, shot selection, pictorial composition, and editing than educators might otherwise do (Roeske 1979). Similarly, given the essentially static nature of much of mental healthcare delivery, thought will need to be given as to how to adapt video content to maximize attentiveness. An option here might be to develop content that replicates the interprofessional collaborative aspects of mental healthcare or to develop videos around service user journeys through complex healthcare systems.

Live Simulation

Simulation has only begun to achieve prominence in mental health education in recent years (Attoe et al. 2016). Where, historically, it has been used mainly for supporting history-taking and mental state examination, mental health educators are now exploring its use in a variety of novel ways. These include the following:

- Replicating difficult clinical situations that require nuanced approaches to communication (e.g., Kowalski and Sathanandan 2015)
- In situ training on mental health wards to enhance interprofessional collaboration and identify environmental and systemic barriers to effective care (e.g., Lavelle et al. 2017)
- Applying ideas around metacognition to explore decision-making in clinical planning and risk management (e.g., Jabur et al. 2020)
- Improving interprofessional collaboration at the mental-physical interface (e.g., Kowalski et al. 2016; Fernando et al. 2017)
- Improving interprofessional working between emergency services (e.g., Fisher et al. 2020)
- Supporting health professionals returning to clinical work after an absence (e.g., Saunders et al. 2020)

Live simulation typically engages human SPs. The technology used primarily comprises video capture tools. These allow live viewing of scenarios remotely and facilitate video playback for use during debriefing. As such, live simulation employs a relatively low level of technological complexity, although adding in mannikins and patient monitors during physical health-related scenarios increases the need for specific technological know-how.

Conceptually, interprofessional simulation is key for the future given the need to educate professionals for cross-specialty and interagency working in mental health. Such interventions can, however, be logistically complicated and require a significant investment of time and resources, as well as sustained development, if they are to be routinely embedded into educational programs. In addition, as with simulation generally, they can be costly in relation to the number of learners that can take part in each activity.

However, the educational potential of interprofessional simulation merits this investment. The combination of experiential, affective, and transformative learning that can be evoked through scenario and debrief may facilitate the achievement of complex learning outcomes – including participation-based outcomes. This requires debriefers to be particularly skilled at eliciting rich discussions about the nature of mental healthcare practice. At the same time, they must develop skills in supporting individuals to recognize their own attitudes toward both mental ill health and collaborative practice.

Unfortunately, current debriefing theory may not adequately outline the structural and facilitative interventions necessary for promoting the interpersonal and intra-psychic change associated with achieving participation-based learning outcomes. There is a role for psychotherapeutic thinking here, such that mental health educators may prove useful in informing simulation debriefing theory in future.

Tele-education

Tele-education, that is the use of video conferencing software for educational purposes, is increasingly being used in mental health – particularly in countries where the combination of a lack of mental health professionals and vast geographical distances between communities necessitates remote learning (e.g., Canada and Australia). Examples of tele-education for mental health include initiatives aimed at:

- Improving rural workers' competence and confidence for working with child mental health (Fahey et al. 2003; Mitchell et al. 2001)
- Teaching psychiatry residents about managed care (Walter et al. 2004)
- Teaching medical students about transcultural psychiatry (Ekblad et al. 2004)
- Meeting the continuing professional development needs of rural psychiatrists (Greenwood and Williams 2008)
- Building capacity for the treatment and management of complex mental health disorders in primary care (Sockalingam et al. 2018)

Learners' acceptance of this modality is often high though the inherent difficulties seen in tele-education generally have been highlighted – e.g., difficulty maintaining learner engagement; preference for a physical presence; technical issues; and problems with not being able to gauge learner reactions. This latter issue is particularly relevant given the nature of much mental health case material. In the future, consideration will need to be given as to how to manage strong emotional reactions to difficult material remotely. This might involve ensuring the presence of a site coordinator who can follow-up in person with learners.

Similarly, developing initiatives that involve multiple healthcare professionals and agencies will be important in ensuring effective interprofessional collaboration in future. This is likely to be logistically complicated. In addition, the difference that having learners physically meeting one another makes for achieving such outcomes, as compared to only viewing each other via video-link, will need to be explored.

Virtual SPs

Virtual SPs, sometimes referred to as avatars, have been used in a number of different ways in mental health education. These include to:

- Improve assessment skills for specific conditions – including PTSD, major depressive disorder, conduct disorder, and autism spectrum disorder (Kenny et al. 2007, 2008; Pataki et al. 2012; Randell et al. 2007; Shah et al. 2012)
- Enhance therapeutic competencies – e.g., cultural competence (Lambert and Watkins 2013); ethical care (Guise et al. 2012); working with trauma (Kenny et al. 2008)
- Analyze clinicians' implicit biases in relation to patient interactions (Parsons et al. 2009)
- Expose learners to decision-making and critical reasoning (Lambert and Watkins 2013)

Technically speaking, the majority of virtual SPs are generated using carefully scripted, pre-programmed dialogue. With this, it is often the case that either learner choices or avatar responses are restricted to a specific range. The breadth of this range can vary according to the complexity of the script itself, but responses are almost uniformly pre-programmed. This may result in a mismatch in SP response where learners adopt unpredictable approaches.

To allow complete freedom to the learner, virtual SPs would need to incorporate sophisticated artificial intelligence (AI) so that avatars can respond and adapt to a variety of unexpected prompts. AI of this level is not generally possible currently; however, the expectation would be that this technology will become available in the not-too-distant future. At this time, educators will need to work hard to ensure the psychological fidelity of AI-powered virtual SPs' recreations of mental health difficulties.

Online Worlds

On occasion, virtual SPs are embedded into more in-depth online worlds, such as *Second Life*®. Often this is for the same purposes listed above (Sweigart et al. 2014; Vallance et al. 2014; Yellowlees and Cook 2006).

A unique benefit to utilizing an online world over virtual SPs in isolation is that it allows environmental factors to be replicated. Where service users' homes or public spaces are recreated, educators can begin to imply some of the situational aspects of healthcare delivery – e.g., how to ensure personal safety in unfamiliar environments or how to tackle environmental barriers when assessing service users in public (e.g., lack of privacy) (Kidd et al. 2012). This may be significant for supporting appreciation of the practical aspects of healthcare delivery in the community.

Educational Games

Computer-based educational games can be used to take the concept of virtual SPs and online worlds a step further by embedding them into a gamified context, thereby stimulating engagement and motivation. Despite their popularity in the treatment of various mental health difficulties, their use in mental health education is somewhat limited.

The concept of gamifying aspects of mental illness, and the ethics of doing so, may act as a barrier to the development of educational games in mental health education. As such, educators will need to adopt a sensitive and ethical approach to their design if they are to be taken up routinely. One means of doing this might be by focusing on narrative-centered learning environments where learners are able to engage in guided exploratory learning (Andrews 2011). Games of this type could be a useful means of improving understanding of the challenges faced by those suffering with mental ill health. Incorporating service users into game development will be crucial in ensuring fidelity to sufferers' lived experience.

Virtual Reality

Where virtual reality (VR) is already being used in some treatments in mental healthcare – notably, post-traumatic stress disorder – its use in education is sparse. Possible applications for VR include the following:

- Development of communication and psychotherapy skills (Elliman et al. 2016; Moran et al. 2018)
- Improving attitudes and empathy toward those with mental illness (Yee and Bailenson 2006; Kalyanaraman et al. 2010)
- Teaching about side effects of psychotropic medication, delirium, and drug intoxications (Moran et al. 2018)

It is important to make a distinction here between interventions with virtual SPs and online worlds, which are observed via a computer or tablet, and VR, which employs headsets to immerse participants into simulated environments. Pedagogically speaking, it is this immersion which may improve the achievement of specific learning outcomes. Improved motivation, the opportunity for visualization and reification, and the activation of experiential and active learning are all felt to be important here (Mantovani et al. 2003).

Practically, VR can safely simulate expensive and/or potentially dangerous activities in an accessible manner, e.g., where the presence of more severe mental health difficulties on inpatient units compromises learner safety.

Where the fidelity and acceptability of computer-generated environments may be an issue for virtual SPs and online worlds, VR may circumvent this, to a degree, by directly displaying real-world environments as opposed to computer-generated ones. This might allow learning outcomes related to situational factors in mental healthcare delivery to be achieved in a more acceptable way to learners.

An interesting area that may gain further traction in the future is the use of augmented reality (AR). This involves the superimposition of computer-generated imagery onto a user's view of the real world. The educational benefits of AR are similar to those of VR (Diegmann et al. 2015). However, the opportunity for real-world involvement may improve learners' engagement further due to the activity being better integrated into their actual lived experience. AR has been used in mental health education to reduce stigma related to schizophrenia by simulating the psychotic symptoms that sufferers may experience in day-to-day life (Silva et al. 2017).

Box 4 outlines some existing examples of technology-enhanced learning initiatives in mental health education.

Box 4 Case Studies of Technology-Enhanced Mental Health Education

(i) *Video-based interventions*

Wilkening et al. (2017) developed an interprofessional education programme to enhance learning of advanced psychopharmacology. Using branched-narrative interactive patient scenarios, and complementing these with debriefing sessions led by a psychiatric pharmacist and psychiatrist, the researchers were able to demonstrate statistically significant improvements in knowledge along with high learner satisfaction with the format.

(ii) *Tele-education*

Sockalingam et al. (2018) developed an educational programme for primary care teams working in rural and underserved regions of Ontario, Canada. They delivered 64 hours of continuing education via videoconferencing technology. This included didactic lectures alongside case reviews. Evaluation demonstrated improvements in knowledge and perceived competence for managing mental health and substance use disorders. The programme received high engagement and satisfaction ratings.

(iii) *Live simulation*

Jabur et al. (2020) developed an interprofessional simulation course focusing on cognitive bias in decision-making processes. Participants voted on whether to compulsorily admit a service user in acute mental health crisis and were supported to understand the cognitive processes underpinning their decisions via debriefing. An adaptive "choose your adventure" style approach was taken whereby alternative scenarios were observed depending on the group's collective decision.

(iv) *Virtual SPs*

Lambert and Watkins (2013) developed a virtual SP named Mohammed which they used to introduce first year mental health students to a service user's journey on an acute psychiatric inpatient ward. Over a period of 2 weeks, students experienced nursing processes and were encouraged to make clinical decisions around appropriate interventions to support Mohammed. This was incorporated into a blended learning approach which enhanced students' critical thinking skills, cultural competency and communication skills.

(v) *Online worlds*

(continued)

Box 4 (continued)

Kidd et al. (2012) developed a Second Life® simulation to teach undergraduate mental health nursing students about home-based assessment and planning for service users with schizophrenia and major depressive disorder. They found that students found online worlds to be a moderately effective learning tool - appreciating, in particular, the opportunity to practice assessing the safety of home environments in a secure way.

(vi) *Educational games*

Andrews (2011) describes the development of an educational game to enhance awareness of the psychological health challenges faced by military personnel. *"Walk in My Shoes"* is a narrative-centric guided exploratory game in which learners encounter a number of decision-making activities and cognitive exercises within a virtual "mini-world." Learners are able to practice the coping strategies that may be beneficial in managing such psychological health challenges.

(vii) *Virtual reality*

Kalyanaraman et al. (2010) developed a VR simulator with the aim of improving empathy for, and reducing stigma towards, those suffering from schizophrenia. Learners assumed the position of a service user and undertook a number of everyday experiences - all the while accompanied by auditory and visual hallucinations characteristic of schizophrenia. By encouraging learners to consider how it must feel to have such symptoms, the researchers were able to demonstrate increased empathy and improve attitudes towards people with the condition.

TEL offers considerable advantages to mental health educators. These include the opportunity to:

- Supplement learner experiences where clinical placements may be difficult to facilitate or where there may be particular safety issues, e.g., in forensic settings
- Increase the accessibility of mental health training for remote rural communities, particularly where there is a lack of mental health professionals
- Increase the variety of clinical scenarios that learners are exposed to where some presentations may be relatively rare, e.g., culture-bound syndromes

However, just as there are often difficulties in implementing new clinical interventions in mental healthcare, there will also be numerous challenges to seeing TEL methods adopted routinely in mental health education.

In particular, questions about the validity of learners' experiences will remain, even as the capabilities of virtual environments to recreate mental health difficulties improve. Even where human SPs are engaged in live simulation, reticence is expressed about the psychological fidelity of their portrayals (Abramowitz and

Rollhaus 2013). As such virtual SPs, online worlds and VR scenarios will need to be extremely persuasive if they are to be adopted more routinely in the future.

Similarly, the use of "machine" portrayals of mental health difficulties raises specific ethical dilemmas. In particular, what are we communicating about our attitude toward those with mental health needs if we believe that we can recreate their suffering using a computer?

Generally, though, skepticism exists when considering the potential for TEL to teach a specialty which is, at its heart, rooted in the interpersonal and the intimate (Brenner 2009). In particular, there are concerns about the ability of such technologies to replicate the unconscious dynamics that occur during mental healthcare. This may be between service user and clinician or between professionals themselves. Understanding such processes is fundamental to the practice of mental healthcare and is, therefore, privileged in the minds of many educators.

While this skepticism may reflect generational differences in attitudes toward new technologies, there is a reality that there is not yet enough evidence to demonstrate that TEL methods can replicate such complexity. As such, there remains a fundamental barrier to their uptake that must be addressed if educators are to use such methods as more than curiosities in the future.

The converse of this attitude is the enthusiastic embracing of TEL methods' teaching potential without sufficient evidence of their pedagogical value. A middle ground is needed where healthy skepticism is maintained but where TEL activities continue to be developed and researched in order to establish their effectiveness.

Here there is a practical aspect to contend with – namely, that most healthcare professionals are not skilled enough to develop TEL activities themselves. The development of such activities may rely on external parties, e.g., app developers, computer programmers, and game designers. This brings additional costs and time commitments since such parties may not have specialist medical knowledge and, thus, may require considerable input in order to create relevant and realistic educational tools.

In reality, while TEL opens up exciting new possibilities for teaching, we are not currently at a stage in mental health education where it will supersede more conventional teaching methods. As such, a blended approach is likely to emerge – one that combines the potential of TEL with more established teaching methods.

Regardless of the technological bounds that new methods bring, it is helpful to employ some guiding principles by which to operationalize new technologies. These include the following:

- Maintaining a solid pedagogical justification for any choice of TEL method – in particular what specific learning outcome it is being used to achieve and what mechanisms of change it mobilizes
- Addressing the range of learning outcomes that are salient to the provision of mental healthcare in the modern age – i.e., participation-based outcomes as well as acquisition-based ones
- Ensuring that TEL methods invoke the complex interpersonal dynamics involved in mental health treatment

- Retaining service users at the heart of development
- Using TEL to move away from hospital-based teaching to distributed learning in a flexible and blended way

Conclusion

An increasing burden of mental ill health globally coupled with a deficit in the number of mental health professionals required to meet this need has necessitated major changes to healthcare systems. This creates unique challenges for those seeking to equip future generations with the requisite knowledge, skills, and attitudes for working with those with mental health difficulties. Add in the wider responsibility that educators have to skill up all those in society in the pursuit of improving population mental health and you have a huge task with several unique educational conundrums to solve.

At the same time, we need to consider the dominant discourses that are informing the current development of mental health education and assess whether there is a need to reframe our overarching purposes in mental healthcare – moving away from disease-centered models to strengths-based approaches.

By harnessing the key learning of the past and employing some of the core principles outlined above, it is possible to develop a roadmap for the future of mental health education. For this to be successful, a cohesive, considered approach with solid theories of change is required. This approach should be grounded in the philosophies and paradigms that reflect current thinking in mental healthcare itself. At the same time, educational initiatives must be pragmatically delivered in line with contemporary clinical and educational contexts and be in step with technological advances.

Thinking differently about how we approach mental health education – the pedagogical paradigms we adopt, the learning outcomes we are aiming for, and the techniques we use – is key to ensuring that we prepare healthcare professionals, and indeed others, to deliver care that improves the experience of service users *and* their health outcomes.

As with many educational initiatives, there are a number of challenges to embedding new ways of educating in mental health. First and foremost, there is a pressing need to instill a common educational ethos within the mental health community – one that recognizes the importance of ongoing educational initiatives permeating the field as well as the need to educate those outside of mental healthcare.

Educators will need to be skilled up in relation to both the design and delivering of interventions that target complex learning outcomes and that incorporate elements of interprofessional design, co-production, as well as technological components.

In tandem with this, institutions that are willing to integrate new ways of teaching into everyday practice are required. Such institutions need to demonstrate a readiness to develop services and systems that facilitate the implementation of the learning that comes from educational practice. Only in this way can people action the learning they acquire.

There is also an imperative to address the comparative lack of research into mental health education in order that we might better understand its unique nature. In particular, expanding our understanding of how to achieve complex learning outcomes related to mental health practice is key. This will require increased opportunities for education scholars to undertake such research as well as increased funding and resources.

Ultimately, what is required going forward is an ongoing commitment from professionals, healthcare institutions, and government, despite challenging financial and political landscapes globally, to advocate for excellent mental healthcare and to invest in the infrastructure and resourcing required to support educational programs seeking to promote this.

Key Learning Points

- Mental health education must be developed in response to contemporary clinical and educational contexts in order to maximize its impact on improving population mental health.
- Future initiatives must adapt to include non-mental health professionals and be informed by the need for better integration of care pathways.
- New educational paradigms and learning outcomes are required to effect changes within complex healthcare systems in order to promote improved population mental health.
- Current trends such as IPE, co-production, and TEL may provide the tools through which to achieve necessary learning outcomes.

Cross-References

- ▶ Debriefing Practices in Simulation-Based Education
- ▶ Focus on Theory: Emotions and Learning
- ▶ Interprofessional Education (IPE): Trends and Context
- ▶ Medical Education: Trends and Context
- ▶ Reflective Practice in Health Professions Education
- ▶ Simulation as Clinical Replacement: Contemporary Approaches in Healthcare Professional Education
- ▶ Technology Considerations in Health Professions and Clinical Education
- ▶ Transformative Learning in Clinical Education: Using Theory to Inform Practice

References

Abbass A. Small-group videotape training for psychotherapy skills development. Acad Psychiatry. 2004;28(2):151–5.

Abramowitz MZ, Rollhaus ED. The case against standardized patients' simulating psychotic disorders. Acad Psychiatry. 2013;37(6):444.

Andrews A. Serious games for psychological health education. In: International Conference on Virtual and Mixed Reality. Heidelberg: Springer, Berlin; 2011. pp. 3–10.

Attoe C, Kowalski C, Fernando A, Cross S. Integrating mental health simulation into routine healthcare education. Lancet Psychiatry. 2016;3(8):702–3.

Attoe C, Billon G, Riches S, Marshall-Tate K, Wheildon J, Cross S. Actors with intellectual disabilities in mental health simulation training. J Ment Health Train Educ Pract. 2017;12:272.

Attoe C, Lillywhite K, Hinchliffe E, Bazley A, Cross S. Integrating mental and physical health care: the mind and body approach. Lancet Psychiatry. 2018;5(5):387–9.

Bailey KG, Deardorff P, Nay WR. Students play therapist: relative effects of role playing, videotape feedback, and modeling in a simulated interview. J Consult Clin Psychol. 1977;45(2):257.

Bateman A, Brown D, Pedder J. Introduction to psychotherapy: an outline of psychodynamic principles and practice. Routledge; 2010.

Billon G, Attoe C, Marshall-Tate K, Riches S, Wheildon J, Cross S. Simulation training to support healthcare professionals to meet the health needs of people with intellectual disabilities. Adv Ment Health Intellect Disabil. 2016;10(5):284.

Brenner AM. Uses and limitations of simulated patients in psychiatric education. Acad Psychiatry. 2009;33(2):112–9.

Cahn ES. No more throw-away people: the co-production imperative. Edgar Cahn; 2000.

Christianson SA, editor. The handbook of emotion and memory: research and theory. Psychology Press; 2014.

Clark M. Co-production in mental health care. Ment Health Rev J. 2015;14:213–9.

Colham T, Roberts A, Springham N, Karlin L, Nettle M, Pierri P, Patel M, Watts R. Are mainstream mental health services ready to progress transformative co-production? National Development Team for Inclusion, Bath. 2016. https://www.ndti.org.uk/assets/files/MH_Coproduction_position_paper.pdf

Davies J, Sampson M, Beesley F, Smith D, Baldwin V. An evaluation of Knowledge and Understanding Framework personality disorder awareness training: can a co-production model be effective in a local NHS mental health trust? Personal Ment Health. 2014;8(2):161–8.

DeCarvalho RJ. The humanistic paradigm in education. Humanist Psychol. 1991;19(1):88–104.

Delaney KR, Carlson-Sabelli L, Shephard R, Ridge A. Competency-based training to create the 21st century mental health workforce: strides, stumbles, and solutions. Arch Psychiatr Nurs. 2011;25(4):225–34.

Diegmann P, Schmidt-Kraepelin M, Eynden S, Basten D. Benefits of augmented reality in educational environments-a systematic literature review. Benefits. 2015;3(6):1542–56.

Ditton-Phare P, Loughland C, Duvivier R, Kelly B. Communication skills in the training of psychiatrists: a systematic review of current approaches. Aust N Z J Psychiatr. 2017;51(7):675–92.

Eaton J, McCay L, Semrau M, Chatterjee S, Baingana F, Araya R, Ntulo C, Thornicroft G, Saxena S. Scale up of services for mental health in low-income and middle-income countries. Lancet. 2011;378(9802):1592–603.

Ekblad S, Manicavasagar V, Silove D, Bärnhielm S, Reczycki M, Mollica R, Coello M. The use of international videoconferencing as a strategy for teaching medical students about transcultural psychiatry. Transcult Psychiatry. 2004;41(1):120–9.

Ekblad S, Mollica RF, Fors U, Pantziaras I, Lavelle J. Educational potential of a virtual patient system for caring for traumatized patients in primary care. BMC Med Educ. 2013;13(1):110.

Elliman J, Loizou M, Loizides F. Virtual reality simulation training for student nurse education. In: 2016 8th international conference on games and virtual worlds for serious applications (VS-games). IEEE; 2016. p. 1–2.

Engeström Y. Expansive learning at work: toward an activity theoretical reconceptualization. J Educ Work. 2001;14(1):133–56.

Fahey A, Day NA, Gelber H. Tele-education in child mental health for rural allied health workers. J Telemed Telecare. 2003;9(2):84–8.

Fairlie S. Coproduction: a personal journey. Ment Health Rev. 2015;20(4):267.

Fenwick TJ. Experiential learning: a theoretical critique from five perspectives. Information series no. 385. ERIC Clearinghouse on Adult, Career, and Vocational Education and Training for Employment, Ohio State University; 2001.

Fernando A, Attoe C, Jaye P, Cross S, Pathan J, Wessely S. Improving interprofessional approaches to physical and psychiatric comorbidities through simulation. Clin Simul Nurs. 2017;13(4):186–93.

Finch D, Peacock M, Lazdowski D, Hwang M. Managing emotions: a case study exploring the relationship between experiential learning, emotions, and student performance. Int J Manag Educ. 2015;13(1):23–36.

Fisher M, Vishwas A, Cross S, Attoe C. Simulation training for Police and Ambulance Services: improving care for people with mental health needs. BMJ Simul Technol Enhanc Learn. 2020;6 (2):121.

Frenk J, Chen L, Bhutta ZA, Cohen J, Crisp N, Evans T, Fineberg H, Garcia P, Ke Y, Kelley P, Kistnasamy B. Health professionals for a new century: transforming education to strengthen health systems in an interdependent world. Lancet. 2010;376(9756):1923–58.

Garralda ME. The use of videos to illustrate child psychopathology to medical students. Psychiatr Bull. 1989;13(2):69–72.

Gorrindo T, Baer L, Sanders KM, Birnbaum RJ, Fromson JA, Sutton-Skinner KM, Romeo SA, Beresin EV. Web-based simulation in psychiatry residency training: a pilot study. Acad Psychiatry. 2011;35(4):232–7.

Gorrindo T, Goldfarb E, Birnbaum RJ, Chevalier L, Meller B, Alpert J, Herman J, Weiss A. Simulation-based ongoing professional practice evaluation in psychiatry: a novel tool for performance assessment. Jt Comm J Qual Patient Saf. 2013;39(7):319–23.

Grech JD, Brandt R, O'Boyle-Duggan M. Effectiveness of live simulation of patients with intellectual disabilities. J Nurs Educ. 2012;51(6):334–42.

Greenwood J, Williams R. Continuing professional development for Australian rural psychiatrists by videoconference. Australas Psychiatry. 2008;16(4):273–6.

Guise V, Chambers M, Conradi E, Kavia S, Välimäki M. Development, implementation and initial evaluation of narrative virtual patients for use in vocational mental health nurse training. Nurse Educ Today. 2012;32(6):683–9.

Hall I, Hollins S. Changing medical students' attitudes to learning disability. Psychiatrist. 1996;20 (7):429–30.

Happell B. Moving in circles: a brief history of reports and inquiries relating to mental health content in undergraduate nursing curricula. Nurse Educ Today. 2010;30(7):643–8.

Henderson M, Brooks SK, del Busso L, Chalder T, Harvey SB, Hotopf M, Madan I, Hatch S. Shame! Self-stigmatisation as an obstacle to sick doctors returning to work: a qualitative study. BMJ Open. 2012;2(5):e001776.

Horgan A, Manning F, Bocking J, Happell B, Lahti M, Doody R, Griffin M, Bradley SK, Russell S, Bjornsson E, O'Donovan M. 'To be treated as a human': using co-production to explore experts by experience involvement in mental health nursing education–the COMMUNE project. Int J Ment Health Nurs. 2018;27(4):1282–91.

Horton-Deutsch S, McNelis AM, Day PO. Developing a reflection-centered curriculum for graduate psychiatric nursing education. Arch Psychiatr Nurs. 2012;26(5):341–9.

Illingworth P, Chelvanayagam S. Benefits of interprofessional education in health care. Br J Nurs. 2007;16(2):121–4.

Jabur Z, Lavelle M, Attoe C. Improving decision-making and cognitive bias using innovative approaches to simulated scenario and debrief design. BMJ Simul Technol Enhanc Learn. 2020;6 (1):49–51.

Kalyanaraman SS, Penn DL, Ivory JD, Judge A. The virtual doppelganger: effects of a virtual reality simulator on perceptions of schizophrenia. J Nerv Ment Dis. 2010;198(6):437–43.

Karagiannopoulou E. Revisiting learning and teaching in higher education: a psychodynamic perspective. Psychodyn Pract. 2011;17(1):5–21.

Kenny P, Parsons TD, Gratch J, Leuski A, Rizzo AA. Virtual patients for clinical therapist skills training. In: International workshop on intelligent virtual agents. Berlin/Heidelberg: Springer; 2007. p. 197–210.

Kenny P, Parsons T, Pataki C, Paton M, St George C, Sugar J, Rizzo A. Virtual Justina: a PTSD virtual patient for clinical classroom training. Annu Rev Cyber Ther Telemed. 2008;6(1):111.

Kidd LI, Knisley SJ, Morgan KI. Effectiveness of a second life® simulation as a teaching strategy for undergraduate mental health nursing students. J Psychosoc Nurs Ment Health Serv. 2012;50 (7):28–37.

Kinderman P. A psychological model of mental disorder. Harv Rev Psychiatry. 2005;13(4):206–17.

Kowalski C, Sathanandan S. The use of simulation to develop advanced communication skills relevant to psychiatry. BMJ Simul Technol Enhanc Learn. 2015;1(1):29–32.

Kowalski CM, Attoe C, Fisher M, Cross S. G85 Interprofessional simulation to improve collaborative working for young people with physical and mental health needs. Arch Dis Child. 2016;101(Suppl 1):A49.

Kristensen MM, Sølvhøj IN, Kusier AO, Folker AP. Addressing organizational barriers to continuity of care in the Danish mental health system–a comparative analysis of 14 national intervention projects. Nord J Psychiatry. 2019;73(1):36–43.

Lake J, Turner MS. Urgent need for improved mental health care and a more collaborative model of care. Perm J. 2017;21:17–24

Lambert N, Watkins L. Meet Mohammed: using simulation and technology to support learning. J Ment Health Train Educ Pract. 2013;8:66.

Lamont S, Brunero S. 'eSimulation' part 1: development of an interactive multimedia mental health education program for generalist nurses. Collegian. 2013;20(4):239–47.

Lavelle M, Attoe C, Tritschler C, Cross S. Managing medical emergencies in mental health settings using an interprofessional in-situ simulation training programme: a mixed methods evaluation study. Nurse Educ Today. 2017;59:103–9.

Lawlis TR, Anson J, Greenfield D. Barriers and enablers that influence sustainable interprofessional education: a literature review. J Interprof Care. 2014;28(4):305–10.

Lewis L. User involvement in mental health services: a case of power over discourse. Sociol Res Online. 2014;19(1):1–5.

Liese BH, Gribble RS, Wickremsinhe MN. International funding for mental health: a review of the last decade. Int Health. 2019;11(5):361–9.

Longley M, Williams R, Furnish S, Warner M, Owen JW. Promoting mental health in a civil society: towards a strategic approach. London, UK: The Nuffield Trust; 2001.

Maher A. Learning outcomes in higher education: implications for curriculum design and student learning. J Hosp Leis Sport Tour Educ. 2004;3(2):46–54.

Mantovani F, Castelnuovo G, Gaggioli A, Riva G. Virtual reality training for health-care professionals. Cyber Psychol Behav. 2003;6(4):389–95.

Marcus ER. Empathy, humanism, and the professionalization process of medical education. Acad Med. 1999;74(11):1211–5.

Maslow AH. A theory of human motivation. Psychol Rev. 1943;50(4):370.

Mezirow J. Transformative dimensions of adult learning. San Francisco: Jossey-Bass; 1991.

Miller PR, Tupin JP. Multimedia teaching of introductory psychiatry. Am J Psychiatr. 1972;128 (10):1219–23.

Minghella E, Linsky K. Co-production in mental health: not just another guide. London: Skills for Care; 2018. https://www.skillsforcare.org.uk/Documents/Topics/Mental-health/Co-production-in-mental-health.pdf

Mitchell JG, Robinson PJ, McEvoy M, Gates J. Telemedicine for the delivery of professional development for health, education and welfare professionals in two remote mining towns. J Telemed Telecare. 2001;7(3):174–80.

Moran J, Briscoe G, Peglow S. Current technology in advancing medical education: perspectives for learning and providing care. Acad Psychiatry. 2018;42(6):796–9.

National Survivor User Network. 4PI National Involvement Standards. London. 2015. http://www.nsun.org.uk/assets/downloadableFiles/4PINationalInvolvementStandards-A4ExecutiveSummary-201532.pdf

Naylor C, Taggart H, Charles A. Mental health and new models of care. Lessons from the vanguards. Kings Fund and Royal College of Psychiatrists; 2017.

Needham C. Realising the potential of co-production: negotiating improvements in public services. Soc Policy Soc. 2008;7(2):221–31.

Neumann TP. Critically reflective learning in a leadership development context. Unpublished doctoral dissertation, University of Wisconsin, Madison. 1997.

Owen K, Hollins S, Butler G. A new kind of trainer: how to develop the training role for people with learning disabilities. RCPsych Publications; 2004.

Pantziaras I, Fors U, Ekblad S. Training with virtual patients in transcultural psychiatry: do the learners actually learn? J Med Internet Res. 2015;17(2):e46.

Paris SG, Winograd P. How metacognition can promote academic learning and instruction. In: Dimensions of thinking and cognitive instruction, vol. 1. Lawrence Erlbaum Associates; 1990. p. 15–51.

Parkin A, Dogra AP. Making videos for medical undergraduate teaching in child psychiatry: the development, use and perceived effectiveness of structured videotapes of clinical material for use by medical students in child psychiatry. Med Teach. 2000;22(6):568–71.

Parsons TD, Kenny PG, Cosand L, Iyer A, Courtney CG, Rizzo AA. A virtual human agent for assessing bias in novice therapists. In: MMVR. 2009. p. 253–8.

Pataki C, Pato MT, Sugar J, Rizzo AS, Parsons TD, George CS, Kenny P. Virtual patients as novel teaching tools in psychiatry. Acad Psychiatry. 2012;36(5):398–400.

Patel V, Saxena S, Lund C, Thornicroft G, Baingana F, Bolton P, Chisholm D, Collins PY, Cooper JL, Eaton J, Herrman H. The Lancet Commission on global mental health and sustainable development. Lancet. 2018;392(10157):1553–98.

Perkins R, Meddings S, Williams S, Repper J. Recovery colleges 10 years on. Nottingham: ImROC; 2018. https://yavee1czwq2ianky1a2ws010-wpengine.netdna-ssl.com/wp-content/uploads/2018/03/ImROC-Recovery-Colleges-10-Years-On.pdf

Pilgrim D. The biopsychosocial model in Anglo-American psychiatry: past, present and future? J Ment Health. 2002;11(6):585–94.

Priest HM, Roberts P, Dent H, Blincoe C, Lawton D, Armstrong C. Interprofessional education and working in mental health: in search of the evidence base. J Nurs Manag. 2008;16(4):474–85.

Randell T, Hall M, Bizo L, Remington B. DTkid: interactive simulation software for training tutors of children with autism. J Autism Dev Disord. 2007;37(4):637–47.

Rao H, Mahadevappa H, Pillay P, Sessay M, Abraham A, Luty J. A study of stigmatized attitudes towards people with mental health problems among health professionals. J Psychiatr Ment Health Nurs. 2009;16(3):279–84.

Ravitz P, Silver I. Advances in psychotherapy education. Can J Psychiatry. 2004;49(4):230–7.

Ringness TA. The affective domain in education. Little, Brown; 1975.

Roeske, NC. The medium and the message: development of videotapes for teaching psychiatry. Am J Psychiat. 1979;136 (11):1391–1397.

Rose D, Fleischmann P, Tonkiss F, Campbell P, Wykes T. User and carer involvement in change management in a mental health context: review of the literature. Report to the National Co-ordinating Centre for NHS Service Delivery and Organization R & D. London: Service User Research Enterprise, Institute of Psychiatry, De Crespigny Park; 2002.

Saunders A, Brooks J, El Alami W, Jabur Z, Laws-Chapman C, Schilderman M, Tooley C, Attoe C. Empowering healthcare professionals to return to work through simulation training: addressing psychosocial needs. BMJ Simul Technol Enhanc Learn. 2020;6:371. bmjstel-2019.

Saxena S, Thornicroft G, Knapp M, Whiteford H. Resources for mental health: scarcity, inequity, and inefficiency. Lancet. 2007;370(9590):878–89.

Schrank B, Slade M. Recovery in psychiatry. Psychiatr Bull. 2007;31(9):321–5.

Severinsson EI. The phenomenon of clinical supervision in psychiatric health care. J Psychiatr Ment Health Nurs. 1995;2(5):301–9.

Sfard A. On two metaphors for learning and the dangers of choosing just one. Educ Res. 1998;27(2):4–13.

Shah AA, Beinecke RH. Global mental health needs, services, barriers, and challenges. Int J Ment Health. 2009;38(1):14–29.

Shah H, Rossen B, Lok B, Londino D, Lind SD, Foster A. Interactive virtual-patient scenarios: an evolving tool in psychiatric education. Acad Psychiatry. 2012;36(2):146–50.

Silva RD, Albuquerque SG, Muniz AD, Pedro Filho PR, Ribeiro S, Pinheiro PR, Albuquerque VH. Reducing the schizophrenia stigma: a new approach based on augmented reality. Comput Intell Neurosci. Volume 2017.

Slay J, Stephens L. Co-production in mental health: a literature review. London: New Economics Foundation; 2013. https://b.3cdn.net/nefoundation/ca0975b7cd88125c3e_ywm6bp3ll.pdf

Sockalingam S, Arena A, Serhal E, Mohri L, Alloo J, Crawford A. Building provincial mental health capacity in primary care: an evaluation of a project ECHO mental health program. Acad Psychiatry. 2018;42(4):451–7.

Sturgeon DA. Videotapes in psychiatry: their use in teaching observation techniques. Med Educ. 1979;13(3):204–8.

Sunnqvist C, Karlsson K, Lindell L, Fors U. Virtual patient simulation in psychiatric care–a pilot study of digital support for collaborate learning. Nurse Educ Pract. 2016;17:30–5.

Sweigart L, Burden M, Carlton KH, Fillwalk J. Virtual simulations across curriculum prepare nursing students for patient interviews. Clin Simul Nurs. 2014;10(3):e139–45.

Tajfel H, Turner JC. The social identity theory of intergroup behavior. In: Worchel S, Austing WG, editors. Psychology of intergroup relations. Chicago: Nelson-Hall Publishers; 1986. p. 7–24.

Taylor E. Fostering Mezirow's transformative learning theory in the adult education classroom: a critical review. Can J Study Adult Educ. 2000;14(2):1–28.

Thacker A, Crabb N, Perez W, Raji O, Hollins S. How (and why) to employ simulated patients with intellectual disabilities. Clin Teach. 2007;4(1):15–20.

Thomas B, Courtenay K, Hassiotis A, Strydom A, Rantell K. Standardised patients with intellectual disabilities in training tomorrow's doctors. Psychiatr Bull. 2014;38(3):132–6.

Topol E. The Topol review: preparing the healthcare workforce to deliver the digital future. Health Education England. Feb 2019. https://topol.hee.nhs.uk/

Turner JC. Some current issues in research on social identity and self-categorization theories. In: Social identity: context, commitment, content, vol. 3, no. 1. Blackwell; 1999. p. 6–34.

Vallance AK, Hemani A, Fernandez V, Livingstone D, McCusker K, Toro-Troconis M. Using virtual worlds for role play simulation in child and adolescent psychiatry: an evaluation study. Psychiatr Bull. 2014;38(5):204–10.

Walter DA, Rosenquist PB, Bawtinhimer G. Distance learning technologies in the training of psychiatry residents: a critical assessment. Acad Psychiatry. 2004;28(1):60–5.

Whiteford HA, Degenhardt L, Rehm J, Baxter AJ, Ferrari AJ, Erskine HE, Charlson FJ, Norman RE, Flaxman AD, Johns N, Burstein R. Global burden of disease attributable to mental and substance use disorders: findings from the Global Burden of Disease Study 2010. Lancet. 2013;382(9904):1575–86.

Wilkening GL, Gannon JM, Ross C, Brennan JL, Fabian TJ, Marcsisin MJ, Benedict NJ. Evaluation of branched-narrative virtual patients for interprofessional education of psychiatry residents. Acad Psychiatry. 2017;41(1):71–5.

Woodside-Jiron H, Jorgenson S, Strolin-Goltzman J, Jorgenson J. "The glue that makes the glitter stick": preliminary outcomes associated with a trauma-informed, resiliency-based, interprofessional graduate course for child welfare, mental health, and education. J Publ Child Welfare. 2019;13(3):307–24.

World Health Organization. Mental health: facing the challenges, building solutions. Report from the WHO European Ministerial Conference. 2005. http://www.euro.who.int/__data/assets/pdf_file/0008/96452/E87301.pdf

World Health Organization. Mental health action plan 2013–2020. 2013. https://www.who.int/mental_health/publications/action_plan/en/

Yee N, Bailenson JN. Walk a mile in digital shoes: the impact of embodied perspective-taking on the reduction of negative stereotyping in immersive virtual environments. Proc Presence. 2006;24:26.

Yellowlees PM, Cook JN. Education about hallucinations using an internet virtual reality system: a qualitative survey. Acad Psychiatry. 2006;30(6):534–9.

Zeivots S. Emotional highs in adult experiential learning. Aust J Adult Learn. 2016;56(3):353–73.

Zigmont JJ, Kappus LJ, Sudikoff SN. Theoretical foundations of learning through simulation. Semin Perinatol. 2011;35(2):47–51.

Dental Education: A Brief History

14

Andrew I. Spielman

Contents

Introduction 252
A Brief History 252
   Dental Practitioners 252
   Written Record 253
   The Dental Practitioner-Author 255
   Early Attempts to Regulate the Practice of Dentistry 256
   Apprenticeship as a Form of Training 257
   The First Dental School, Professional Publication, and Dental Society 259
   Regulating the Practice of Dentistry 263
   Reforming Dental Education 263
Conclusions 265
Cross-References 265
References 265

Abstract

Throughout its long history, dental education evolved considerably. Instead of a traditional, linear, and temporal description, this chapter will focus on the elements that constitute dental education today and their evolution from the solo, anonymous practitioner, to the first scrolls ("textbooks"), to apprenticeship, to the first dental schools, to legislation to regulate the practice and the complex network of elements and the highly regulated profession that is today.

Keywords

Dental education · History · Dentistry · Dental school · Fauchard

---

A. I. Spielman (✉)
New York University College of Dentistry, New York, NY, USA
e-mail: ais1@nyu.edu

© Springer Nature Singapore Pte Ltd. 2023
D. Nestel et al. (eds.), *Clinical Education for the Health Professions*,
https://doi.org/10.1007/978-981-15-3344-0_17

Introduction

Dental education today is far from a simple undertaking. It requires specialized textbooks and publications, specialized facilities for anatomy dissection, preclinical laboratories and simulation centers, intramural clinical practice, hospital rotations, regional or national board exams along with licensing and accreditation bodies. Dependent on the country, formal dental education can range from 4–9 years until one is fully licensed and recognized.

A Brief History

The path that brought us to this point, however, was not a linear progression by any means. Indeed, the history of dental education can be viewed like a river that meandered in a rather haphazard fashion. Beginning from its unremarkable and narrow scope, this river was continuously widened over the centuries by additional "tributaries," each confluence representing an aspect of education, all of which played their respective roles in creating major "waterway" that we know as modern dentistry.

Dental Practitioners

The oldest incarnation of dental education was the self-taught practitioner, who learned his trade and honed his craft through trial and error. The earliest dental interventions date back some 13,000 years to the Late Upper Paleolithic Era in what is today Tuscany (Oxilia et al. 2017), where archaeologists have retrieved several teeth showing signs of human manipulation to enlarge the pulp chambers, along with the presence of vegetal fibers and bitumen inside, presumably placed on purpose. Similarly, Early Neolithic evidence from 7,500–9,000 years ago from Pakistani graveyards indicates effective use of drills to remove decayed tissue from teeth (Coppa et al. 2006). The first sign of restoration of tooth decay dates from a 6,500 year-old specimen found in what is today Slovenia, in which beeswax was used to restore a cracked tooth (Bernardini et al. 2012). These interventions were carried out by anonymous practitioners, whose knowledge was likely passed on to others through observation.

The first dental practitioner whose name was recorded was a man named *Hesy-Ra*, an Egyptian in the employ of Pharaoh Djoser, who reigned during the first half of the third millennium B.C.E. For his service to the king, Hesy-Ra was accorded the title, "Great One of the Dentists" or *Wer-ibeh-senjw*, as shown in this photograph from his mastaba tomb in Sakkara, Egypt. Hesy-Ra was a master ivory carver, who doubtless acquired his knowledge by observing other practitioners whose names are now lost to history. As writing evolved, some practitioners eventually saw fit to share their knowledge by reducing it to writing. Such written records are the second oldest element of dental education (Fig. 1).

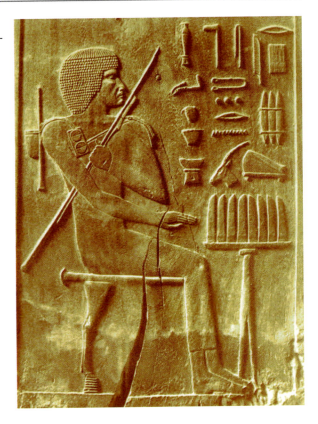

Fig. 1 Relief of Hesy-Ra from his mastaba, photo Hesy-Ra_CG1426.jpg: User:GDK: James Edward Quibell. (Image in public domain)

Written Record

The earliest written record related to teeth was a *Sumerian clay tablet* dating to 3,000 B.C.E., with a cuneiform inscription referring to the legend of the "tooth worm," which was thought to be the cause of tooth decay (Hoffmann-Axthelm 1981). This legend persisted in many countries until the beginning of the twentieth century.

The Assyro-Babylonian civilization had extensive written observations on how to treat diseases of the mouth and teeth. In fact, there are numerous references to teeth found in many of the 660 cuneiform medical tablets of King Ashurbanipal (seventh century B.C.E.) discovered by Henry Layard in 1847 in Nineveh. According to R. Campbell Thompson, a noted Oxford University scholar of Mesopotamian history, these tablets are at least 3,800 years old and date from the period of Enlil-Bani, King of Isin (Thompson 1923). Two of the tablets contain curative incantations for diseases of the mouth, teeth, bad breath, and salivation (Thompson 1926; Paulissian 1991, 1993). In addition, toothpicks are known to have been used by the Assyro-Babylonians (Paulissian 1991).

One of the best-known texts describing treatment for head and neck trauma is the *Edwin Smith Papyrus* from the sixteenth century B.C.E. Purchased in 1862 by its

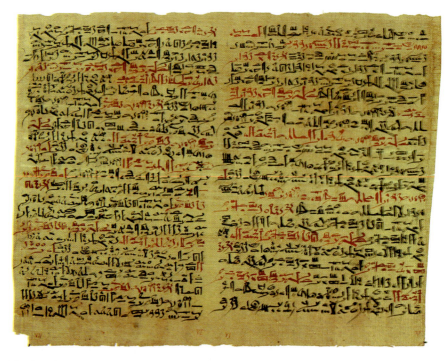

Fig. 2 Edwin Smith Papyrus. (Image in public domain)

namesake, who was an American Egyptologist, the 4.68 m papyrus describes 48 trauma cases including seven referring to the head. It is considered to be the first medical "textbook." Interestingly, the level of sophistication indicated by the Edwin Smith Papyrus far exceeded the knowledge that even Hippocrates could call upon more than a millennium later (Fig. 2).

Up until the dawn of the Renaissance in the sixteenth century, no text had ever been exclusively dedicated to the subject of the oral cavity or teeth. Instead, the medical texts of renowned ancient and early medieval physicians such as *Galen of Pergamon* or *Avicenna* made only tangential reference to treating oral and dental conditions that were known to them.

The invention of the moveable printing press around 1450, however, created an opportunity to disseminate the classical works of such noted physicians. But perhaps, more importantly, the printing press also led to the publication of newer works containing the accumulated scientific knowledge from the Arab World. It can scarcely be overstated how much the printing press popularized information and made knowledge accessible en masse.

A case in point was the first dental book dedicated exclusively to the subject of teeth, *Zene Artzney* (*Medicine for the Teeth*) (Zene Artzney 1981). Published in Leipzig in 1530 and written in German, the book was intended for itinerant dentists. Within its 44 pages, basic information was provided on dentition along with practical advice on how to deal with loose, decayed, or painful teeth. The book proved so popular that between 1530–1576 it was reprinted in no less than 15 editions. The first English edition was published in 1541 (Zene Artzney 1981).

A mere 2 years later, in 1543, arguably the most influential medical text of its day was published. *Andreas Vesalius*, a young Belgian professor of anatomy at the University of Padua published his seminal work, *De Humanis Corporis Fabrica* (*On the Workings of the Human Body*), a remarkably accurate (from a science standpoint) and artistically extraordinary atlas and text (Vesalius 1543). The copper-etched illustrations were the work of Jan Van Calcar, a fellow Belgian and a student of Titian. Van Calcar observed cadaver dissections performed by Vesalius, who served three roles at once: reader, pointer, and dissector, which had until then been assigned to three different persons.

Just 20 years later, in 1563, *Bartolomeo Eustachi*, an anatomist and contemporary of Vesalius, published the first comprehensive work on teeth, a 96-page pamphlet entitled *Libellus de Dentibus* (*A Treatise on the Teeth*) (Eustachio 1563). Unlike *Zene Artzney*, Eustachi's book was intended for the more educated practitioner and was, in fact, republished later that year as part of a larger work, *Opuscula Anatomica* (*A Small Anatomical Study*), a comprehensive volume by Eustachi which included his observations on the kidneys and the auditory system. This set the stage for the appearance of the first true textbook on teeth.

The Dental Practitioner-Author

The next step in the evolution of dental education occurred near the end of the sixteenth century with the emergence of renowned practitioners who also boasted equally famous published works. The first to do so was *Ambroise Paré*, a surgeon-barber to four French Kings; Paré was a practicing barber-surgeon, who dedicated three chapters to dentistry in his *Oeuvres* (Paré 1575). Written in French rather than the usual Latin, these chapters dealt with treatment of mandibular subluxation, traumas to the tongue and provided a detailed description of the barber-surgeon's instruments (Paré 1595a, b). Paré accumulated his experience during the Italian and the French Wars of Religion, which wracked both countries for much of the 1500s. When not on the battlefield, Paré busied himself by perfecting various techniques including cauterization of caries and re-implantation of teeth. Much of his practical knowledge was incorporated into his book, which, by way of example, provided illustrations of forceps for extraction, files to smooth out sharp-edged teeth, and obturators for cleft palates. In addition to his inventive mind, Paré also displayed a concern for the patient's comfort, to whatever extent such a thing was feasible in the sixteenth century. For instance, instead of using hot oil to cauterize open wounds, the standard treatment at the time, Paré substituted with a gentler wound dressing made of egg yolk, rose oil, and turpentine (Fig. 3). Indeed, his use of ligature to stop bleeding instead of hot iron cauterization earned him the nickname, "the gentle surgeon."

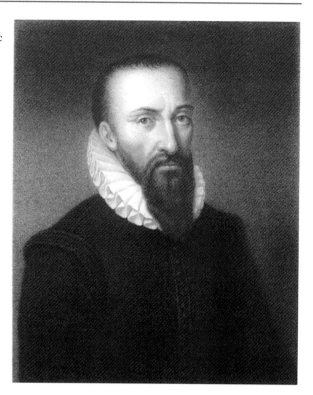

Fig. 3 Paré, Ambroise, 1510?–1590. (Image in public domain)

Early Attempts to Regulate the Practice of Dentistry

The publication of textbooks on teeth facilitated the dissemination of knowledge to those wishing to learn the craft of dentistry. These books served as a useful supplement to simple observation and/or formal apprenticeship. In the early days of the profession, both training and practice were unregulated and virtually unrestricted. This situation naturally led to a broad range of "expertise" among practitioners, many of whom were woefully unqualified. This was exacerbated by the fact that both barbers *and* surgeons laid claim to the title of standard-bearers of the profession.

As long as barbers and surgeons coexisted in dentistry, there had been tensions between trained and nontrained practitioners. Practicing dentistry became regulated at different times in different countries. These regulations served two purposes: to restrict admission to the profession and to ensure safe, knowledgeable practice. For instance, in England, the earliest form of professional regulation dates back to 1308, when the Company of Barbers of London was established. A few decades later, in 1369, the Fellowship of Surgeons was established and was later formally incorporated in 1462. Nearly a century later, by act of Parliament, Henry VIII granted a charter to the Company of Barbers and Surgeons of London. Even though they were part of the same company, the act expressly stipulated that barbers were to restrict their practice to dentistry, haircutting, wig making, or shaving whereas surgery was reserved to physicians. This union of the barbers and surgeons was eventually dissolved in 1745, when the two trades were finally split into their own respective companies.

Other countries took rather different routes to the professionalization of dentistry. In Prussia, for example, Duke Frederick William, Elector of Brandenburg, issued an edict in 1685 mandating that all dentists sit for an exam before a commission in order to demonstrate their knowledge. A similar edict was issued by Louis XIV of France in 1699 whereby dentists were required to undergo an examination with three masters of surgery at the Collège du Saint Côme in Paris before they could call themselves "experts." Additional restrictions were added in 1766 when a 2–3 year apprenticeship became compulsory, and members were prohibited from engaging in the trade of barbers.

Apprenticeship as a Form of Training

Practicing dentistry was never a full-time profession until it became formally regulated. During the early medieval period, dental practice was generally the domain of *barbers* and *dentatores* as first described in the influential medical treatise, *Chirurgia Magna*, written by Guy de Chauliac in 1363. They performed a variety of procedures including extractions, bloodletting, shaving, cutting hair, and even the occasional limb amputation, thereby living up to their title of barber-surgeon. It was quite customary in those days for barber-surgeons to move from town to town like itinerant tradesman performing their craft in public spaces. These early practitioners went by many monikers depending on where they lived: In medieval France, they were termed "arracheurs des dents" (snatchers of teeth), in Prussia they were called "zahnbrecher" (tooth-breakers), in England they were dubbed "operators for the teeth," and in Italy they advertised themselves as "cavadenti" (tooth-drawers). Those that proved more skillful would often give up this itinerant lifestyle, opting instead to be directly employed by wealthy patrons, or in some cases, aristocrats and even kings. Endowed with a fixed place, their craft was passed on to their descendants, or any students seeking an apprenticeship who were willing to pay a fee for their specialized training.

The term *chirurgien-dentiste*, or surgeon-dentist, was first coined by *Pierre Fauchard*, a famous French dentist and the author of *Le Chirurgien Dentiste*, a comprehensive overview of the dentistry (Fauchard 1728). Published in 1728, this work stands as a milestone in the history of dental education and marks the beginning of dentistry as a specialized profession (Fig. 4). Perhaps as a result of this, Fauchard is often regarded as the "father of modern dentistry."

Within its two volumes, *Le Chirurgien Dentiste* covered all that was known in the craft of dentistry at the time. It included a description of the "structure, relations and mechanics of the teeth, … the disease of the teeth and its conservation" along with common instruments, treatment options, and descriptions of typical oral and dental

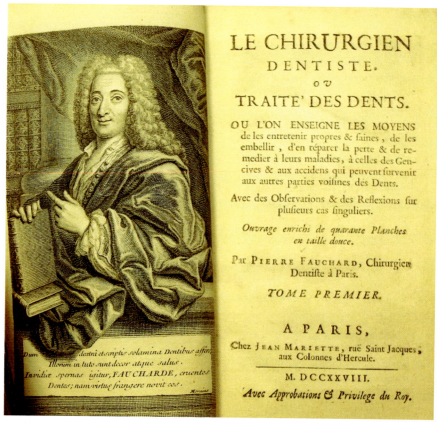

Fig. 4 Pierre Fauchard's masterpiece, *Le Chirurgiene Dentiste*, 1728. Photo taken of the first edition in the NYU College of Dentistry Rare Book Collection. (With permission from AI Spielman)

pathologies. Additionally, the work included Fauchard's own professional observations gleaned from his long years of practice in the French Royal Navy, in the cities of Angers and Paris. Before publishing, Fauchard secured the endorsement of 19 of the most prominent physicians, scientists, surgeons, and dentists of the day, thereby ensuring broad acceptance of his work and cementing his legacy (Spielman 2007). Fauchard's publication spurred a flurry of over 40 French publications related to dentistry over the next 50 years. *Le Chirurgien Dentiste* was translated into German within 5 years of its initial publication, though the English edition would not be published for more than two centuries (1946).

With the availability of such published texts on dentistry, apprenticeship became the generally accepted form of education in the eighteenth and early nineteenth centuries. For a fee, students could learn the trade while practicing under the supervision of an established barber-surgeon typically for a period of 1–3 years.

14 Dental Education: A Brief History

Upon completion, the newly minted practitioner was usually barred from opening up shop within a specified distance of his teacher in order to avoid undue competition.

In 1728, the same year that Fauchard published his seminal work, the most influential surgeon and dentist of eighteenth century Scotland, *John Hunter* was born. Hunter enjoyed a reputation as an outstanding surgeon, anatomist, and dentist. And through his appointment to St. George's Hospital, he became not only the leading surgeon of his time but also one of the foremost educators of young surgeons in England. This form of learning the trade was far more advanced. It involved apprenticeship in a hospital. Hunter's influence on English dental publishing was similar to that of Fauchard some 40 years earlier in France.

While apprenticeship was necessary to practice at that time, an official license was not yet required. This next step in the development of the profession did not occur until 1771, when Benjamin Fritsche, a Mecklenburg dentist, received permission from the faculty of medicine at Christian Albrecht University in Kiel to formally practice dentistry. Twelve years later, in 1783, a second dentist, Philipp Frank from Würzburg was issued a certificate by Karl Caspar Siebold, a professor of surgery. Such developments eventually led to the appointment of certified dentists to teach medical students in universities, thereby marking the next step in the evolution of dental education.

The first formal series of lectures on dentistry in England were given to medical students in 1799 at Guy's Hospital in London. Their teacher was a dentist named Joseph Fox who had been a student of Hunter and had authored the 1803 treatise "The Natural History of the Human Teeth." Not surprisingly, Guy's Hospital became the first to appoint a dental-surgeon to its staff (Gelbier 2016). Around that time in Germany, a dentist by the name of Karl Joseph Ringelmann, became the first professor permitted to teach dentistry at the University of Würzburg beginning in 1825. Such dental education was limited to medical students, who generally performed dental work only within the context of their medical practices.

These modest progressions foreshadowed the era of simultaneous education of entire cohorts of dental students within an academic setting: In other words, what we would today call, a dental school. The next step was the opening of such formal dental schools. These schools provided the education necessary to enter into the profession but not the subsequent lifelong learning needed to keep up with the growing body of medical knowledge. That role would come to be filled by medical/dental publications and professional societies.

The First Dental School, Professional Publication, and Dental Society

Dental Schools

During the eighteenth and early nineteenth centuries, France and England were the most advanced nations in the field of dentistry. But by midcentury as the Industrial Revolution got underway and a market for more sophisticated dental care began to emerge, the United States took center stage in dental education.

Formal dental education in the United States first appeared at the beginning of the 1800s. It grew out of two main necessities. First, there was a lack of opportunity to be formally trained for those who wished to enter the profession. Second, partly due to this lack of training opportunities, there was a proliferation of untrained and often shady practitioners who naturally brought disrepute to the dental profession. As the overall number of dentists in America grew, dentistry's reputation became increasingly worse. While the initial number of dentists in the United States around 1800 was insignificant, by 1825 there were close to 200 practicing dentists in the country, and by 1847 there were 120 dentists in New York alone.

It was a vicious cycle: There were not enough well-trained dentists, and there were insufficient teachers to resolve the shortage. Many physicians and surgeons practiced dentistry on the side. They had learned the trade by apprenticeship. A number of practitioners offered formal training courses for private pupils. Such courses were neither cheap nor adequate to accommodate all those wishing to enter the profession. Private apprenticeship was traditionally 12–18 months and cost anywhere from $500 to $1,000. Others went as far as to open private schools for more than one pupil at a time. One such school was operated by *John Harris* in Bainbridge, Ohio. Harris was a physician and the older brother of Chapin Harris, a cofounder of the Baltimore College of Dental Surgery, whose impact will be discussed later.

Some, like Horace Hayden, another cofounder of the Baltimore College of Dental Surgery, saw the need to extend dental education to medical students in an effort to elevate the status of dentistry. *Horace Hayden* and *Chapin Harris* emerged as the leaders of the nineteenth century movement to modernize dental education.

Both Hayden and Harris, along with their colleague *Eleazar Parmly*, envisioned a four-step approach to enhance the profession of dentistry. First, they sought to establish dental departments within medical schools. These were to be based on a curriculum that would provide formal training to physicians, treating dentistry as a subspecialty of medicine. Second, they advocated for the establishment of professional publications to serve as a medium for sharing knowledge and clinical experience. As a third step, they worked to set up professional societies where dentists could meet regularly and share their experiences. Up until then, dentists had mostly operated in isolation without the benefit of the collective wisdom of their peers. And finally, realizing that the profession desperately needed a legislative framework within which the practice of dentistry could be properly regulated, they lobbied state and local politicians to pass laws that would ultimately protect the public from unskilled and unscrupulous practitioners.

Though they are mostly known for their professional contributions to dentistry, on a personal level, Hayden and Harris also led intellectually rigorous lives. Both travelled widely and had distinguished careers outside of dentistry. They had met at a time when American society was changing rapidly due to the industrialization. Indeed, their backgrounds neatly complemented each other. Hayden was a learned man of science with much wisdom gleaned from long age which he gladly shared with his colleague who was 37 years his junior. Harris, in contrast, was relatively youthful and dynamic. Indeed, he was responsible for a great deal of the organizational impetus behind the changes to dental education.

Horace Hayden had originally studied geology and was the author of several notable papers on the topic including the *Geological Sketch of Baltimore* published in 1810. His interest in dentistry came about by accident. In 1795, Horace Hayden was in New York and in need of dental care. During an appointment with John Greenwood, one of George Washington's dentists, Hayden became fascinated with the field. He requested Greenwood's help in procuring dental books in order to broaden his knowledge and to receive training in dentistry. Of the several available textbooks at the time, Greenwood suggested John Hunter's book, *The Natural History of the Human Teeth*. Hayden ended up staying in New York for an apprenticeship with Greenwood before finally returning to Baltimore in 1800. Hayden opened his own practice and became a successful dental surgeon. His reputation earned him the respect of educators from the University of Maryland Medical School, where he was invited to give a course in dentistry to the medical students in 1837. In recognition of his numerous contributions to medical education, he was eventually awarded one of the few honorary medical degrees ever given to a dentist from both the University of Maryland and Jefferson College of Medicine in Philadelphia.

Chapin Harris had initially studied medicine and established a practice in Greenfield, Ohio. Like many of his physician colleagues, he also performed occasional dental extractions. His focus shifted primarily to dentistry, however, when his brother, John (mentioned earlier), invited him to attend his school in Bainbridge, Ohio, that had operated out of his home from 1823–1828. Chapin Harris graduated from the school in 1828 and settled in Bloomfield, Ohio where he practiced medicine, surgery, and dentistry.

Hayden and Harris originally sought to develop dental education within an existing institution of higher education. In 1837, they approached the University of Maryland administration with a request to establish a Dental Department with a full course in dental training as part of the medical school. Their request was denied on the grounds that medical students already have plenty to study and that a single training course would not make them proficient in dentistry.

As an alternative, in 1839, they submitted a petition to the Maryland Legislature to establish an independent dental school. In spite of opposition and lobbying from the medical establishment, on February 1, 1840, their charter was granted. Later that year, the first dental school in the world, Baltimore College of Dental Surgery, was opened with a faculty of just four professors. On November 3, 1840, Chapin Harris delivered his introductory lecture to the college's inaugural class of five students. In its first 10 years, Baltimore College of Dental Surgery graduated 84 students and awarded 151 honorary degrees. The principal requirement for graduation was completion of either two sessions or 2 years of preceptorship (apprenticeship). Each session lasted no less than 4 months but facilities were rather inadequate. It was not until 1846 that the first practical instruction in a dental infirmary was added to the curriculum. Horace Hayden became the first president of the dental college and remained in that post until his untimely death in 1844 after which Harris took over the position.

In contrast, dental education in Europe took a rather different path. Even though dental practice in France and England had been more advanced during the 1700s, the establishment of formal dental education was much slower to take place in these countries. The usual form of education in England involved a lengthy apprenticeship under the tutelage of surgeons and physicians that practiced dentistry on the side.

The Company of Surgeons of London became the Royal College of Surgeons in 1843 whose jurisdiction included the whole of England. There is no doubt that the establishment of scientific societies along with the first dental school in the United States served as a source of inspiration for the dental-surgical establishment in Great Britain. In 1845, *John Tomes* gave a series of lectures to medical students at Middlesex Hospital. Later, under his leadership, the *Odontological Society of London* was formed in 1856. It had become obvious that there was a need for formally recognized dentists whose training included much more than a single medical school course. Tomes asked the Royal College of Surgeons to issue a dental diploma as a means of formal certification. Two years later, the Odontological Society created what would become the Royal Dental Hospital in Soho Square, and in 1859, the first dental school in the UK, the *London School of Dental Surgery* was opened. Very soon after, other dental hospitals opened including the National Dental Hospital in 1861 (Gelbier 2016).

In 1834, the noted French physician and author of *Traite sur les Dents* (1820), *Joseph Jean-Francois Lemaire*, offered a theoretical and practical course in dentistry at the University of Paris. He charged a fee of 10 francs (Manuel 2009). The first formal dental school in Paris *(L'École Dentaire)* opened in 1879 while the first German dental school opened in 1884 in Berlin. In Canada, similar to the British dental schools, the *University of Toronto* was established in 1858.

Dental Journals

Soon after establishing the first dental school in the world, Hayden and Harris set about establishing a professional dental publication, a step which they hoped would enhance the profession through lifelong dental education for practitioners. In 1839, along with Eleazar Parmly and a group of other visionary dentists, Harris began publishing the first scientific journal for dentistry, *The American Journal of Dental Science*. After all, dentistry was a profession that was expanding, and knowledge needed to be shared. By 1840, the journal had grown to a circulation of 317 subscribers located in 22 US states and foreign countries, including England, Scotland, France, Holland, and the West Indies. Soon, other trade publications began to crop up, such as *The New York Dental Recorder* (1847), *The British Journal of Dental Sciences* (1856), and *Dental Cosmos* (1859).

Dental Societies

On August 18, 1840, around the same time that the first dental journal appeared, Hayden, Harris, and 40 of the brightest dentists of the time gathered in New York to cofound the *American Society of Dental Surgeons* with Harris as its first president.

14 Dental Education: A Brief History

This had been an integral part of their plan to enhance the overall reputation of the profession. Although the society had become defunct by the mid-1850s, it was the forerunner to the American Dental Association (ADA), a name that was assumed in 1859. Over in Canada, the Royal College of Dental Surgeons of Ontario was created in 1868. England followed suit in 1880 with the establishment of the British Dental Association.

Regulating the Practice of Dentistry

During the mid-nineteenth century, there were several attempts to enact legislation to regulate the profession in the United States. One of the earliest examples of this was in Alabama. In 1841, the Alabama State Legislature passed an act regulating the practice of dental surgery. The law in effect mandated that anyone wishing to become a dentist had to be licensed as a physician first and formally approved by the medical board to practice. This law remained in effect until the beginning of the American Civil War. In 1868, New York, Kentucky, and Ohio became the next three states in the United States to legislatively regulate the practice of dentistry. The minimum age limit was set at 16 along with a minimum requirement of 4 years of apprenticeship under a licensed dentist. Those meeting these criteria were then permitted to sit for an examination by the State Board of Censors.

In early nineteenth century England, except for London and the immediate area around it, there were effectively no restrictions on who could practice dentistry. In the City of London, the College of Surgeons and the College of Physicians set specific rules for practicing. In response to this situation, the Parliament passed The Dentists Act of 1878 which aimed to regulate the practice of dentistry in the UK. Up until then, this had been the task of the Royal College of Surgeons of England, which was the sole diploma-granting body.

Reforming Dental Education

Limiting the practice of dentistry was a critically necessary step to control widespread abuse by unqualified individuals. However, the opening and running of dental schools remained unregulated. With few exceptions, early dental schools were essentially for-profit trade schools. Curriculum and educators were not standardized. Dental education was in dire need of reform.

After the opening of Baltimore College of Dentistry, many other schools, primarily in the United States were established in the years that followed. Most of these were modeled after the school in Baltimore. However, many of these early schools folded, merged, or were absorbed into other dental schools. Criticism of dental curricula led to some improvements in educational requirements and length of education. An 1872 ADA report on the status of education argued that no dental student should be admitted until they have at least a minimum of 1 year private dental apprenticeship in an office. The report indicated that "there are in this country some twelve or fourteen thousand dentists, of various grades of ability or dis-ability. Among these are hundreds, yes thousands, who have had little or no preliminary instruction. Probably not one quarter of this number read the current dental literature of the day, and are strangers to dental or medical text books of any description" (Francis 1872). As a result, eventually the ADA established a minimum of 2 years for the course of instruction of a dentist. In spite of such advances, uneducated dentists far outnumbered those that graduated from a dental school. For instance, between 1840 and 1850, a total of 115 graduated with a DDS degree in the United States. That number in the United States rose to 532 by 1860. Nevertheless, they represented only 3.9% of those practicing in 1850 and 9.5% of those in 1860. In comparison, an 1850 survey in the UK showed that there were "300 dentists in London and 400 in the provinces" some with medical degrees but none with a formal dental school diploma (Hillam 1990).

Overall, during the 40 years from 1840–1880, a total of 24 dental schools opened in the United States, all but five were proprietary and independent. Europe and Canada followed suit with schools in London, Glasgow, Toronto, Montreal, etc. A handful of schools established dental departments as part of a major university medical school, starting with Harvard in 1867, followed by University of Michigan in 1875 and University of Pennsylvania in 1878. These decisions were in response to ongoing criticism from the medical establishment of the proprietary nature of most dental schools. As dental education formally took off, most institutions initially had two-session programs. But gradually, the length of dental education increased to three, and eventually four sessions over the subsequent decades.

A critical juncture in dental education occurred when William J. Gies, a biochemist from Columbia University, was tasked by the Carnegie Foundation to review the status of dental education (Gies 1926). The 5-year study undertaken by a committee chaired by Gies examined the critical lack of science and standardization in dental education. The 692-page document changed the profession, established standards, and set the stage for formal nationwide board examinations that began in 1934. The Gies Report, as it became known, was published in 1926 and marked another milestone in the history of dental education. Mirroring the 1910 Flexner Report (on the rather poor state of medical education) (Flexner 1910), the Gies Report argued, among other things, for greater cooperation between dentistry and medicine, the inclusion of dental research findings in school curricula, as well as the need for basic science courses for dental students, all in order to meet the demands for dental healthcare in the future.

William Gies' influence was also felt in other ways. In 1919, Gies chaired an editorial board made up of 70 distinguished dentists and scientists that was instrumental in establishing the Journal of Dental Research. He stated in the editorial of the journal: "Research in its highest expression is open-minded inquiry for truth, to be found and revealed unreservedly for the information, instruction, advantage, and welfare of all" (Gies 1919). Around that same time, he helped found the American Association of Dental Schools, the predecessor to the American Dental Educators Association (ADEA), a leading international institution that heavily influenced dental education in the decades that followed.

Conclusions

In the 95 years since the Gies Report was issued, dental education has expanded in its sophistication, requirements, content, and scope. Today, dentistry is a highly regulated profession. There are close to 2000 dental schools worldwide, to say nothing of dental therapy, dental nursing, and dental hygiene programs. The explosion of knowledge and the types of treatments is constantly driving change in our profession. Dental education must adapt and follow suit. During the next few decades, dental schools will find themselves at a crossroads. Technological advances in information delivery (online, virtual, simulation), scientific advances, and newer, less invasive procedures will impact the format, content, timing, and location of education. These will inexorably alter the way we interact with students and patients. Ultimately, this will benefit society and the oral health of our patients.

Cross-References

- ▶ Clinical Education in Nursing: Current Practices and Trends
- ▶ Competencies of Health Professions Educators of the Future
- ▶ Dental Education: Context and Trends
- ▶ Interprofessional Education (IPE): Trends and Context
- ▶ Learning and Teaching in the Operating Theatre: Expert Commentary from the Nursing Perspective
- ▶ Medical Education: Trends and Context
- ▶ Nursing and Midwifery Education: Historical Perspectives
- ▶ Surgical Education and Training: Historical Perspectives

References

Bernardini F, Tuniz C, Coppa A, Mancini L, Dreossi D, Eichert D, et al. Beeswax as dental filling on a Neolithic human tooth. PLoS One. 2012;7:e44904. https://doi.org/10.1371/journal.pone. 0044904.

Coppa A, Bandioli L, Cucina A, Frayer DW, Jarrige C, Jarrige JF, et al. Palaeontology: early Neolithic tradition of dentistry. Nature. 2006;440:755–6. https://doi.org/10.1038/440755a.

Eustachio B. Libellus de dentibus. Venice; 1563.

Fauchard P. Le Chirurgien Dentiste. Paris: Pierre-Jean Mariette; 1728. p. 1728.

Flexner A. Medical education in the United States and Canada. New York City: The Carnegie Foundation for the Advancement of Teaching; 1910.

Francis CE. Report of the (newly appointed) Committee on Dental Education. In: Transactions of the American Dental Association. Wabash Steam Printing House, Chicago, IL, 1872. p. 111.

Gelbier S. Origins of dental education and training in the USA and UK. J Hist Dent. 2016;64:112–20.

Gies WJ. J Dent Res. 1919;1:1–7.

Gies WJ. Dental education in the United States and Canada. The Carnegie foundation for the advancement of teaching, Waverley Press, Baltimore, 1926.

Hillam C. The roots of dentistry. The Lindsay Society for the History of Dentistry, BDK, Amsterdam, New York, 1990.

Hoffmann-Axthelm W. History of dentistry. Quintessence Publishing; 1981.

Manuel DE. Dental education in Paris in the 1830s. Dent Hist. 2009;49:4–15.

Oxilia G, Fiorillo F, Boschini F, Boaretto E, Apicella SA, Mateucci C, et al. The dawn of dentistry in the late upper Paleolithic: an early case of pathological intervention at Riparo Fredian. Am J Phys Anthropol. 2017;163:446–61. https://doi.org/10.1002/ajpa.23216.

Paré A. Les oeuvres, Gabriel Buon, Paris, 1575.

Paré A. Chapter XXV - Les instruments propres pour archer et rompre les dents (The instruments appropriate to pull and break up teeth), 1595a. p 513–516. https://gallica.bnf.fr/ark:/12148/bpt6k53757m/f488.item.r=bouche

Paré A. Chapter VIII-X - Cure particuliere des luxations: Et premierement de la Mandibule inferieure (Chapter VIII), Maniere de reduire la mandibule luxeé en la partie anterieure des deux costez (Chapter IX) and Maniere de reduire la mandibule luxeé seulment d'un costé. (Chapter X), 1595b, p 463–465. https://gallica.bnf.fr/ark:/12148/bpt6k53757m/f488.item.r=bouche

Paulissian R. Medicine in Ancient Assyria and Babylonia. J Assyr Acad Soc. 1991;V:3–51. http://www.jaas.org/edocs/v5n1/Paulissian.pdf. Accessed 15 July 2019.

Paulissian R. Dental care in Ancient Assyria and Babylonia. J Assyr Acad Soc. 1993;VII:96–116. http://www.jaas.org/edocs/v7n2/Paulissian2.pdf. Accessed 15 July 2019.

Spielman AI. The birth of the most important 18th century dental text: Pierre Fauchard's Le Chirurgien Dentiste. J Dent Res. 2007;86:922–6. https://doi.org/10.1177/154405910708601004.

Thompson RC. Assyrian medical texts. Humphrey Milford Oxford University Press; 1923.

Thompson, RC. In: Assyrian medical texts; 1926. https://journals.sagepub.com/doi/pdf/10.1177/003591572601901703. Accessed 15 July 2019.

Vesalius A. De Humanis Corporis Fabrica Libri Septem. Basel: Ioanni Oporino; 1543.

Zene Artzney. The classics of dentistry library; Leslie B. Adam Publisher, Birmingham, AL, 1981.

Surgical Education and Training: Historical Perspectives

15

John P. Collins

Contents

Introduction	268
Origins of Surgeons, Physicians, and Apothecaries	269
Introduction	269
Royal Charters for Physicians, Surgeons, and Apothecaries	270
Separation of the Surgeons from the Barbers	270
Surgeon-Apothecaries, "Pure" Surgeons, and Their Practices	272
The Evolution of Surgical Education and Training	272
The Apprenticeship System	272
New Opportunities for Learning	273
Medical Education and the Universities	274
Transformations in Teaching and Learning	275
Learning to Cope with the Patients' Pain and Suffering	276
Milestones in Surgical Education and Training After 1850	277
Introduction	277
William Halsted's and Edward Churchill's Surgical Training in America	277
Changes in Surgical Education and Training in Great Britain and Ireland	278
The Tipping Point in Surgical Education and Training	280
Conclusion	281
Cross-References	281
References	281

Abstract

Surgeons trace their origins to the barber-surgeons, from whom they separated in the mid-eighteenth century to develop the art and science of surgery. It would take them another 100 years to transform themselves from the manual workers of

---

J. P. Collins (✉)
University Department of Surgery, University of Melbourne, Melbourne, Australia

Nuffield Department of Surgical Sciences, University of Oxford, Oxford, UK

Green Templeton College, Oxford, UK
e-mail: john.collins@hillviewlodge.co

© Springer Nature Singapore Pte Ltd. 2023
D. Nestel et al. (eds.), *Clinical Education for the Health Professions*,
https://doi.org/10.1007/978-981-15-3344-0_18

medicine into a professional medical elite. The defining learning experience for aspiring surgeons was the apprenticeship. Originating in community settings, apprentices supplemented their education at the new hospitals and their adjoining learning facilities and private amenities and ultimately at the expanding Universities. The newly formed surgical colleges and corporations remained predominantly as examination bodies for a further century.

The first formal surgical training program originated in Germany. Introduced into North America in the late nineteenth century with initial acclaim, it was later considered too autocratic, pyramidal, and wasteful, and replaced in many centers by a more efficient system. Surgical apprenticeship in the United Kingdom remained unchanged until the latter half of the twentieth century when it was acknowledged as excessively long, wasteful, and ruinous for the many trainees unsuccessful in obtaining consultant hospitals posts.

It was the developments at the end of the twentieth century that led to a tipping point in surgical training and a search for a new educational model. Advances in educational theory, operating room efficiency, sicker hospital patients, emphasis on reducing medical errors, shorter residents' working hours, and new surgical techniques such as minimally invasive surgery, changed the learning environment forever. In response, surgical skills laboratories were developed where the teaching, learning, and practice of technical and other skills could take place with immediate feedback prior to the resident performing surgery on patients. Efforts continue to ensure that a patient-centered and resident-orientated surgical education is available worldwide.

Keywords

Historiography · Apothecaries · Surgeons · Surgery · Education · Apprenticeship · Simulation

Introduction

Although the history of surgery dates back to its medieval origins, it was not until the second half of the eighteenth century that a turning point occurred in its development. Commencing with the eighteenth-century Enlightenment, a transformation occurred across Europe leading to new concepts in thought, science, education, and healing programs, the combination of which influenced the practice of surgery and medical education. The previous order and structure of medical studies broke down and were replaced by less arbitrary training of medical practitioners including surgeons (Bonner 1995).

Despite its long history, it was not until the years between 1750 and 1850 that surgery developed from a manual craft into a scientific medical discipline, and surgeons transformed themselves from the manual workers of medicine into a professional medical elite. Furthermore, it would take another quarter of a century (1846–1873) before pain, hemorrhage, and infection, "the great evils which had always embittered the practice of surgery and checked its progress … were robbed of their terrors," and the practice of surgery was enabled to advance (Halsted 1904). With each major advance in surgery, improvements became necessary in the methods used to prepare surgeons for independent surgical practice.

The aims of this chapter are to provide a historical perspective on the evolution of the education and training of surgeons from the beginning of the professionalization of surgery around 1750 to the end of the twentieth century. Commencing with an overview of the origins of surgeons, their corporations, and of surgical practice, the major developments in surgical education, training, and learning will be discussed. Although the major focus will be on surgical education in English-speaking countries, references will be made where relevant to developments on the Continent of Europe.

Origins of Surgeons, Physicians, and Apothecaries

Introduction

By the end of the eighteenth century, British law recognized three official orders of medical practitioners, namely, physicians, surgeons, and apothecaries, although it was common for individuals to practice across these categories (Willcock 1830). There were of course many others then plying their trade to the sick including chemists, druggists, and various irregular "healers." Because the development of the three major medical groups was so interconnected, their origins are best understood when considered together.

The physicians or practitioners of internal medicine traced their medieval ancestry to learned clerics and were recognized as the educated elite and knowledgeable about theory in the medical world. The medieval origins of modern surgery lie elsewhere – in the institutional separation of head and hand. Although there were learned surgeons in the Middle Ages, the rank and file surgeons traced their origins to the guilds of barbers, apothecaries, and grocers. While internal medicine was regarded as a book learned profession and occurred in places of higher learning, the procedural practices of surgery were fostered in the civic world of trades and guilds. Significant contributions were also made to the development of surgery as well as to internal medicine by Arab-Islamic medicine (Conrad 1995). The apothecaries originated as grocers who collected provisions for culinary and medicinal purposes and later began to manufacture and sell medicines based on prescriptions mainly from physicians.

A decision by the Roman Catholic Church in the Edict of Tours in 1163 forbade monks from shedding blood, and the resulting void in the practice of surgery was filled by the barbers who had been their previous assistants. Throughout the medieval period, much of the manual medical practice notably bloodletting, drawing teeth, and lancing abscesses was carried out by the barbers who had learned their skills from the clerics. The medieval surgeons or craftsmen very occasionally performed more major operations such as amputations, lithotomy, and trepanation.

Royal Charters for Physicians, Surgeons, and Apothecaries

Royal Charters from various monarchs enabled the physicians, surgeons, and apothecaries to become formally established. The physicians were incorporated into a College of Physicians by a Charter from Henry VIII in 1518. Five years later, an Act of Parliament gave them the right to practice medicine in all its branches including surgery, although they rarely performed practical procedures. The College bylaws mostly restricted its license to those who had first obtained a university medical degree from Oxford or Cambridge and this limited its numbers and eventually its influence.

The Barber-Surgeons of Dublin were incorporated in 1446 by a Royal Charter from Henry VI for the promotion and exercise of the Art of Surgery (Widdess 1984). In 1506 James IV granted a Charter or Seal of Cause that incorporated the Barbers and Surgeons of Edinburgh, establishing them as the guardians and teachers of surgical practice (Society of Barbers of Edinburgh Archive 1722–1846). In London, those barbers who performed surgical procedures as well as barbering were united to the group of surgeons who had confined their practice to surgery, through an Act of Parliament and the granting of a Charter by Henry VIII in 1540, forming a trade guild and livery company (not a college), known as the Barber-Surgeons of London (Young 1890). The barber-surgeons of Glasgow were incorporated by James IV in 1599 and referred to as a "Facultie" (Geyer-Kordesch and Macdonald 1999).

The apothecaries who had formed themselves into one of the ancient companies of the City of London received a Charter of Incorporation from James I in 1617 (Willcock 1830). This enabled them to separate from the Grocers Company, extend their role, formalize their apprenticeship training, and reduce the previous overriding authority and power of supervision by the College of Physicians of London. Apothecaries are an important consideration in the history of surgery and surgical education as a high proportion of them practiced as surgeon-apothecaries from the second half of the eighteenth century.

Separation of the Surgeons from the Barbers

The growing role of surgeons in contemporary military campaigns and their greater knowledge of anatomy and increasing application to new learning, including natural history and the experimental sciences, raised their medical and social status and gradually expanded their power. Those surgeons among the Barber-Surgeons of London who wished to expand the art and science of surgery sought to sever what they perceived to be a restrictive union with the barbers. An Act of Parliament in 1745 dissolved this union and incorporated the surgeons under the commonly known name of The Company of Surgeons of London (Willcock 1830). This action was a significant milestone, as it was the first major statement by a group of surgeons in England that they wished to be recognized as legitimate medical practitioners, committed to the development and teaching of the art and science of surgery. It was for similar reasons that surgeons separated from the barbers in Berlin in 1725 and in Paris in 1743. The founding of the Academy of Surgery in Paris in 1731 replaced the French barber surgeons' guild. This event has been referred to as the "turning stake in the history of surgery, as the starting line in its scientific labours and of its true career" (Halsted 1904).

In Edinburgh, the barbers separated from the barber-surgeons in 1772. This was due to their resentment to the favoritism shown by the surgeons to the apothecaries and surgeon-apothecaries. The Edinburgh surgeons obtained a Royal Charter in 1778, which incorporated The Royal College of Surgeons of the City of Edinburgh and recognized the College as a learned and academic corporation. A subsequent Charter in 1851 separated the College from the Town Council and changed its title to The Royal College of Surgeons of Edinburgh (Dingwall 2005). In Dublin, the surgeons separated from the Barber-Surgeon's guild for the same reasons as the London surgeons, and obtained a Royal Charter, which established The Royal College of Surgeons in Ireland in 1784. Education was named in the application as one of its primary objectives, and in 1884 the College instituted a medical school as part of its corporation (Widdess 1984).

Despite the aspirations of its founders, the Company of Surgeons of London failed to reach the status and influence they had envisaged and after an uninspired existence was dissolved in 1797 (Minutes of The Company of Surgeons 1797). Its demise was not unexpected and perhaps foreshadowed by John Gunning, Master of the Company, in his damming retirement speech in 1790. He remarked that "your theatre is without lectures, your library room without books is converted to an office for your Clerk, and your committee room is become his eating parlour, . . . you have instituted lectures neither in surgery, nor indeed in anatomy of any degree of importance." He concluded that those responsible "on the least reflection must see & feel a great indecency in all of this" (Minutes of The Company of Surgeons 1790).

The failure of the Company was most likely due to its leaders being more preoccupied with the financial rewards generated by their private surgical practices and the income received from their students, rather than on the development and teaching of anatomy and surgery under the Company's patronage (Lawrence 1992). Following the dissolution of Company, the Royal College of Surgeons of London was established by Royal Charter in 1800. Its name was later changed to that of the Royal College of Surgeons of England in 1843, and which expanded its remit to the whole of England and Wales (Cope 1959).

Apothecaries began to provide advice to patients by way of consultation and prescribed the medicines which they manufactured and sold. The Royal College of Physicians of London objected to this practice in what is known as the Rose Case but the House of Lords ruled it appropriate for the Apothecaries to do so in 1704 (Hunting 1998). This decision marked the formal recognition of apothecaries' right to offer advice and prescribe as well as dispense medicines. In so doing, they became the forerunners of general practitioners. By the end of the eighteenth century, apothecaries had become fully entrenched and this was acknowledged by the prominent St Thomas's physician William Charles Wells, who referred in his 1799 letter to "the complete establishment of the apothecary as medical practitioners" (Wells 1799).

Surgeon-Apothecaries, "Pure" Surgeons, and Their Practices

From the middle of the eighteenth century, surgeon-apothecaries and apothecaries took on an increasing role in treating the sick, performing surgical procedures, and delivering babies. The London surgeon-apothecary James Parkinson observed in 1800 that few practitioners could survive financially by limiting their practice to either medicine (physic) or surgery, unless they had private means, or a hospital appointment, which brought them greater status and enhanced their reputation (Parkinson 1800). In 1795, the medical writer, reformer and previous surgeon-apothecary John Mason Good, observed that "there are few apothecaries in the country who do not engage in the practice of surgery and by far the greatest number in London do the same" (Good 1795). This was confirmed by the 1783 Medical Register of medical practitioners in provincial England, which showed that surgeon-apothecaries made up 82.3%, apothecaries 3.3%, physicians 11.4%, and "pure" surgeons 2.8% (Loudon 1986).

By the early nineteenth century this had begun to change, particularly in the large cities. Although the celebrated English surgeon William Lawrence told his students in 1830 that 'in the great majority of instances physic and surgery are both practised … by one set of persons, the surgeons and apothecaries; probably nineteen-twentieths of disease are under their care, …' (he added that) "in the metropolis and some large towns, they are exercised by two different classes of persons, whose education differs widely in important points." Lawrence noted these two classes were taught in separate courses by different teachers and their regulation was entrusted by law to two distinct public bodies, namely, the Royal College of Physicians of London and the Royal College of Surgeons of London (Lawrence 1829–1830).

Surgeon-apothecaries were mostly occupied with consultations, prescribing, and dealing with non-surgical problems. In addition, they performed blood-letting, drawing teeth, delivering babies in difficult labors, managing infections including lancing of abscesses, trussing ruptures, dressing wounds and burns, dealing with injuries including fractures and dislocations, and managing venereal disease (Porter 1995). Less commonly, they performed procedures such as hernia reduction, surgery on the testicle and the breast, and occasionally amputations.

A "pure" surgeon in the metropolis and large cities attended to the same surgical problems and performed similar procedures to the surgeon-apothecary. They also carried out more major operations such as mastectomy, amputation, and cutting for bladder stones, and with greater frequency. However, major surgery was not common. A review of the surgical cases admitted to Nottingham Hospital between 1795 and 1797 confirms that most of the surgical cases managed were minor (Loudon 1986).

The Evolution of Surgical Education and Training

The Apprenticeship System

The seeds of a surgical career are planted in the earliest stages of a student's medical education and it is here that the vital elements of the building blocks of a surgical identity begin to be acquired (Leppaniemi 2006). Unlike today where these foundations are built in universities, those who wished to become surgeons in the early eighteenth century had to rely on what they could learn during an apprenticeship in the community.

In contrast to some European countries like Germany where the universities had a prominent role in medical education, the defining experience for most medical practitioners in Great Britain and America was the apprenticeship (Bonner 1995). It was also the entry point to a full surgical career from the middle of the eighteenth century. In Great Britain and Ireland, boys as young as 14 undertook an apprenticeship of 5–7 years with an experienced medical practitioner and lived in their master's residence where he acted as their loco parentis. A certified contract outlined the education they were to receive, and the financial cost varied from 50 to 200 pounds or more, depending on the reputation of the master and on whether he had a hospital appointment.

In North America, a significant number of medical practitioners lacked an apprenticeship or formal training until late in the eighteenth century. Once the apprenticeship system became established it remained the pattern throughout the eighteenth century and part of the nineteenth. Those who embarked on an apprenticeship usually spent 3 years with a practitioner for which they paid the annual sum of around 100 dollars (Bonner 1995). The apprenticeship system slowly began to change when some of the American students who had traveled to study medicine in places like Leyden, Paris, London, and Edinburgh returned with an ambition to share the learning experiences they had enjoyed in hospitals and lecture-halls.

New Opportunities for Learning

Although apprenticeship system remained the mainstay of medical education throughout the eighteenth century and into the nineteenth, the original arrangements became insufficient for the needs of the expanding medical workforce and the medical marketplace apprentices were about to enter. These external factors were accentuated by the growing dissatisfaction among apprentices at the variable level of their teaching, and a lack of direct contact with patients until late in their apprenticeship. There were few opportunities to learn anatomy and the new and evolving subjects then becoming important for future medical practice. At the same time, some practicing surgeons had begun to consider the existing apprenticeship model as no longer fit for purpose. The London-based surgeon-apothecary James Parkinson, wrote in 1800 that "of all the modes which could be devised for a medical and chirurgical education, this is the most absurd" (Parkinson 1800). As the second half of the eighteenth century progressed, students became masters of their own learning. In addition to selecting apprenticeships with practitioners whose practice focus was similar to that of their own career aspirations, they began to seek new educational opportunities.

The development and expansion of hospitals and the transformation of their purpose into places of teaching as well as healing and research, provided new locations for learning outside the traditional apprenticeships and the universities. Apprentices began to supplement their education by undertaking a period "walking the wards" of a hospital and learning first-hand about different diseases and their management, as well as observing surgical operations. These students were referred to as apprentices, dressers, or pupils depending on their origin and nature of their hospital attachments. The apprentices and dressers acted as assistants to the surgeons and the money they paid was the sole property of the surgeon to whom they were attached (Wilks and Bettany 1892).

In addition to the scope of medical experience provided by the expanding hospitals, facilities were added to these institutions for students to learn anatomy and to attend lectures in surgery, medicine, physiology, midwifery, and other new and expanding subjects. Developed predominantly by the surgeons who carried out most of the teaching, many of these institutions went on to become important medical schools in London and the provinces. Independent private facilities for learning anatomy and other subjects were also established to cater for the growing population of medical students. The most prestigious was the Great Windmill Street School in London, which was founded in 1768 by the noted Scottish anatomist, physician, obstetrician, and teacher William Hunter. Here, he and his brother John offered students instruction in anatomy and opportunities for cadaver dissection. They also provided lectures in surgery, physiology, pathology, midwifery, and diseases of women and children (Thompson 1942).

The arrangements for apprenticeships at some of the London hospitals were however not without their critics. One anonymous medical practitioner wrote to *The Lancet* in 1824 on how the cost of 500 guineas for an apprenticeship to a hospital surgeon limited such opportunities to those whose parents could afford to pay this large fee. Furthermore, he claimed they usually did so in the expectation of their son's subsequent appointment to the staff of that hospital, thereby limiting such prospects to others. This correspondent also referred to the absence of formal teaching and the students having to fend for themselves "as a wild colt is turned to grass" (Anonymous 1824).

Medical Education and the Universities

Unlike some countries on the continent of Europe, the early universities in Britain and America were indifferent to the needs of higher medical education. Few medical practitioners graduated from the existing English universities of Oxford and Cambridge during the eighteenth century and those who did so, were usually destined to practice as physicians. Following the establishment of medical schools in Scotland at the University of Edinburgh in 1726 and the University of Glasgow in 1751, new and more accessible opportunities for a university-based medical education became available. The secular University of Edinburgh in particular, became popular with students from the United Kingdom and the English-speaking world. Between the years 1750 and 1800, the combined Scottish Universities of Edinburgh and Glasgow graduated 2600 medical practitioners (Calman 2007). During the same period, the amalgamated number who graduated from Oxford and Cambridge, was 246 or an average of five per year (Robb-Smith 1966).

However, it should be noted that despite the large numbers of medical students milling around in Edinburgh in 1805, only 21% of them took the MD degree (Lawrence 1988). This may have been due to a combination of the perceived loss of status of the Edinburgh MD degree among the students, their dissatisfaction with their teaching, or the alternative opportunities to complete their education in universities like Leiden. It was here that the Dutch physician Herman Boerhaave had earlier established his celebrated form of clinical teaching, and whose ongoing legacy accounted for Leiden's popularity.

American medical schools commenced as a supplement to the apprenticeship system. On their return from their overseas studies, John Morgan and William Shippen became highly influential in the establishment of America's first medical school at the University of Pennsylvania in 1765. Morgan was appointed as professor of medicine and Shippen as professor of anatomy and surgery. Medical schools were founded also at Kings College (Columbia University) in 1768 and Harvard Medical School in 1783, but the outbreak of the Revolution brought interruption and confusion during their early years (Flexner 1910). Despite the call from Morgan and others for those contemplating a medical career to renounce the apprenticeship system in favor of a more systemic study of the learned branches of medicine, most medical practitioners continued to train by apprenticeship. By the early nineteenth century, only a third of even prominent medical practitioners held a medical degree (Bonner 1995).

Transformations in Teaching and Learning

By 1800, surgical students were seeking to learn a curriculum, which best equipped them for their future practice, and which university professors seemed unable to provide (Lawrence 1988). The increasing focus on practical medical education as opposed to book learning had already led university medical students to spend part of their time "walking the wards" of major hospitals in search of this experience. Furthermore, the form of anatomy being taught by the surgeons had become radically different from that by the universities. In the late eighteenth century, French surgeons discovered when performing postmortems that many internal disorders were due to local pathological changes in the same way as external disorders. Moreover, these disorders could be managed by them, rather than by the physicians as was previously the practice (Temkin 1951). This led surgeons to dismantle the old anatomy and recreate it into a more surgically focused subject, and which they demonstrated was best learned by individual students performing dissection, rather than by demonstration (Lawrence 1988).

Similarly, the emerging generation of surgeons who were campaigning for science-based surgery, began to shape the newly established disciplines of physiology, pathology, and clinical surgery along their interests which were "cognitively quite different from the traditional bodies of knowledge over which university professors presided" (Lawrence 1988). This led to a multitude of extramural surgical teachers offering popular alternative courses to the universities as well as those being offered by the Royal Colleges of Surgeons in London, Edinburgh, and Dublin. A mixed pattern of medical education and training therefore emerged, and students could avail from a combination of learning opportunities depending on their financial circumstances and career aspirations.

The content of the curriculum was defined by the surgical teachers and clinical experience was dependent on the case-mix of patients encountered by students on the hospital wards. Familiarity with surgery was learned by observing procedures being performed in the operating theater. The famous English surgeon Sir Astley Cooper, reminded his surgical students of the importance to the surgeon of studying both medicine and surgery (Cooper 1823). This was reinforced by the London surgeon Sir William Lawrence, who highlighted the importance of a surgeon knowing about the local as well as the general treatment of a disease and stated that a surgeon who is "ignorant of the latter, is incompetent to the duties of the profession" (Lawrence 1829–1830).

In 1800, the Leeds surgeon James Lucas, recommended that those wishing to become surgeons should complete an appropriate education and training and acquire a qualification in surgery by formal examination, before being allowed to commence independent surgical practice (Lucas 1800). In terms of assessment, surgeons entering the army or navy were traditionally required to pass an examination for Membership of the Company of Surgeons of London and subsequently for Membership of one of the Royal Colleges of Surgeons. Those wishing to practice as hospital surgeons were also required to pass a similar examination. An increasing number of surgeon-apothecaries did likewise although this was not strictly necessary for those in smaller towns or rural areas. After the different Royal Colleges of Surgeons in the United Kingdom and Ireland established the Fellowship (FRCS) examination, this diploma gradually became a requirement for all surgeons seeking hospital appointments.

The Apothecaries Act of 1815 required those who wished to practice as apothecaries in England and Wales to undertake an apprenticeship including a period in a hospital and a qualification through examination. The Society of Apothecaries became responsible for carrying out the provisions of the Act and awarded a Licence of the Society of Apothecaries (LSA) to those who were successful in their examination (Hunting 1998). A significant proportion of surgeon-apothecaries were already in possession of the Diploma of the Royal Colleges of Surgeons of London. Although the Diploma of the Royal College of Surgeons of Edinburgh entitled the holder to practice as a surgeon-apothecary in Scotland, it was not recognized by the Act.

Learning to Cope with the Patients' Pain and Suffering

In the era prior to the advent of inhalation anesthesia, certain methods were used in the expectation of equipping trainee surgeons to cope with the emotional strains they would experience when inflicting pain on their patients during surgery and the changing of wound dressings. These included the dissection of cadavers, exposure to and becoming accustomed to the smells of infected wounds and ulcers on hospital wards, and observing operations being performed on awake and screaming patients. William Hunter informed his students that dissection "informs the head, gives dexterity to the hand, and familiarises the heart with a sort of necessary humanity, the use of cutting instruments upon our fellow-creatures" (Hunter 1784). Similarly, the London surgeon William Lawrence informed his students in 1830 "to prepare yourselves for operating on the living by cutting the dead" (Lawrence 1829–1830).

One example of the expectations placed upon surgical students by their teachers and occasionally by a medical family, is illustrated in the letters of Hampton Weeks. Weeks was a surgeon-apothecary dresser at St Thomas's hospital between 1801 and 1802. In a letter to his father and brother – both apothecary-surgeons – he describes how after first feeling "too great a tenderness" for his patient who was having his leg amputated, he had rapidly become "callous" and accustomed to the suffering, and had "seen several operations . . . and mind nothing about it, the more the poor devils cry, the more I laugh with the rest of them" (Ford 1987). That Weeks accomplished this dispassion within a period of 3 weeks raises questions about its authenticity. Historian Michael Pernick claimed that "the emotional ability to inflict huge suffering was a prerequisite for those wishing to consider surgery as a career," at that time (Pernick 1983). Although this must have been partly true, surgeons taught their students about the importance of compassion for their patients. The Scottish surgeon John Bell wrote that the attributes of humanity, mercy, and tenderness toward patients were to be prized in a surgeon (Bell 1801). Sir Benjamin Brodie stated that "he who can look with indifference on the agonies of a fellow creature is not a person to practise surgery" (Brodie 1824).

Milestones in Surgical Education and Training After 1850

Introduction

In the second half of the nineteenth century surgical practice began to undergo rapid changes. The introduction of inhalation anesthesia in 1845 (Bigelow 1846), antisepsis in 1867 (Lister 1867), and better surgical instruments to control bleeding, resulted in painless surgery and a significantly reduced risk of infection and hemorrhage. Surgery rapidly expanded and new and more complex operations became possible on every part of the human body. However, no formal systems were yet in place to train surgeons, who remained mostly self-taught and dependent on what they had been able to learn during their apprenticeships. The first formal surgical training program was introduced in Berlin in the 1860s by the famous German surgeon Bernard von Langenbeck, sometimes referred to as the "father of the surgical residency." This system was further developed in Vienna by Theodor Billroth who had been his former surgical resident.

William Halsted's and Edward Churchill's Surgical Training in America

The influential American surgeon William Halsted studied in Austria and Germany for 2 years and observed for himself these training arrangements. He was so impressed by what he saw that he introduced a comparable university-directed system at Johns Hopkins Medical School in 1889. This was later adopted by several other major centers in the United States and remained the cornerstone of much of American surgical training for almost a century. In his presentation of "The Annual Address in Medicine" at Yale University (his alma mater) in 1904, Halsted described his first 15 years' experience with this new training scheme. His overt confidence in his new system was reflected by his statement that, "we need a system, and we will surely have it, which will produce not only surgeons but surgeons of the highest type, men who will stimulate the first youths of our country to study surgery and to devote their energies and their lives to raising the standards of surgical science" (Halsted 1904).

Although Halsted's residency system was admired for ensuring residents were given graduated responsibility, it was however considered autocratic, pyramidal, and wasteful. It was primarily aimed to produce just one outstanding individual from the eight residents admitted to the first year of the program. Of these eight, four occupied 1-year positions, another became a house surgeon, and the remaining three spent prolonged periods of time with no guarantee of being appointed as staff surgeons. Halsted dismissed the objections that his system was too long, and that "the young surgeon will be stale, his enthusiasm gone before he has completed his arduous term of service" (Halsted 1904).

In 1931, Edward Churchill, surgeon at the Massachusetts General Hospital introduced what has been referred to as the "rectangular structure" of surgical training (Grillo 2004). Churchill was critical of the Halsted model mainly because of the number of poorly trained surgeons it inadvertently produced. He remarked that "half a surgical training is about as useful as half a billiard ball." Furthermore, he considered the system depended on a single individual or principal surgeon and that the relationship established between a dominant master and a docile apprentice was anti-intellectual and antiscientific (Grillo 2004). In its place, Churchill proposed that six residents be admitted instead of the eight in Halsted's system. Four of these would receive the 4 years of training with built-in flexibility tailored to the individual resident's needs. He believed this length of training was required for a surgical resident to be prepared for independent surgical practice. The remaining two residents were destined by their superior performance for higher surgical careers. Churchill also proposed there would be a group of "masters," with no single personality dominating the institution.

One aspect of the Halsted training system which remained a concern to some surgeons for many years was that, if the "resident-teach-resident tradition founded in the days of Halsted ... is not viewed critically, it will be a fertile source not only of good surgery but sometimes of poor surgical habits" (Woodhall 1965). This reflected the growing awareness of the need for greater supervision of residents by more senior staff members. The "rectangular" system of Churchill and remnants of Halsted's arrangements remained the core of surgical residency training in North America until the end of the twentieth century.

Changes in Surgical Education and Training in Great Britain and Ireland

Although the education of medical students had undergone a number of advances including time spent in a laboratory, the traditional apprenticeship system for training surgeons remained mostly unchanged until the second half of the twentieth century. Postgraduate surgical training was by then divided into two formal stages followed by a third prior to selection for appointment as a consultant. Those hoping to be surgeons applied in large numbers for what were predominantly service positions. The selection process took into account the applicant's record of academic and other achievements recorded in their curriculum vitae, comments made in testimonial letters or "references" from those with whom they had previously worked, the impression given during interview, and a combination of opportunity and luck (Gough et al. 1988).

After completing their internship and commonly another year, trainees sat the Part 1 or Primary Fellowship Examination of a Royal College of Surgeons in the basic sciences, which had a pass rate at each examination of around 25%. The second stage involved a minimum period of 3 years including at least one spent in a surgical post which carried clinical responsibilities and continuous operative experience in an approved hospital. The trainee then sat the Part 2 or Fellowship examination which included a written component; clinical examination of patients; and an oral examination in pathology, operative surgery, and surgical science. The pass rate in each Fellowship examination was between 25% and 30% (Wells 1966). Successful admission to Fellowship was not regarded as a mark of surgical competence and was followed by a further stage which could last anywhere from 4 to 8 years before the person obtained a hospital consultant post. Gaining a university higher degree improved the candidate's chance of obtaining one of these scarce positions.

At a meeting of the International Federation of Surgical Colleges on Surgical Education and Training held in 1965, it was noted that too little attention had been paid to this long period of training. In the report of the meeting it was noted that training could "occupy anything up to or even beyond a half of a man's useful lifetime and, in some cases, all of his best and potentially most creative years" (Wells 1966). This was the same criticism that had been leveled at Halsted's scheme some 75 years earlier. Despite the willingness of delegates to address these concerns, little changed. In 1973, Ian McColl, professor of surgery at Guy's Hospital in London, described a new comprehensive surgical training program recently introduced at that hospital. In his damning critique of contemporary surgical training in the United Kingdom, he pointed out that the "lack of security for the surgical trainee is quite unacceptable, and the number in training is greatly in excess of the consultant requirements for the United Kingdom." He also drew attention to the disruption the current system had on the individual trainee and their family life (McColl 1973). At that particular time, the likelihood of a surgical registrar in general surgery with 2 or more years' experience, obtaining a senior-registrar post within the next year was one in seven. This increased to one in nine if those working in academic units were added (Health Trends 1972). McColl observed that "those entering the consultant surgical ranks today are too old, over trained, and demoralised" (McColl 1973).

Notwithstanding these serious issues, large numbers of medical graduates continued to embark on surgical training. The enormous wastage was compounded by the reluctance of other medical colleges to recognize prior learning in a different discipline to their own, adding further to the time many medical graduates spent in training before joining the medical workforce. In 1993, the Chief Medical Officer at the Department of Health, Sir Kenneth Calman, produced a report on medical training, partly to comply with European Union directives including the requirement to reduced working hours (Calman 1993). This report eventually led to some changes in training and which were better suited to cope with the demands of high technology surgery.

The Tipping Point in Surgical Education and Training

Toward the end of the twentieth century, several developments led to a tipping point in the traditional methods for training surgeons. Advances in educational theory, emphasis on operating room efficiency and therefore less time for training, sicker hospital patients with more complex problems, new surgical techniques such as minimally invasive surgery, greater emphasis on reducing medical errors, and shorter working hours for residents led to a search for a new and more appropriate educational model for training surgeons (Reznick and MacRae 2006).

The educational theories developed by Fitts and Posner in 1967, and accepted in the surgical literature (Kopta 1971), demonstrated that motor skills are acquired, and expertise developed through cognitive, integrative, and autonomous stages. Furthermore, it was argued that it is the number of hours a resident spends in deliberate practice, rather than the hours spent in surgery, which determines the level of expertise acquired (Ericsson 1996).

In response to these developments, facilities were organized outside the operating room, where the teaching and learning of technical skills could take place and the resident could progress through each of these stages. Deliberate practice with immediate feedback became an integral part of this process. To enable this to take place, different materials and simulators were developed varying from simple mechanical trainers to those which were computer based. The goal was to ensure that residents demonstrated a required level of surgical proficiency before being allowed to operate on patients.

One by-product of greater familiarity with these skills laboratories was to examine their potential role in testing the innate skills of those applying for surgical training. The current opinion at this time is that it is not sufficiently developed, validated, and feasible for inclusion (Collins et al. 2019). Whether skills laboratories can be integrated into the selection process and further developed as part of the existing surgical education programs, remains the focus of ongoing research.

A major educational concern in the history of training surgeons has been the ongoing reliance on a traditional method for assessment. This has been historically based on a combination of the end-of-rotation reports from the surgeons with whom the resident had worked, a logbook record of the resident's operative experience, followed by knowledge-testing, and the assessment of clinical skills in formal examinations. The reliability and validity of this form of assessment as the sole marker of the overall competence of a surgeon has been seriously challenged on basic educational principles. Although formal examinations do have their place, the various forms of continuous in-training assessment, including multisource feedback on the resident's everyday performance in the workplace, are now an integral part of education and training. The conundrum that remains is striking a balance between the undoubted benefits of in-training assessment to learning and the dangers of a preoccupation with evaluation (Collins 2013). These pitfalls were well summarized in the words of William Osler who wrote, "we make the examination the end of education, not an accessory in its acquisition, ... the spirit is taken out of instruction and teacher and taught alike go down into the valley of Ezekiel – where they stay among the dry bones" (Osler 1913).

Conclusion

The history of the education and training of surgeons for independent practice has witnessed many changes. From a slow and meandering beginning during which the apprentices became masters of their own education, and sought new opportunities for learning, its journey has followed the developments in surgery and in medicine. It would however take several years and a number of external factors to bring about the changes required to develop an educational system, which would ensure the safety of patients was center stage, the contribution of trainees was valued, and their right to a more balanced lifestyle respected.

Cross-References

▶ Dental Education: A Brief History
▶ Learning and Teaching in the Operating Theatre: Expert Commentary from the Nursing Perspective

References

Bell J. The principles of surgery, vol. 1. Edinburgh: T. Cadell & W. Davies; 1801. p. 12–4.
Bigelow H. Insensibility during surgical operations produced by inhalation. Boston Med Surg J. 1846;35:309–17.
Bonner TN. Becoming a physician: medical education in Great Britain, France, Germany, and the United States 1750–1945. Oxford/New York: Oxford University Press; 1995. p. 6–7, 20, 44, 45–6. Reference cited by Bonner, Hudson RF. Patterns in medical education in nineteenth century America. Master's thesis, Johns Hopkins University; 1966. p. 51.
Brodie B. Introductory lecture. Lancet. 1824;3(54):23.
Calman K. Hospital doctors: training for the future: the report of the working group on specialist medical training. London: Health Publications Unit; 1993.
Calman KC. Medical education: past, present and future, handing on learning. Edinburgh: Churchill Livingstone Elsevier; 2007. p. 150–1.
Collins JP. In-training assessment at the Royal Australasian College of Surgeons. ANZ J Surg. 2013;83(6):404–8.

Collins JP, Doherty EM, Traynor O. Selection into surgical education and training. In: Nestel D, Dalrymple K, Paige JT, Aggarwal R, editors. Advancing surgical education: theory, evidence and practice. Singapore: Springer Nature; 2019. p. 157–70.

Conrad L. The Arab-Islamic medical tradition. In: Conrad LN, Nutton M, Porter V, Weir RA, editors. The Western tradition, 800 B.C.–1800 A.D. Cambridge: Cambridge University Press; 1995. p. 115–21.

Cooper A. Surgical lectures. Lancet. 1823;1(1):3–10.

Cope Z. The history of The Royal College of Surgeons of England. London: Anthony Blond; 1959. p. 21 & 70.

Dingwall H. A famous and flourishing society: the history of the Royal College of Surgeons of Edinburgh, 1505–2005. Edinburgh: Edinburgh University Press; 2005. p. 89 & 145.

Ericsson KA. The acquisition of expert performance: an introduction to some of the issues. In: Ericsson KA, editor. The road to excellence: the acquisition of expert performance in the arts and sciences, sports, and games. Mahwah: Lawrence Erlbaum Associates; 1996. p. 1–50.

Fitts PM, Posner MI. Human performance. Belmont: Brooks/Cole; 1967.

Flexner A. Medical education in the United States and Canada. New York: Carnegie Foundation for the Advancement of Education; 1910. p. 3–5.

Ford J. A medical student at St. Thomas's Hospital, 1801–1802, The Weekes family letters. Med Hist Suppl. 1987;7:39–49.

Geyer-Kordesch J, Macdonald J. Physicians and surgeons in Glasgow. The history of the Royal College of Physicians and Surgeons of Glasgow, 1599–1858. London: The Hambledon Press; 1999.

Good JM. op. cit., Appendix L, p. 10; Good JM. The history of medicine, so far as it relates to the profession of the apothecary. 1795. p. 146–7. Cited by Holloway SWF. The Apothecaries Act 1815: a reinterpretation, Part 1: the origins of the Act. 1966. p. 108. http://www.ncbi.nim.nih.gov.pdf.medhis00151-0005. Accessed 27 May 2020.

Gough MH, Holdsworth R, Bell JA, et al. Personality assessment techniques and aptitude testing aids to the selection of surgical trainees. Ann R Coll Surg Engl. 1988;70:265–79.

Grillo HC. Edward D. Churchill and the "rectangular" surgical residency. Surgery. 2004;136: 947–52.

Halsted WS. The training of the surgeon. Bull Johns Hopkins Hosp. 1904;15(162):267–75.

Health Trends. 1972;4:49.

Hunter W. Two introductory lectures, delivered by Dr William Hunter, to his last course of anatomical lectures at the Theatre in Windmill Street; as they were left corrected for the press by himself. London: J. Johnson; 1784. p. 67.

Hunting P. A history of the Society of Apothecaries. London: Society of Apothecaries; 1998. p. 55, 198–9.

Kopta JA. The development of motor skills in orthopaedic education. Clin Orthop Relat Res. 1971;75:80–5.

Lawrence W. Lectures on surgery, medical and operative. Lecture 1: introduction. Lancet. 1829–1830;1:33–42.

Lawrence C. The Edinburgh medical school and the end of the 'old thing' 1790–1830. Hist Univ. 1988;7:262, 263, 265–6.

Lawrence C. Democratic, divine and heroic: the history and historiography of surgery. In: Lawrence C, editor. Medical theory, surgical practice: studies in the history of surgery. London/New York: Routledge; 1992. p. 20.

Leppaniemi A. Wanted: surgical education. Scand J Surg. 2006;95:3.

Letter to the Editor. The Lancet. 1824. p. 275.

Lister J. On a new method of treating compound fracture, abscess, etc., with observations on the conditions of suppuration. Lancet. 1867;1:336–9.

Loudon I. Medical care and the general practitioner 1750–1850. Oxford: Clarendon Press; 1986. p. 26, 75.

15 Surgical Education and Training: Historical Perspectives

Lucas J. A candid inquiry into the education, qualifications and offices of a surgeon-apothecary. Bath: S. Hazard; 1800. p. 12.

McColl I. Comprehensive surgical training programme. Lancet. 1973;1(7797):254–5.

Minutes of The Company of Surgeons of London, Royal College of Surgeons of England Library & Archives, COS/1/2. 1790. p. 214–7.

Minutes of The Company of Surgeons of London, Royal College of Surgeons of England Library & Archives, COS/1/2. 1797. p. 271.

Osler W. An introductory address on examinations, examiners and examinees. Lancet. 1913;182:1047–50.

Parkinson J. The hospital pupil; or an essay intended to facilitate the study of medicine and surgery. London: H.D. Symonds; 1800. p. 26, 29. https://archive.org/details/TheHospitalPupil. Accessed 19–21 July 2018.

Pernick M. The calculus of suffering in nineteenth-century surgery. Hastings Cent Rep. 1983;13 (2):26–36.

Porter R. The eighteenth century. In: Conrad L, Neve M, Nutton V, Porter R, Wear A, editors. The Western medical tradition: 800 B.C.–1800 A.D. Cambridge: Cambridge University Press; 1995. p. 434–5.

Reznick RK, MacRae H. Teaching surgical skills – changes in the wind. N Engl J Med. 2006;355:2664–9.

Robb-Smith A. Medical education at Oxford and Cambridge prior to 1850. In: Pointer F, editor. The evolution of medical education in Britain. London: Pitman; 1966. p. 49.

Society of Barbers of Edinburgh Archive, Ref: GB 779 SB1:1722–1846. Royal College of Surgeons of Edinburg Archives. https://archiveshub.jisc.ac.uk/data/gb779-sb. Accessed 13 June 2020.

Temkin O. The role of surgery in the rise of modern medical thought. Bull Hist Med. 1951;25: 248–59.

Thompson S. The Great Windmill Street School. Bull Hist Med. 1942;12:383–5.

Wells WC. A letter to Lord Kenyon, 1799, footnote to pp. 83–5. Cited by Holloway SWF. The Apothecaries Act 1815: a reinterpretation, Part 1: The origins of the Act. 1966. p. 108. http://www.ncbi.nim.nih.gov.pdf.medhis00151-0005. Accessed 27 May 2020.

Wells C. Surgical education and training. Ann R Coll Surg Engl. 1966;39(5):267–98.

Widdess J. The Royal College of Surgeons in Ireland and its medical school 1784–1984. 3rd ed. Dublin: Publications Department/Published by the College; 1984. p. 14–5.

Wilks S, Bettany G. A biographical history of Guy's Hospital. London: Ward, Lock, Bowden & Co.; 1892. p. 88–9.

Willcock J. The laws relating to the medical profession; with an account of the rise and progress of its various orders. London: A. Strahan, W. Clarke; 1830. p. ccxxx, 30, 60.

Woodhall B. The training of the surgical specialist. Am J Surg. 1965;110(1):73–7.

Young S. The annals of the Barber-Surgeons of London, compiled from their records and other sources. London: Blades, East & Blades; 1890. p. 78–81. https://archive.org/details/annalsofbarbersu00youn. Accessed 13 June 2020.

Nursing and Midwifery Education: Historical Perspectives

16

Lisa McKenna, Jenny Davis, and Eloise Williams

Contents

Introduction	286
Nursing Education	287
Early Nurse Education: The Nightingale Model	287
Hospital-Based Training	288
Emergence of Specialty Education	289
The Second-Level Nurse	291
Evolution of Higher Education in Nursing	293
Future Challenges for Nurse Education	295
Midwifery Education	296
Early Midwifery Education	296
Evolution of Higher Education in Midwifery	297
Conclusion	298
References	299

Abstract

Nursing and midwifery are old and well-established professions. While some of their history has intersected at different points, they are distinct professions underpinned by different philosophies. They have also developed in different ways as a result of complex political and social influences. Furthermore, midwifery in particular has developed in a variety of models globally and hence its education varies internationally. This chapter provides an overview of the historical development of professional education for nurses and midwives. It describes early historical approaches to the training of each discipline through apprenticeship-style models to subsequent education delivery in higher education

L. McKenna (✉) · J. Davis
School of Nursing and Midwifery, La Trobe University, Melbourne, VIC, Australia
e-mail: l.mckenna@latrobe.edu.au; j.davis@latrobe.edu.au

E. Williams
Northern Health, La Trobe University, Melbourne, VIC, Australia
e-mail: Eloise.williams@latrobe.edu.au

© Springer Nature Singapore Pte Ltd. 2023
D. Nestel et al. (eds.), *Clinical Education for the Health Professions*,
https://doi.org/10.1007/978-981-15-3344-0_19

institutions. In doing so, it explores some of the resulting international variations through local influences on evolution of the professions. It also describes how the two professions have at times intersected in their histories.

> **Keywords**
>
> Apprenticeship · Direct-entry · Midwifery · Nursing · Education · History

Introduction

Nursing and midwifery have often been described as being the same or variations of one profession. While there have been intersections, they are distinctly different disciplines underpinned by differences in philosophy and focus. These differences have been unclear at times in their respective evolutions, so it seems pertinent to begin by clarifying the distinctions. Hence, this section provides an overview of the professions that are nursing and midwifery. It describes the underpinning philosophies and practices as a foundation to understanding historical development of their education systems and some of the resulting tensions.

Nursing is among the oldest professions. The International Council of Nurses (ICN) defines nursing as a role that:

> …encompasses autonomous and collaborative care of individuals of all ages, families, groups and communities, sick or well and in all settings. Nursing includes the promotion of health, prevention of illness, and the care of ill, disabled and dying people. Advocacy, promotion of a safe environment, research, participation in shaping health policy and in patient and health systems management, and education are also key nursing roles. (ICN 2019)

To use the title, a nurse must have completed a recognized general nursing program and be authorized to practice nursing in his/her country (ICN 2019). The term "midwife" literally means to be "with woman," and the midwifery profession is also one of the world's oldest. The International Confederation of Midwives (ICM) recognizes a midwife as:

> a person who has successfully completed a midwifery education programme that is based on the ICM Essential Competencies for Basic Midwifery Practice and the framework of the ICM Global Standards for Midwifery Education and is recognized in the country where it is located; who has acquired the requisite qualifications to be registered and/or legally licensed to practice midwifery and use the title 'midwife'; and who demonstrates competency in the practice of midwifery. (ICM 2017)

Unlike nurses, midwives work predominantly in a framework underpinned by wellness, rather than illness (Nordby 2016, 2017; Yates et al. 2020), and midwives have also existed throughout recorded history. They work with women throughout childbearing including: pregnancy, labor, childbirth, and the postnatal period. In doing so, they monitor maternal and fetal well-being, provide support and education,

16 Nursing and Midwifery Education: Historical Perspectives

health counseling, and refer when required. Their scope of practice also extends across the lifespan of women incorporating sexual and reproductive health. Hence, they work under a framework of woman-centered care (McKenna 2009; Yates et al. 2020). However, models of midwifery care vary around the world as education and practice have evolved locally.

Nursing Education

Early Nurse Education: The Nightingale Model

Florence Nightingale is credited with transformation of nursing from an unrespectable vocation to a highly organized and paid profession for women. However, she was not the first or only person to contribute to the reform of nursing (Jensen 1965; Nightingale 2009b). Nightingale achieved reform by elevating moral and ethical standards of the women practicing nursing, improving hospital administration, and by creating a formalized training program (Russell 1990).

As a young woman, Florence Nightingale recognized a calling to serve humanity (Roux and Halstead 2009). She accompanied her parents on overseas trips to visit the poor, which influenced her desire to become a nurse (Hunt 2017). Nursing at that time was not considered to be a suitable career for a lady, and thus her parents would not allow her to pursue it (Jensen 1965). Eventually, she came across a reputable nurse training school for deaconesses in Kaiserswerth, Germany, and her family gave her permission to train there in 1851 (Kalisch and Kalisch 1995).

Following training, Nightingale returned to London in 1853 to assume a position as superintendent of a home for sick gentlewomen, and the next year she was summoned to Scutari in the Crimea to set up a hospital for the wounded (Nightingale 2009a). It was during this time that she became known as the "lady with the lamp," completing nightly rounds by lamp light (Zerwekh 2015). Nightingale's work during the Crimean war became renowned. She recognized that nurses' work needed to occur alongside the work of doctors, and nurses needed to receive adequate training (Nightingale 2009b). In recognition of Nightingale's work, a fund was set up in her name in 1855 for the purposes of supporting nursing training (Jensen 1965).

Based on years of observation, experience of nursing the sick and wounded, nursing training and research, Nightingale created a set of principles which she published in her book, *Notes on Nursing: What It Is and What It Is Not,* in 1859 (Hunt 2017; Kalisch and Kalisch 1995). These focused on improving sanitation of the environment; however, the book was originally written for women caring for the sick in the home (Nightingale 1946). Nightingale identified that fresh air, clean water, effective drainage, and cleanliness were most important in preventing disease, and identified that warmth, light, quiet, and good nutrition contributed to people's general health (Nightingale 2009b). She applied these principles in the reform of hospitals and to improve welfare of the sick and wounded (Nightingale 1863).

Following the Crimean war, Nightingale returned to London and established a nurse training school at St Thomas's Hospital in London in 1860, financed by the

Nightingale fund (Jensen 1965). She developed her own system of hospital administration which included appointing a matron or lady superintendent who was the most senior and highly skilled nurse in the hospital, acting as a nursing leader and setting an example for other nurses to follow (Russell 1990). Nightingale developed a formal 1-year training program for student nurses, then called probationers, who were a minimum of 25 years of age and selected based on their moral standards and attitudes (Nightingale 2009b). Probationers were provided with training, food, accommodation, uniforms, and a minimum wage and they were expected to board in the nurse's home under care of the home sister who supervised their behavior, provided moral and spiritual guidance, and disciplined them if necessary (Nightingale 2009b; Russell 1990).

Probationers were trained utilizing an apprenticeship style of teaching involving an experienced nurse teaching the craft of nursing on the job with trainees rotated through various clinical areas to gain an array of experience (Roux and Halstead 2009; Russell 1990). The ward sister (charge nurse) provided practical, hands-on instruction regarding personal care of patients including bathing and feeding; clinical tasks such as dressings and giving enemas; application of Nightingale principles particularly cleanliness, ventilation, and observing the sick; and other domestic tasks like cooking and making beds (Nightingale 2009b). The probationer was expected to take notes and keep a journal, which would be checked by the home sister (Nightingale 2009b). Probationers were provided with theoretical training from medical instructors who delivered lectures in physiology, chemistry, and medical/surgical topics and the matron reinforced teaching (Kalisch and Kalisch 1995). Detailed records were kept regarding the probationer's clinical and theoretical training and they needed to pass several written and oral examinations throughout the year (Nightingale 2009b).

Towards the end of training, Nightingale organized a meeting with the graduating nurse and would use information gained to write a recommendation for their future appointment (Nightingale 2009b). It was expected that Nightingale nurses would work for several more years after completing their training, taking up positions in other hospitals around the country and overseas to reform nursing and train others (Russell 1990).

The Nightingale system of nurse training at St Thomas's Hospital in London was very successful, resulting in requests for Nightingale nurses to be sent to establish hospital training schools globally (Nightingale 2009a). Demand for trained nurses was great and Nightingale was challenged to keep up with demand, however she did succeed in sending nurses to many countries, including Australia and Canada (Nightingale 2009a). Other countries, for example, North America, adopted Nightingale principles in their reform of nursing (Russell 1990).

Hospital-Based Training

Prior to the introduction of modern Nightingale-style hospital-based nurse training in many countries, inpatient care was delivered by a largely untrained, if not poorly trained, workforce. Post-Nightingale models, there were calls for formalization of nursing education around the world (Ousey 2011). As a result, many nursing education systems, such as those in Australia and Singapore, resembled their British colonial origins, historically public hospital-based apprenticeship programs (Goh et al. 2019). The system of training nurses on-the-job, predominant throughout the nineteenth and twentieth centuries, was based on students exchanging their labor for nursing instruction (Grehan 2017).

Nursing education during the nineteenth and twentieth centuries was dominated by the medical profession, with doctors directly involved in teaching students how to care for patients, and the student demographic was predominantly young, single, and female (Jinks et al. 2014). This system of training primarily focused on meeting service workforce needs and characterized as "...instilling obedience and discipline and nursing practice was characterised by rituals and routines that had been passed down from one generation to the next" (Jinks et al. 2014, p. 641).

Historically, nursing education was provided at hospital level; in Australia, for example, this occurred across multiple sites and jurisdictions, largely developed to meet local needs and content, delivered with varying theory and practical require-ments. With increased focus on content and quality of nurse education and minimum standards, smaller nursing schools were closed, as they could no longer meet these standards; nursing education then became centralized at larger health services. Ultimately, increasing demands to raise nurse education and professional practice standards and to provide increasingly complex care to patients were behind decisions to move nurse education into higher education – focusing on education of nurses by nurses and less on the supply of a nursing workforce (Jinks et al. 2014).

Hospital-trained nurses, in countries such as Australia, were supported to upgrade their qualifications to a Bachelor of Nursing (post-registration) as part of the transition of nurse education to higher education in the early 1990s (Gill et al. 2015). Similar schemes existed elsewhere, with the profession having advanced to graduate entry-level requirement through minimum bachelor qualifi-cation in most countries (Jokiniemi et al. 2019). Remaining countries are either transitioning or maintain multiple education pathways dependent on local circum-stances (White 2017).

Emergence of Specialty Education

Transfer of specialty postgraduate nursing education from hospitals to higher educa-tion began in the early to late 1990s. Even in specialty education, international variations exist (Marshall 2019) in addition to questions about poorly reported practice and patient impacts of postgraduate education (Gullick et al. 2019; Ng et al. 2014). Most post-registration education in critical care existed as ad-hoc training for nurses and doctors together until the 1960s, when more formalized post-registration education was developed in Australia and the UK (Marshall 2019). In some settings today, hospitals and health services offer specialist nurse education as part of partnership arrangements with tertiary institutions (Gullick et al. 2019).

The emergence of specialty, or postgraduate, education occurred largely due to advances in medicine and healthcare technology, opportunities for nursing scope of practice expansion, changing models of care and provision of a workforce that could care for patients with increasingly complex care needs and who would previously have not survived (Darcy Associates 2015). The development of specialist nurse education and advancing of nursing practice is largely dependent on changing community healthcare needs and expectations, expanding professional practice knowledge, and increased access to emerging technologies (Zahran et al. 2012). Specialty practice also improves workforce planning and supports development of educational programs that align nursing skill development with community needs (National Nursing and Nursing Education Taskforce (N3ET) 2006).

Advanced practice roles, such as nurse practitioners, have emerged and vary across countries with roles and titles not universally well-defined nor understood (Masso and Thompson 2017). International variance in specialist and/or advanced practice nursing role titles and levels of education contributes to continued lack of clarity in role recognition and scope of practice (Casey et al. 2019), particularly in countries without national regulation. Barriers and enablers to implementing nurse practitioner roles are multilevel and further complicated when perceived to challenge traditional professional boundaries or involve task shifting Masso and Thompson 2017).

Established nurse practitioner or advanced practice nursing roles are primarily found in high-income countries (Schober and Stewart 2019). In the United States (USA), advanced practice nurses are recognized as Advanced Practice Registered Nurses (APRN) with titles such as clinical specialist, certified nurse-midwife, nurse-anesthetist, and nurse-practitioner (Parker and Hill 2017). Nurses in Australia can secure specialized practice endorsement in two areas: Nurse Practitioner and Endorsement for Scheduled Medicines Registered Nurses (Rural and Isolated Practice) (Birks et al. 2019), these being the only advanced practice roles regulated in Australia. New Zealand has two established advanced practice roles – nurse practitioners who are regulated and have defined scope of practice and clinical nurse specialists whose role is not regulated nor defined – both roles are expected to be masters-level educated (Carryer et al. 2018).

In Australia, the national regulator has distinguished Advanced Practice Nursing (APN) from Advanced Nursing Practice (ANP). APN includes a prescribed educational level, specified advanced nursing practice experience, and continuing professional development, whereas the ANP is a level of practice rather than a role, is specific to the individual, and does not specify an educational level (Nursing and Midwifery Board of Australia 2016). In many countries, such as the USA and Australia, nurse practitioners work autonomously in advanced and extended clinical roles and are authorized to perform some specified functions traditionally the realm of medical practitioners (e.g., prescribing some medications, ordering diagnostic tests, and making referrals) (Traczynski and Udalova 2018).

Specialist nurses practice within competency frameworks. These are professionally established, have acceptable level of clinical knowledge and skills for [specialist] nurses, and allow for competence to be measured and evaluated. Specific frameworks for specialist (critical care, mental health) nurses have been established to facilitate clinical practice and education development in many developed countries (e.g., the UK, the USA, Europe, and Australia) (Gullick et al. 2019) and other settings (e.g., China) (Zhang et al. 2019). Competency frameworks enable professionals to provide safe and effective nursing practice for the public and adapt to complex, ever-changing healthcare environments (Zhang et al. 2019).

Clinical nurse specialities and areas of practice can include but not limited to anesthetics, burns, cardiac care, community health, critical care, diabetes education, dialysis, disaster, education, emergency, family health, gerontology/aged care, infection control, intensive care, management, medical nursing, mental health, neonatal intensive care, occupational health, oncology/palliative care, pediatric, perioperative, reconstructive/plastic surgical, rehabilitation, remote area nursing, renal, rural nursing, school nursing, surgical nursing, and wound management.

Advancing nursing knowledge and dynamic practice requires research knowledge and skills. There is an assumption that postgraduate specialist and research education translate to practice based on "best available evidence and research"; however, this has been challenged (Bressan et al. 2016). An Australian review examining the need for regulation of specialty areas within nursing identified a variety of mechanisms used internationally to recognize and regulate specialty practice, including licensure, endorsement, credentialing, validation, and certification (Nursing and Midwifery Board of Australia 2016). The review also identified that "...formal regulation of specialty groups for purposes of registration did not reduce the risk to the public, and there was a lack of significant evidence that regulation of specialty practice improves patient/client outcomes" (NMBA 2016, p. 1).

Speciality areas within nursing and organizations representing specialist nursing groups have developed processes (e.g., competency standards) for recognizing specialty practice. In Australia, "...this provides sufficient means of acknowledging specialist nursing practice...and may be recognised by employers and the health industry at large" (Nursing and Midwifery Board of Australia 2016).

The Second-Level Nurse

From the middle of the nineteenth century, at the time of Florence Nightingale, there was only one level of trained nurse who eventually became regulated and registered with the professionalization of nursing (Schwirian 1998). Between the middle of the nineteenth and twentieth centuries, global demand for nurses increased significantly, primarily in response to war, including the American Civil War, World War I and II, and Korean and Vietnam Wars (Hunt 2017). There were insufficient registered nurses to send to the battlefields and consequently increased demand for nurses was met by using untrained or minimally trained volunteers (Hunt 2017; Kalisch and Kalisch 1995).

During the Great Depression of the 1930s, registered nurses became too expensive to employ so hospitals sought cheaper options, resulting in training assistant nurses to deliver some care (Brown 1994). Post-World War II there remained a huge shortage of trained nurses in civilian hospitals globally, due to large numbers of casualties which increased demand for nurses (Bassett 1993; Kalisch and Kalisch 1995). Many nurses returning from wars chose to leave nursing because of poor pay and working conditions, or pursued more diverse career opportunities that had arisen for women (Bassett 1993). Some also chose to marry, and at that time, nurses were required to be single; they were thus forced to leave nursing, which further contributed to nursing shortages (Kalisch and Kalisch 1995).

Introduction of the second level of nurse occurred internationally at different times with the aim of relieving nursing shortages, to replace untrained or minimally trained nursing assistants with qualified nurses and reduce costs of employing more registered nurses (Seccombe et al. 1997). The first training school in America for second-level nurses, known as practical nurses, began in 1897 (Kalisch and Kalisch 1995). In the United Kingdom, the updated Nurses Act in 1943 paved the way for state-enrolled assistant nurses to begin training (Edwards 1945). In 1947, a school for nursing aides opened in Alberta, Canada (Tarnowski et al. 2017), and Australia followed in 1950 with the opening of the first school for nursing aides in Melbourne (Bassett 1993). Other countries also began training second level nurses at varying times including New Zealand, Singapore, South Africa, Japan, Canada, and several European countries (Robinson and Griffiths 2007; Seccombe et al. 1997).

Second-level nurses were originally trained in hospitals utilizing a similar apprenticeship model used for that of first-level (registered) nurses (Clarke 2016). They worked as assistant nurses under supervision of registered nurses who taught them the practical skills of nursing on the job (Edwards 1945). The role of the second-level nurse was to assist with basic nursing tasks which would free up the registered nurse to complete more complex patient care (Jacob et al. 2013). Training generally took place within hospitals; however, there was considerable variation in length of the courses which were as short as 9 months in Canada and America, 12 months in Australia, and 18 months to 2 years in the United Kingdom (Bassett 1993; Edwards 1945; Kalisch and Kalisch 1995; UKCC 1986).

Second-level nurses continued to be trained and worked in their respective healthcare services throughout the twentieth century; however, the United Kingdom and New Zealand were exceptions. A review of nursing led by Asa Briggs in the UK concluded it was unnecessary to have two levels of nurse (United Kingdom Central Council for Nursing 1986). In the mid-1980s as part of Project 2000 which saw reform of nursing education, second-level nurse (state enrolled nurse, SEN) training courses began being phased out and were discontinued by 1995 (Le Var 1997). Existing SENs could continue working, however, were encouraged to convert to registered nurses, and were replaced with healthcare assistants (Le Var 1997). A similar situation occurred in New Zealand where excessive numbers of enrolled nurses in hospitals influenced ceasing of courses by 1994. However, training was recommenced from 2002 (Dixon 2001; NCNZ 2004) due to nursing shortages. A more recent review of nursing conducted in the UK by Francis (2013) concluded that the model created by Project 2000 consisting of first-level nurses and healthcare assistants was not ideal resulting in revival of a second-level nurse in England only, ensuring this time that they had solid career structures (Francis 2013). The first cohort of nursing associates began in 2017 (Department of Health 2017).

Today, second-level nurses continue to be known by many different names depending on the country in which they work (Currie and Carr-Hill 2013). Titles include licensed practical nurse and licensed vocational nurse in America; registered practical and licensed practical nurse in Canada; enrolled nurse in Australia and New Zealand; and nursing associate in England (Butcher and Mackinnon 2015). Training has evolved substantially in response to changing roles and expanding scope of practice for second-level nurses, and is conducted outside the healthcare environment in vocational institutions and some universities (Clarke 2016). Courses are typically at diploma level, conducted over 18 months to 2 years and include medication administration and acute care subjects (Jacob et al. 2013).

Evolution of Higher Education in Nursing

Nurses and nursing have increasingly become specialized in the past two decades and thus able to take on roles historically performed by others (Bressan et al. 2016). They represent the largest health professional group within healthcare, and there are sustained calls for nurses to take on greater roles in healthcare systems to meet global healthcare challenges (Institute of Medicine 2011; Wong et al. 2015). Expectations for dynamic global roles and expanding scope of nursing practice are influenced by needs of individuals, communities, populations, and healthcare services, reflecting changing and pluralistic societies and a need for academically prepared nurses (Bressan et al. 2016; Jokiniemi et al. 2019).

Education and professional development are natural enablers of expanded scope of practice (Birks et al. 2019); however, lack of organized and available education can act as barriers to advanced nursing practice (McKenna et al. 2015). Ongoing health workforce reform will be required to meet needs from chronic and complex conditions in ageing populations, amid existing workforce shortages, to enable health professionals to work at optimum scope of practice (McKittrick and McKenzie 2018).

The level of nurse education has changed significantly from its early vocational and service ethos, transitioning into higher education with expectations of high academic rigor and expanding practice (Ousey 2011). Theories of learning relevant to nursing have also changed. Schools of nursing and healthcare organizations have a global responsibility to prepare nurses to become lifelong learners by teaching them how to learn and be reflective and critical thinking practitioners (Davis et al. 2014).

The World Health Organization (WHO) set a global standard for professional preparation of nurses (World Health Organization 2009); however, all nurses practice in local contexts, and different countries have different healthcare and nursing workforce priorities. While global standards establish priorities for countries to work toward university-level nurse education, this must be strategically relevant to regional/national/local setting and sustainable (Morin 2012). Five key components of global standards include program graduates, program development and revision, program curriculum, academic faculty and staff, and program admission (World

Health Organization 2009). Systems that articulate regulation and minimum standards for entry-level and specialist nurse education and professional practice are well established in many countries.

The evolution and maturity of nursing can be measured by presence of specialties, levels of nursing education, policies specific to nursing, extent of nursing research, and nursing leadership (Schober and Stewart 2019). Continuing professional practice development in nursing, and the education that underpins it, is dependent upon specific sociopolitical and cultural contexts and sustainable resources (Zahran et al. 2012). For example, the USA has set targets for the percentage of nurses who hold bachelor degrees to be increased to 80% by 2020 (Institute of Medicine 2011), and Australian ICU workforce standards have recommended proportions of nursing staff working in ICUs who must hold specialist critical care qualifications (Chamberlain et al. 2018).

Higher education and specialization in nursing, such as at master's level, is seen as a strategy for internationalization and professionalization of nursing, and underpins provision of quality healthcare. This is particularly so in less educationally developed countries such as Jordan (Zahran et al. 2012) and China (Zhang et al. 2019), as well as in Singapore (Goh et al. 2019) and Eastern Europe (Wong et al. 2015). Such strategies are underpinned by reports of better patient outcomes associated with more educated nurses (Aiken et al. 2011), however, remain context-driven. Nurses in parts of Africa, for example, provide care to a wide range of people with very few resources and where there is a need for many thousands more nurses with good generalist skills, together with specialty-based nurses (APPG 2016). Well-resourced parts of the world such as the UK, the USA, Europe, Canada, Australia, and NZ have varying but relatively well-established specialty nurse education and practice models, in contrast to low- to middle-income countries, such as India, parts of Asia and Latin America, where specialty education in nursing continues to develop (APPG 2016; Sripathy et al. 2017).

Despite global education standards, migration of nurses has highlighted continuing variation in education of nurses. This is more evident in low- to middle-income countries with growing numbers of privately operated and largely unregulated nursing and medical schools (Sripathy et al. 2017). Provision of transnational nursing education, increasingly within strategic business models that include education providers in developed countries delivering a variety of pre-registration and post-registration programs in partnership with developing country providers (Morin 2012) is growing. Lack of oversight of nursing education curricula in some countries, however, means minimum standards may be difficult to determine.

Specialty nursing roles are suggested as ideal for addressing healthcare disparities in less developed countries and underserved populations, e.g., primary care and specialties (Scanlon et al. 2019). In China, the health system remains hospital and acute care focused and with less well-developed primary healthcare systems (Parker and Hill 2017). This situation reflects global challenges of increasing complex chronic disease, ageing populations, and healthcare demand, and highlights critical gaps in both service delivery and education of the nursing workforce. A review of APN roles in low-income countries identified wide variation in educational preparation (duration: 48 h to 3 years; type: continuing professional development (CPD), nonaccredited post-registration diploma to masters inside and/or outside of country), and lack of education standards and endorsement (Scanlon et al. 2019). Advanced practice-based, interprofessional collaborative roles and team approaches to care can lead to positive changes in healthcare, including improving sustainability and safety, and decreased costs (Andregård and Jangland 2015).

There is no internationally recognized, nor consensus, definition or model of advanced practice nursing (Zahran et al. 2012). Different role titles, legal requirements, and scope of practice are established according to context (Andregård and Jangland 2015). Reasons for introducing these roles are commonly to improve access, flexible, innovative, continuity, and quality of care and benefits reported as reduced length of stay and improved cost efficiency (Andregård and Jangland 2015).

The utility of specialist or generic fields of nursing has been being debated (ANMF 2019; Zahran et al. 2012) amid concerns that specializations in nursing may lead to practice "silos" and limit transferability (O'Connor et al. 2018). Conversely, a specialist nurse (e.g., postgraduate/masters level) with advanced knowledge, cognitive and research skills may have increased capacity to transfer these skills/qualities to nonspecialist or generalist integrated practice areas (O'Connor et al. 2018; Zahran et al. 2012).

Future Challenges for Nurse Education

Barriers to nurse education and training and continuing professional development are common across the globe, yet more critical in some parts of the world. These can be financial, technological, lack of availability, geographic limitations (e.g., rural/ remote areas), shortage of teaching/education staff, and heavy workloads. Appropriate skill mix and care is among the biggest staffing challenges in healthcare globally. Measures to address ongoing global nursing workforce shortages have included "…changing education programs, creating new categories of nurse, adjusting public expectations of what a nurse is and what a nurse does" (Grehan 2017, p. 37).

Skilled migration schemes, that include nurses, are established workforce management strategies in many developed countries (Grehan 2017). Migration of nurses impacts the distribution healthcare workers globally and health of populations, and there are calls for richer countries to adopt more responsible approaches to workforce planning (APPG 2016). In other countries, measures to address workforce shortages include task shifting, role substitution, and increasing use of unqualified workers (APPG 2016).

Domains and models of care continue to evolve. Historically, concepts of care emerged in the community, moved into hospitals, and are now shifting back into the community, the locus of control shifting more to patients and social models of care (Grehan 2017). There is increasing emphasis on building the primary healthcare workforce in response to chronic and complex disease. Internationally, increased emphasis is on building primary healthcare nursing workforce in response to chronic and complex disease (Halcomb et al. 2016); however, historic professional hierarchies still act as barriers to advancing practice roles in some settings (e.g., medicine) (APPG 2016).

Competition for, and quality of, clinical learning environments are ongoing challenges for nursing education, apart from disparity across global preregistration programs in the number of clinical experience hours (White 2017). These challenges have increased interest and debate about the utility of simulation and other embedded technologies in nursing education and practice (Grehan 2017). Furthermore, a shortage of nursing faculty, whereby there will be insufficient numbers of appropriately qualified nurses to educate the future nursing workforce, has been flagged as part of overall global nursing workforce shortage predictions (Nardi and Gyurko 2013; White 2017).

Clinical practice and healthcare technologies are dynamic, and therefore education needs to be ongoing at all levels to support maintenance and advancement of specialist nursing knowledge and skills (Gullick et al. 2019). More flexible and innovative approaches to nursing education are among many issues that will challenge the sustainability of current approaches to entry-level and specialist nurse education, including how best to optimize the contribution of nursing to global health.

Midwifery Education

Early Midwifery Education

Historically, education of midwives was delivered through apprenticeship-style training with an older midwife, or from around the eighteenth century, a physician (Litoff 1982). These midwives, also known as "lay midwives," provided care for women in their homes, which was where childbirth traditionally occurred (Barclay 2008). In a vast number of countries, increased medicalization of childbirth led to it being largely managed in hospital settings with medical oversight. Hence, the nature of midwifery practice changed, although in different ways globally. The evolution of formal midwifery education followed a very different trajectory to that of nursing, even though at times was closely connected in many countries.

To understand the early education of midwives, it is necessary to understand some of the evolutionary influences regionally. In Australia, as well as other countries, in the late 1800s, lay midwives providing childbirth support to women were discredited by medical practitioners as unsafe (Fahy 2007). Resulting medicalization brought the introduction of regulation through state-based legislation, with midwifery training being made available to nurses, initially via 6- or 12-month courses (Trembath and Hellier 1987). In New Zealand, a very similar trajectory has been described, where the *Nurses and Midwives Registration Act* of 1925 moved midwifery into a post-registration nursing qualification. Existing midwives were reclassified as maternity nurses with limited scope of practice (Stojanovic 2008). With the move of midwifery education to a post-registration nursing qualification, these programs became hospital-based certificate programs in both Australia and New Zealand, resulting in individuals holding two qualifications, namely Registered Nurse and Registered Midwife.

In Canada, as in other countries, traditional midwives received no formal education. As other professions began to assume care during childbearing in the nineteenth century, midwifery disappeared from the country (Kaufman 1998). It was not until 1984 that the first direct-entry midwifery program emerged in British Columbia; however, there was no formal regulation of midwives until 1994. Hence, that program could not be recognized (Relyea 1992). In 1993, the first university-based, bachelor degree in midwifery commenced in Ontario, with others following soon after (Butler et al. 2016).

In the USA, education of midwives took a very different direction but was still linked closely to nursing. In the early 1900s, midwifery was reportedly practiced, largely by immigrants from Europe or Mexico, or African Americans born in the south (Dawley 2003), some without any formal midwifery education. Burst (2005) argues that in a trade-off between having practice autonomy and credibility, the profession of nurse-midwifery emerged despite heavy opposition. Midwifery was "allowed to come into being *only* attached to nursing and *under* the auspices of medical supervision and control." The first school was established to offer midwifery education to nurses in New York City in 1925 (Burst and Thompson 2003). Since that time, the nurse-midwife has continued to flourish in that country but does vary state by state.

Evolution of Higher Education in Midwifery

Higher education in midwifery has varied across jurisdictions and introduction of midwifery baccalaureate qualifications has been a relatively recent trend in many countries. From the transfer of nursing and midwifery education to the higher education sector in Australia, midwifery was initially, and continues to be, offered at postgraduate diploma level as a specialty qualification available to Registered Nurses who wish to register as midwives. In 2002, the first Bachelor of Midwifery, also sometimes referred to as "direct-entry midwifery" program was offered in the States of Victoria and South Australia (Leap et al. 2002), and these soon became available in other states. For the first time, students did not have to be nurses before they could become midwives (McKenna and Rolls 2007). There has been a similar trend elsewhere towards bachelor-level degrees in midwifery. In Jordan, midwifery degrees were introduced in 2002 as existing nurse-midwifery programs were reportedly not producing required numbers of midwives for the country's needs (Abushaikha 2006).

In the United Kingdom, direct-entry midwifery was introduced in 1989. Prior to that time, whilst not a specific requirement, most entrants were nurses first (Maggs 1994). With the establishment of the European Union, midwifery education developed in a number of central and eastern European countries. In Slovenia, midwifery was able to be moved from being offered in a nursing department to its own department, while in Slovakia and the Czech Republic, midwifery moved to being offered at bachelor's degree level in 2003, after which a master's degree was made available (Mivšek et al. 2016).

In China, midwifery education followed a different path. Formal midwifery education was introduced in 1929 in Beijing with a 2-year midwifery degree (Gao et al. 2019). Midwifery curriculum guidelines were released in the 1920s, The Cultural Revolution saw a halt to midwifery education between 1966 and 1972 (Cheung 2009). In 1983, a 3-year secondary direct-entry midwifery program commenced, followed by a Diploma in Midwifery in 2000 and Bachelor degree in 2014 (Gao et al. 2019). From 2008, midwifery students have been permitted to apply for the professional nursing examination in order to practice in hospitals (Zhu et al. 2018) and register as nurses, not midwives (Gao et al. 2019).

Midwifery and midwifery education are not recognized in all countries to the full extent of the ICM definition. This has influenced development of the profession and its education in these locations. In a study of six South Asian countries (Afghanistan, Bangladesh, Bhutan, India, Nepal, and Pakistan), it was identified that while all offered some type of midwifery education, even though all except Afghanistan, included this as part of nursing education courses (Bogren et al. 2012). In a number of countries, midwifery education in offered at diploma level, sometimes as a post-registration qualification for nurses and in others, as a standalone qualification. For example, in Singapore, midwifery is available to Registered Nurses as a post-registration qualification, Advanced Diploma in Nursing (Midwifery), offered by a polytechnic institution (Singapore Nursing Board 2019). In Turkey, midwifery education is available as a 4-year program through vocational high schools or as a BSc in Midwifery in universities. In that country, the midwife's scope of practice includes care of children up to 6 years of age (Sogukpinar et al. 2007).

Over recent years, higher level qualifications have been developed in the midwifery discipline across many countries, with some universities offering master's degrees in midwifery, and more recently, professional doctorates have become available for those wishing to pursue research careers but remain in clinical practice. Increasingly, midwives are also undertaking Doctor of Philosophy degrees, furthering the professional knowledge base.

Conclusion

Nursing and Midwifery are two distinct professions, with their own philosophies and bodies of knowledge, and both have long and established histories. While they began very separately in different contexts, the two professions and their education have intersected in many countries at different times of their evolution. Midwifery, in particular, has encountered a range of challenges in its practice and educational offerings as a result of political and social influences. Today, in many countries, each has its own academic pathway, while in other countries, midwifery continues to struggle to be recognized as an autonomous profession.

References

Abushaikha L. Midwifery education in Jordan: history, challenges and proposed solutions. J Int Womens Stud. 2006;8:185–93.

Aiken LH, Cimiotti JP, Sloane DM, Smith HL, Flynn L, Neff DF. Effects of nurse staffing and nurse education on patient deaths in hospitals with different nurse work environments. Med Care. 2011;49:1047–53.

Andregård A-C, Jangland E. The tortuous journey of introducing the Nurse Practitioner as a new member of the healthcare team: a meta-synthesis. Scand J Caring Sci. 2015;29:3–14.

APPG. All-Party Parliamentary Group on global health: triple impact – how developing nursing will improve health, promote gender equality and support economic growth. London: All-Party Parliamentary Group; 2016.

Australian Nursing and Midwifery Federation. Educating the nurse of the future – independent review of nursing education. ANMF submission. Melbourne: Australian Nursing and Midwifery Federation; 2019.

Barclay L. A feminist history of Australian midwifery from colonisation until the 1980s. Women Birth. 2008;21:3–8.

Bassett J. Nursing aide to enrolled nurse: a history of the Melbourne School for Enrolled Nurses. South Yarra: Melbourne School for Enrolled Nurses; 1993.

Birks M, Davis J, Smithson J, Lindsay D. Enablers and barriers to registered nurses expanding their scope of practice in Australia: a cross-sectional study. Policy Polit Nurs Pract. 2019;20:145. https://doi.org/10.1177/1527154419864176.

Bogren MU, Wiseman A, Berg M. Midwifery education, regulation and association in six South Asian countries: a descriptive report. Sex Reprod Health. 2012;3:67–72.

Bressan V, Tolotti A, Barisone M, Bagnasco A, Sasso L, Aleo G, Timmins F. Perceived barriers to the professional development of modern nursing in Italy – a discussion paper. Nurs Educ Pract. 2016;17:52–7.

Brown GD. Enrolled nurses: where do they go from here? J Nurs Manag. 1994;2(5):213–6.

Burst HV. The history of nurse-midwifery/midwifery education. J Midwifery Womens Health. 2005;50:129–37.

Burst HV, Thompson JE. Genealogic origins of nurse-midwifery education programs in the United States. J Midwifery Womens Health. 2003;48:464–72.

Butcher DL, Mackinnon KA. Educational silos in nursing education: a critical review of practical nurse education in Canada. Nurs Inq. 2015;22:231–9.

Butler MM, Hutton EK, McNiven PS. Midwifery education in Canada. Midwifery. 2016;33:28–30.

Carryer J, Wilkinson J, Towers A, Gardner G. Delineating advanced practice nursing in New Zealand: a national survey. Int Nurs Rev. 2018;65(1):24–32.

Casey M, O'Connor L, Cashin A, Fealy G, Smith R, O'Brien D, Glasgow ME. Enablers and challenges to advanced nursing and midwifery practice roles. J Nurs Manag. 2019;27:271–7.

Chamberlain D, Pollock W, Fulbrook P. ACCCN Workforce Standards for Intensive Care Nursing: systematic and evidence review, development, and appraisal. Aust Crit Care. 2018;31:292–302.

Cheung NF. Chinese midwifery: the history and modernity. Midwifery. 2009;25:228–41.

Clarke L. Foundations of nursing: enrolled division 2 nurses, ANZ ed. South Melbourne: Victorian Cengage Learning Australia; 2016.

Currie EJ, Carr-Hill RA. What is a nurse? Is there an international consensus? Int Nurs Rev. 2013;60:67.

Darcy Associates. Review of postgraduate nursing and midwifery education in Victoria. Final report. St Kilda: Darcy Associates; 2015.

Davis L, Taylor H, Reyes H. Lifelong learning in nursing: a Delphi study. Nurs Educ Today. 2014;34:441–5.

Dawley K. Origins of nurse-midwifery in the United States and its expansion in the 1940s. J Midwifery Womens Health. 2003;48:86–95.

Department of Health. Regulation of nursing associates in England: have your say. Br J Healthc Assist. 2017;11:553–5.

Dixon A. Second-level nurse. Int J Nurs Pract. 2001;7:360.

Edwards MM. State-enrolled assistant nurses. Am J Nurs. 1945;45:893–4.

Fahy K. An Australian history of the subordination of midwifery. Women Birth. 2007;20:25–9.

Francis R. Report of the mid Staffordshire NHS foundation trust public inquiry. 2013. https://assets. publishing.service.gov.uk/government/uploads/system/uploads/attachment_data/file/279121/0898_iii.pdf. Accessed 02 Oct 2019.

Gao L-L, Lu H, Leap N, Homer C. A review of midwifery in mainland China: contemporary developments within historical, economic and socio-political contexts. Women Birth. 2019;32:e279–83.

Gill FJ, Leslie GD, Grech C, Latour JM. An analysis of Australian graduate critical care nurse education. Collegian. 2015;22:71–81.

Goh HS, Tang ML, Lee CN, Liaw SY. The development of Singapore nursing education system: challenges, opportunities and implications. Int Nurs Rev. 2019;66:467. https://doi.org/10.1111/inr.12539.

Grehan M. Visioning the future by knowing the past. In: Daly J, Speedy S, Jackson D, editors. Contexts of nursing: an introduction. 5th ed. Chatswood: Elsevier; 2017.

Gullick J, Lin F, Massey D, Wilson L, Greenwood M, Skylas K, Gill FJ. Structures, processes and outcomes of specialist critical care nurse education: an integrative review. Aust Crit Care. 2019;32:331–45.

Halcomb E, Stephens M, Bryce J, Foley E, Ashley C. Nursing competency standards in primary health care: an integrative review. J Clin Nurs. 2016;25:1193–205.

Hunt DD. Fast facts about the nursing profession: historical perspectives in a nutshell. New York: Springer; 2017.

Institute of Medicine. The future of nursing: leading change, advancing health (978-0-309-48319-3). Institute of Medicine. 2011. https://www.nap.edu/catalog/12956/the-future-of-nursing-leading-change-advancing-health. Accessed 2 Oct 2019.

International Confederation of Midwives. 2017. https://www.internationalmidwives.org/assets/files/definitions-files/2018/06/eng-definition_of_the_midwife-2017.pdf. Retrieved 23 Sept 2019.

International Council of Nurses. Nursing definitions. 2019. https://www.icn.ch/nursing-policy/nursing-definitions. Retrieved 24 Sept 2019.

Jacob R, Barnett A, Sellick K, McKenna L. Scope of practice for Australian enrolled nurses: evolution and practice issues. Contemp Nurse. 2013;45:155–63.

Jensen DM. Jensen's history and trends of professional nursing. 5th ed. Saint Louis: Mosby; 1965.

Jinks AM, Richardson K, Jones C, Kirton JA. Issues concerning recruitment, retention and attrition of student nurses in the 1950/60s: a comparative study. Nurs Educ Pract. 2014;14:641–7.

Jokiniemi K, Suutarla A, Meretoja R, Kotila J, Axelin A, Flinkman M., . . . Fagerström L. Evidence-informed policymaking: modelling nurses' career pathway from registered nurse to advanced practice nurse. Int J Nurs Pract. 2019. https://doi.org/10.1111/ijn.12777

Kalisch PA, Kalisch BJ. The advance of American nursing. 3rd ed. Philadelphia: J.B. Lippincott; 1995.

Kaufman KJ. A history of Ontario midwifery. J SOGC. 1998;20:976–81.

Le Var RMH. Project 2000: a new preparation for practice – has policy been realized? Part 2. Nurs Educ Today. 1997;17:263–73.

Leap N, Barclay L, Nagy E, Sheehan A, Brodie P, Tracy S. Midwifery education: literature review and additional material. In: National review of nursing education. Canberra: Commonwealth of Australia; 2002.

Litoff JB. The midwife throughout history. J Nurse Midwifery. 1982;27:3–11.

Maggs C. Direct but different: midwifery education since 1989. Br J Midwifery. 1994;2:612–6.

Marshall AP. Educating the critical care nurse of the future. Aust Crit Care. 2019;32:273–4.

Masso M, Thompson C. Australian research investigating the role of nurse practitioners: a view from implementation science. Collegian. 2017;24:281–91.

McKenna L. The emergence of midwifery as a distinct discipline. In: Willis E, Reynolds L, Keleher H, editors. Understanding the Australian health care system. Sydney: Elsevier; 2009.

McKenna L, Rolls C. Bachelor of midwifery: reflections on the first 5 years from two Victorian universities. Women Birth. 2007;20:81–4.

McKenna L, Halcomb E, Lane R, Zwar N, Russell G. An investigation of barriers and enablers to advanced nursing roles in Australian general practice. Collegian. 2015;22:183–9.

McKittrick R, McKenzie R. A narrative review and synthesis to inform health workforce preparation for the Health Care Homes model in primary healthcare in Australia. Aust J Prim Health. 2018;24:317–29.

Mivšek P, Baškova M, Wilhelmova R. Midwifery education in Central-Eastern Europe. Midwifery. 2016;33:43–5.

Morin KH. Evolving global education standards for nurses and midwives. MCN: Am J Matern Child Nurs. 2012;37:360–4.

Nardi DA, Gyurko CC. The global nursing faculty shortage: status and solutions for change. J Nurs Scholarsh. 2013;45:317–26.

National Nursing & Nursing Education Taskforce (N3ET). A national specialisation framework for nursing and midwifery. Melbourne: The Department of Human Services; 2006.

Ng LC, Tuckett AG, Fox-Young SK, Kain VJ. Exploring registered nurses' attitudes towards post graduate education in Australia: instrument development. J Nurs Educ Pract. 2014;4(3):20.

Nightingale F. Notes on hospitals. 3rd ed. London/Ann Arbor: Longman, Green/University Microfilms; 1863.

Nightingale F. Notes on nursing: what it is and what it is not. Philadelphia: J.B. Lippincott; 1946.

Nightingale F. Florence Nightingale extending nursing. Waterloo: Wilfrid Laurier University Press; 2009a.

Nightingale F. Florence Nightingale: the Nightingale school. In: McDonald L, editor. The Nightingale school. Waterloo: Wilfrid Laurier University Press; 2009b.

Nordby H. The meaning of illness in nursing practice: a philosophical model of communication and concept possession. Nurs Philos. 2016;17:103–18.

Nordby H. Concept communication and interpretation of illness. Holist Nurs Pract. 2017;31: 158–66.

Nursing and Midwifery Board of Australia. Fact sheet: advanced nursing practice and specialty areas within nursing. NMBA. 2016. https://www.nursingmidwiferyboard.gov.au/Codes-Guidelines-Statements/FAQ/fact-sheet-advanced-nursing-practice-and-specialty-areas.aspx. Accessed 2 Oct 2019.

Nursing Council of New Zealand. New Zealand registered nurses, midwives and enrolled nurses workforce statistics 2002. NCNZ. 2004. https://www.nursingcouncil.org.nz/Public/Publications/Workforce_Statistics/NCNZ/publications-section/Workforce_statistics.aspx?hkey=3f3f39c4-c909-4d1d-b87f-e6270b531145. Accessed 02 Oct 2019.

O'Connor L, Casey M, Smith R, Fealy GM, Brien DO, O'Leary D, . . . Cashin A. The universal, collaborative and dynamic model of specialist and advanced nursing and midwifery practice: a way forward? J Clin Nurs. 2018;27:e882–94.

Ousey K. The changing face of student nurse education and training programmes. Wounds UK. 2011;7:70–5.

Parker JM, Hill MN. A review of advanced practice nursing in the United States, Canada, Australia and Hong Kong Special Administrative Region (SAR), China. Int J Nurs Sci. 2017;4:196–204.

Relyea MJ. The rebirth of midwifery in Canada: an historical perspective. Midwifery. 1992;8: 159–69.

Robinson S, Griffiths P. Nursing education and regulation: international profiles and perspectives. London: National Nursing Research Unit, Kings College; 2007. http://eprints.soton.ac.uk/348772/1/NurseEduProfiles.pdf. Retrieved 05 Oct 2019.

Roux GM, Halstead JA. Issues and trends in nursing: essential knowledge for today and tomorrow. Sudbury: Jones and Bartlett Publishers; 2009.

Russell RL. From Nightingale to now: nurse education in Australia. Sydney: Harcourt Brace Jovanovich; 1990.

Scanlon A, Murphy M, Smolowitz J, Lewis V. Low- and lower middle-income countries advanced practice nurses: an integrative review. Int Nurs Rev. 2019;67:19. https://doi.org/10.1111/inr.12536.

Schober M, Stewart D. Developing a consistent approach to advanced practice nursing worldwide. Int Nurs Rev. 2019;66:151–3.

Schwirian PM. Professionalization of nursing: current issues and trends. 3rd ed. Philadelphia: J.B. Lippincott; 1998.

Seccombe I, Smith G, Buchan J, Ball J. Enrolled nurses: a study for the UKCC (344). Brighton; 1997. https://www.employment-studies.co.uk/system/files/resources/files/344.pdf. Retrieved 05 Oct 2019.

Singapore Nursing Board. Post-registration programmes. 2019. https://www.healthprofessionals.gov.sg/snb/accreditation-of-nursing-education-programmes/accredited-nursing-programmes/post-registration-programmes

Sogukpinar N, Saydam BK, Bozkurt ÖD, Ozturk H, Pelik A. Past and present midwifery education in Turkey. Midwifery. 2007;23:433–42.

Sripathy A, Marti J, Patel H, Sheikh JI, Darzi AW. Professional education and universal health coverage: a summary of challenges and selected case studies. Health Aff. 2017;36:1928–36.

Stojanovic J. Midwifery in New Zealand 1904–1971. Contemp Nurse. 2008;30:156–67.

Tarnowski GJ, Bateman T, Stanger L, Phillips LA. Update of licensed practical nurse competencies in Alberta. J Nurs Regul. 2017;8:17–22.

Traczynski J, Udalova V. Nurse practitioner independence, health care utilization, and health outcomes. J Health Econ. 2018;58:90–109.

Trembath R, Hellier D. All care and responsibility: a history of nursing in Victoria 1850–1934. Melbourne: The Florence Nightingale Committee; 1987.

United Kingdom Central Council for Nursing. Project 2000: a new preparation for practice. London: UKCC; 1986.

White E. A comparison of nursing education and workforce planning initiatives in the United States and England. Policy Polit Nurs Pract. 2017;18:173–85.

Wong FKY, Liu H, Wang H, Anderson D, Seib C, Molasiotis A. Global nursing issues and development: analysis of World Health Organization documents. J Nurs Scholarsh. 2015;47:574–83.

World Health Organization. Global standards for the initial education of professional nurses and midwives. Geneva: WHO; 2009.

Yates K, Birks M, Coxhead H, Zhao L. Double degree destinations: nursing or midwifery. Collegian. 2020;27(1):135–40.

Zahran Z, Curtis P, Lloyd-Jones M, Blackett T. Jordanian perspectives on advanced nursing practice: an ethnography. Int Nurs Rev. 2012;59:222–9.

Zerwekh J. Nursing today: transition and trends. 8th ed. Saint Louis: Elsevier Health Sciences; 2015.

Zhang X, Meng K, Chen S. Competency framework for specialist critical care nurses: a modified Delphi study. Nurs Crit Care Nurs. 2019;25:45. https://doi.org/10.1111/nicc.12467.

Zhu X, Yao J, Lu J, Pang R, Lu H. Midwifery policy in contemporary and modern China: from the past to the future. Midwifery. 2018;66:97–102.

Health Sciences and Medicine Education in Lockdown: Lessons Learned During the COVID-19 Global Pandemic

17

Suzanne Gough, Robin Orr, Allan Stirling, Athanasios Raikos, Ben Schram, and Wayne Hing

Contents

Introduction	304
The Impact of COVID-19 on Accredited Programs Within Health Sciences and Medicine	304
The Context of Transitioning to Multimodal Delivery	306
Case Study 1: Doctor of Physiotherapy Multimodal Delivery Approach	309
Case Study 2: Adapting Anatomy Learning and Teaching Methods During COVID-19	321
Reimagining Medical and Health Professional Education beyond the COVID-19 Pandemic	327
Conclusion	327
Cross-References	328
References	328

Abstract

The global COVID-19 pandemic has initiated an immediate and rapid digital upskilling of students, academics, and professional staff to enable transitions from more traditional face-to-face (F2F) learning to remote and/or multimodal delivery methods. This chapter provides an overview of the impact of COVID-19 on accredited medicine, nursing, and allied healthcare programs worldwide. We provide methods and flexible strategies that can be incorporated into the delivery of modern health science curricula during the current COVID-19 pandemic and beyond, as universities and programs undergo a digital transformation within learning and teaching. Two case studies illustrate the ability to harness technology to develop and deliver high-quality inclusive educational experiences for students during the pandemic. Top tips to optimize learner engagement, provision of multiple modes of participation, equity, and equivalency of experience, and

---

S. Gough (✉) · R. Orr · A. Stirling · A. Raikos · B. Schram · W. Hing
Faculty of Health Sciences and Medicine, Bond University, Gold Coast, QLD, Australia
e-mail: sgough@bond.edu.au; rorr@bond.edu.au; astirlin@bond.edu.au; araikos@bond.edu.au; bschram@bond.edu.au; whing@bond.edu.au

© Springer Nature Singapore Pte Ltd. 2023
D. Nestel et al. (eds.), *Clinical Education for the Health Professions*,
https://doi.org/10.1007/978-981-15-3344-0_141

enhancing the reusability of learning materials and artifacts for assessment or clinical placement preparation, are shared. Each case study highlights the transferability to other disciplines and legacy of these adaptations beyond COVID-19.

Keywords

Cognitive load · Digital technology · Inclusivity · Instructional design · Multimodal delivery

Introduction

The global coronavirus pandemic (COVID-19) has resulted in unprecedented health, financial, and socioeconomic turmoil around the globe. As a result of illness, restriction of movement, social and physical distancing requirements, the education of 1.5 billion students has been impacted across 191 countries (UNESCO 2020). In November 2020, a report from a nonprofit organization on learning and teaching reimagined (Maguirem et al. 2020), explored how COVID-19 has fundamentally changed approaches and delivery of learning and teaching. Prior to March 2020, the overwhelming majority of university programs in the UK favored on-campus delivery, with the exception of the Open University. The report identified the expectations of a greater shift over the next 10 years to a blended learning approach comprising of online lectures, online and in-person tutorials, and seminars, to give rise to priority to in-person workshops, laboratory/studio-based practical work (Maguirem et al. 2020).

In this chapter we share our collective experiences through two case studies and provide methods and flexible strategies that can be incorporated into the delivery of modern health science curricula, during the current COVID-19 pandemic and beyond. The context of the chapter is drawn from a university approach that used theory, empirical research, and practical guidance to dynamically respond to the evolving situation. The two case studies illustrate the ability to harness technology to develop and deliver high-quality educational experiences for students during the disruption of the global COVID-19 pandemic. Each case study highlights the lasting legacy of these adaptations beyond COVID-19.

The Impact of COVID-19 on Accredited Programs Within Health Sciences and Medicine

Health sciences and medicine programs have not been spared from the disruption generated by the COVID-19 pandemic. In response, universities have been required to continually accommodate social and physical distancing measures that have never before impacted the delivery of learning, teaching, and assessment (Parkin 2020). For many healthcare professions, the ramifications of the disruption to on-campus and clinical placement-based education have led to a delay in the entry of the next generation of health professionals into the workforce (APHRA 2020; Carolan et al.

2020; World Physiotherapy 2020c). The extent to which university programs have requested changes to entry-level programs in response to COVID-19 disruption for graduating cohorts has varied across professional disciplines, universities, and countries worldwide (AHPRA 2020; AMC 2020; HCPC 2020; World Physiotherapy 2020c). For example, in April 2020, World Physiotherapy (2020a) surveyed key stakeholders involved in education, regulation, and accrediting organization, to establish the impact and consequences of COVID-19 to entry to practice education. Key findings related to the ongoing uncertainty of the impact of COVID-19 on entry-level programs, flexibility in regulatory body ability to allow emergency response has been a barrier and an enabler. Acknowledging that these findings are focused on global physiotherapy programs, parallels are being drawn to other medical and allied health professional education providers.

For some university programs, the onset of COVID-19 created the need to rapidly redesign the delivery of both coursework subjects and/or clinical placements (Cleland et al. 2020; Gordon et al. 2020; Keegan et al. 2020; Torda et al. 2020; World Physiotherapy 2020a). Primarily the redesign has been due to the restrictions on national and international travel affecting students' ability to study on campus, and those students whose clinical education was impacted by the cancellation of placements (Gordon et al. 2020). The World Physiotherapy briefing papers (2020a, b, c) reported the most frequently reported challenge facing entry-level programs has been the availability of clinical placement opportunities. Similarly, the impact on clinical placement availability (e.g., cancellation, partial cancellation, and decreased activity) has also impacted medical, nursing, and allied health programs across the globe (AHPRA 2020; Kapila et al. 2020; Lynch 2020; MacDougall et al. 2020; White 2020). Changes to the clinical environment and delivery of consultations/patient management conducted via telehealth, reductions to Emergency Department attendance, reduced hospital admissions for non--COVID-19 illnesses, cancellation of nonurgent elective surgery, workforce capacity, risk, and appropriateness of settings have also shaped placement availability and opportunities (AHPRA 2020; CSP 2020a, b; Iacobucci 2020; Lynch 2020; MacDougall et al. 2020; World Physiotherapy 2020a, b, c). Similarly, across medicine and allied healthcare, the requirements of employees to work in different clinical areas from normal pre-COVID-19 practice and a greater shift towards relocating to acute medical wards, has also impacted placement availability (Chartered Society of Physiotherapy 2020a, b; Royal College of Physicians 2020a, b). To enable continuation of academic studies, medical and allied healthcare programs have responded on an individual basis, re-sequencing academic, and placement elements of the curriculum as the pandemic situation changed, while ensuring accreditation requirements were maintained (AHPRA 2020; CSP 2020a; GMC 2020; MacDougall et al. 2020; Torda et al. 2020; World Physiotherapy 2020a, b, c).

The following section presents an example of a university-wide approach that used theory, empirical research, and practical guidance to dynamically respond to the need to pivot from face-to-face teaching to remote delivery, followed by a further transition to multimodal delivery.

The Context of Transitioning to Multimodal Delivery

The global pandemic initiated the immediate digital up skilling of students, academics, and professional staff to enable the transition from face-to-face (F2F) learning to remote learning followed by a multimodal delivery (MMD) approach. These approaches enabled the commitment to students to provide flexible study options through a multimodal approach. In this approach, students who were physically able to attend on-campus tutorials, seminars, workshops, clinical skills, and laboratory sessions face-to-face in the physical classroom were united with their peers accessing synchronously via the virtual classroom.

Four MMD scenarios were developed by the University for Adoption by academics according to the location of students. These options are presented in Fig. 1 (Bond University 2020b). Multimodal delivery is a technologically enhanced teaching approach to support learner engagement through multiple communication and learning platforms (Bond 2020b). These MMD approaches combine best practices of online learning and face-to-face delivery, creating a "hybrid" educational experience for learners (Bond 2020b; Clay 2020), irrespective of their geographical location. These MMD approaches allow all students to engage in learning activities both synchronously (e.g., via tutorial, clinical skills, workshops, and simulation-based education, and asynchronously (e.g., via flipped classroom or self-directed learning activities or review of classroom recordings). They were developed to ensure effective and efficient delivery of coursework content for programs across the University, during a period of time when academics and professional staff were able to return to deliver content on-campus. At this time, teaching rooms were subject to constraints on room capacity due to social distancing requirements set by the Australian Government. The adoption of this MMD approach required the development of short, medium, and long-term strategic plans, to harness technology as the vehicle to develop and deliver high-quality multimodal learning experiences, irrespective of the students' geographical location. Equity of experience and group cohesion were positioned at the forefront of design considerations and the learner remained at the heart of all activity.

A review of digital and teaching skills required by students, academics, and professional staff utilizing the MMD approach was undertaken and a university-wide training program was developed. The "3-P" ("plan, prepare and practice") training program was developed to ensure that all academics and professional staff felt fully prepared to use the enhanced in-class technologies in advance of engaging with students. All MMD rooms were equipped with pan-tilt-zoom (PTZ) front and rear-cameras, enhanced audio capture, lapel microphones and/or roving microphones, and dual-screen tech-desks. Additional specialist audio-visual technologies were also added for laboratories, simulation, and specialist teaching areas, to capture the intricacies of clinical skills. The Blackboard Collaborate web conferencing platform within the Blackboard Learning Management System enabled digital recording of real-time teaching activities on-campus within the classroom as well as outdoor and specialist

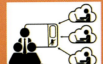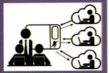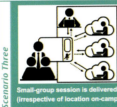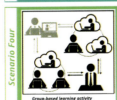

Fig. 1 Multimodal delivery pedagogy (Bond 2002b) NB: high-resolution image supplied. (Courtesy of Bond University, Australia. Consent was gained from the Doctor of Physiotherapy students featured in the photographs)

teaching facilities. Additional digital platforms such as Microsoft TEAMS and Zoom video communications were integrated within the suite of digital conferencing facilities, each selected dependent on need, for example, video sharing, and number of digital break-out rooms allowed by the digital platform.

In addition, comprehensive videos, TALK (teaching and learning knowledge) sheets and and eGuide were developed by the Office of Learning and Teaching to continually support preparedness for MMD (Bond 2020b, c). Videos and top tips were provided for staff and students to optimize the MMD (Fig. 2). Digital technology "netiquette" tip sheets were also developed to optimize learner engagement,

MULTI-MODAL DELIVERY – REMINDERS FOR STAFF

Remember to...

- ✓ Set up equipment/desktop/laptop and test audio volumes
- ✓ Enable microphone (lapel) for Mediasite (lecture recording) if applicable
- ✓ Outline expectations, 'plan B' and 'housekeeping' for your session

For example:
(i) Identify what platform you are using for class (e.g. Collaborate / Teams)
(ii) Outline how you want students to engage (e.g. raise hand / chat feature; turn camera on when speaking)
(iii) Explain when and how will you respond to student questions/comments (e.g. as they occur or by pausing every 20 minutes to check questions/comments etc)
(iv) Explain what students need to do if they experience a technology fail/network outage during 'live' session (e.g. wait 2 mins and attempt to log back in, contact subject tutor/Assistant Teaching Fellow, call IT Service desk, refer to recording post-session etc)

- ✓ Record your session
- ✓ Conclude session 5 minutes prior to scheduled class finish time to enable next class and instructor adequate set-up time

MULTI-MODAL DELIVERY – REMINDERS FOR STUDENTS

 On-campus students   **Off-campus students**

 Turn off notifications – avoid multitasking during the session    Turn off notifications – avoid multitasking during the session

🔇 Turn off computer audio and speakers to avoid feedback noise   🎤 Mute microphone unless you are speaking

🎧 Use headphones if working in groups with off-campus students while in the physical classroom   🔊 Turn on camera and microphone when speaking

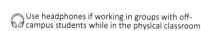 To take care of yourself and others, if you are feeling unwell please do not attend the physical class but you may consider joining virtually   🎧 Use headphones if you are not in a quiet space

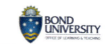

Fig. 2 Multimodal delivery top tips for staff and students (NB: high-resolution image supplied). (Courtesy of Bond University, Australia. Consent was gained from the Doctor of Physiotherapy students featured in the photographs)

through the development of optimal working environments and minimizing distractions for others.

The following section presents two case studies that illustrate the ability to harness technology to continue to deliver high-quality educational experiences during the disruption of a global pandemic.

Case Study 1: Doctor of Physiotherapy Multimodal Delivery Approach

The Doctor of Physiotherapy (DPHTY) program at Bond University is an intensive, six semester program which admits cohorts of 60 students (Bond University 2020a). Traditionally, students attended campus for theory, small group learning, simulation-based education, and clinical skills activities, for six or more hours per day. Australian physiotherapists are first-contact practitioners who upon graduation often need to be completely independent and function on their own. As such, the teaching approach strives to progress the students along the Pedagogy–Andragogy–Heutagogy continuum, from student-centered learner to reflective learner (Halupa 2015). The entry-level physiotherapists, along with allied health professional and medicine graduates, are required to continually engage in critical thinking, clinical reasoning practices, and operate within highly complex healthcare environments (Gough et al. 2016; Thackray and Roberts 2016; Higgs 2020).

Traditional Delivery Approaches

To optimize learning over this 2-year, six semester intensive period, multiple teaching approaches are blended and applied to meet student requirements. During periods of heavy knowledge and clinical skills-based content (e.g., completing core musculoskeletal, cardiorespiratory, and neurological physiotherapy content), dedicated consideration is given to reducing extraneous load while enhancing germane load, in order to mitigate excessive cognitive load (Van Merriënboer et al. 2006; Reedy 2015; Sewell et al. 2018; Sweller 2020). Approaches used to achieve this strategy include adopting "chunking" (Miller 1956) and "scaffolding" (Vygotsky 1978) and employing an adapted cognitive learning model to redesign the resources and key themes, aligning them with subsequent and preceding program subjects and within subject sessions. For example, in the Foundations of Physiotherapy subject, chunks are grouped into themes like the clinical physiotherapist and the physiotherapist in action. These "chunks" are then scaffolded to progressively reinforce knowledge at an individual resource subject level and at a curriculum level. Subjects are also augmented with small group learning sessions (e.g., problem-based leaning) with a focus on not only learning but critical thinking (Gunn et al. 2012; Zhou 2018; Seibert 2020).

In addition to direct learning theory, indirect factors that can impact on learning are considered, notably those that can lead to excessive levels of stress and reductions in attention, engagement, and knowledge retention. The former is given particular attention, as students undertaking a physiotherapy degree both in the Bond University DPHTY program (Brooke et al. 2020) and across the profession as a whole report high levels of stress and burnout due to their studies (Wilski et al.

2015; Afridi and Fahim 2019; Beltran-Velasco et al. 2019). Examples of the practical application adopted to optimize learning (Box 1) will be explored in more detail throughout this chapter. The program delivery was constantly fine-tuned through a rigorous quality assurance cycle. This approach was effective, with negligible student attrition, extremely low overall failure rates and the Good Universities Guide rating Bond University first in Australia for "Overall student experience" (95.9%) for postgraduate health services education. However, the program was originally predicated on students attending class in person.

The Impact of the Pandemic and Teaching Adaptation

With the closure of state and international borders in Australia, due to the pandemic, the ability for students to attend on-campus face-to-face classes was notably impacted. As over 40% of the cohort were overseas, and another 20% were inter-state, three different student sub-cohorts arose: (1) physically on-campus students, (2) remote students engaging in teaching delivery in real time (synchronous); and at times (3) remote students engaging with the materials after delivery (asynchronously) due to time zone differences.

The physical separation potentially added to the already notably high levels of perceived stress and burnout, associated with the higher educational demands of entry-level *(Bachelors, Masters and Doctor of Physiotherapy)* programs (Frank and Cassady 2005; Lin and Huang 2012; Afridi and Fahim 2019; Beltran-Velasco et al. 2019; Brooke et al. 2020). Key risk factors in the development of stress, burnout, and anxiety, for example, lack of engagement, support, and feelings of isolation, were acknowledged, and the subdivision of a cohort coupled with remote/MMD had the potential for exacerbation during the pandemic. As such, a key strategy to deliver education to a DPHTY cohort, who had never met each other as they commenced their program during the pandemic, was to harness student engagement through a paradigm shift that focused on blending the human and technological aspects of education. This was to ensure that all students felt part of a dynamic learning community throughout all methods of content delivery. It was essential that our multimodal approach enabled content to be delivered in an equitable manner for all students. Sessions were still conducted in real-time for on-campus students. However, often the on-campus (face-to-face) students were simultaneously logged into the University's Learning Management System, enabling group connection and cohesion with those students joining remotely. Sessions were broadcast via the digital conferencing platform Blackboard Collaborate and were also recorded to allow for asynchronous student learning and revision for the summative assessments. Additionally, the design of multimodal tutorial and small group learning activities also promoted group and cohort cohesion.

Multimodal Lectures: Traditional lecture-style delivery was augmented with edutainment and strategies to increase learner engagement (Box 1). Lectures and small group learning activities were delivered F-2-F for both on-campus and remote students (Fig. 1, scenario three) via Blackboard Collaborate. The lead educator presented the content, while another staff member (typically the subject convener or a teaching assistant) monitored the live feed and chat functions. Active engagement of the entire cohort was promoted by purposely designed and impromptu sharing of questions from within the on-campus classroom and remote students providing comments via the video conferencing and chat function (Fig. 3). The chat comments and audio were also accessible when reviewing the classroom recording asynchronously. This way, the student class was maintained as one cohort, regardless of location. Similarly, this approach allowed the academics to monitor and facilitate student engagement ensuring discussions were active and equitable, irrespective of the geographical location.

This approach also allowed academics to maintain regular and supportive presence for both on-campus and remote students, as they are visible throughout the entire learning process.

Box 1: Examples of Indirect Factors that Can Influence Student Learning

Indirect factors influencing student learning	Observation	Practical applications adopted to optimize learning
Selye's General Adaption Syndrome (GAS) details how a body responds to stress, which can be derived from a multitude of sources outside of the learning environment (Selye 1950). Initially, the body moves into an alarm reaction phase, synonymous with nomenclature like culture shock, before beginning to adapt and then to thrive. However, if the stress is prolonged or continues to increase it can lead to burnout	This pattern is seen during the DPHTY program when the course commences with students arriving from various states in Australia and from around the globe. Students transition from an undergraduate to a postgraduate program and are required to attend classes daily for around 6-h per day. In addition, with the majority of students having never met before, they transition through the initial stages of "group dynamics." These initial stresses led to a shock phase (i.e., culture shock). However, the students do recover after around 4–6 weeks (counter-shock) and then begin to thrive in the "new normal." However, the intensive nature of the program predisposes students to fatigue and staleness towards the end of the 14-week semesters. With limited holidays, no more than 2 weeks between most semesters, the continued intensity has the potential to lead to burnout and fatigue (Brooke et al. 2020)	Staffs who convene cover the theory of "GAS" in a short informal session, highlighting to students that what they are feeling is normal. Strategies to mitigate this new stress, such as taking breaks, optimizing nutrition, sleep, and exercise are discussed and access to support services provided, should the need arise Staffs are cognizant of the volume of new knowledge imparted in the first few weeks while students are adapting to other stressors (e.g., moving, transition to postgraduate, new groups, and friendships) Where possible, half-day breaks are included later in the semester to provide short "brain breaks."

(continued)

Box 1: Examples of Indirect Factors that Can Influence Student Learning
(continued)

Indirect factors influencing student learning	Observation	Practical applications adopted to optimize learning
Circadian rhythms are characterized by periods of alertness and drowsiness (NIGMS 2020). Adenosine is also higher in the afternoon than the morning, which contributes to tiredness (HMSDSM 2007)	Students typically return from lunch breaks tired, particularly after covering long theoretical sessions in the morning. Sessions which are heavy in theoretical content are more difficult to digest for students and deliver for staff when they are scheduled in the afternoon	Highly theoretical contact delivered during arousal periods (morning) with practical sessions delivered during lull periods (e.g., after lunchtime) For afternoon sessions which are of a theoretical nature, sessions are shorter with more breaks and, where possible, include small group work Highly theoretical assessments (e.g., written examinations) are conducted in the morning
Yerkes–Dodson law (1908), represents an inverted "U" that suggests that learning is optimized when there is sufficient stimulation but decreases if the stimulation is too great	Having a vibrant, dynamic online platform where the course resources are accessed, in conjunction with additional activities such as discussion boards, riddle of the day, and other optional engagement activities, can enhance students' interest in the program. However, if the learning materials are already excessive these additional media may negatively impact on learning Acutely, this law can also be considered in conjunction with circadian rhythms. During periods of alertness stimulatory materials and experiences (e.g., interactive simulations) are increased while during circadian lulls stimulation is decreased (e.g., basic practical still revision) Chronically, this law can be	Content volume and presentation need to be carefully balanced to engage the student but not overwhelm them with considerations given to time of day (micro) and time of semester (macro) considerations of importance Be clear in setting expectations, explaining how students will navigate their learning, seek feedback, and manage issues Ensure all learners have equal access and opportunity to engage with learning regardless of the mode of delivery Changes in teaching delivery (Visual, Aural, Read/write, and Kinesthetic sensory modalities) and format (e.g., lectures, small group work, practical simulations, etc.) can be manipulated to increase or

(continued)

Box 1: Examples of Indirect Factors that Can Influence Student Learning (continued)

Indirect factors influencing student learning	Observation	Practical applications adopted to optimize learning
	considered in conjunction with GAS. Following commencement of a program or after a semester break, stimulation is progressively increased and maintained before being reduced as the semester progresses to avoid staleness	decrease stimulation to suit requirements
Group dynamics follows the progression of the cohort's development, interactions, and adopting a system of behaviors and typically follows a 5-stage model, being forming-storming-norming-performing- adjourning model (Maples 1988)	The initial stages are tied to the GAS. Integration of technology-enhanced learning can magnify physical and mental wellbeing manifestations. Awareness of the challenges of establishing group dynamics through learning environments, particularly the hybrid of remote and on-campus students engaging in the same learning activities is essential (Clay 2020), to enable inclusivity rather than segregation	MMD has meant that the opportunity for the informal naturally occurring interactions between students (e.g., after sessions, during lunch, at the library, etc.) are reduced (esp. for remote students). Furthermore, students engaging remotely may find it difficult to build friendships and bond with their peers. To develop a virtual learning community: Rules for group interactions (esp. for MMD) need to be established early on to provide a feeling of safety and facilitate acceptance. The educators need to be highly visible and present during initial stages as students will look to them for what is normal, seeking guidance and direction Development of in-class and extra-curricular activities to engage students to develop social groups and peer-support/learning buddies, irrespective of geographical location. For example, using intentionally plan interactions (online/

(continued)

Box 1: Examples of Indirect Factors that Can Influence Student Learning (continued)

Indirect factors influencing student learning	Observation	Practical applications adopted to optimize learning
		synchronous/F-2-F) of interactive activities (e.g., quick trivia challenges in groups before class. Team names can be based on specific treatment techniques, anatomical landmarks, etc.)
		In the initial stages constantly change groups to allow as wide an exposure to other students as possible with each session drawing out commonalities in students (e.g., Who has had a knee operation? Who is in Canada? Who owns a dog?) assisting students to find like-minded members in their cohort
		When using TEAMs, Collaborate, or Zoom software applications, encourage students to use their camera where bandwidth allows and to have a photo uploaded as their icon. Also encourage students to change this photo regularly and again include in engaging activities (e.g., "socks-for-docs" days where profile photos have them wearing their favorite socks).
		Practical applications across subjects include early inclusion of large (e.g., cultural immersion camp) group activities progressing to a smaller group (e.g., problem-based learning) interactions to facilitate group dynamic development.

(continued)

Box 1: Examples of Indirect Factors that Can Influence Student Learning
(continued)

Indirect factors influencing student learning	Observation	Practical applications adopted to optimize learning
Light exposure (especially blue-enriched white) enhances alertness (Sleegers et al. 2012; Rodríguez-Morilla et al. 2018)	Sessions conducted in the evenings and reading online resources late into the night can impact on the student's sleep patterns	Encourage students to increase their exposure to natural sunlight (i.e., window shades drawn up) in the morning sessions Use blue light themes on PowerPoint slides and presentations to increase attention during sessions For evening work switch electronic media to "night mode" (orange tinge) and avoid electronic work in the evenings before going to sleep
Use of handwritten notes - Despite being able to take more notes utilizing a laptop, research has shown that taking notes using a pen and paper, allows students to put ideas in their own words, enhancing individual interpretation of ideas and enhancing performance on tests (Mueller and Oppenheimer 2014)	Most students tend to use a laptop for taking notes, attempting to transcribe everything which was being said verbatim. This does not allow digestion of the information and requires revisiting the information at a later date	Embed triggers in digital content (e.g., asking for a student's thoughts on a topic) with accompanying paper workbooks, full of white space for taking handwritten notes

Enhancing Learner Engagement through Edutainment: Edutainment is the merging of education and entertainment, to allow the learner to acquire knowledge in an interesting, exciting, engaging, and entertaining format (Anikina and Yakimenko 2015). Ellaway (2016) introduced a conceptual framework of game-informed principles for health professions education. This framework challenges educators to consider how simulation, games, and serious game facets may be used to effect desirable educational outcomes, through consideration of instructional design principles (Ellaway 2016). To enrich student engagement with the learning environment, learning materials, and their peers; interaction points were added into sessions which could be completed both in real time and asynchronously. Purposefully designed videos with questions and countdown timers before answers appeared, added variety and challenges throughout learning activities. Edutainment examples included inviting students to physically act out complex health processes,

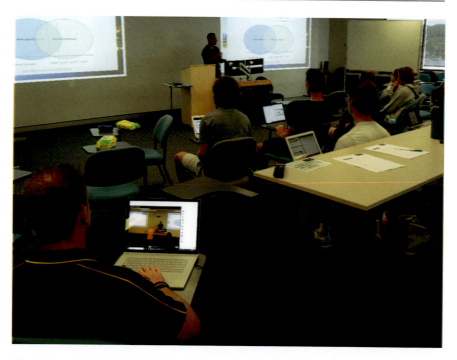

Fig. 3 The educator delivering content to on-campus students, while the remote students, monitored by another staff member, watches, and engages with the remote students. (Courtesy of Bond University, Australia. Consent was gained from the Doctor of Physiotherapy students featured in the photographs)

either in real-time or asynchronously; "choose your own adventure" quests; and "who wants to be a physio student" game shows, with questions and answer revision exercises. Coursework was integrated across platforms, from student workbooks to interactive videos to digital research papers, allowing the student to extend themselves or seek guided clarification on content.

Multimodal small group learning: Small group learning activities were similarly delivered via the Learning Management System to simultaneously engage the on-campus and remote students (Fig. 1, scenario 3). Students were either randomized or small groups were formed for students to discuss learning activities. Figure 4 illustrates how feedback of a group activity to the larger group was enacted, with participation from both on-campus and remote students.

Throughout the small group learning activities, the remote operation of the PTZ cameras enabled close-up live viewing and recording of the whiteboard. The close-up capture of illustrations augmented the audio delivery for both on-campus and remote students. Again, this method enabled equitable visibility of class notes and peer feedback, which promoted engagement from the entire cohort. The screen-sharing functionality within the Blackboard Collaborate digital platform also permits on-campus and remote students to share groupwork developed in "breakout rooms,"

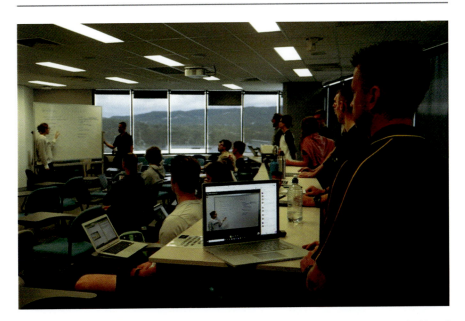

Fig. 4 Close up capture of the small group learning feedback to all students via Blackboard Collaborate. (Courtesy of Bond University, Australia. Consent was gained from the Doctor of Physiotherapy students featured in the photographs)

again removing geographical boundaries. Throughout the session, both on-campus and remote students contributed to the live chat function and posted questions/ responses. These were simultaneously monitored and integrated into the groups' discussions via the lead educator, subject convener, or teaching assistant monitored the live feed and chat functions (Fig. 4).

Multimodal practical skills sessions: Digital technology integration using a hand-held phone or video camera, similarly, enabled integration of a live video-feed within the Learning Management System, to engage remote students with a practical learning activity (Fig. 5). Using this MMD approach (Fig. 1, scenario three), the on-campus students completed practical sessions with the lead educator, while a teaching assistant was responsible for a live-stream video recording from various angles. In this instance, a mobile phone was integrated as the live video feed via Blackboard Collaborate, while the subject convener facilitated active engagement and questions from the remote students via the live chat and video functionality. This is perhaps one of the more challenging learner engagement activities to deliver using a multimodal approach. However, careful consideration was given to the video capture angle, for example, whether a wide-angle view or close-up filming was undertaken to optimize learning (Fig. 5). Prior dissemination of the requirements to obtain and utilize learning artifacts such as practical equipment (tape measures, goniometers to measure join angles, patient-reported outcome measurement tools) was important. Thus, despite being remote, students could participate in practical components of the skills sessions from their own home. Additionally, a

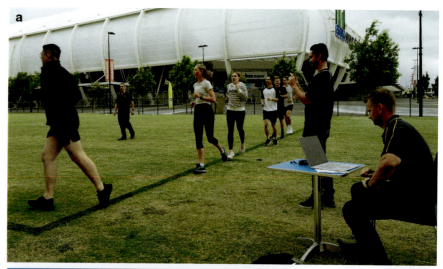

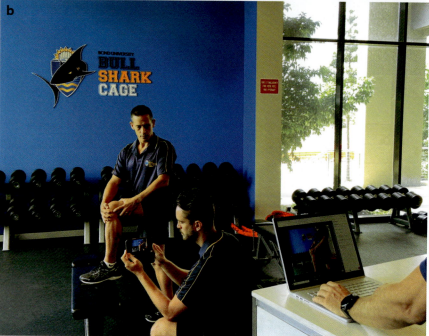

Fig. 5 (**a**) Wide angle and close-up live stream video feed of an outdoor practical session. (**b**) Close-up live stream video feed of an indoor practical session. (Courtesy of Bond University, Australia. Consent was gained from the Doctor of Physiotherapy students featured in the photographs)

prepared and considered approach was required to ensure that remote students accessing the learning activities felt involved as opposed to detached from the learning activity and or group.

Optimizing learner engagement despite geographical location in various time zones: Within the DPHTY program, international students were geographically located across seven different time zones. The ability to deliver content in real time meant that there were limited times in which the delivery could occur. To optimize daylight learning, live learning activities were scheduled from 800 to 1200 h in Australia, meaning that for the majority of overseas students in the United States and Canada, classes ran in the early evenings for the eastern coast but mid-afternoon for the western coast. These time zone variations meant differences in circadian rhythms and the impact of blue-enriched light on sleep for students watching prior to going to sleep likewise needed to be considered (Box 1). To increase student engagement and informal learning, discussion board competitions were held with topics that were designed to be enjoyable yet pertinent. For example, "Name movies or television series with physiotherapists in them." Or *"If you could have a superpower to use an advanced scope in your treatment, what would it be?"* (X-ray vision was an example answer.) These informal approaches allowed students to engage with the program at times of their choosing.

Additional challenges arose, including group dynamics and equity of internet access/broadband speed, which are less prevalent when all students are geographically located on-campus. Naturalistic opportunities for group dynamic evolution were hampered, as not all students were engaged in real time for every session. Also, there were fewer opportunities for informal group development (e.g., opportunistic talking to each other after class, during lunch, or at the library).

Given that students studying remotely did not have the opportunity to take advantage of the on-campus "open-door" access to academic staff, "digital open-door" sessions were scheduled to provide students with the opportunity for ad hoc, as required meetings with academics. Likewise, to increase informal engagement of all students, a virtual classroom, "the Oasis Coffee Lounge," was opened for the duration of subjects. This virtual space was used to build an active, participatory, and social learning community to further strengthen student engagement. An accompanying noticeboard was added to the discussion board to allow students to coordinate more formal digital study sessions. The popularity of the virtual "Oasis Coffee Lounge" led to excessively large groups, and as such, additional virtual VIP lounges were added which students could "break out to" if the lounge became too busy.

Connectivity Challenges: For those studying remotely, the impact of the students' learning environment is beyond the control of the academic. For some students, the household living room/bedroom became an office. While online netiquette rules have been developed (Fig. 2), often competing influences of family members also having to work remotely from home or siblings also being home-schooled, created a significant demand for internet bandwidth. This was particularly of note for those in opposite time zones, whereby family members may be socializing and using video and game streaming services in the early evenings. Having an awareness of the potential impact of family situations was imperative, and academics needed to be mindful of this when requesting students to engage with video. This is of particular note, as different video conferencing platforms give preference to video or audio feed. Knowledge of the video conferencing application's quality of service requirements can provide insight into students' complaints of latency, jitter, and video/audio loss during sessions as well as allowing the academic to provide immediate assistance to a student should these arise during a session.

Top Tips for Livestreaming of Practical Skills

The following top tips have been developed based on lessons learned from several DPHTY coursework subjects featuring clinical skills that have been delivered multimodally and guidance from the Office of Learning and Teaching (Bond 2020c):

1. The learning outcomes for multimodal delivery remain unchanged. The challenge is to ensure inclusivity for all learners. Use instructional design principles for multimodal delivery which include providing learner choice through multiple modes of participation, ensuring equivalency, reusability, equity, and accessibility.
2. Established consent from students to be filmed throughout the semester during practical sessions. *This will help streamline organization of the session activities and ensure close-up recording is only undertaken featuring students who feel comfortable doing so.*
3. Operation and positioning of the iPhone/Camera used for close-up video capture requires careful consideration, to optimize the angle and intricacy of the details required for the remote audience.
4. Consider using a plug-in Bluetooth microphone that connects to the iPhone/ Camera, in order to optimize sound quality when streaming/filming close-up demonstrations or when high quality room microphones are not available *(e.g., outside venues)*
5. Ensure students are aware of any equipment they require in order to participate and practice any skills at home that mirror classroom provisions *(e.g., stethoscope, tape measures, stop watches, to maximize engagement, equivalency, and equity of experience as much as practically possible).*
6. High video and audio quality capture promotes reusability of the recording by students to recap/re-visit content *(which can be especially useful for revision for assessment or clinical placement preparation).*
7. Recording skills sessions via the Learning Management System promote equity, reusability, and accessibility to all students, irrespective of the geographical location of the campus. *Often, these are saved and titled by presentation date/ time and, as such, need to be renamed to facilitate student access.*

Summary

Case study one has provided a brief overview of innovative MMD approaches that can be adapted for use across a wide variety of academic programs, as well as health sciences and medicine. The examples from the Doctor of Physiotherapy program illustrate, how modifications were made to the delivery to optimize inclusivity for all students commencing studies in seven geographical time zones during COVID-19. Examples of curriculum design adaptations to reduce academic stress, and accommodate the impact of circadian rhythm on learning, knowledge retention, and assessment performance. These students focused MMD modifications to learning experiences have enabled the program to deliver a high-quality program that provides equivalency, reusability, and accessibility of learning materials and while maintaining accreditation requirements.

Case Study 2: Adapting Anatomy Learning and Teaching Methods During COVID-19

Within the health sciences and medicine, many subjects are, by their very nature, clinical and competency-based. Face-to-face teaching remains a cornerstone of clinical skills education, simulation-based skills, and basic science subjects like anatomy and physiology. The current pandemic has limited or in some cases prohibited the access to cadaveric dissection laboratories and on-campus live delivery, which is a deviation from the principal method of learning anatomy since the seventeenth Century (Iwanaga et al. 2020). Case study two provides examples as to how clinical anatomy learning and teaching can be modified for delivery using a MMD approach.

Clinical Anatomy Context: Anatomy is often considered to be one of the foundation studies in healthcare education, a solid grounding providing a platform for clinical examination, decision-making, and treatment methods later in a student's studies (and future practice). It is therefore imperative for students to grasp these concepts prior to graduating to ensure safe clinical practice (Estai and Bunt 2016; Losco et al. 2017; Chen et al. 2020). For over a decade, programs have reduced the proportion of time within health science and medical curricula for learning and teaching of clinical anatomy. This is partly due to the transition to more problem-based learning or case-based curricula, and a greater importance placed on self-directed learning (Asad and Nasir 2015; Losco et al. 2017) and rising operating costs associated with traditional dissection (Bergman et al. 2014). While academics are challenged with the significant reduction in anatomy contact hours over recent decades, the growth of multimedia and electronic resources has offered new possibilities for anatomy education, and a way to address the decreased face-to-face time (Asad and Nasir 2015; Barry et al. 2016; Losco et al. 2017).

Effective methods of learning and teaching anatomy include computer-assisted learning; computer-assisted instruction; 3D visualization technologies (including virtual reality and laparoscopic dissection models); simulation; and use of traditional dissection; prosection; models; and textbooks (Losco et al. 2017). Anatomists continually seek to develop innovative, engaging, and creative methods of delivering proactive learning, while stimulating long-term memory development (Iwanaga et al. 2020; Saverino 2021).

The challenge during the global COVID-19 pandemic has been how to utilize these effective methods of anatomy learning and teaching with students who are geographically located off-campus. Similarly, for those anatomists who were able to teach with students' on-campus, social distancing restrictions also limited the physical capacity in anatomy laboratories and associated teaching spaces. While social distancing requirements have previously impacted education during the Severe Acute Respiratory Syndrome-associated coronavirus (SARS-CoV) outbreak in 2003, the scale during the current COVID-19 pandemic is unprecedented (Parkin 2020).

Previous research investigating the ideal practices for anatomy education found that multiple pedagogical resources combined within a teaching session provided students with the best learning outcomes and importantly led to greater student engagement (Estai and Bunt 2016; Losco et al. 2017). Although its merits are widely debated, human body dissection remains a valuable method of education for the anatomical sciences (Asad and Nasir 2015; Losco et al. 2017). In addition to being useful to demonstrate anatomical relationships and spatial understanding of structures, it allows students to develop discipline-independent skills such as teamwork, leadership, and professionalism. There is also strong evidence that the act of learning with human prosections or cadavers provides students with valuable insights into human frailty and mortality: students can gain a greater appreciation of the value of human life (Leboulanger 2011). Including the use of prosection and cadavers for learning was therefore felt to be important, but not without its issues. One other important consideration is the relative costs associated with purchasing alternative methods of delivering anatomy content if these had not previously been adopted. Procurement of additional digital technologies, 3D visualization technologies, simulation models, and associated upskilling of academic staff during the economic constraints of the current pandemic, have also contributed to the redesign or hybrid approach to anatomy education.

Challenges Associated with the Use of Anatomical Material: Use of anatomical material is highly regulated and all educational institutions within Australia must abide by their respective State Government legislation, for example, Transplantation and Anatomy Act 1979 (Queensland Government 2019). Handling and use of the material must be undertaken in a respectful manner and, within Bond University, is governed by strict rules about photography and dissemination of any material involving cadaveric tissue (Queensland Government 2019). Although regarded as one of the cornerstones of medical education (Orsbon et al. 2014), cadaveric anatomy dissection is decreasing around the globe, oftentimes replaced with multi-modal and computer-based teaching modalities. Within many countries, such as Australia, the United Kingdom, Canada, and the United States of America, teaching time allocated to anatomy has decreased together with the time spent dissecting (Rockarts et al. 2020). In some countries, this reduction in cadaveric dissection is due to the financial cost and regulatory challenges of maintaining a dissection-based program, and in other locales it is due to factors such as educators' perceptions of the value of dissection and access to appropriately trained staff (Estai and Bunt 2016).

In our Faculty, permission was granted to allow the livestreaming of anatomy lesson content via the secure Blackboard Collaborate platform. This allowed livestreaming within a secure infrastructure, to which dedicated access was permitted to the respective student cohorts, academics, and teaching assistants.

Redesign of Clinical Anatomy Delivery

The presentation of clinical anatomy to a remote or multimodal cohort of students was approached in much the same way as planning a traditional on-campus, face-to-face anatomy laboratory session. Instructional design principles were used to ensure the appropriate selection and use of technology, matched with the best modality to achieve the anatomy-learning outcomes (Snell et al. 2018). While certain topics naturally lend themselves to PowerPoint presentations, such as histology or embryology, other areas require visual representation using live video or with 3D virtual reality (Fig. 6).

The delivery of the anatomy content was designed to be able to be delivered in two MMD approaches:

- Session delivered live on-campus to face-to-face learners and streamed live to remote learners (Fig. 1, Scenario 1)
- Session delivered live on-campus to and streamed live with all students engaging online via the Blackboard Collaborate, to students engaging online regardless of location, for example, on-campus in collaborative learning spaces or remote locations. Additional support from academic staff was required to facilitate active engagement of learners and real-time exchange of questions and answers (Fig. 1, Scenario 2)

Key Consideration for Remote or Multimodal Delivery

Several key factors were essential for the delivery of the remote and MMD of anatomical content, including appropriate selection of digital technologies, connectivity optimization, environmental considerations, provision of additional digital technology set up time, content volume and cognitive load, flipped practical, post-session considerations, and constructive alignment of learning activities and assessment.

Appropriate Selection of Digital Technologies to optimize Delivery: As the COVID-19 pandemic started to cause disruptions around the world, many educators shifted to using online video conferencing applications such as Zoom, Skype, or Microsoft Teams to run remote teaching sessions. As these tools gained prominence around the world, questions surrounding their security were raised. The media featured stories with high-profile examples of classes being disrupted by troublemakers or, in some more serious cases, racist or anti-semitic individuals. Care must therefore be taken in selecting which application to use and to ensure robust password protection. This is particularly important when dealing with human body donors as all care must be taken to be respectful, and only allow the relevant students to view and handle the material (Queensland Government 2019; Queensland Health 2019).

Connectivity Optimization: Live streaming of video with the inclusion of 3D anatomy, PowerPoint presentations, and narration is contingent on a seamless production without any audio or video dropouts. A strong internet bandwidth and

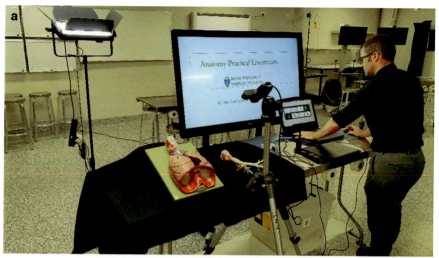

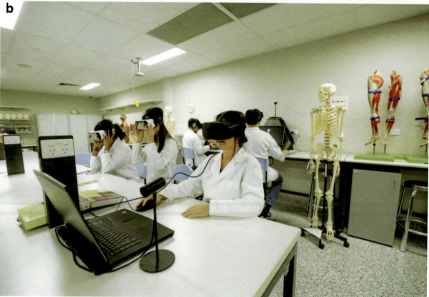

Fig. 6 (**a**) An educator preparing to deliver a virtual anatomy practical on the respiratory system. (**b**) Students learning anatomy using virtual reality. (Courtesy of Bond University, Australia. Consent was gained from the Doctor of Physiotherapy students featured in the photographs)

high-quality video feed are vital for those hosting the live stream. Careful consideration of vital technology is required, so not to pose as a distractor to learning. Additional technological operational demands have the potential to overcomplicate the delivery and detract from the key learning activities or outcomes.

Optimize the Live Stream Environment: While every educator preference and needs may be different, the optimal environmental set up requires careful consideration. Our suggestions were based on experience and also supported by a wealth of research associated with digital technologies and digital ethnography (for example, Pink et al. 2015). Pink and colleagues (2015) encourage the rethinking of pre-digital practices, media, and environments from a research perspective, which is directly transferable to the educational setting. In particular, filming/livestreaming from an isolated environment, free from interruptions, and high-quality internet connections are a bare minimum (Fig. 2).

Additional Digital Technology Set-up Time: A key factor that became evident in the initial delivery was just how crucial the setup phase was to produce a seamless experience for the students and to avoid additional stress for the educator. Careful selection of the most appropriate prosection and/or dissection specimens, and models need to take place in advance (ideally several days before the planned session). Pre-testing of digital equipment set up and live-stream practice was advocated for all teaching sessions as part of the 3P training model. Such testing of anatomical digital technologies, livestreaming connectivity, and optimization of audio-visual equipment was essential. This allowed for time to set the parameters and, on one occasion, swap out any malfunctioning equipment.

Content Volume and Cognitive Load: The utilization of multiple modes of anatomical representation meant that it was also important to consider the volume of content being disseminated. Being cognizant of how the students interact with the material, and the amount of information being shared is critical to allow the students to feel engaged without feeling overwhelmed. Therefore, as in case study one, considerations of cognitive load were essential to the success of the delivery (Van Merriënboer et al. 2006; Reedy 2015; Sewell et al. 2018; Sweller 2020).

Flipped Practical Approach: To maximize the time spent during the multimodal sessions, a "flipped practical" approach to the learning was utilized. The idea of the flipped classroom, or inverted classroom, has been studied at length with the major benefit generally accepted as being improved student-learning performance (Honeycutt 2016; Akcayir and Akcayir 2018). Akcayir and Akcayir's systematic review of the literature confirmed this general belief but cautioned its benefits for students with low self-regulation behaviors and poor time management skills (Akcayir and Akcayir 2018). Pre-recorded voice-over PowerPoint (VoPP's) lectures and videos relating to that week's content were generated to form the flipped element of the class. This proved vital in ensuring students attending the session were primed with the relevant baseline knowledge in advance and the live stream anatomy class was positioned to further strengthen their knowledge, clarify difficult topics, and apply their learning to the clinical anatomy context.

Each session was accompanied by a digital workbook that the students could annotate in and complete short, structured questions. To facilitate the question-and-answer dynamic that would take place in a normal F-2-F laboratory session, the synchronous chat function in Blackboard Collaborate was used. One major learning point that came from this interaction is that having a co-presenter in the teaching room to act as the chat facilitator was crucial to ensure the session was more efficient and engaging for the students.

Post-session Considerations: Equally important to the live sessions were the affordances put in place to ensure the students had a way of contacting the faculty staff following the teaching session. It is not unreasonable to expect that once the students have had time to consolidate their knowledge and reflect on the session, they will have follow-up questions. Ordinarily this could be remedied by having office visiting hours and laboratory drop-in sessions. With students accessing content remotely, digital drop-in sessions were timetabled and the email addresses of the lecturers were made known should the students have a question outside of regular hours.

Constructive Alignment of Learning and Assessment

Constructive alignment of learning outcomes, learning and teaching activities and assessment tasks was essential (Biggs 2003). This is particularly important in health education programs where graduates are required to meet the societal expectations of healthcare workers in their respective professions. It was essential to review the assessment requirements, especially when cohorts may not all be geographically located with access to the physical anatomy laboratory. Thus, it is essential when re-designing delivery modes to review the authenticity and alignment of assessment tasks/formats and ensure compliance with accreditation requirements (Ashford-Rowe et al. 2014; Villarroel et al. 2018). Some online exam platforms have the functionality to integrate the use of multiple assessment formats including video, 3D anatomy, and clickable "hotspot" type questions that can be delivered within formats that are accessible to students undertaking exams/assessments remotely. The potential impact of assessment changes on academic integrity was also crucial to ensure compliance with University and Tertiary Education Quality and Standards Agency requirements (TEQSA 2019). While remote proctoring of assessments and/or examination is growing, it raises digital security and transparency requirements. It is essential that students and academics are clearly aware of the nature, purpose, and intent of the use of artificial intelligence for remote proctoring.

Summary

The academic year in 2020 has brought with its unprecedented changes in the anatomy educational landscape. Adoption of the 3P training principles, "plan, prepare and practice" helped to minimize disruptions and develop action plans for the just-in-case moments. As academics navigate the evolving digital educational landscape, the goal remains to design and deliver high-quality educational experiences despite the physical disruption of the learning environment. Additionally, key principles remain to position the student at the heart of all learning, teaching, and assessment within the constraints of accreditation requirements. Despite the disruption to teaching, learning, and assessment, anatomists, and educators alike, will continue to discover novel new teaching strategies that will likely continue to be embedded beyond the current pandemic. The strategies posed in case study two have application beyond the discipline of anatomy. Evaluation of the effectiveness of the hybrid/blending of computer-assisted instruction/computer-assisted learning, simulation, models, and traditional prosection/dissection to remote and multimodal cohorts is now warranted.

Reimagining Medical and Health Professional Education beyond the COVID-19 Pandemic

In March, the 2020 EDUCAUSE Horizon report identified six emerging technologies and practices: *elevation of instructional design, adaptive learning technologies, open educational resources, artificial intelligence and machine learning, extended reality* referred to as XR (which includes augmented reality, virtual reality, mixed reality, or haptic technologies), and *analytics for student success* (Brown et al. 2020a, b). While this report profiles the key trends and emerging technologies, it was published at the onset of the COVID-19 pandemic affecting the majority of the world. The report acknowledged the challenges associated with anticipating the future, the five influential factors that purportedly would shape global higher education, teaching, and learning. Brown and colleagues (2020a, b) aptly describe these influential trends in *technology* (artificial intelligence, next-generational digital learning environments, analytics, and privacy questions), *higher education* (changes in student populations, alternative educational pathways, and online education), *politics* (decrease in higher education funding, value of higher education, and political polarization), *economics* (cost of education, future skills and work, and climate change), and *social* (wellbeing, mental health, demographical changes, equity, and fair practice). All of which are highly influential in the current pandemic circumstances.

Since the initial outbreak, research focusing on the impact of the COVID-19 pandemic has exponentially grown in relation to healthcare. Literature documenting the impact of the pandemic on education is emerging and will continue to shape the educational landscape for medical and allied health professional education for years to come (Goh and Sandars 2020; Gordon et al. 2020; Sandars and Goh 2020). Key messages arising from these early medical education systematic reviews and commentaries relate to the rapid deployment of remote synchronous and asynchronous educational strategies, are likely to remain beyond the pandemic (Bond 2020c; Goh and Sandars 2020; Gordon et al. 2020; Sandars and Goh 2020). Currently, there is limited published literature pertaining to faculty development related to the rapid transition to digital platforms to support healthcare education (Cleland et al. 2020; Finn et al. 2020; Keegan et al. 2020) and the impact on student health and wellbeing (Blake et al. 2020; Brown et al. 2020a, b). Additionally, the economic implications of learning during the disruption of the COVID-19 pandemic have yet to be reported from multiple stakeholder perspectives (students, education providers, placement providers, and accrediting bodies).

Conclusion

This chapter has presented an overview of the significant and rapid transition from F-2-F to remote learning, and multi-modal delivery in medical and allied health profession education. The global COVID-19 pandemic has required educational institutions and clinical placement providers to rapidly adopt and effectively utilize available or new technology to optimize learning and teaching despite geographical distance of the students from the classroom. This transition has initiated digital enhancements, infrastructure investment and upgrades, and rapid up skilling of academic and professional staff to allow programs to develop high-quality, fully inclusive, and accessible learning. The extent to which universities and programs will need to continue to deliver components of the coursework subjects and placements in remote/multimodal format is unknown, and will likely be highly variable and governed by outbreaks and respective government restrictions and guidance. As higher educational institutions emerge from the COVID-19 era, and transition from what is becoming known as "COVID-19-normal" to the "post-COVID-19" era, it is imperative that educational designers/academics examine and share the lessons learned in respect to their specific curriculum and circumstances and accreditation requirements.

Cross-References

▶ Practice Education in Occupational Therapy: Current Trends and Practices

Acknowledgments Daniel Maupin, Assistant Teaching Fellow, Bond University, for his contribution to the delivery of the Doctor of Physiotherapy subjects and photographs.

References

Afridi A, Fahim MF. Identification of stressors and Perceptional difference of stress in first and final year Doctor of Physical Therapy students; a comparative study. JPMA. 2019;69(4):572–5.

Akçayır G, Akçayır M. The flipped classroom: A review of its advantages and challenges. Comput Educ. 2018;126:334–45.

Anikina OV, Yakimenko EV. Edutainment as a modern technology of education. Proc Soc Behav Sci. 2015;166:475–9.

Asad MR, Nasir N. Role of living and surface anatomy in current trends of medical education. International Journal of Advance Research and Innovative Ideas in Education. 2015;1:203–210.

Ashford-Rowe K, Herrington J, Brown C. Establish the critical elements that determine authentic assessment. Assess Eval High Educ. 2014;39(2):205–22. https://doi.org/10.1080/02602938.2013.819566.

Australian Health Practitioner Regulation Agency (AHPRA). National principles for clinical education during COVID-19. 2020. Available from: https://www.ahpra.gov.au/News/COVID-19/National-principles-for-clinical-education-during-COVID-19.aspx. Accessed 18 Nov 2020.

Australian Medical Council (AMC). COVID-19. Accreditation requirements in 2020 in response to COVID-19. 2020. Available from: https://www.amc.org.au/covid-19/. Accessed 18 Nov 2020.

Barry DS, Marzouk F, Chulak-Oglu K, Bennett D, Tierney P, O'Keeffe GW. Anatomy education for the YouTube generation. Anat Sci Educ. 2016;9(1):90–6.

Beltran-Velasco AI, Ruisoto-Palomera P, Bellido-Esteban A, Garcia-Mateos M, Clemente-Suarez VJ. Analysis of psychophysiological stress response in higher education students undergoing clinical practice evaluation. J Med Syst. 2019;43(3):68. https://doi.org/10.1007/s10916-019-1187-7.

Bergman EM, Verheijen IWH, Scherpbier AJJA, Van der Vleuten CPM, Bruin ABH. Influences on anatomical knowledge: the complete arguments. Clin Anat. 2014;27:296–303.

Biggs JB. Teaching for quality learning at university. Open University Press, Buckingham. 2003.

Blake H, Bermingham F, Johnson G, Tabner A. Mitigating the psychological impact of COVID-19 on healthcare workers: a digital learning package. Int J Environ Res Public Health. 2020;17(9):2997.

Bond University. Doctor of physiotherapy program. 2020a. Available from: https://bond.edu.au/program/doctor/physiotherapy. Accessed 18 Nov 2020.

Bond University. Talk-sheet: multi-modal delivery pedagogy. Gold Coast: Bond University Office of Learning and Teaching; 2020b.

Bond University. eGuide: multi-modal teaching and learning. Gold Coast: Bond University Office of Learning and Teaching; 2020c.

Brooke T, Brown M, Orr R, Gough S. Stress and burnout: exploring postgraduate physiotherapy students' experiences and coping strategies. BMC Med Educ. 2020;20:433. https://doi.org/10.1186/s12909-020-02360-6.

Brown ME, Archer RL, Finn GM. A virtual postgraduate community of practice. Med Educ. 2020a. https://onlinelibrary.wiley.com/doi/full/10.1111/medu.14214

Brown M, McCormack M, Reeves J, Brook DC, et al. Educause horizon report teaching and learning edition. Louisville: EDUCAUSE; 2020b. Available at: https://library.educause.edu/resources/2020/3/2020-educause-horizon-report-teaching-and-learning-edition#materials. Accessed 18 Nov 2020.

Carolan C, Davies CL, Crookes P, McGhee S, Roxburgh M. COVID 19: disruptive impacts and transformative opportunities in undergraduate nurse education. Nurse Educ Pract. 2020;46:102807. https://doi.org/10.1016/j.nepr.2020.102807.

Chartered Society of Physiotherapy (CSP). COVID-19 guidance for higher education institutions (updated October 2020) London: Chartered Society of Physiotherapy. 2020a. Available from: https://www.csp.org.uk/system/files/documents/2020-10/COVID_19%20Guidance%20Oct%202020_0.pdf

Chartered Society of Physiotherapy (CSP). COVID-19 information for physiotherapy students (Updated 06 May 2020). London: Chartered Society of Physiotherapy. 2020b. Available from: https://www.csp.org.uk/system/files/documents/2020-10/COVID_19%20Guidance%20Oct%202020_0.pdf. Accessed 18 Nov 2020.

Chen S, Zhu J, Cheng C, Pan Z, Liu L, Du J, Shen X, et al. Can virtual reality improve traditional anatomy education programmes? A mixed-methods study on the use of a 3D skull model. BMC Med Educ. 2020;20(395). https://doi.org/10.1186/s12909-020-02255-6.

Clay J. JISC guide: digital learning in higher education. A primer created for university leaders as part of the learning and teaching reimagined initiative. Bristol: JISC; 2020. Available from: https://www.jisc.ac.uk/guides/digital-learning-in-higher-education. Accessed 18 Nov 2020.

Cleland J, McKimm J, Fuller R, Taylor D, Janczukowicz J, Gibbs T. Adapting to the impact of COVID-19: sharing stories, sharing practice. Med Teach. 2020;42(7):1–4. https://doi.org/10.1080/0142159X.2020.1757635.

Ellaway RHA. Conceptual framework of game-informed principles for health professions education. Adv Simul. 2016;1(28):1–9. https://doi.org/10.1186/s41077-016-0030-1.

Estai M, Bunt S. Best teaching practices in anatomy education: a critical review. Ann Anat Anatomischer Anzeiger. 2016;208:151–7.

Finn GM, Brown MEL, Laughey W, Due~nas A. #pandemicpedagogy: using twitter for knowledge exchange. Med Educ. 2020. https://onlinelibrary.wiley.com/doi/full/10.1111/medu.14242

Frank LM, Cassady SL. Health and wellness in entry-level physical therapy students: are measures of stress, anxiety, and academic performance related? Cardiopulmon Phys Therapy J. 2005;16(4):5–13.

General Medical Council (GMC). Information for medical students. 2020. Available from: https://www.gmc-uk.org/news/news-archive/coronavirus-information-and-advice/information-for-medical-students. Accessed 18 Nov 2020.

Goh PS, Sandars J. A vision of the use of technology in medical education after the COVID-19 pandemic. MedEdPublish. 2020;9:1–8.

Gordon M, Patricio M, Horne L, Muston A, Alston SR, Pammi M, Thammasitboon S, Park S, Pawlikowska T, Rees EL, Doyle AJ, Daniel M. Developments in medical education in response to the COVID-19 pandemic: A rapid BEME systematic review: BEME guide no. 63. Med Teach. 2020;42(11):1202–15. https://doi.org/10.1080/0142159X.2020.1807484.

Gough S, Yohannes AM, Murray J. Using video-reflexive ethnography and simulation-based education to explore patient management and error recognition by pre-registration physiotherapists. Adv Simul. 2016;1(9):1–17. https://doi.org/10.1186/s41077-016-0010-5.

Gunn H, Hunter H, Haas B. Problem based learning in physiotherapy education: a practice perspective. Physiotherapy. 2012;98(4):330–5.

Halupa CM. Chapter 5: Pedagogy, andragogy, and heutagogy. In: Halupa CM, editor. Transformative curriculum design in health sciences education. 2015. pp. 143–58. https://doi.org/10.4018/978-1-4666-8571-0.ch005.

Harvard Medical School Division of Sleep Medicine (HMSDSM). Healthy sleep: external factors that influence sleep. 2007. Available from: http://healthysleep.med.harvard.edu/healthy/science/how/external-factors. Accessed 30 Nov 2020.

Health Care and Professions Council (HCPC). Joint statement on how we will support and enable the student allied health professional workforce to respond to the COVID-19. 06 April 2020. Available from: https://www.hcpc-uk.org/news-and-events/news/2020/joint-statement-on-how-we-will-support-and-enable-the-student-allied-health-professional-workforce-to-respond-to-the-covid-19/. Accessed 18 Nov 2020.

Higgs J. Developing clinical reasoning capabilities. In: Nestel D, Reedy G, McKenna L, Gough S, editors. Clinical education for the health professions. Singapore: Springer; 2020. https://doi.org/10.1007/978-981-13-6106-7.

Honeycutt B. FLIP it! Whitepaper: 10 strategies to encourage students to actually DO the pre-class work in flipped & active learning classrooms. North Carolina: FLIP IT Consulting LLC; 2016.

Iacobucci G. Covid-19: all non-urgent elective surgery is suspended for at least three months in England. BMJ. 2020;368:m1106. https://doi.org/10.1136/bmj.m1106.

Iwanaga J, Loukas M, Dumont M, Tubbs RS. A review of anatomy education during and after the COVID-19 pandemic: revisiting traditional and modern methods to achieve future innovation. Clin Anat. 2020; 1–7. https://doi.org/10.1002/ca.23655.

Kapila V, Corthals S, Langhendries L, Kapila AK, Everaert K. The importance of medical student perspectives on the impact of COVID-19. BJS. 2020;107:e372–3. https://doi.org/10.1002/bjs.11808.

Keegan DA, Chan M, Chan T. Helping medical educators worldwide pivot their curricula online: PivotMedEd.com. Med Educ. 2020;54(8):766–7. https://doi.org/10.1111/medu.14220.

Leboulanger N. First cadaver dissection: stress, preparation, and emotional experience. Eur Ann Otorhinolaryngol Head Neck Dis. 2011;128(4):175–83.

Lin S, Huang Y. Investigating the relationships between loneliness and learning burnout. Act Learn High Educ. 2012;13(3):231–43. https://doi.org/10.1177/1469787412452983.

Losco CD, Grant WD, Armson A, Meyer AJ, Walker BF. Effective methods of teaching and learning in anatomy as a basic science: A BEME systematic review: BEME guide no. 44. Med Teach. 2017;39(3):234–43. https://doi.org/10.1080/0142159X.2016.1271944.

Lynch C. Nearly half of physicians expect to be working under capacity for at least a year, RCP survey finds. BMJ. 2020;369:m2634. https://doi.org/10.1136/bmj.m2634.

MacDougall C, Dangerfield P, Katz D, Strain W. The impact of COVID-19 on medical education and medical students. How and when can they return to placements? MedEdPublish. 2020;9(1):159. https://doi.org/10.15694/mep.2020.000159.1.

Maguirem D, Dales L, Pauli M. Learning and teaching reimagined. A new dawn for higher education? Bristol: JISC; 2020. Available from: https://repository.jisc.ac.uk/8150/1/learning-and-teaching-reimagined-a-new-dawn-for-higher-education.pdf. Accessed 18 Nov 2020.

Maples MF. Group development: extending Tuckman's theory. J Special Group Work. 1988;13(1):17–23.

Miller GA. The magical number seven plus or minus two. Psychol Rev. 1956;63:81–97.

Mueller P, Oppenheimer D. The pen is mightier than the keyboard: advantages of taking longhand notes over laptop note taking. Assoc Psychol Sci. 2014;25(6):1159–68. https://doi.org/10.1177/0956797614524581.

National Institute of General Medical Sciences. Circadian rhythms. 4 March 2020. Available from: https://www.nigms.nih.gov/education/fact-sheets/Pages/circadian-rhythms.aspx. Accessed 30 Nov 2020.

Orsbon CP, Kaiser RS, Ross CF. Physician opinions about an anatomy core curriculum: A case for medical imaging and vertical integration. Anat Sci Educ. 2014;7(4):251–61. https://doi.org/10.1002/ase.1401.

Parkin D. Advance HE: socially distanced on campus education: the next big question. York: Advance HE; 2020. Available from: https://www.advance-he.ac.uk/news-and-views/socially-distanced-campus-education-next-big-question. Accessed 18 Nov 2020.

Pink S, Leder-Mackley K, Hackett PMW. Visual and sensory ethnography. In: Hackett, P. (Ed.). Qualitative research methods in consumer psychology: ethnography and culture (1st ed.). Psychology Press, 2015. https://doi.org/10.4324/9781315776378.

Queensland Government. Transplantation and Anatomy Act 1979. 1 September 2021. 2019. Available from https://www.legislation.qld.gov.au/view/html/inforce/current/act-1979-074. Accessed 23 Nov 2020.

Queensland Health. School of anatomy compliance process audit checklist and evaluation tool 4.1. July 2019. Available from https://www.health.qld.gov.au/__data/assets/pdf_file/0032/692276/school-audit-eval-tool-form.pdf. Accessed 23 Nov 2020.

Reedy G. Using cognitive load theory to inform simulation design and practice. Adv Simul. 2015;11(8):355–60.

Rockarts J, Brewer-Deluce D, Shali A, Mohialdin V, Wainman B. National survey on Canadian undergraduate medical programs: the decline of the anatomical sciences in Canadian medical education. Anat Sci Educ. 2020;13(3):381–9.

Rodríguez-Morilla B, Madrid JA, Molina E, Pérez-Navarro J, Correa Á. Blue-enriched light enhances alertness but impairs accurate performance in evening chronotypes driving in the morning. Front Psychol. 2018;9:688. https://doi.org/10.3389/fpsyg.2018.00688.

Royal College of Physicians. COVID-19 and its impact on NHS workforce. London: Royal College of Physicians; 2020a. Available from: https://www.rcplondon.ac.uk/news/covid-19-and-its-impact-nhs-workforce. Accessed 18 Nov 2020.

Royal College of Physicians. C tracking the impact of COVID-19 on the workforce. London: Royal College of Physicians; 2020b. Available from: https://www.rcplondon.ac.uk/news/tracking-impact-covid-19-workforce. Accessed 18 Nov 2020.

Sandars J, Goh P-S. Design thinking in medical education: the key features and practical application. Journal of Medical Education and Curricular Development. 2020. https://doi.org/10.1177/2382120520926518.

Saverino D. Teaching anatomy at the time of COVID-19. Clinical anatomy (New York, N.Y.), 2021;34(8):1128. https://doi.org/10.1002/ca.23616.

Seibert S. Problem-based learning: a strategy to foster generation Z's critical thinking and perseverance. Teach Learn Nurs. 2020. https://doi.org/10.1016/j.teln.2020.09.002.

Selye H. The physiology and pathology of exposure to stress: a treatise based on the concepts of the general-adaptation-syndrome and the diseases of adaptation. Montreal: Acta; 1950.

Sewell JL, Maggio L, ten Cate O, van Gog T, Young JQ, O'Sullivan PS. Cognitive load theory for training health professionals in the workplace: a BEME review of studies among diverse professions: BEME guide no. 53. Med Teach. 2018;41(3):256–70. https://doi.org/10.1080/0142159X.2018.1505034.

Sleegers PJC, Moolenaar NM, Galetzka M. Lighting affects students' concentration positively: findings from three Dutch studies. Light Res Technol. 2012;45(2):159–75. https://doi.org/10.1177/1477153512446099.

Snell L, Son D, Onishi. Instructional design: applying theory to teaching practice. In: Swanwick T, Forrest T, O'Brien BC, editors. Understanding medical education: evidence, theory and practice. 3rd ed. Wiley; 2018. https://doi.org/10.1002/9781119373780.ch6.

Sweller J. Cognitive load theory and educational technology. Educ Technol Res Dev. 2020;68(1):1–16.

Tertiary Education Quality and Standards Agency (TEQSA). Australian government tertiary education quality and standards agency. Guidance note: academic integrity. 28 March 2019. Available from: https://www.teqsa.gov.au/sites/default/files/guidance-note-academic-integrity-v1-2-web.pdf?v=1581307285. Accessed 23 Nov 2020.

Thackray D, Roberts L. Exploring the clinical decision-making used by experienced cardiorespiratory physiotherapists: a mixed method qualitative design of simulation, video recording and think aloud techniques. Nurse Educ Today. 2016;49:96–105. https://doi.org/10.1016/j.nedt.2016.11.003.

Torda AJ, Velan G, Perovic V. The impact of the COVID-19 pandemic on medical education. MJA. 2020;23(4):1187–8.e1.

United Nations Educational, Scientific and Cultural Organization (UNESCO). COVID-19 educational disruption and response. Paris: UNESCO; 2020. Available from: https://en.unesco.org/covid19/educationresponse. Accessed 23 Nov 2020.

Van Merriënboer JJG, Kester L, Paas F. Teaching complex rather than simple tasks: balancing intrinsic and germane load to enhance transfer of learning. J Appl Cogn Psychol. 2006;20(3):343–52.

Villarroel V, Bloxham S, Bruna D, Bruna C, Herrera-Seda C. Authentic assessment: creating a blueprint for course design. Assess Eval High Educ. 2018;43(5):840–54. https://doi.org/10.1080/02602938.2017.1412396.

Vygotsky LS. Mind in society: the development of higher psychological processes. Harvard: Harvard University Press; 1978.

White C. Student placements. What makes a great placement? Frontline, Issue 9. 2020. Available from: https://www.csp.org.uk/frontline/article/student-placements. Accessed 18 Nov 2020.

Wilski M, Chmielewski B, Tomczak M. Work locus of control and burnout in polish physiotherapists: the mediating effect of coping styles. Int J Occup Med Environ Health. 2015;28(5):875–89.

World Physiotherapy. World physiotherapy response to COVID-19 briefing paper 1: immediate impact on the higher education sector and response to delivering physiotherapist entry level education. London: World Physiotherapy; 2020a. Available from: https://world.physio/sites/default/files/2020-07/Education-Briefing-paper-1-HEI.pdf. Accessed 18 Nov 2020.

World Physiotherapy. World physiotherapy response to COVID-19, briefing paper 3: immediate impact on students and the response to delivering physiotherapy entry level education. London: World Physiotherapy; 2020b. Available from: https://world.physio/sites/default/files/2020-07/Education-Briefing-paper-3-Students-24-June-2020.pdf. Accessed 18 Nov 2020.

World Physiotherapy. World physiotherapy response to COVID-19, briefing paper 4: the impact on entry level education and the reponses of regulators. 2020c. Available from: https://world.physio/sites/default/files/2020-08/Education_Briefing_4_Regulation.pdf. Accessed 18 Nov 2020.

Yerkes RM, Dodson JD. The relation of strength of stimulus to rapidity of habit-formation. J Comp Neurol Psychol. 1908;18:459–82.

Zhou Z. An empirical study on the influence of PBL teaching model on college students' critical thinking ability. Engl Lang Teach. 2018;11(4):15–20. https://doi.org/10.5539/elt.v11n4p15.

Part II

Philosophical and Theoretical Underpinning of Health Professions Education

Cognitive Neuroscience Foundations of Surgical and Procedural Expertise: Focus on Theory

18

Pamela Andreatta

Contents

Introduction	336
Expertise and Experts	336
Neural Implementation of Expertise	338
Cognitive Mechanisms of Expertise	339
Cognitive Expertise	339
Perceptual Expertise	340
Psychomotor Expertise	341
Other Factors Associated with Expertise	343
Synthesis/Summary	344
References	345

Abstract

This chapter describes the cognitive processes and associated neuroscientific manifestations of expertise in surgery and other specialties where procedural acumen encompasses a component of expertise, and considers the processes by which health professions' educators may leverage this knowledge to support the development of expertise in procedural domains. Three primary dimensions of procedural performance are considered, including perceptual expertise (the ability to accurately recognize and differentiate patterns from perceptual inputs), cognitive expertise (the ability to accurately interpret, differentiate, and render decisions in complex environments), and psychomotor expertise (the ability to anticipate and execute accurate motor responses). The foundational elements of expertise are embedded in long-term memory, and the development of expertise requires significant investment by individuals to rigorously engage in the content

---

P. Andreatta (✉)
The Norman M. Rich Department of Surgery, Uniformed Services University & the Walter Reed National Military Medical Center "America's Medical School", Bethesda, MD, USA
e-mail: pamela.andreatta1@gmail.com

© Springer Nature Singapore Pte Ltd. 2023
D. Nestel et al. (eds.), *Clinical Education for the Health Professions*,
https://doi.org/10.1007/978-981-15-3344-0_22

domain for significant periods of time. Once acquired, expertise appears to be effortless; however, neuroscience confirms that experts' brains are highly stimulated; they are simply stimulated in different areas than novices, because they have developed different strategies for working within their expertise domain. Importantly, expertise in one domain does not transfer to another domain, primarily because of the very neuroscientific mechanisms by which expertise is developed. If domain patterns alter (e.g., open surgical procedures become laparoscopic procedures), expertise may need to be reacquired to accommodate the changes in the performance domain.

Keywords

Cognitive processing surgical expertise · Cognitive neuroscience surgical expertise · Acquisition of surgical expertise · Developing surgical expertise · Expert surgeons · Surgical performance acquisition · Maintenance of surgical expertise · Procedural expertise · Developing procedural expertise · Cognitive neuroscience procedural expertise · Cognitive processing procedural expertise · Procedural performance acquisition · Procedural mastery · Surgical mastery

Introduction

The aim of all procedurally based health professions education programs is to facilitate the development of all participating learners to acquire and master professional expertise in those requisite procedures. The cognitive processes involved in developing expertise have been studied for decades, with a rich literature describing both theoretical and empirical foundations for understanding the overarching construct of expertise, as well as its constituent components. In this chapter, I will explore those processes and how they manifest through neural implementation in the brain by examining the differences between novice and expert practitioners in the primary performance dimensions of surgical and procedural care: cognitive, perceptual, and psychomotor. I will begin with an overview of expertise and performance domains, then describe the processes of examining neural implementation before discussing the processes associated with cognitive, perceptual, and psychomotor expertise. I will then consider the transfer of expertise between performance domains and the effects of diminished practice and aging on expert performance over time.

Expertise and Experts

Expertise describes a constellation of abilities (knowledge, skills, etc.) within a specific performance domain that are acquired through active engagement in a relatively stable environment. Expertise domains are extremely complex and achieving domain mastery can take years of dedicated practice (Shanteau 1992). The stability of the environment is essential for the dedicated practice required to develop expertise because it enables performance acquisition through consistent regularity. Expertise domains have performance markers that enable practitioners to consciously or unconsciously understand the consistencies and predictabilities within the environment, which will facilitate their performance when managing new and novel situations. Although changes may occur in the expertise domain, they typically do not radically change the environment to the extent that previously acquired abilities become irrelevant. For example, the expertise domain of cardiothoracic surgery is a stable environment, where if changes happen (new equipment, surgical device, scheduling system, etc.), it does not destabilize previously acquired abilities in the domain. The foundational elements of the expertise domain of cardiothoracic surgery (anatomical, physiological, pathological, procedural, etc.) remain largely intact. However, the introduction of a significant disruptor to an expertise domain's stability may shift the acumen of individuals who mastered performance in the domain prior to the disruption. For example, endovascular technologies and procedures were a significant disruptor to the domain of cardiothoracic surgery because the stability of the operative environment changed to the extent that prior knowledge was only partially useful in the performance space and a constellation of new abilities were required to develop mastery.

In the context of this chapter, an expert is an individual who performs in a way that is consistently excellent, exceptional, or extraordinary (Ericsson 2008). Consistent and reliable performance excellence is made possible because experts develop the ability to perceive and analyze the features of the performance environment differently from novices. Experts have developed deep knowledge structures within a domain that allow them to employ completely different strategies than novices, who lack that necessary knowledge. Where novices may inefficiently implement rudimentary strategies with inconsistent quality, expert performance is accurate and efficient, with the execution of the discrete components seemingly automatic.

Expert performance is not dependent on external circumstances, rather it is the consequence of extensive exposure to a domain in which stability produces regularities that experts encode into memory. Therefore, the key contributor to expert performance in any domain is long-term memory (LTM). LTM stores acquired domain-specific knowledge, which enables highly efficient interaction between the cognitive processes of attention and perception that results in outstanding performance (Bilalić 2017). Experts' deep knowledge in LTM enables them to reduce the complexity of any domain situation by using pattern recognition and selective attention to focus on its salient aspects. The content of experts' memory guides attention to the most relevant information, whether it is perceptual or kinetic, to produce outstanding performances. Cognitive expertise primarily engages memory and mental processes that are initiated by environmental stimuli. Perceptual expertise relies on information captured through our visual, auditory tactile, and olfactory senses. Psychomotor expertise pertains to domains where physical responses represent the principle performance markers.

Ideally, the aim of health professions education is to create expert practitioners in all surgical and procedural expertise domains. To optimally accomplish this goal, we need to understand how experts achieve extraordinary outcomes in their respective domains. Despite content differences, all expertise domains rely on similar, if not identical, cognitive mechanisms. Therefore, we will examine the literature from complementary expertise domains related to the primary performance dimensions of surgical and procedural practice (cognitive, perceptual, psychomotor) and consider how they describe the processes by which surgical and procedural expertise are developed.

Neural Implementation of Expertise

To understand the development of expertise from a neuroscientific perspective, we need to examine how the brain works to facilitate the cognitive mechanisms of ability acquisition. Neuroscientists employ functional neuroimaging techniques to measure brain activity that provides insight into the brain's functioning. Functional magnetic resonance imaging (fMRI) provides an indirect measure of brain activation by capturing how much blood was present in particular areas of the brain at a certain point in time. However, the precision of fMRI techniques is marginally hindered by the temporal lag between brain activation and the moment blood reaches the engaged areas. Electroencephalography (EEG) captures electrical currents around the scalp with more temporal precision but does not provide for localization accuracy. Magnetoencephalography (MEG) measures magnetic fields produced by electrical currents in the brain and captures activation with more temporal and localization precision. Voxel-based morphometry (VBM) is a structural neuroimaging technique that measures the anatomical properties of the brain by converting its volume into voxels, small three-dimensional structures. The morphological characteristics of the brain can then be compared between groups, including the connections within the brain where neurons (gray matter) connect to each other through white matter. This connectivity can be captured using diffusion tensor imaging (DTI).

The brain's ability to adapt to any environment (neuroplasticity) can be captured through these neuroimaging techniques, and evidence confirms functional reorganization allows the brain to accommodate different cognitive mechanisms in the development of expertise (Sadato 2005). For example, at the onset of expertise development that requires visual discrimination, both the frontal areas, which are responsible for manipulation of information in memory, and the parietal lobe, which is important for multisensory integration and spatial cognition, may be activated (Schneider and Chein 2003). As expertise develops, less attentional resources will be required to perform, because practice acquired proficiency will lead to a considerably reduced activation pattern. Over time, experts' performance becomes almost automatic, because the brain adapts to the constraints of the environment and they enact qualitatively different strategies that require fewer neural resources to perform (Bilalić et al. 2010, 2011, 2012) Through the development of expertise, experts' brains accommodate the processes of perceiving, retrieving stored information from LTM to match patterns, and focusing attention where it is most relevant. When compared with the brains of novices performing the same work, the brains of experts demonstrate a phenomenon of functional expansion, which describes how experts have more activation in the same brain area as novices, and may also engage different brain areas. This brain expansion aligns with the cognitive mechanism behind experts' performance, wherein the brain accommodates all the knowledge-related processes that underlie their expertise.

Observed functional expansion in perceptual and cognitive domains associated with visual discrimination expertise will occur in the temporal lobe, which carries visual information about discrete and interconnected elements in an environment (Guida et al. 2012, 2013; Mishkin et al. 1983). The fusiform gyrus (FG) and the parahippocampal gyrus (PHG) within the temporal lobe, which are important for memory and perception, also differentiates experts from novices in visual discrimination abilities (Kanwisher et al. 1997; Schwarzlose 2005; Epstein and Kanwisher 1998; McCandliss et al. 2003). In other words, the brain reacts by expanding its activation and engaging additional brain areas in the temporal lobe to make domain-specific knowledge available and facilitate the more efficient strategies of experts. During the development of expertise, the brain rearranges activation patterns from the frontal areas that are responsible for general processes to temporal ones that store domain-specific knowledge, and the neural implementation reflects a shift from general strategies used by novices to knowledge-based strategies enacted by experts. Functional reduction may also be observed in the improvement of task execution that requires no change in strategy, which is more typical of the skill acquisition approach in psychomotor expertise. The brain's implementation of expertise closely follows the cognitive strategies that are responsible for experts' outstanding performance, with the differences between novice and expert strategies reflected in the different neural signatures.

Cognitive Mechanisms of Expertise

Cognitive Expertise

As discussed previously, all expertise domains feature systems and attributes that are stable, and situations that routinely arise in one form or another. Experts acquire knowledge about these domain consistencies through years of exposure and practice, and this knowledge is stored in LTM (Chase and Simon 1973; Gobet et al. 2001; Gobet and Simon 1996). Experts do not perform better than novices because they can examine all the aspects of situation more quickly. Rather, experts discriminate incoming sensory information by matching it to the contents of LTM through a process called pattern recognition. The ability to rapidly discriminate information allows experts to automatically focus their attention on the important aspects of the environment, reduce complexities by disregarding less informative elements, and thereby adeptly employ qualitatively different strategies from those used by novice, with fewer cognitive resources. Pattern recognition also enables experts to interpret situations inferentially, including other situational aspects that may or may not be obvious to nonexperts. For example, experts in interpreting radiological images are able to successfully identify lesions in a fifth of second because they are automatically able to access a rich knowledge base of visual patterns, which enables them to quickly decipher any problem, immediately focus on the salient details, and ignore irrelevant ones (Kundel and Nodine 1975). Experts have a perceptual advantage because they process the environment differently.

Overtime, experts develop elaborate knowledge structures in LTM. The best experts have such sophisticated knowledge structures that they can grasp the essence of a complex situation within seconds. For example, expert surgeons and proceduralists will be able to grasp the essence of structures and pathological variations much more accurately and efficiently than their weaker colleagues. They will be able to focus their analytic search efforts immediately towards promising solutions, while weaker performers may investigate irrelevant paths that delay or obfuscate an optimal approach. As expertise develops and performance difficulty increases, the brain recruits additional resources from the opposite hemisphere through a process referred to as the double take of expertise (Guida et al. 2013; Bilalić et al. 2011). Neural expansion and double take of expertise enable the more sophisticated and complex strategies implemented by experts.

If an expert encounters a novel situation in their domain, they will automatically activate the domain-specific knowledge stored in LTM to compare the new situation with previously encountered situations (Richman et al. 1995; Feigenbaum and Simon 1984). Acquired knowledge structures in LTM enable experts to orient themselves quickly in a new situation as long as the foundational environment remains stable and automatically facilitates optimal methods for dealing with the new situation. For example, an unexpected bowel perforation during abdominal surgery creates an unpredictable situation that is easily corrected by an expert colorectal surgeon, but likely unnerving for a novice. On the other hand, experts will typically have a preconceived idea about how to manage almost any situation relating to their expertise domain, which may make them somewhat inflexible and dismissive of new alternatives. An example of this phenomenon, called satisfaction of search, is when surgical environments rapidly uptake substantial technological advancements that may eclipse the abilities of experts to accommodate the new knowledge in LTM with comparable speed. An illustration of this is the introduction of robotic surgical platforms, which required many hours of ancillary training before expert surgeons in traditional or laparoscopic techniques were sufficiently adept at its implementation in surgical procedures. Some traditionalists dismissed the value of robotic surgery, while others reorganized their knowledge structures to accommodate robotic techniques as an expansion of practice in their expertise domain.

Perceptual Expertise

The processes of human perception are both active and constructive. That is, the brain processes information from different sensory modalities and interprets it based on our previous experiences, developed knowledge structures, and associated expectations. The brain devotes numerous cortical areas to processing sensory information from the environment; however, because we interpret the information based on these individual internal factors, the image we create in our brain is not an exact replica of the stimuli in the environment. Therefore, perceptual expertise is a direct result of abilities honed through experience and practice in an environment. For example, the more experience a surgeon has in interpreting radiological images, the more efficient and accurate their perceptions of radiological images will be.

Expert interpretation of radiological images illustrates how previously discussed cognitive mechanisms come together in a circular fashion to enable outstanding perceptual performance. Perception from sensory input activates experience from memory that is then used to focus attention, which again influences perception. This circularity between new sensory input and memory activation describes holistic processing. Holistic processing enables experts to grasp the relationships between individual parts of a visual stimulus immediately, as a whole. Novices will not process the necessary domain knowledge to holistically process the visual input and consequently need to inspect the parts of the stimulus separately.

Holistic processing activates a part of the fusiform gyrus (FG) at the inferior side of the brain's temporal lobe, called the fusiform face area (FFA), because it is particularly responsive to faces (Kanwisher et al. 1997). Although the FFA has an important role in holistic processing of all visual stimuli, the temporal areas, the limbic system (hippocampus), and the frontal areas of the brain also contribute to other stimuli-driven and attentional processes involved experts interpreting and acting upon perceived input. For example, an expert radiologist will use holistic processing to perceive a radiological image, but that perception must then be integrated with other information from memory to determine a diagnosis. For many specialties, in addition to visual perception, interpretation of tactile sensory input is an important component of expertise, as is auditory input. Perceptual inputs from palpation (tactile) are used across the health professions for identifying optimal vessels for cannulation. Physiotherapists use palpation for patient assessment, neural mobilization, and other therapeutic neuromuscular treatments. Nurses will holistically consider perceptual cues from multiple modalities (visual, tactile, auditory, olfactory) to assess patient status. The mapping between cognitive mechanisms and their neural implementation that enable visual perceptual expertise is the same for the other sensory modalities (auditory, tactile, olfactory).

Psychomotor Expertise

A large component of all surgical and procedural expertise is associated with the ability of clinicians to adeptly and appropriately use their hands, and in some situations, other parts of their bodies, to complete operative procedures. Tactile perceptual expertise is a part of this performance construct, but the predominant contributor is psychomotor control. Psychomotor expertise is comprised of domain-specific knowledge acquired through practice and exposure in the performance environment. Deliberate practice that consists of focused activities in a single performance aspect and includes corrective feedback is instrumental in the development of psychomotor expertise. These skill development activities may take place in any environment that facilitates the foundations of deliberate practice, including simulated contexts that represent the expertise domain.

During training, surgeons and proceduralists acquire psychomotor abilities through focused and timely practice, to which their bodies adapt despite any initial anatomical and physiological differences. A common topic in surgical education is the contribution of innate biological factors relative to external environmental factors in the development of surgical proficiency. Through training, those innate and environmental factors intertwine in such a complex manner that it is difficult to speak of their isolated influence on development of proficiency. In the end, surgical and procedural expertise is the result of both factors, with focused practice having the greatest impact on performance abilities. For example, after only 1 week of performing a short practice exercise moving the fingers of one hand in a predictable pattern, the functional properties of the brain areas responsible for voluntary control of movements changed (Pascaual-Leone et al. 1995). Like surgeons, musicians also use the fingers of both dominant and nondominant hands to perform, and studies of musicians reveal structural differences between right-hand dominant musicians and nonmusicians in the right motor cortex, which is responsible for voluntary movement of the left side of the body (Amunts et al. 1997). The structural representation of the left hand was underdeveloped when compared to musicians who routinely use their left hand to perform. Colloquially referred to as "muscle memory," it is actually brain motor memory that commands all voluntary actions involved with psychomotor performance. The cortical areas (primary and secondary motor areas) and the parietal areas are important for the execution of movements. The subcortical areas (basal ganglia and cerebellum) are also involved in psychomotor expertise, particularly with regard to its acquisition. The brain reorganizes its structural and functional properties to accommodate the environmental demand made by psychomotor performance. Cortical representations of the body parts involved in psychomotor expertise become more pronounced and their structural properties change through the development of new connections between functional areas.

The kinematic information that comprises motor knowledge is stored in the brain as a series of individual complex movements that enable execution of domain-specific actions. This kinematic information is packed together as a motor program, where a number of isolated elements have been grouped together as a unit, or chunk. The term motor program is a cognitive construct but mirror neurons give it a neural basis. Mirror neurons are found in the prefrontal areas (the inferior frontal gyrus), premotor areas, and parietal areas (the inferior and superior parietal lobe together with the dividing intraparietal sulcus), but also in the temporal lobe (posterior middle temporal gyrus) and cerebellum. They are collectively called the action observation network (AON) because their motoric and perceptual properties work together to send information about what needs to be enacted to the primary motor areas, which then engage the muscles of the limbs via the spine. Mirror neurons fire when people execute movements and are therefore extremely important for voluntary control of movements, the essence of any psychomotor expertise. Experts activate the AON to a much larger extent than novices because they have developed substantial motor knowledge, which becomes activated even when experts anticipate the need for psychomotor implementation. This surprising property of the AON's mirror neurons has been linked with prediction performance in motor expertise and provides information about how the uses of simulation in the development and maintenance of surgical and procedural expertise leverages the anticipation and prediction opportunities afforded by the AON to enable outstanding psychomotor performance (Rizzolatti and Craighero 2004). One of the hallmarks of experts' exceptional performance is the use of qualitatively different strategies based on domain-specific knowledge, and this is also evident in neural implementation of psychomotor expertise.

Other Factors Associated with Expertise

There are two factors associated with surgical and procedural expertise that are frequently discussed, because they are integral to professionalism, quality, and safety in the context of patient care. The first is the transfer of acquired abilities between expertise domains. For example, surgeons with acquired expertise performing operative procedures using traditional open techniques will not necessarily demonstrate equivalent expertise performing laparoscopic procedures, and gastroenterologists with expertise in gastrointestinal endoscopic procedures will not demonstrate equivalent expertise performing urological endoscopic procedures. The second is the decline of acquired surgical and procedural abilities with age or lack of practice.

It is extremely rare for experts in one domain to be able to transfer their mastered abilities to another expertise domain, no matter how similar the domain is. Two domains will have different environmental constraints and produce different situations, which constitute the core of the knowledge stored in expert memory. The knowledge may be of different kinds, perceptual or kinetic, which then influences the way the brain implements the knowledge-based processes typical of experts. For example, open surgical procedures require different techniques, instruments, equipment, and visual and tactile perceptions than robot-assisted minimally invasive surgical procedures, despite common dimensions (i.e., anatomy, procedural aims, etc.) associated an intended surgery. The abilities of expert pathologists to rapidly differentiate microscopic cell patterns does not facilitate equivalent expertise in differentiating the details of a radiological image, because despite the common neuroscientific mechanisms of perceptual differentiation, the content domains of pathology and radiology are sufficiently distinct to render acquired pattern recognition processes ineffectual between the two domains. Expertise in airway management of adult critical care patients may not transfer to pediatric infant critical care patients because the anatomical and physiological domain knowledge is distinct in many dimensions. The palpation expertise of physiotherapists to perform neuro-mobilization techniques would not readily transfer to determining an optimal vein for cannulation, despite their commonality in requiring holistic processing of multiple modalities to perform well.

Paradoxically, it is this underlying mechanism common to all types of expertise that renders transfer remarkably difficult. As previously discussed, all experts, without exception, leverage their LTM to circumvent inherent cognitive and neural limitations. The deep knowledge structures in LTM enable experts to efficiently reduce the information load that the expertise environment places on the cognitive and neural system. Accomplished practitioners in one expertise domain may be able to develop proficiency in another expertise domain, but those abilities will be the outcome of further development in the second domain, not the transfer of acquired abilities from the first expertise domain.

The decline of acquired abilities through diminished use or with age is also an important consideration for surgeons and proceduralists because of the clear implications for patient care quality and safety. Research on expertise provides insight into how domain-specific knowledge influences the aging process, where practice and the accumulation of knowledge may lessen the effects of general, age-related decline. Physical prowess and reaction times decline with aging in the general population, as do cognitive abilities such as learning in general, reasoning, and spatial ability (Mireles and Charness 2002; Salthouse 2009). These changes are often attributed to the general deterioration of the brain structure that occurs as part of the aging process, particularly in the prefrontal and parietal cortex, which is believed to be responsible for a wide range of phenomena related to cognitive control (Fjell et al. 2009; Sullivan and Pfefferbaum 2006). Older adults can achieve comparable performance to that of younger adults by scaffolding neural activation in a way that the aging brain compensates for diminishing neural power (Park and Chun 2009). Experts, on the other hand, usually engage symmetric brain areas in the temporal and inferotemporal lobe to enable the knowledge retrieval necessary for any domain-specific tasks at hand. Therefore, unlike older adults in the general population, experts involve additional task-specific processes, based on domain-specific knowledge, for their outstanding performance. It remains unclear if older experts also demonstrate similar compensatory patterns, such as the scaffolding of neural resources, to maintain performance as they age.

Examining the potential impact of aging on work performance is a dynamic area of research that thus far has revealed variable and inconclusive outcomes. There are studies that show work performance does not decline with age, that the aging brain is more than adaptable enough if exposed to continued stimulation and engagement, and that performance may actually improve with age in some domains (Sturman 2003; Vaci et al. 2015). There are currently no studies that definitively shed light on professional concerns and inquiries about the interaction between expertise and aging in surgery or procedural medicine.

Synthesis/Summary

Experts are individuals who consistently produce outstanding performance in their domains of specialization. Although experts have the same neuronal and cognitive limitations as nonexperts, the abilities they have acquired through structured exposure and practice enables them to see and interpret situations in their domain differently. There are numerous cognitive processes that enable experts' highly efficient performance, including the automatic matching of perceptions with knowledge stored in LTM that allows experts to focus attention on the important situational aspects, thereby biasing their perceptions of the environment. Experts regularly engage additional brain areas to implement their complex cognitive strategies, which link directly to neural implementation. Although the general cognitive and neural principles are essentially the same for all expertise domains, the areas engaged by experts in psychomotor domains (prefrontal and parietal areas) may differ from perceptual and cognitive domains (inferotemporal cortex), depending on which brain region the actual knowledge has been stored.

Experts in different domains may engage different brain areas, but in all instances, they engage a greater amount of brain area than novices and often require a completely different brain network than novices. The differences in neural implementation are a direct consequence of the knowledge-based cognitive strategies used by experts, which novices are unable to depend on because they lack the necessary domain-specific knowledge. Novice performance may appear comparably awkward and inefficient, because it relies on crude strategies that demand fewer neural resources. The aim of surgical, medical, and health professions educators is to facilitate activities during training that enable novices to develop the deep knowledge-based reserves in LTM that lead to neural expansion and the effectually efficient cognitive strategies indicative of expertise.

References

Amunts K, Schlaug G, Jäncke L, Steinmetz H, Schleicher A, Dabringhaus A, Zilles K. Motor cortex and hand motor skills: structural compliance in the human brain. Hum Brain Mapp. 1997;5(3):206–15.

Bilalić M. The neuroscience of expertise. New York: Cambridge University Press; 2017. p. 225–8.

Bilalić M, Langner R, Erb M, Grodd W. Mechanisms and neural basis of object and pattern recognition: a study with chess experts. J Exp Psychol Gen. 2010;139(4):728–42.

Bilalić M, Kiesel A, Pohl C, Erb M, Grodd W. It takes two – skilled recognition of objects engages lateral areas in both hemispheres. PLoS One. 2011;6(1):e16202.

Bilalić M, Turella L, Campitelli G, Erb M, Grodd W. Expertise modulates the neural basis of context dependent recognition of objects and their relations. Hum Brain Mapp. 2012;33(11):2728–40.

Chase WG, Simon HA. Perception in chess. Cogn Psychol. 1973;4(1):55–81.

Epstein R, Kanwisher N. A cortical representation of the local visual environment. Nature. 1998;392(6676):598–601.

Ericsson KA. Deliberate practice and acquisition of expert performance: a general overview. Acad Emerg Med. 2008;15(11):988–94.

Feigenbaum EA, Simon HA. EPAM-like models of recognition and learning. Cogn Sci. 1984;8(4):305–36.

Fjell AM, Westlye LT, Amlien I, Espeseth T, Reinvang I, Raz N, Dale AM, Walhovd KB. High consistency of regional cortical thinning in aging across multiple samples. Cereb Cortex. 2009;19(9):2001–12.

Gobet F, Simon HA. Templates in chess memory: a mechanism for recalling several boards. Cogn Psychol. 1996;31(1):1–40.

Gobet F, Lane PCR, Croker S, Cheng PCH, Jones G, Oliver I, Pine JM. Chunking mechanisms in human learning. Trends Cogn Sci. 2001;5(6):236–43.

Guida A, Gobet F, Tardieu H, Nicolas S. How chunks, long-term working memory and templates offer a cognitive explanation for neuroimaging data on expertise acquisition: a two-stage framework. Brain Cogn. 2012;79(3):221–44.

Guida A, Gobet F, Nicolas S. Functional cerebral reorganization: a signature of expertise? Reexamining Guida, Gobet, Tardieu, and Nicolas' (2012) two-stage framework. Front Hum Neurosci. 2013;7:590.

Kanwisher N, McDermott J, Chun MM. The fusiform face area: a module in human extrastriate cortex specialized for face perception. J Neurosci. 1997;17(11):4302–11.

Kundel HL, Nodine CF. Interpreting chest radiographs without visual search. Radiology. 1975;116(3):527–32.

McCandliss BD, Cohen L, Dehaene S. The visual word form area: expertise for reading in the fusiform gyrus. Trends Cogn Sci. 2003;7(7):293–9.

Mireles DE, Charness N. Computational explorations of the influence of structured knowledge on age-related cognitive decline. Psychol Aging. 2002;17(2):245–59.

Mishkin M, Ungerleider LG, Macko KA. Object vision and spatial vision: two cortical pathways. Trends Neurosci. 1983;6:414–7.

Park S, Chun MM. Different roles of the parahippocampal place area (PPA) and retrosplenial cortex (RSC) in panoramic scene perception. NeuroImage. 2009;47(4):1747–56.

Pascaual-Leone A, Nguyet D, Cohen LG, Brasil-Neto JP, Cammarota A, Hallet M. Modulation of muscle responses evoked by transcranial magnetic stimulation during the acquisition of new fine motor skills. J Neurophysiol. 1995;74(3):1037–45.

Richman HB, Staszewski JJ, Simon HA. Simulation of expert memory using EPAM IV. Psychol Rev. 1995;102(2):305–30.

Rizzolatti G, Craighero L. The mirror-neuron system. Annu Rev Neurosci. 2004;27:169–92.

Sadato N. How the blind "see" Braille: lessons from functional magnetic resonance imaging. Neuroscientist. 2005;11(6):577–82.

Salthouse T. Major issues in cognitive aging. New York: Oxford University Press; 2009.

Schneider W, Chein JM. Controlled & automatic processing: behavior, theory, and biological mechanisms. Cogn Sci. 2003;27(3):525–59.

Schwarzlose RF. Separate face and body selectivity on the fusiform gyrus. J Neurosci. 2005;25(47):11055–9.

Shanteau J. Competence in experts: the role of task characteristics. Organ Behav Hum Decis Process. 1992;53(2):252–66.

Sturman MC. Searching for the inverted U-shaped relationship between time and performance: meta-analyses of the experience/performance, tenure/performance, and age/performance relationships. J Manag. 2003;29(5):609–40.

Sullivan EV, Pfefferbaum A. Diffusion tensor imaging and aging. Neurosci Biobehav Rev. 2006;30(6):749–61.

Vaci N, Gula B, Bilalić M. Is age really cruel to experts? Compensatory effects of activity. Psychol Aging. 2015;30(4):740–54.

Mastery Learning in Health Professions Education

19

Raymond Yap

Contents

Introduction	348
History and Definitions	348
Essential Elements of Mastery Learning	350
Mastery Learning Requires a Clearly Articulated Curriculum	350
Mastery Learning Requires Individual Tailoring of Education to each Learners' Ability and Rate of Progression	352
Models of Mastery Learning	354
Review of Empirical Research on Mastery Learning in Health Professions Education	355
Strengths	357
Weaknesses	357
Conclusion	359
References	359

Abstract

Mastery learning is the concept that all learners are able to achieve a certain set level of aptitude, and the variation is the method and time that is required for each learner to attain this level of mastery. There has been relatively slow uptake of its use across health professions educations, and until recently, most of the literature has focused on the learning of procedural skills within a medical education context. Nonetheless, mastery learning has excellent promise as a useful tool and framework in the area of health professions education.

Keywords

Mastery learning · Health professions education · History of · Deliberate practice · Learning objectives

R. Yap (✉)
Department of Surgery, Cabrini Hospital, Cabrini Monash University, Malvern, Melbourne, VIC, Australia
e-mail: raymondjyap@crsurgery.com.au

© Springer Nature Singapore Pte Ltd. 2023
D. Nestel et al. (eds.), *Clinical Education for the Health Professions*,
https://doi.org/10.1007/978-981-15-3344-0_24

Introduction

Mastery learning is an education framework that premises that the main marker in the progression of learning is mastery, rather than time. In other words, to progress within a learning plan, students must gain mastery of the previous level of material before being allowed to continue to the next level of learning. At its heart, it is a competency-based education philosophy that expects that all learners can achieve excellence (McGaghie et al. 1978). Competency-based learning is the concept that learning should be centered around the attainment of certain levels of ability (or competence)(Dubois 1993). Therefore, the instruction of learners, their assessment and grading, and the report and evaluation of learning programs should be centered on this concept. Mastery learning is a rather exacting version of competency-based learning, where progression is only measured by levels of competence, and all attention is placed on moving between levels of competency until "mastery" is attained in the stated area. One of its central tenets is that instead of variation between outcomes of particular students, mastery learning posits that the variation in education is the amount of time and resources that individual students take to attain a certain outcome. Like many education concepts, it originated in primary and secondary school contexts, but has been rapidly adopted in medical education over the last decade, largely due to its promise of allowing all learners to gain competency and mastery over a particular area (McGaghie 2015a). Uptake outside of medical education in other areas of health professions has been quite limited.

This chapter aims to take the reader through the historical basis of mastery learning, looking at its roots within primary and secondary education, and then its translation into medical education and health professions education more widely. It will then move on to a discussion of the essential elements of mastery learning and discuss different models being used today. Finally, a review of the literature surrounding mastery learning looking at strengths and weaknesses will be conducted.

History and Definitions

The earliest recorded use of a form of mastery learning was conceived by Carleton Washburne, who developed the "Winnetka Plan" in 1919 for the elementary schools of District 36 in Winnetka, Illinois, USA. Each student would learn different topics at different grade levels, according to their demonstrated previous ability. Learners would not progress in their grade level for a particular topic until mastery or 100% achievement had been attained. This was in response to the highly structured curriculums at the time which treated all students as the same in their ability to learn. Although widely imitated in different forms across the United States, it probably has not received the academic recognition that it should have.

Bloom, as many readers will know, was a famous professor of education at the University of Chicago and perhaps is most famous for publishing the influential Bloom's taxonomy which had been written by a committee he chaired (Bloom 1956). In 1963, John Carroll had presented his Model of School Learning which postulated that there were both individual learner differences and instructional variables that predicted achievement (Carroll 1963). Around the same time, Bloom and his graduate students had been conducting research into individual student differences in learning. In the course of their research, observations were made that despite little variation in teaching practices, student end achievement was highly variable. Combining his observations with Carroll's model, Bloom hypothesized that by using aptitude to predict learning ability and adjusting the time and quality of instruction to each student on this basis, it would be possible for most students (approximately 90%) to achieve mastery. Finally in 1968, Bloom published his seminal paper on mastery learning (Bloom 1968). Although these two developments may seem unrelated, mastery learning depends upon a clearly articulated curriculum, and without a method of categorizing learning objectives into their domains and levels of complexity, this task is essentially impossible. This is further explored below in "Mastery learning requires a clearly articulated curriculum." All of this was conducted in the shadow of the development in the concepts surrounding programmed instruction and instructional system designs, exploring the idea that education could be highly organized and built along theories of how information is processed.

Carroll's model had predicted that with a normal distribution of aptitude, uniform teaching methods would result in an identical distribution of achievement (Fig. 1). By individualizing instruction to each student, Bloom's proposal would lead to a skewed distribution in achievement despite a normal distribution of aptitude. Bloom introduced the concept of five variables that influence mastery learning:

1. Aptitude as a predictor of the rate of learning, rather than a predictor of final ability.
2. Quality of instruction on individual students, rather than a group.
3. Ability for learner to receive instruction.

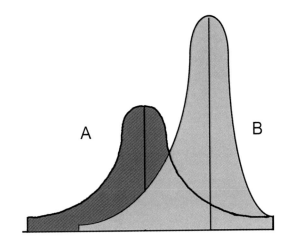

Fig. 1 (a) Uniform teaching methods will result in similar normal distribution curves for aptitude and achievement. (b) By tailoring instruction to individual students according to their aptitude, Bloom hypothesized that many more students would be able to attain mastery

4. Perseverance, i.e., management of the student's motivation to enhance learning.
5. Time allowed for learning.

Through the manipulation of these five variables, Bloom claimed that the learning of most students could be enhanced to the level that would allow mastery of a given topic. He went on to describe his "Learning for Mastery" system. Similarly, around the same time, Keller described his "Personalized System of Instruction," which drew on similar concepts to provide a different model of mastery learning (Keller 1967).

It took until 1978 for these concepts to be introduced into medical education literature. William McGaghie saw the potential for medical education in the models of mastery learning, in particular when combined with deliberate practice (McGaghie et al. 1978), based on his own experience when learning statistics (McGaghie 2015b). This realization was part of a greater movement that recognized that time-delineated learning where knowledge was gained through clinical experience in an apprenticeship model was not sufficient to teach medical students in the modern era. As McGaghie himself acknowledges, mastery learning is a form of competency-based education, where the aim of the learner is to reach certain levels of ability (competence), rather than using clinical time or experience as a guide (McGaghie 2015a). One of the earliest published examples in healthcare was its use in teaching registered nurses to manage stable hypertensive patients (Pinkney-Atkinson 1980). However, its mention in the literature in the 1980s and 1990s was fairly sporadic. It was only in the last 20 years that its tenets have been applied to health professions literature, especially to the area of simulation-based education (McGaghie et al. 2014).

Essential Elements of Mastery Learning

McGaghie, as mentioned previously, a driving force behind mastery learning within health professions, summarizes the following seven features as being essential to mastery learning (McGaghie et al. 2009). In Table 1, these elements are listed as well as an accompanying worked example of teaching laparoscopic suturing skills.

From these elements, several key themes can be elucidated. These include the need for a clear curriculum with structured learning objectives, tailoring of educational activities to learners, and the monitoring of progress of learners through accurate and timely assessment. Each of these elements will be explored below.

Mastery Learning Requires a Clearly Articulated Curriculum

For mastery learning to be effective, clear learning objectives need to be stated. Without clear goals to aim for, learning where progression is only through the attainment of mastery can often be frustrating as both educators and learners become

Table 1 Essential elements of mastery Learning

Element	Example
1. Baseline, or diagnostic testing.	Use of the fundamentals of laparoscopic surgery program (objective structured assessment of technical skill measurement) to look at laparoscopic skill domains
2. Clear learning objectives, sequenced as units usually in increasing difficulty.	• Describe the optimal port placements for laparoscopic instruments and suture material. • Demonstrate the ability to load the needle on a needle driver in a stereoscopic environment. • Discuss the methods of tying knots in a laparoscopic environment.
3. Engagement in educational activities (e.g., deliberate skills practice, calculations, data interpretation, reading) focused on reaching the objectives.	• Watching of a video demonstrating and describing laparoscopic suturing. • Deliberate skills practice of suturing in stereoscopic and laparoscopic environments. • Using Peyton's model to demonstrate suturing between learners (active description of the task at hand while performing it).
4. A set minimum passing standard (e.g., test score) for each educational unit.	Scoring more than 80% in a test format regarding the principles of laparoscopic suturing
5. Formative testing to gauge unit completion at a preset minimum passing standard for mastery.	Testing students' ability to manipulate the needle within a laparoscopic environment and to load it correctly three times a row
6. Advancement to the next educational unit given measured achievement at or above the mastery standard.	Once the needle has been correctly loaded, to then move onto the step of suturing the dummy model
7. Continued practice or study on an educational unit until the mastery standard is reached.	Allowing take-home kits for continued deliberate practice followed by weekly assessment of suturing skill

lost in the material of the curriculum. Although a full coverage of the construction of curriculum is outside the scope for this chapter, a brief summary key to the application of mastery learning is discussed.

Identifying the need and likely aptitude of learners is an essential aspect to curriculum in mastery learning (Guskey 2012). Mastery learning focuses on progression from point to point of achievement, and recognizing the starting point of learners is vital. Assessment strategies will be covered more fully below; however, some form of pre-learning assessment will be important. This can come in the form of a formal assessment before the commencement of classes, review of previous assessment material from other related subjects, or the use of introductory classes or initial assessments to gauge aptitude.

An advantage of mastery learning is that it is possible to fit it, with some adjustment, into current curricular models (Block and Burns 1976). Often curriculum has been designed to fit around a particular timeframe, such as a school year or over a course length (e.g., 3 or 4 years). If the objectives within that curriculum have

Table 2 Intravenous cannulation mastery learning objectives

1. Discuss the principles of sterile preparation and demonstrate their technique.
(a) Discuss why sterile preparation is important and provide examples of sterile and non-sterile technique.
(b) Demonstrate hand-washing and sterile gloving procedures.
(c) Perform a sterile preparation of the skin in preparation for cannulation.
2. Identify suitable veins for cannulation and explain their reasoning.
(a) Discuss which veins would be suitable for cannulation and their reasoning.
(b) Demonstrate the identification of a suitable vein.
3. Demonstrate safe and successful cannulation of a superficial vein.
(a) Perform a sterile procedure where a vein is successfully cannulated.
4. Show a method of securing the intravenous cannula in place.

been written in a clear and concise manner, it is merely the progression through the curriculum that needs to be adjusted to allow for mastery learning. The essential defined objectives can often remain the same, or need only minor adjustment to tailor them toward a mastery learning approach.

Objectives may need to be restructured and broken down to allow grouping into discrete achievement levels. Each level should cover a small amount of material that can be easily covered. These should then be ordered into a logical sequence where one objective leads to the next. An example is covered in Table 2, looking at how teaching of a procedural skill such as intravenous cannulation might be performed.

In this simple example, each objective is an important aspect in the entire process, but its mastery also leads to the next objective in a logical, stepwise fashion. Mastery of one aspect leads to the next level which then can be worked upon, until mastery of all aspects and the procedure has been attained. Individual assessment of each level to measure mastery, as well as supplemental instruction and material, is needed to ensure students meet each level of mastery. These concepts are more fully expanded in the next two sections.

Mastery Learning Requires Individual Tailoring of Education to each Learners' Ability and Rate of Progression

At the heart of mastery learning is the concept that each student progresses at a different rate and requires different amounts and methods of instruction to progress. It cannot be understated that for mastery learning to succeed, each individual student needs to develop, in conjunction with their teacher, their own path to the required objective. In an ideal setting, each student would have an individual learning plan that they would help develop and would progress completely at their own pace. Unfortunately, within the constraints of most modern courses and teaching environments, this is simply impossible.

Technology can bridge some of these gaps. Allowing for the free access of course materials and assessments online allows students to tackle them within their own preferred order and timeframes. The delivery of these materials can be replicated from course to course, allowing teachers more time to spend on individualized teaching. Remote voice and video-conferencing abilities can cut down on travel time and allow teachers to meet more students in the same amount of time. Programs can be developed to track students' progress in real-time and allow for possible near-instantaneous correction. Care must be taken however, as the progression of technology to online classrooms has often led to less class engagement and completion rates (Katy 2015). Healthcare education benefits in particular from technological advancement in simulator technology (Barsuk et al. 2012a, b; Wayne et al. 2008). Simulators allow students to practice and progress at their own pace, without the usual constraints of patient and instructor time. These can be extended to domains such as communication and teamwork, although in health education, they have been limited to the teaching of procedural skills.

Referring back to Table 2, in the example regarding intravenous cannulation, it may become apparent that the learner identifies unsuitable veins for cannulation due to their size (objective 2). A supplementary approach might look at the reasoning behind vein size in relation to cannula size, and exercises to be able to practice the identification of vein size using simple eyesight alone to correct this specific deficiency. This may include the use of landmarks such as the width of the needle or other markers to help with this endeavor.

Mastery Learning Requires Regular, Accurate, and Timely Assessment of Learners Assessment within the mastery learning format has different goals to traditional, high-stakes testing (Zimmerman and Dibenedetto 2008; Biggs 1998). Instead of using assessment for an external decision such as university placement or rank within a course, assessment here is primarily to drive the next step of learning. Therefore, assessments are formative, rather than summative in nature. The primary conclusion from these assessments is to provide feedback to learners and teachers as to whether a particular mastery of an objective has been met. A secondary conclusion is discovery where the learner is still deficient and what needs further practice or correction to meet that level of mastery.

To continue driving the education process, it is vital that these assessments are both frequent and targeted. Frequency allows for more data points on the progress of a student, as well as highlighting to teachers where further instruction may be required. Targeting of the assessment both in terms of the objective and the student both creates more accurate data as to current aptitude of the student and their current limitations, as well as the possibility of charting progression through a specific level before mastery. As can be expected, this can be quite a time-consuming task, especially if more formal methods of testing are conducted.

Referring again to Table 2, depending on the stage of the learners, this can include formal assessments like demonstration of the cannulation of a vein (objective 3) in a practice OSCE format. However, informal assessments such as observation of learners' ability to wash their hands as they prepare for their lesson (objective 1) or students critiquing each other as they practice together are also part of this process.

Models of Mastery Learning

Bloom named his method as "Learning for Mastery" (LFM). In this approach, the curriculum or subject matter is first divided into discrete topics. Students within a given learning group all start at the same level with a baseline level of instruction. After this instruction has been performed, which Bloom envisaged as happening over a week or two, a formative assessment is then undertaken to assess mastery of the topic with each individual student. If mastery is demonstrated, students are given additional tasks to enrich their understanding of the topic and further develop their mastery in this given area. Students who have not yet achieved mastery are given further instruction and teaching in areas that were shown to be deficient by their formative assessment.

This further instruction is called alternative learning resources. It may include small group work, extra assignments, individual tutoring, review of the instructional material, or the use of alternative textbooks and sources of information. The use of information technology allows for more specialized methods of further instruction as previously discussed.

In contrast, Keller came up with a Personalized System of Instruction (PSI). While Bloom envisaged his work within the classroom setting, Keller saw his work being utilized within undergraduate and postgraduate education. The epitome of PSI is best summed up by Keller himself: "This is a course through which you may move, from start to finish, at your own pace. You will not be held back by other students or forced to go ahead until you are ready. At best, you may meet all the course requirements in less than one semester; at worst, you may not complete the job within that time. How fast you go is up to you" (Keller, p80)(Keller 1968).

Keller argued for five essential components: (1) written texts that would allow students the maximum freedom in how they chose to cover the learning, although the advent of technology has meant that many forms of communication and teaching can be now be presented in a delayed fashion; (2) division of the curriculum into discrete units that should have relationships to each other; (3) that students should have the freedom to progress at their own speed; (4) mastery of a unit through demonstration of multiple assessments, of which redirection back to course material if mastery was not achieved; and (5) the use of instructors as proctors who would certify mastery, explain and discuss areas of weakness, give individualized tuition as required, and act as guides through a given subject.

As can be seen, both models are reflective of the time that they were envisaged and also their intended setting. Neither is completely analogous to most of health professions education today. Students rarely spend only time in a classroom format and often tackle multiple different areas of curriculum at the same time. A completely time-free model of learning is also difficult to implement within our time-based society, especially in the context of university semesters or limits to the length of specialty training. Nonetheless, elements of both models have numerous applications and examples that will be examined below.

Finally, the concepts of mastery learning and deliberate practice are impossible to separate. The role and usefulness of deliberate practice in the medical education literature as first described by Ericsson (Ericsson et al. 1993) is well established (Duvivier et al. 2011). Many of the concepts within deliberate practice have near-identical counterparts within mastery learning: well-defined learning objectives, level of difficulty individualized to the learner, precise measurements of learning, informative feedback, self-regulation, and constant evaluation to reach a mastery standard to advance to the next unit. Concepts of deliberate practice should be seen as complementary to mastery learning, and educators should not quibble too much on separating these two similar domains.

Review of Empirical Research on Mastery Learning in Health Professions Education

The study of mastery learning within health professions is relatively recent, with all published systematic reviews since 2010. The largest, and probably most comprehensive, was published in 2013. This paper reviewed 82 papers that evaluated simulation-based mastery learning (Cook et al. 2013). They looked for papers that both compared mastery learning to no instruction, but also mastery learning to non-mastery learning methods. The majority of these studies were within the medicine profession at the postgraduate level (49/82, 60%), while 26 (32%) of the studies involved medical students. Only 17 (21%) studies were of other health professions, which included nursing, dentistry, and emergency medicine technicians. Due to the simulation-based inclusion criteria, only two of studies on physical examination were in contexts other than the acquisition of a specific procedural skill. A significant proportion (49%) of these were in some aspect of minimally invasive surgery, usually in the form of laparoscopic surgery.

Cook et al. divided their evaluation of outcome into three main areas: speed of procedure, process (ratings of a task, either from instructor or learner), and product (a result observable from the task such as knot integrity). Unsurprisingly, against no instruction, mastery learning had a positive effect on process ratings, although the effect size was highly variable (pooled 1.29 but ranged from 0.22 to 4.56). On results, the effect size was 0.73 and again inconsistent (ranging from 0.09 to 1.68). An effect size of greater than 0.8 is considered large. These numbers were also reflected in the smaller amount of studies (8) that had an alternate teaching model in the second arm, with pooled effect sizes greater than 0.8.

Even accounting for publication bias, these results would point to the effectiveness of mastery learning in health professions education. Nonetheless, significant limitations exist. Only 8 (10%) of the studies made the comparison between mastery learning and another active form of instruction. Mastery learning took longer in all instances, and the total learning time was longer. The question raised is that if other instructional methods were given the same amount of time, would they have achieved the same results? The studies themselves were of highly variable quality, and their lack of consistency hampers any attempt at systematic review and meta-analysis. Although the authors attempted to reveal factors that may lead to the success or failure of the mastery learning model, they failed to do so.

Other types of reviews into mastery learning have been conducted such as a realist synthesis review (Griswold-Theodorson et al. 2015). The aim of this review was an attempt to uncover when mastery learning might be effective for which types of learners under what circumstances. Only 14 articles were found to adhere to all 7 principles of mastery learning as previously defined which included some of results outcome (patient or healthcare system). Again, most of these studies look at some type of procedural skill, and all of these studies were within the medical profession. All but two focused on postgraduate trainees, and none of the studies looked at non-technical skills such as teamwork or communication. Although they found that mastery learning was effective in delivering real-world outcomes, caution must be taken in interpreting these results as the comparator group was often no-intervention, and details about the alternative instruction, where applied, are relatively scarce.

To demonstrate some of the difficulties found in the literature in regard to mastery learning, a close examination of one of the trials is conducted below. Zendejas et al. ran a randomized control trial of mastery learning versus standard practice in the learning of laparoscopic inguinal hernia repair (Zendejas et al. 2011). The learners in the mastery learning group were superior in all three areas: they were operatively faster (time), had higher performance scores (process), and had lower intraoperative complications (product). However, they also received intensive instruction, time on simulators, additional course materials, and immediate tailored feedback which the other group did not receive. Essentially, the other group did not receive any kind of formal instruction, nor was their educational journey considered in any structured fashion. Many of the trials described in these reviews are similar to this study and thus do not provide a fair comparison between mastery learning and other forms of instruction or teaching. In addition, the participation rate was only 50% in this study, similar to other studies in the areas, which introduces the possibility of selection bias. In addition, adherence to all seven principles of mastery learning outlined above was not covered.

As can be seen in this brief literature review, there is evidence within the health professions education of the advantages and benefits of mastery learning. If nothing else, mastery learning can provide a spur to encourage the development of comprehensive learning models, providing the framework to drive implementation of curriculum that can benefit students. Nonetheless, questions in regard to its superiority to a more traditional form of learning still remain. Its benefits outside a technical or procedural domain are not yet proven, and its effectiveness in learners that are not postgraduate medical trainees has scant evidence. Which elements of mastery learning are effective, and the success of specific aspects such as high repetitions, method of feedback, self-regulation, and cognitive interactivity, is also unfortunately not clear. Further research is needed to clarify these areas of enquiry and to further broaden the case of evidence in mastery learning.

Strengths

The clearest advantage of mastery learning is the focus on the fact that students are individuals with different abilities of learning and different learning paces. Bloom's concept that achievement is constant while learning time is variable is probably best encapsulated within postgraduate learners acquiring a specific skill. These are learners that have already proven their ability to learn and master other areas, and thus with the right training methods, should be able to achieve mastery at the same level across the entire group.

In addition, mastery learning focuses instructors on the curriculum at hand and provides a learner-centric focus toward educational objectives. The breakdown of teaching subjects into more manageable, smaller units of instruction allows learners to focus on one aspect of subject material and gain mastery before moving on. This is likely to lead to increased satisfaction with learning and, therefore, higher progression and completion rates.

It is well known that teachers who expect their students to pass and teachers that tolerate higher levels of failure are their own self-fulfilling prophecy (Brophy 1982). Unfortunately, there is no literature in the health professions literature that look at this specific aspect of mastery learning, but the fact that mastery learning provides a basis to the belief that all students are able to attain a level of mastery despite apparent ability is surely seen as an advantage by giving teachers the confidence that their learners will succeed.

One often overlooked derivative of mastery learning is the development of self-regulation. While mastery learning does not specifically have self-regulation as one of its tenets, the goal-orientated nature of progression naturally leads toward self-direction and reflection in one's own mastery of a given subject. The literature in this particular area is conflicting with two studies showing contrasting results. One study by Brydges et al. (2010) found no difference in self-regulation, while Gauger et al. (2010) pointed that those learners that were encouraged toward self-regulation attained better results. The divergence in these studies probably proves the point; those in Brydges et al. were studied over 1 day where their self-regulation was essentially a one-off affair, while learners in Gauger et al.'s study were allowed to develop their self-regulation capacities over a longer period of time (4 months). This difference is likely explained by the development of self-regulation over a longer period of time, which presumably would follow these learners after the study is completed. The ability for self-regulation and self-reflective practice are seen as important aspects of life-long learning.

Weaknesses

Perhaps the largest barrier to entry for mastery learning is the amount of curriculum work that is needed to make it succeed. Firstly, a comprehensive curriculum of the subject matter needs to be developed with definable learning objectives. Secondly, these learning objectives must then be divided into domains of learning with specific units of learning. Thirdly, methods of initial teaching and assessment as well as alternative teaching methods to help attain mastery need to be developed so that students can succeed. Finally, these elements must then be synthesized within a framework that is practically achievable within the constraints of the teaching program. This is probably the single largest barrier that has stopped the spread of mastery learning across health professions and across the greater educational field. It is one of the reasons that Winnetka Plan did not progress to all districts across the United States despite its seeming success. This curriculum and subject development are simultaneously time and resource consuming. Technological aids can help with some aspects as recording lectures for future listening as well as providing platforms for self-learning and assessment that can be more easily be formatted from existing material. Nonetheless, it remains a significant barrier to embedding mastery learning. Indeed, it is probably why most of the literature surrounding mastery learning in health professions are centered around the acquisition of a single procedural skill; this provides for a contained curriculum and subject matter which is usually achievable in a timeframe of weeks.

As part of the curriculum issue, specifically stated instructional goals need to be set. This is easy at the individual group level where teachers have ultimate freedom to decide what their pupils learn. However, at the institutional level, it may be difficult for faculty to agree to what goals should be set. Broad learning outcomes are usually straightforward to agree upon, but specific objectives may clash as different faculty have different viewpoints on the importance of different objectives. Instructors will themselves often need instruction as to how to teach to these specific goals and techniques in meeting and correcting deficiencies in their students. In the same way, rigorous assessment and feedback loops are required for mastery learning to succeed. These are often areas that clinicians who are asked to teach are lacking in.

Teaching a mixed cohort is also challenging. Instructors must be able to meet the needs to different learners, at different levels. There is a tendency that learners who acquire mastery quickly are often neglected, having "run out of things to do." Curriculums must have room for high achievers to pursue lest they disconnect due to boredom. One method is to use those who enter mastery quickly to teach and coach other learners. In the healthcare environment, where teaching is often seen as a part of clinical duties, this can expose learners to this aspect of their education and future career. However, this needs to be carefully managed, as those who attain mastery quickly may not understand why their peers are not as quick. Similarly, those learners who have not achieved mastery may feel resentment toward their peers.

There is no doubt that mastery learning requires an increase in time and effort. In our current health professions educational systems, teachers and clinicians already feel overburdened with their current workloads. As can be seen by any of the trials in the literature, the time investment into mastery learning is substantial, even once the curriculum, study plan, and materials have been set. These extra time and resource requirements may make it prohibitive in some situations.

Conclusion

Mastery learning is quickly gaining acceptance within health professions education as a powerful tool for learning. The promise of allowing all students the ability to gain mastery is a powerful concept in healthcare, where competency for all is the desired goal, rather than excellence of a few. Nonetheless, there are numerous barriers in the area of time and resourcing that impede its further implantation in health education. Caution must be made of the widespread applicability of its benefits as these have mainly been tested in the postgraduate medical education sphere within the context of procedural skill teaching. Further work is required to confirm its use in broader health professions education contexts and also to find innovative ways to implement within the current education resourcing constraints.

References

Barsuk JH, Cohen ER, Caprio T, McGaghie WC, Simuni T, Wayne DB. Simulation-based education with mastery learning improves residents' lumbar puncture skills. Neurology. 2012a;79: 132–7.

Barsuk JH, Cohen ER, Vozenilek JA, O'connor LM, McGaghie WC, Wayne DB. Simulation-based education with mastery learning improves paracentesis skills. J Grad Med Educ. 2012b;4:23–7.

Biggs J. Assessment and classroom learning: a role for summative assessment? Assess Educ: Princ Policy Pract. 1998;5:103–10.

Block JH, Burns RB. 1: mastery learning. Rev Res Educ. 1976;4:3–49.

Bloom BS. Taxonomy of educational objectives: the classification of educational goals. *Cognitive domain*. New York: David McKay. C; 1956.

Bloom BS. Learning for mastery. Instruction and curriculum. Regional education Laboratory for the Carolinas and Virginia, topical papers and reprints, number 1. Eval Comment, 1968; 1, n2.

Brophy J. Successful teaching strategies for the inner-city child. The Phi Delta Kappan. 1982;63: 527–30.

Brydges R, Carnahan H, Rose D, Dubrowski A. Comparing self-guided learning and educator-guided learning formats for simulation-based clinical training. J Adv Nurs. 2010;66:1832–44.

Carroll JB. A model of school learning. Teach Coll Rec. 1963;64:723–33.

Cook DA, Brydges R, Zendejas B, Hamstra SJ, Hatala R. Mastery learning for health professionals using technology-enhanced simulation: a systematic review and meta-analysis. Acad Med. 2013;88:1178–86.

Dubois DD. Competency-based performance improvement: a strategy for organizational change. Amherst: ERIC; 1993.

Duvivier RJ, VAN Dalen J, Muijtjens AM, Moulaert VR, VAN DER Vleuten CP, Scherpbier AJ. The role of deliberate practice in the acquisition of clinical skills. BMC Med Educ. 2011;11:101.

Ericsson KA, Krampe RT, Tesch-Römer C. The role of deliberate practice in the acquisition of expert performance. Psychol Rev. 1993;100:363–406.

Gauger PG, Hauge LS, Andreatta PB, Hamstra SJ, Hillard ML, Arble EP, Kasten SJ, Mullan PB, Cederna PS, Minter RM. Laparoscopic simulation training with proficiency targets improves practice and performance of novice surgeons. Am J Surg. 2010;199:72–80.

Griswold-Theodorson S, Ponnuru S, Dong C, Szyld D, Reed T, McGaghie WC. Beyond the simulation laboratory: a realist synthesis review of clinical outcomes of simulation-based mastery learning. Acad Med. 2015;90:1553–60.

Guskey TR. Mastery learning. Encyclopedia of the Sciences of Learning, 2097–2100. New York: Springer; 2012.

Katy J. Massive open online course completion rates revisited: assessment, length and attrition. Int Rev Res Open Dist Learn. 2015;16

Keller FS. Engineering personalized instruction in the classroom. Rev Int Psicol. 1967;1:144–56.

Keller FS. Good-bye, teacher.... J Appl Behav Anal. 1968; 1, 79–89.

McGaghie WC. Mastery learning: it is time for medical education to join the 21st century. Acad Med. 2015a;90:1438–41.

McGaghie WC. When I say . . . mastery learning. Med Educ. 2015b;49:558–9.

McGaghie WC, Miller GE, Sajid AW, Telder TV. Competency-based curriculum development on medical education: an introduction. Public Health Pap. 1978;68:11–91.

McGaghie WC, Siddall VJ, Mazmanian PE, Myers J. Lessons for continuing medical education from simulation research in undergraduate and graduate medical education: effectiveness of continuing medical education: American College of Chest Physicians Evidence-Based Educational Guidelines. Chest. 2009;135:62S–8S.

McGaghie WC, Issenberg SB, Barsuk JH, Wayne DB. A critical review of simulation-based mastery learning with translational outcomes. Med Educ. 2014;48:375–85.

Pinkney-Atkinson VJ. Mastery learning model for an inservice nurse training program for the care of hypertensive patients. J Contin Educ Nurs. 1980;11:27–31.

Wayne DB, Barsuk JH, O'leary KJ, Fudala MJ, McGaghie WC. Mastery learning of thoracentesis skills by internal medicine residents using simulation technology and deliberate practice. J Hosp Med. 2008;3:48–54.

Zendejas B, Cook DA, Bingener J, Huebner M, Dunn WF, Sarr MG, Farley DR. Simulation-based mastery learning improves patient outcomes in laparoscopic inguinal hernia repair: a randomized controlled trial. Ann Surg. 2011;254:502–11.

Zimmerman BJ, Dibenedetto MK. Mastery learning and assessment: implications for students and teachers in an era of high-stakes testing. Psychol Sch. 2008;45:206–16.

Threshold Concepts and Troublesome Knowledge

20

Sarah E. M. Meek, Hilary Neve, and Andy Wearn

Contents

Introduction: What Are Threshold Concepts? 363
Threshold Concept Theory 363
    Troublesome Knowledge: A Key Feature of a Threshold Concept 366
    Defining a Threshold Concept: Issues 367
    Can Threshold Concepts Be Skills or Capabilities? 368
    How Do Threshold Concepts Link to Other Pedagogic Theories? 368
Proposed Threshold Concepts in Medical and Healthcare Professional Education 370
    Metacognitive Thresholds 371
    Professional Identity Thresholds 371
    Thresholds for Medical Educators 372
Moving Forward 372
    Who Can Best Identify Threshold Concepts in the Health Professions? 372
    Pedagogical Approaches for Supporting Students to Cross Thresholds 372
    Supporting Students Through the Liminal Space 373
    Helping Students Tackle Troublesome Knowledge 373
    Facilitating Threshold Crossing 375
    Relevance to Curriculum Design and Assessment 376
Conclusions 377
References 378

S. E. M. Meek (✉)
School of Medicine, Dentistry and Nursing, University of Glasgow, Glasgow, UK
e-mail: Sarah.Meek@glasgow.ac.uk

H. Neve
Peninsula Medical School, Faculty of Medicine and Dentistry, University of Plymouth, Plymouth, UK
e-mail: hilary.a.neve@plymouth.ac.uk

A. Wearn
Medical Programme Directorate, Faculty of Medical and Health Sciences, University of Auckland, Auckland, New Zealand
e-mail: a.wearn@auckland.ac.nz

© Springer Nature Singapore Pte Ltd. 2023
D. Nestel et al. (eds.), *Clinical Education for the Health Professions*,
https://doi.org/10.1007/978-981-15-3344-0_25

Abstract

Threshold concepts, first defined in 2003, are fundamental disciplinary concepts which are transformative, integrative, and irreversible and usually involve troublesome knowledge. A significant body of literature has been published in diverse disciplines from photography to physics, identifying possible threshold concepts and exploring how best to teach, learn, and assess them. Threshold concept research has been undertaken in several health professions and, more recently, within medical education.

In this chapter we introduce and define threshold concepts and examine their relationship to other pedagogic theories. We synthesize and critique current thinking and relevant literature from across the disciplines and discuss how the threshold concept framework can influence curriculum design, learning support, and teaching, including specific pedagogical strategies. We identify and review possible relevant threshold concepts drawing on research in nursing, the allied health professions, and medicine.

We explore the relative lack of critical analysis of the threshold concept framework and acknowledge that further educational research to understand and test potential threshold concepts, particularly empirically based studies, would be valuable for the health profession education community. However, by demonstrating how experts across the disciplines have used the threshold concept framework to research and gain new insights into the learner experience, we aim to encourage readers to consider its relevance and possible application to their work. In addition, we propose that troublesome knowledge is itself an important concept for both educators and researchers in health professions education.

Keywords

Threshold concepts · Medical education · Health professions education · Troublesome knowledge · Self-directed learning

Abbreviations

EPA   Entrustable professional activity
ITCK   Integrated Threshold Concept Knowledge
PBL   Problem-based learning
SOLO   Structure of observed learning outcomes
SRL   Self-regulated learning
TC   Threshold concept
TCF   Threshold concept framework
TCITF   Threshold Capability Integrated Theoretical Framework
WTP   Ways of thinking and practicing
ZPD   Zone of proximal development

Introduction: What Are Threshold Concepts?

As health professions educators, how do we know which concepts are fundamental to medical practice, or central to the grasp of the subject, and which are most likely to be troublesome for learners? Threshold concepts (TCs), first reported in 2003 (Meyer and Land 2003), throw light on these questions and, in doing so, can help us understand how to facilitate learning of these concepts.

This chapter seeks to provide a foundation for educators and educational researchers within medicine and the health professions, who wish to study or apply threshold concept theory in their work. It aims to:

- Introduce, define, and critically review the threshold concept framework (TCF) and highlight recent developments
- Discuss its potential application in medical and health professional education
- Explore TCs identified within, or relevant to, health professional education

Threshold Concept Theory

Threshold concepts (TCs) were theorized during an extensive research study (Land et al. 2005a), which sought to identify factors that led to improved student engagement and high-quality learning across 12 higher education institutions and 4 disciplinary contexts. Threshold concepts were identified as distinct from disciplinary building-blocks or "core concepts" in that they are critical for mastery of a discipline and are **transformative**, leading to "a change in knowing, doing, being, and future learning possibilities" (Barradell and Peseta 2016). A number of additional characteristics, or criteria, define threshold concepts. They are usually **troublesome,** rendering them cognitively or affectively difficult to grasp. Learning them can take time, as students must pass through a transitional **liminal** phase. Crossing the threshold to mastery often involves the **integration** of several strands of knowledge and is usually **irreversible**. The criteria are explained in more depth in Table 1. The case study (Box 1) illustrates these ideas in practice, with several examples of how educators might use TCs theory to conceptualize student learning, in order to improve their teaching practice.

> **Box 1 An illustrative example of implications for teachers: Hormonal control**
> You are running a small group teaching session on hormonal control, as follow-up to a recent lecture. You ask students to apply their learning to a case study about the menstrual cycle. You soon realize that the students, who all attended the lecture, are struggling with the scenario. "I just don't get this" you hear, as you move between the subgroups. "I didn't understand this at
>
> (continued)

Table 1 Meyer and Land's criteria for threshold concepts

Criterion (Meyer and Land 2003, 2005)	Reason for threshold nature (Meyer and Land 2003, 2005)	Comments
Transformative	The learner's understanding or view of a subject or discipline is transformed. A conceptual shift: opens up a new, previously inaccessible way of thinking about the subject. May be an ontological shift	Ontological shift example: the student begins to think like a professional rather than a student ("becoming a doctor")
Troublesome	Involves knowledge that is, for example, counterintuitive, confronting or alien	See later discussion of troublesome knowledge
Irreversible	Once learned, it is difficult to "unlearn" a TC. Subject experts may not recall their own difficulties in grasping a particular concept and may underestimate how problematic it can be for students	Irreversibility intuitively follows from the transformative nature of TCs. However, it is not known if there are qualitative or quantitative differences in memory and retention of threshold and non-threshold concepts
Integrative	Brings together different aspects of the subject that previously did not seem (to the student) to be related. Integration may be between different subject areas or between theory and practice	This integrative aspect of TCs is particularly prominent in TCs in biological sciences (Taylor 2006). The integrating and transformative functions of TCs are closely related and can be hard to disentangle (Land et al. 2018)
Bounded	The concept is limited by boundaries with other concepts and by disciplinary boundaries	Increasingly, it is being acknowledged that there are some generic TCs that transcend disciplines
Discursive	Involves an extension of students' use of language and discipline-specific terminology	For example, learning to use medical terminology
Reconstitutive	The student's prior understanding is reconfigured according to their new understanding	This characteristic in particular places TCF as a constructivist model of learning
Liminal	Learners occupy a transitional "liminal" space where they may oscillate between old and new conceptual understandings, sometimes for a considerable time	Students may "mimic" threshold crossing without true conceptual change, e.g., as ritual knowledge (Land et al. 2006)

Box 1 (continued)

school either" says one student "even though I passed biology." "Let's just give up and get a coffee," says another.

How can this be? You spent hours trying to make your lecture clear and accessible. You don't understand why your teaching is not leading to effective learning.

You share this with Jo, a colleague. She suggests that the threshold concept framework might help. Some concepts, Jo explains, are fundamental to students' understanding of a subject but can be more difficult and take longer for students to grasp, than other concepts, sometimes leading students to disengage. During this time students are said to be in a "liminal" space. We often don't allow for this, she points out, when planning teaching.

You decide to find out more about teaching threshold concepts. You discover that "homeostasis" has been identified as a possible threshold concept in biology. You read about the different kinds of troublesome learning and the benefits of recursiveness (revisiting learning in different ways). Next year you decide to teach hormonal control over three shorter sessions.

You give students some preparatory reading then ask them to work in groups to draw the menstrual cycle. You watch students drawing the hormonal feedback loops and helping each other out – but most groups soon get stuck and start to lose focus. You suggest they set and research questions around the difficult areas and bring their findings back to the second session. In the next session, several students are more positive. "It's coming together" you hear. "There are two kinds of feedback" explains another as they re-draw the cycle on flipcharts. "We've cracked it," laughs one.

The following week you watch the students successfully apply their knowledge of the menstrual cycle to scenarios about the thyroid and lactation. You have helped them finally "get" hormonal control.

This scenario illustrates how the TCF can help teachers, who have often forgotten what they or their peers found difficult to learn. The concept of hormonal control is fundamental to medicine but often troublesome for students. By recognizing that students are finding learning difficult, offering them opportunities to revisit and integrate their learning in different ways, independently and in groups, they reached a transformative moment as they 'got' the menstrual cycle. By asking them, at a later date, to transfer this learning to new scenarios, you ensured this learning was irreversible.

Since 2003, hundreds of papers have been published, across over 259 disciplines (Land et al. 2016), from photography to physics, aiming to identify TCs and exploring how TCs can inform curriculum development, teaching, and assessment. Threshold concept research has been undertaken in a number of health professions and disciplines and, more recently, within medical education (Neve et al. 2016).

It is important to note that despite its wide uptake, much of the current literature is largely uncritical of threshold concept theory. For example, do TCs actually exist, in an empirical sense? Are they the same for every learner? How can they be reliably identified, and by whom (teacher, learner, subject expert)? Furthermore, the field lacks empirical studies testing the effects of TC-based educational strategies on student learning. We pick up these criticisms later.

Troublesome Knowledge: A Key Feature of a Threshold Concept

An important feature of the TCF is the notion of troublesome knowledge. Students may describe their confrontation with troublesome knowledge as stressful, frustrating, and even scary (Felten 2016; Rattray 2016) and may respond in a range of ways, including resisting or avoiding the subject (Box 1). Longer-term, continued difficulty grasping relevant threshold concepts may even be a barrier to students choosing a particular career path (Neve 2019). Knowledge can be troublesome for various reasons; Table 2 illustrates these different categories with practical examples chosen to resonate with educators across multiple contexts.

However, troublesomeness is not necessarily problematic. Savin-Baden (2007) argues that "stuckness" or disjunction in learning can be positive and useful; it can act as a catalyst for provoking new ways of seeing and can lead to transformation.

Table 2 Troublesome knowledge (Perkins 2006; Meyer and Land 2006)

Forms of troublesome knowledge
Counterintuitive knowledge goes against student's current conceptual model of the topic
Knowledge is described as **inert** when the student cannot connect it to the world around them, so then struggles to apply it meaningfully in practice or in new contexts
Alien knowledge does not fit easily into learners' current understanding or may conflict with their world view or beliefs, e.g., a student may not understand why anyone would smoke when they know that smoking causes disease, until the student encounters someone who experiences little power or agency
Ritual knowledge is represented by the routine answers we give in response to commonly asked questions. For instance, students may perform a respiratory examination as they have been taught, without understanding the underlying concepts or why they are carrying out each step
Troublesome language includes medical jargon which may be meaningless to students and render a topic incomprehensible
Conceptually difficult knowledge is complex in nature. Many medical concepts are extremely complex
Tacit knowledge is implicit within a discipline but may not be overtly explained during teaching. Students may come across such knowledge through interactions with experts and may be only peripherally aware or entirely unconscious of it. This includes aspects of professional practice that are often not taught explicitly, such as issues of power and politics in medical practice (Hafferty 1998)
Nettlesome knowledge (Sibbett and Thompson 2008) is knowledge that learners often repress or ignore because grasping it can challenge cultural or individual beliefs and result in an intense emotional response. This form of troublesomeness was identified in studies of palliative care (Wearn et al. 2016)

Different students respond differently to troublesome knowledge, and recent literature highlights the importance of affect, as well as intellectual and pedagogical factors, in determining students' willingness to engage with liminality. Factors such as resilience and optimism appear to be important (Rattray 2016). In addition, students need to accept that important learning can take time and involve struggle and have the psychological strategies to deal with ambiguity (Land and Rattray 2017; Shopkow 2010). Teachers too need to understand that troublesomeness can be useful and that they need to attend to students' emotional responses, to engage their students with uncertainty and support them through the liminal space (Felten 2016) (Table 2).

In the hormonal control example (Box 1), learning was probably troublesome for several reasons, including being conceptually difficult. In addition, while the group understood the notion of negative and positive feedback, the idea that a single hormone could do both was counterintuitive. This key learning step or "bottleneck" (Middendorf and Pace 2004) may have been tacit knowledge, not explicitly or adequately explained during teaching. The students may have passed their previous biology lessons by using ritual knowledge, without fully understanding the underlying principles and concepts. Additionally, the troublesomeness may be affective or "nettlesome": menstruation may have been a taboo topic at home, or emotionally uncomfortable.

Defining a Threshold Concept: Issues

The lack of clarity about which characteristics (Table 1) must be present to define a concept as threshold has generated criticism (Rowbottom 2007; Barradell 2013). Transformation, Land suggests, is "superordinate and non-negotiable" (Land et al. 2016), while other criteria are usually, but not always present. For example, boundedness may not be essential for concepts in "softer" domains such as professionalism and social sciences (Collett et al. 2017). The lack of clear boundaries may even be what defines these concepts; this can also make them more troublesome for students. Barradell (2013) calls for a clearer definition of a TC, including the relative importance of each characteristic. This would enable researchers to test each potential TC for its "threshold nature."

Where only some TC characteristics are met, concepts may represent "core" concepts (of disciplinary importance, but not threshold) or sub-concepts of a higher-level threshold concept. Davies and Mangan (2007), working in the field of Economics, and Ross et al. working in Biology (Ross et al. 2010) have developed hierarchies of concepts, involving increasing levels of troublesomeness, and complexity. "Basic concepts" or "content knowledge" sit at the bottom level, while higher-level concepts meet the TC criteria and lead to transformation. Ross et al. place "threshold epistemes" at the top of their matrix; these link multiple TCs and are similar to major ontological thresholds such as reflective practice.

The case study (Box 1) illustrates the definition problem. What, in this setting, was the threshold concept? Was it hormonal control or students' understanding of feedback loops? Or were these sub-concepts of a broader threshold concept already proposed in the literature – homeostasis? (Ross et al. 2010; Meek and Jamieson 2014). By helping students identify and anchor their learning to higher-level concepts, teachers can help them to see relationships between their new learning and existing understandings (Novak and Canas 2006) (in this case, connecting hormonal control with other forms of homeostasis).

Can Threshold Concepts Be Skills or Capabilities?

Most TC literature focuses on knowledge and understanding, but some studies suggest that discipline skills, such as interpreting electroencephalography in medicine (Moeller and Fawns 2018), or broader skills like reflective practice (Corrall 2017), may display several characteristics of a TC. Baillie, Bowden, and Meyer (Baillie et al. 2013) draw on both TCF and the notion of capability (Neve and Hanks 2016) to develop a "Threshold Capability Theory" (termed Threshold Capability Integrated Theoretical Framework, TCITF). In this model, "threshold capabilities" are transformative and describe what students need to be able to *do* in order to work in new and changing situations. They usually require mastery of one more threshold concepts or skills. Research in media studies has identified critical thinking as a possible threshold capability (Chen and Rattray 2017). In their review of Bhat et al.'s proposed thresholds, Chen and Poole (2018) distinguish between ontological thresholds, such as "working with uncertainty," and skill set thresholds. In an exploration of learning during a palliative care attachment, Wearn et al. propose five TCs that were ontological in nature and would be observable in practice as capabilities (Wearn et al. 2016). These extensions of TCF may be very relevant to health professions disciplines. Indeed, Ray Land has recently expressed a preference for the term "learning thresholds," to encompass all these possibilities (Chen and Poole 2018).

How Do Threshold Concepts Link to Other Pedagogic Theories?

TCF draws on several older educational and philosophical theories (Table 3) and maps onto both behavioral and constructivist views of learning. Learners are confronted, troubled, and drawn to explore and cross a threshold, the payoff being transformation and progress. Learners are also encouraged to reflect on current knowledge, construct new knowledge, and develop new ways of seeing.

While TCF has been criticized as being "old wine in new bottles" (Cousin 2008), it offers educators opportunities to consider these theories in new ways (Table 3).

For educational researchers, perhaps the closest framework commonly used to identify troublesome and possibly threshold learning areas is Middendorf and Pace's "Decoding the Disciplines" approach, where educators use a series of steps to identify and overcome "bottlenecks" in student learning (Middendorf and Pace 2004). However, these "bottlenecks" may not meet all the criteria for threshold concepts in Table 1; instead they likely reflect "troublesome knowledge" (Perkins 2006), with variable potential for student transformation.

Table 3 Relationships between TCF and established learning theories

Threshold concept framework	Related models/theories	Differences
Transformation is an essential feature of a TC and involves conceptual and ontological change	Mezirow's transformative learning (Mezirow 1991) involves transforming "the beliefs, attitudes, opinions and emotional reactions that constitute our meaning scheme" (p223)	The depth of the transformative change arising from most currently proposed TCs is often not on the same scale as Mezirow's "perspective transformation" (Mezirow 1978) or is not as ontologically significant. TCF adds (a) that it is often the integrative element of TCs, when ideas come together, that is transformative, and (b) that letting go of old understandings can be troublesome
When transitioning to new understandings learners pass through a "**liminal space**" associated with being "stuck" which often feels uncomfortable and troublesome. Learners may respond by avoiding, resisting or disengaging with learning, or by increasing engagement and effort (Berg et al. 2016) Liminality can also be a place of creativity, where learners can see things differently (Savin-Baden 2008)	Vygotsky (1978) sees educators as helping students to cross the "Zone of Proximal Development" (ZPD), the gap between student and teacher knowledge Like liminality, the ZPD is transitional, and students cannot cross it without help, becoming "stuck" if left alone Mezirow describes "perspective transformation" in adult education as triggered by a "disorienting dilemma" (Mezirow 1978), and disorientation is a feature of liminality	Vygotsky sees the liminal phase in terms of cognitive difficulty, and advocates teachers "scaffolding" or modelling to lead students across the ZPD. The TCF recognizes affective elements and the importance of educators supporting students emotionally through the liminal space The sociocultural basis of learning in the ZPD is not emphasized in TCF Recursiveness and oscillations in student understanding are present in the TCF but not the original ZPD model
Threshold concepts are often **bounded** within disciplinary contexts Learning to "think like a professional" meets TC criteria (Neve et al. 2017)	McCune and Hounsell describe "ways of thinking and practicing (WTP)" (McCune and Hounsell 2005), where "legitimate peripheral participation" (Lave and Wenger 1991) by students in experts' communities of practice allows them to learn discipline WTPs, e.g., nomenclature, values, and approaches	TCF acknowledges that threshold crossing can involve shifts in learner identity and behavior, as learners grapple with new WTPs (which may include TCs such as "working with uncertainty" (Neve et al. 2017, 2018; Bhat et al. 2018))

Proposed Threshold Concepts in Medical and Healthcare Professional Education

Researchers have used a range of methods to identify and explore TCs: semi-structured interviews with teachers and clinicians (Meek and Jamieson 2014; Moeller and Fawns 2018; Land and Meyer 2011), audio-diaries with medical students (Neve et al. 2018; Collett et al. 2017), focus groups with registrars in palliative care (Wearn et al. 2016) concept mapping with trainers in geriatric medicine (Wilkinson 2018), and accounts of powerful learning experiences with GPs (Vaughan 2016). In medicine, TCs may exist at a generic level (being a doctor or physiotherapist), as well as within each sub-disciplinary area, be this physiology, medical ethics, or mental health nursing.

Studies in medicine, where concepts met all the main TC characteristics include Wearn et al. (2016), who identify "communication management" and "emotional engagement," and Neve et al. who identify "the immune response" and "spatial relationships in anatomy" (Neve et al. 2018) along with "considering the bigger picture," "I don't need to know everything," and "professional culture" (Neve et al. 2017). Managing or embracing uncertainty has been identified as a possible, or even overarching (Neve and Hanks 2016; Smith et al. 2018), TC in multiple medical disciplines (Neve et al. 2018; Wearn et al. 2016; Meek and Jamieson 2014; Bhat et al. 2018; Vaughan 2016; Smith et al. 2015). In related healthcare professions, caring has been identified as a TC for occupational therapy and physiotherapy students (Clouder 2005), while "evidence-based practice," "clinical reasoning," "client-centered approach," "reflective practice," and the "holistic approach" are proposed TCs in Occupational Therapy (Nicola-Richmond et al. 2016). Evidence-based practice meets the liminal, troublesome, and transformative criteria in nursing (Martindale 2015), and clinical (diagnostic) reasoning meets the key criteria of transformative, troublesome, and integrative for medical students (Pinnock et al. 2019). Bhat et al. found that "burden of responsibility," "purposeful action," "contextual care," and "patient-centeredness" meet the transformative and troublesome criteria and may be TCs in clinical rotations (Bhat et al. 2018).

Other potential TCs have weaker evidence. Meek and Jamieson (Meek and Jamieson 2014) provide preliminary evidence that "population perspectives" and "the nature of evidence" are threshold for preclinical medical students. "Empathy," "ethical challenges," (Ryan 2014), the "complexity of medical care" (Wilkinson 2018), "embodied shared care," and "active inaction" (Wearn et al. 2016) may also be TCs. "Health as politically and socially determined" (Neve et al. 2019) and "inequalities in health" (Chittleborough 2013) may be TCs in public health. Indeed, the persistence of poorer health outcomes and healthcare experiences for minority groups (e.g., Institute of Medicine 2003; Elliott et al. 2015) may suggest that thresholds related to unconscious bias may also be troublesome, and possibly threshold, in medical education and practice. These might include "race" (Winkler, quoted in Atherton et al. 2008), "deficit thinking" (Spillane 2015), "inclusionary othering" (Kempenaar and Shanmugam 2018), and "stigma" (McAllister et al. 2015).

TCs identified in non-healthcare disciplines, such as variability, probability, and the cycle of enquiry in biology (Taylor 2006; Taylor and Meyer 2010), may be relevant to the health professions. However, TCs are bounded by context, including disciplinary context; they may even help define the discipline (Nicola-Richmond et al. 2016). Notably, TCs in individual disciplines do not appear to be additive for interdisciplinary subjects, such as Neuroscience (Holley 2018). It is therefore necessary to reexamine whether each of these concepts from the disciplines that contribute to Medicine is also threshold in medicine (or other healthcare disciplines).

Metacognitive Thresholds

Metacognition is critical to effective learning and regulation of learning. Metacognition refers to individuals' higher-order thinking, whereby they are aware of, and take control of, the cognitive processes involved in their learning (Driessen 2014). Perkins distinguishes "proactive" knowledge from "possessive" and "performative" knowledge (Perkins 2008). Proactive knowledge involves recognizing opportunities and having the ability, and disposition, to apply the knowledge in new settings. Proactive knowledge is essential for self-directed learning and has threshold qualities (Perkins 2008). Educators need to help students to become reflective, critically thinking doctors able to manage their own learning. Indeed, self-regulated learning (SRL) (Zimmerman 1989) may itself be a threshold concept/capability. Meek & Neve (Meek et al. 2019) found evidence that SRL can be transformative in allowing medical students to learn well by problem-based learning (PBL). Also, several studies have found improved SRL after PBL, although this result is not always found and may depend on exactly how PBL is implemented (English and Kitsantas 2013).

In the digital age, these metacognitive skills are intertwined with information literacy (IL), an important skill for doctors. Aspects of IL, such as the contextual and constructed nature of expert authority or that good searches use database structure, have threshold characteristics (Hofer et al. 2012), although the nature of TCs in information literacy is much debated (Wilkinson 2014). One topical proposal is that research skills/capability is a vital threshold for all higher education courses, in the current "post-truth" climate (Hughes 2019).

Professional Identity Thresholds

TCs are often troublesome because they involve uncomfortable identity transitions (Savin-Baden 2008). These are perhaps the most transformative TCs, because of their profound and overarching ontological nature. The transition from self-identifying as "healthcare student" to "nurse," "doctor," or "surgeon" fits all the key TC characteristics (Neve et al. 2017, 2018; Land and Meyer 2011).

Thresholds for Medical Educators

Educators may themselves grapple with TCs related to teaching and learning. While addressing these is beyond the scope of this chapter, an example of a threshold concept for educators is "authenticity" as in the context of surgical training and simulation (Kneebone 2009). Specific concepts around assessment were threshold for discipline experts on an initial university teacher development course (Reimann 2018). Authentic role modelling may be crucial for medical students to cross thresholds in practice (Meek and Jamieson 2014).

Moving Forward

Who Can Best Identify Threshold Concepts in the Health Professions?

Many studies employ questionnaires, interviews, or the Delphi process to discover which concepts experts and teachers think are threshold in their discipline (Neve et al. 2019; Cousin 2008). However, the irreversible nature of TCs means that experts may not even remember learning a TC, nor recall what they found troublesome. Staff may not fully appreciate the range of pre-liminal variation in students' prior conceptions of each TC, nor how different students experience threshold crossing differently (Meyer et al. 2008). Furthermore, expert participants often do not agree about TCs within a given discipline (Barradell 2013).

Research with learners often identifies a distinct but overlapping set of potential TCs compared to staff-based studies. Learners may not know what they need to learn, but are able to describe their learning experience (Barradell 2013). Other studies use both staff and student or trainee participants (Bhat et al. 2018); "transactional curriculum enquiry" studies that use dialogue between teachers, students, and educationalists may prove the most fruitful (Cousin 2008). Briefing participants about TCF before data collection may influence results, so using indirect questions about troublesome or perspective-changing topics is usually more appropriate. "Straight after the moment" approaches (e.g., audio-diaries) may overcome concerns about hindsight bias (Collett et al. 2017).

Pedagogical Approaches for Supporting Students to Cross Thresholds

A number of approaches may help students tackle troublesome concepts and facilitate threshold crossing. Examples are included below.

Supporting Students Through the Liminal Space

Liminality can be discouraging and unsettling, so a safe learning environment is essential. Peer support and provision of collaborative learning spaces such as small group learning (Neve et al. 2017) may enable students to share difficulties and challenge their conceptions. In medical education the PBL learning process appears not only to help students tackle troublesome knowledge, but may itself be a threshold concept or capability (Neve et al. 2018). Students will also need support to tolerate uncertainty and the contestable nature of knowledge (Neve et al. 2018; Meek and Jamieson 2014; Bhat et al. 2018; Vaughan 2016; Smith et al. 2015). This may challenge students' sense of identity as learners.

Helping Students Tackle Troublesome Knowledge

Listening to students' language (as in the case studies, (Box 1 and 2)) can help teachers notice where and why students are stuck, confused, or using mimicry. They can then allocate more time and ensure recursiveness (Land et al. 2005b), using different approaches to revisit the same concepts in new ways.

> **Box 2 Researching threshold concepts: an illustrative example**
>
> Illustrative quotes are based on findings in Neve et al. (2018) and (Cousin (2009)
>
> Your school is undertaking a review of their Year 1 Problem-Based Learning Curriculum. The team have recently learned about threshold concepts and how they are fundamental to the understanding of a discipline. They now want to update their PBL cases to focus both on threshold concepts and on concepts which students find particularly troublesome. They ask you, an educational researcher, to help identify which concepts these might be.
>
> You undertake a literature review and find out about transactional curriculum enquiry (Cousin 2009), where a group of different stakeholders engage in dialogue to discuss and propose a set of threshold concepts. You decide to bring together PBL tutors and students with the aim of identifying Year 1 concepts which are likely to be threshold and/or troublesome for students.
>
> You start the session with a workshop, introducing participants to the notions of threshold concepts and troublesome knowledge, and then record the subsequent lively debate. The recording is transcribed and coded, both for the concepts identified and for evidence that threshold concept criteria have been met.
>
> The table below gives illustrative examples of language demonstrating each of the threshold concept criteria:

	Student quotes	PBL tutor quotes
Transformative	"Finally, suddenly, it all made sense" "my understanding changed completely"	"That is often a light bulb moment for them…"
Integrative	"It all came together when…"	"They only understand it when they see how the processes all join up"
Liminal	"We had to go over this again and again until we got it" "I puzzled over it at first but thought I'd got it…but later when I tried the practice questions I realised I hadn't…then I had to work it through again and now I think I've finally got it again"	"They often think they've got it when they haven't… it can take ages" "they can reproduce the graph, but don't know what it actually means in practice"
Troublesome	"I found all the new language really confusing" "It was frustrating as it didn't seem to fit with what we were taught at school"	"It's just so complex, there is so much happening, they really struggle" "They really don't like the fact there is no clear definition"
Bounded	"The difference between the two suddenly clicked for me"	"it's when they realise it is all part of a single process that they can move on.."
Irreversible	"It seems so obvious now"	"I know it has really stuck for them when…"

You identified several concepts with multiple examples meeting all six criteria, suggesting they were likely threshold concepts. These included "blood pressure regulation," "hormonal control," and "the immune response." You also identified a number of additional concepts which did not meet all six criteria, but were particularly troublesome for Year 1 students. Your curriculum team are now designing new PBL cases based around these concepts.

It is also important to be aware of the affective dimensions of threshold crossing. Affective disequilibrium, perhaps more so than cognitive disequilibrium, is important in prompting student transformation (Timmermans 2010). Individual students' affective and psychological characteristics may determine their engagement with liminality and therefore predict whether threshold crossing will occur (Rattray 2016).

Taylor and Meyer suggest asking students to document their reasoning when attempting exercises involving a particular TC, in order to identify misconceptions. They recommend then discussing the concept explicitly (Taylor and Meyer 2010). This recalls the conceptual change literature, where Vosniadou and Ioannides (Vosniadou and Ioannides 1998) recommend openly discussing students' current conceptions and then providing examples where student's current concepts are inadequate. However, the latter strategy has risks – by memorizing explanations, students may mimic threshold crossing, without full understanding.

Mental models and frameworks can aid learning of conceptually difficult material (Perkins 2006) or seemingly "woolly" ideas (Collett et al. 2017). In interviews with experienced teaching staff, mathematical and spatiotemporal models (e.g., graphs, 3D animations), analogies, and scaffolding were identified as teaching methods that help early years medical students grasp TK and TCs (Meek and Jamieson 2014). Spatiotemporal visual models may be particularly effective for understanding the dynamic nature of many physiological concepts (Horrigan 2018) in preclinical medicine. Similarly, visualizing understanding using diagrams or concept maps can promote integration by helping students identify gaps or make links to prior knowledge during PBL (Neve et al. 2018).

Asking students to reframe a topic from the viewpoint of a layperson, scientist, and doctor can render the concept less "alien" and therefore less troublesome (Perkins 2006). Adopting a range of roles (e.g., nurse, patient, relative) in the "troublesome context" of a complex ward-based simulation enables students to enter the liminal space and can be transformative, particularly when taking on the role of patient (Corbally et al. 2018).

Teachers must also appreciate that troublesomeness may lie with themselves, not just learners. For example, tacit knowledge may seem so intuitive to experts (due to threshold irreversibility) that they no longer relate to the conceptual understanding of a learner who has not yet crossed the threshold (Meyer and Land 2006). Approaches such as "decoding the disciplines" (Middendorf and Pace 2004) can help staff identify tacit knowledge, missing steps, or other bottlenecks that students experience in their teaching. Alternatively, Timmermans and Meyer (2017) used the Integrated Threshold Concept Knowledge (ITCK) framework to allow subject experts to both explore thresholds in their own discipline and embed these into their teaching practice.

Facilitating Threshold Crossing

"Compare and contrast" exercises, discussing a concept from multiple perspectives, using examples of the same concept in different contexts, or showing students multiple ways to approach a problem can open up new thresholds (Land et al. 2006; Male 2012). This use of variation to promote conceptual change is central to Marton's variation theory (Meyer et al. 2008; Bowden and Marton 2004) and is also important in Baillie, Bowden, and Meyer's threshold capability model (Baillie et al. 2013) (described above). Openly discussing students' current conceptions, providing examples where these are inadequate (Vosniadou and Ioannides 1998), and encouraging students to discover discrepancies between their current understanding and new evidence (Perkins 2006) can also facilitate conceptual change.

Transformation often occurs when learners integrate different strands of learning. Therefore, encouraging integration is important. Educators can explicitly highlight links between previously acquired concepts, and between theory and practice (Neve et al. 2017), and model the process of making links (Taylor 2008). Directing students toward a variety of complementary resources may encourage students to make connections themselves.

Seeing the relevance of learning to the real world can help students cross thresholds (Neve et al. 2017). A study of general practitioners suggest that some workplace experiences are particularly transformative, leading them to gain new understanding of themselves in relation to their work and patients and to cross "vocational thresholds" (Vaughan 2016). Where concepts are abstract or "unseen," for example, in radiation physics, 'seeing' how these concepts impact on real patients through a virtual learning environment can facilitate transformation (Hudson et al. 2018). The use of narrative is another powerful way to promote transformation. Literature (McAllister et al. 2015), authentic stories from current practitioners in PBL (Treloar et al. 2018), or video stories within a virtual community (Levett-Jones et al. 2015) can provide narrative examples of transformative concepts in nursing, as well as allowing students to experience new perspectives and provoke liminality.

Although there is a sound theoretical basis for each of the above strategies, as yet there is limited empirical evidence that these improve student learning of TCs. This is an important area for further research.

Relevance to Curriculum Design and Assessment

Threshold concept research can help curriculum designers understand which concepts are fundamental to learning (the "jewels in the curriculum" (Land et al. 2005b)) and which are troublesome and may need more time. Streamlining a curriculum around TCs can reduce the tendency to overcrowd it with content (Cousin 2006); teams in Biology (Taylor et al. 2012) and Occupational Therapy (Rodger and Turpin 2011) have redesigned their curricula around TCs. Whether these redesigns improve student learning, however, is still undergoing evaluation.

A rigid, linear curriculum model will not work if different students cross a threshold at different times. Meyer et al. (2008) suggest that in a group of learners there may be variation in understanding at multiple stages: pre-liminal, liminal and post-liminal. Therefore, the same TC must be encountered throughout the curriculum, to maximize threshold crossing (Land and Meyer 2010). Multiple encounters with the same TC promote threshold crossing (Natanasabapathy and Maathuis-Smith 2019), suggesting that a "spiral" curriculum design is optimal.

Differences in threshold crossing also poses problems for assessment (Land and Meyer 2010). Progress testing, where the same test is administered to students at multiple levels of the curriculum (e.g., Freeman et al. 2010), may be more appropriate. Programmatic assessment, which prioritizes "assessment for learning" over "assessment of learning" (Schuwirth and Van der Vleuten 2011), also fits well into the TC framework. In dental education, Hyde et al. (2018) suggest that reflection on learning TCs may be more important than direct assessment: reflective practice and assessment are complementary for student learning. In outcomes-based assessment, Bhat et al. argue that well-designed EPA (Entrustable Professional Activity) assessments could identify students who still experience troublesomeness due to lack of crossing underlying thresholds and support their learning (Bhat et al. 2018).

Increasingly it is recognized that if learning is to be meaningful and reflect the holistic nature of healthcare, curricula must incorporate tools such as concept mapping to help students to make connections between different threshold concepts and ways of thinking and practicing (Barradell and Peseta 2018). Promoting networked, rather than linear, understandings is particularly important in disciplines where patients have multiple conditions and complex, interconnected needs, such as in geriatric medicine (Wilkinson 2018). This can be supported by a spiral curriculum where the revisiting of concepts (recursiveness) is designed, not just to add more information, but to help students see how to link their conceptual understandings and clinical experiences (Kinchin et al. 2011).

Designing assessments that look for evidence of conceptual and ontological transformation (i.e., threshold crossing) remains a challenge. Tests of knowledge application, or providing justification for answers, rather than allowing students to pass by rote memorization or mimicry, align more closely with TCF. Authentic tasks that integrate understandings are useful for both learning and assessment (Springfield et al. 2017). Concept maps can be used to track changes in student learning and for assessment, as well as facilitate links between threshold concepts and ways of thinking and practicing (Barradell and Peseta 2018). The Structure of Observed Learning Outcomes (SOLO) taxonomy (Biggs and Collis 1982) describes learners' understanding at increasing levels of complexity, from understanding the independent elements of a task or subject, to being able to integrate these into a coherent whole, to ultimately being able to generalize these understandings to new and different settings. A modification of SOLO has been used to assess the extent to which a student "thinks like an economist" (Meyer et al. 2016); this could also be applied to the health professions.

Conclusions

Despite some limitations, the threshold concept framework (TCF) can challenge health professions educators to consider which concepts are critical to the mastery of their particular discipline. Perhaps even more useful, threshold concepts offer a new lens for researching, reflecting on and understanding the student learning experience. As an analytical tool, they can play a particularly important role in rendering more visible the ontological changes that occur during healthcare education (Land et al. 2018). Reflecting on possible threshold concepts and areas of troublesome knowledge in their own teaching can help educators incorporate pedagogical techniques that facilitate threshold crossing and conceptual change. As yet, there is little empirical evidence to suggest that the TCF can contribute to improved knowledge, skills, or attitudes or to better patient care or patient outcomes. These are all areas for future research. However, this difficulty of attributing cause and effect in education is not unique to the threshold concept framework.

It is important to recognize that the threshold concept framework can be troublesome for educators; indeed, the threshold concept may itself be a threshold concept! Yet this framework strikes a chord with many educators, both because the identification of threshold concepts involves delving deeper into our own disciplines and because we seek to promote meaningful and transformative change in our students.

References

Atherton J, Hadfield P, Meyers R. Threshold concepts in the wild. In: Expanded version of paper presented at [Internet]. Queen's University, Kingston; 2008 [cited 2018 Apr 25]. Available from: https://www.researchgate.net/publication/228873314_Threshold_Concepts_in_the_Wild.

Baillie C, Bowden JA, Meyer JHF. Threshold capabilities: threshold concepts and knowledge capability linked through variation theory. High Educ. 2013;65(2):227–46.

Barradell S. The identification of threshold concepts: a review of theoretical complexities and methodological challenges. High Educ. 2013;65(2):265–76.

Barradell S, Peseta T. Promise and challenge of identifying threshold concepts: a cautionary account of using transactional curriculum inquiry. J Furth High Educ. 2016;40(2):262–75.

Barradell S, Peseta T. Integrating threshold concepts and ways of thinking and practising: supporting physiotherapy students to develop a holistic view of the profession through concept mapping. Int J Pract-Based Learn Health Soc Care. 2018;6(1):24–37.

Berg T, Erichsen M, Hokstad LM. Stuck at the threshold: which strategies do students choose when facing liminality within certain disciplines at a business school? In: Land R, JHF M, Flanagan MT, editors. Threshold concepts in practice, Educational futures rethinking theory and practice. Rotterdam/Boston/Taipei: Sense Publishers; 2016. p. 107–18.

Bhat C, Burm S, Mohan T, Chahine S, Goldszmidt M. What trainees grapple with: a study of threshold concepts on the medicine ward. Med Educ [Internet]. 27 Feb 2018 [cited 2018 Apr 26]; Available from: https://doi.org/10.1111/medu.13526.

Biggs JB, Collis KF. Evaluating the quality of learning: the SOLO taxonomy. New York: Academic; 1982.

Bowden J, Marton F. The university of learning: beyond quality and competence in higher education. 1. paperback ed. London: Routledge; 2004. p. 310.

Chen LYC, Poole G. Grappling with troublesome knowledge. Med Educ. 2018;52(6):584–6.

Chen D-L, Rattray J. Transforming thinking through problem-based learning in the news media literacy class: critical thinking as a threshold concept towards threshold capabilities. Pract Evid Scholarsh Teach Learn High Educ. 2017;12(2):272–93.

Chittleborough C. Threshold concepts in a flipped classroom to facilitate learning about health inequalities. In: Adelaide; 2013 [cited 2016 Aug 16]. Available from: http://www.herga.com.au/uploads/2/2/1/2/22122258/herga_conference_book_sept_2013.pdf

Clouder L. Caring as a 'threshold concept': transforming students in higher education into health (care) professionals. Teach High Educ. 2005;10(4):505–17.

Collett T, Neve H, Stephen N. Using audio diaries to identify threshold concepts in 'softer' disciplines: a focus on medical education. Pract Evid Scholarsh Teach Learn High Educ. 2017;12(2):99–117.. Rattray J, Land R, editors.

Corbally M, Kirwan A, O'Neill C, Kelly M. Simulating troublesome contexts: how multiple roles within ward-based simulations promote professional nursing competence. Int J Pract-Based Learn Health Soc Care. 2018;6(1):18–23.

Corrall S. Crossing the threshold: reflective practice in information literacy development. J Inf Lit. 2017;11(1):23.

Cousin G. An introduction to threshold concepts. Plan Theory. 2006;17(1):4–5.

Cousin G. Threshold concepts: old wine in new bottles or new forms of transactional inquiry? In: Land R, JHF M, Smith J, editors. Threshold concepts within the disciplines, Educational futures: rethinking theory and practice. Rotterdam/Taipei: Sense Publishers; 2008. p. 261–72.

Cousin G. Transactional curriculum inquiry: researching Threshold concepts. In: Cousin G, editor. Researching learning in higher education: an introduction to contemporary methods and approaches [Internet]. New York: Routledge; 2009. p. 201–12. Available from: http://blogs.elon.edu/elontc/files/2011/06/Transactional-Curriculum-Inquiry.docx.

Davies P, Mangan J. Threshold concepts and the integration of understanding in economics. Stud High Educ. 2007;32(6):711–26.

Driessen E. When I say...Metacognition. Med Educ. 2014;48:561–2.

Elliott MN, Kanouse DE, Burkhart Q, Abel GA, Lyratzopoulos G, Beckett MK, et al. Sexual minorities in England have poorer health and worse health care experiences: a national survey. J Gen Intern Med. 2015;30(1):9–16.

English MC, Kitsantas A. Supporting student self-regulated learning in problem- and project-based learning. Interdiscip J Probl-Based Learn [Internet]. 5 Sept 2013 [cited 2019 Jun 15];7(2). Available from: https://docs.lib.purdue.edu/ijpbl/vol7/iss2/6.

Felten P. On the threshold with students. In: Land R, JHF M, Flanagan MT, editors. Threshold concepts in practice, Educational futures rethinking theory and practice. Rotterdam/Boston/Taipei: Sense Publishers; 2016. p. 3–9.

Freeman A, Van Der Vleuten C, Nouns Z, Ricketts C. Progress testing internationally. Med Teach. 2010;32(6):451–5.

Hafferty FW. Beyond curriculum reform: confronting medicine's hidden curriculum. Acad Med. 1998;73(4):403–7.

Hofer AR, Townsend L, Brunetti K. Troublesome concepts and information literacy: investigating threshold concepts for IL instruction. Portal Libr Acad. 2012;12(4):387–405.

Holley KA. The role of threshold concepts in an interdisciplinary curriculum: a case study in neuroscience. Innov High Educ. 2018;43(1):17–30.

Horrigan LA. Tackling the threshold concepts in physiology: what is the role of the laboratory class? Adv Physiol Educ. 2018;42(3):507–15.

Hudson L, Engel-Hills P, Winberg C. Threshold concepts in radiation physics underpinning professional practice in radiation therapy. Int J Pract-Based Learn Health Soc Care. 2018;6(1):53–63.

Hughes G. Developing student research capability for a 'post-truth' world: three challenges for integrating research across taught programmes. Teach High Educ. 2019;24(3):394–411.

Hyde S, Flatau A, Wilson D. Integrating threshold concepts with reflective practice: discussing a theory-based approach for curriculum refinement in dental education. Eur J Dent Educ. 2018;22 (4):e687–97.

Institute of Medicine (US) Committee on understanding and eliminating racial and ethnic disparities in health care. Unequal treatment: confronting racial and ethnic disparities in health care [Internet]. Smedley BD, Stith AY, Nelson AR, editors. Washington (DC): National Academies Press (US); 2003 [cited 2019 Jun 15]. Available from: http://www.ncbi.nlm.nih.gov/books/NBK220358/.

Kempenaar LE, Shanmugam S. Inclusionary othering: a key threshold concept for healthcare education. Med Teach. 2018;40(9):969–70.

Kinchin IM, Cabot LB, Kobus M, Woolford M. Threshold concepts in dental education. Eur J Dent Educ. 2011;15(4):210–5.

Kneebone R. Perspective: simulation and transformational change: the paradox of expertise. Acad Med. 2009;84(7):954–7.

Land R, Meyer JHF. Threshold concepts and troublesome knowledge (5): dynamics of assessment. In: JHF M, Land R, Baillie C, editors. Threshold concepts and transformational learning, Educational futures: rethinking theory and practice. Boston: Sense Publishers; 2010. p. 61–80.

Land R, Meyer JHF. The scalpel and the 'mask': threshold concepts and surgical education. In: Fry H, Kneebone R, editors. Surgical education: theorising an emerging domain, Advances in medical education. Dordrecht: Springer Netherlands; 2011. p. 91–106.

Land R, Rattray J. Guest editorial – special issue: threshold concepts and conceptual difficulty. Pract Evid Scholarsh Teach Learn High Educ. 2017;12(2):63–80.

Land R, Reimann N, Meyer JHF. Enhancing learning and teaching in economics: a digest of research findings and their implications. [Internet]. 2005 ETL project; 2005a [cited 2017 Aug 21]. Available from: http://www.etl.tla.ed.ac.uk/docs/EconomicsDigest.pdf.

Land R, Cousin G, Meyer JHF, Davies P. Threshold concepts and troublesome knowledge: implications for course design and evaluation. In: Rust C, Oxford Centre for Staff and Learning Development, editors. Improving student learning: diversity and inclusivity. Oxford: Oxford Centre for Staff & Learning Development; 2005b. p. 53–64.

Land R, Cousin G, Meyer JHF, Davies P. Conclusion: implications of threshold concepts for course design and evaluation. In: Meyer J, Land R, editors. Overcoming barriers to student understanding: threshold concepts and troublesome knowledge. London/New York: Routledge; 2006. p. 195–206.

Land R, Meyer JHF, Flanagan MT. Preface: threshold concepts in practice. In: Land R, JHF M, editors. Threshold concepts in practice, Educational futures rethinking theory and practice, vol. 68. Rotterdam/Boston/Taipei: Sense Publishers; 2016. p. xi–xxxiv.

Land R, Neve H, Martindale L. Threshold concepts, action poetry and the health professions: an interview with ray land. Int J Pract-Based Learn Health Soc Care. 2018;6(1):45–52.

Lave J, Wenger E. Situated learning: legitimate peripheral participation. Cambridge: Cambridge University Press; 1991.

Levett-Jones T, Bowen L, Morris A. Enhancing nursing students' understanding of threshold concepts through the use of digital stories and a virtual community called 'Wiimali'. Nurse Educ Pract. 2015;15(2):91–6.

Male S. Engineering thresholds: an approach to curriculum renewal: guide for engineering educators on curriculum renewal using threshold concepts. An outcome report of the ALTC project "Engineering thresholds: an approach to curriculum development". [Internet]. Australian government office for learning and teaching; University of Western Australia; 2012 [cited 2018 Apr 26]. Available from: https://www.academia.edu/3045367/Guide_for_Engineering_Educators_on_Curriculum_Renewal_Using_Threshold_Concepts.

Martindale L. Threshold concepts in research and evidence-based practice: investigating troublesome learning for undergraduate nursing students [Internet] [Ph.D.]. [Durham]: Durham University; 2015 [cited 2016 Jul 20]. Available from: http://etheses.dur.ac.uk/10998/.

McAllister M, Lasater K, Stone TE, Levett-Jones T. The reading room: exploring the use of literature as a strategy for integrating threshold concepts into nursing curricula. Nurse Educ Pract. 2015;15(6):549–55.

McCune V, Hounsell D. The development of students' ways of thinking and practising in three final-year biology courses. High Educ. 2005;49(3):255–89.

Meek SEM, Jamieson S. Threshold concepts and troublesome knowledge in the first year curriculum at a UK Medical School. 2014. In: From personal practice to communities of practice [Internet]. Dublin: NAIRTL; p. 122–3. Available from: http://www.nairtl.ie/documents/BookofAbstracts_ONLINE.pdf.

Meek SEM, Gilbert K, Neve H. Using the threshold concept framework to explore student learning by PBL in two UK medical schools. Abstract in: Toward a learning culture. Bergen; ISSOTL; 2019.

Meyer JHF, Land R. Threshold concepts and troublesome knowledge (1) – linkages to ways of thinking and practising. In: Rust C, editor. Improving student learning – ten years on. Oxford: OCSLD; 2003. p. 412–24.

Meyer JHF, Land R. Threshold concepts and troublesome knowledge (2): epistemological considerations and a conceptual framework for teaching and learning. High Educ. 2005;49(3):373–88.

20 Threshold Concepts and Troublesome Knowledge

Meyer JHF, Land R. Threshold concepts and troublesome knowledge: an introduction. In: Meyer J, Land R, editors. Overcoming barriers to student understanding: threshold concepts and troublesome knowledge. London/New York: Routledge; 2006. p. 3–18.

Meyer JHF, Land R, Davies P. Threshold concepts and troublesome knowledge (4): issues of variation and variability. In: Land R, JHF M, Smith J, editors. Threshold concepts within the disciplines, Educational futures: rethinking theory and practice. Rotterdam/Taipei: Sense Publishers; 2008. p. 59–74.

Meyer JHF, Knight DB, Baldock TE, Callaghan DP, Mccredden J, O'Moore L. What to do with a threshold concept. In: Land R, Meyer JHF, Flanagan MT, editors. Threshold concepts in practice. Rotterdam: Sense Publishers; 2016. p. 195–209.

Mezirow J. Perspective transformation. Adult Educ Q. 1978;28(2):100–10.

Mezirow J. Transformative dimensions of adult learning. San Francisco: Jossey-Bass; 1991.

Middendorf J, Pace D. Decoding the disciplines: a model for helping students learn disciplinary ways of thinking. New Dir Teach Learn. 2004;2004(98):1–12.

Moeller JJ, Fawns T. Insights into teaching a complex skill: threshold concepts and troublesome knowledge in electroencephalography (EEG). Med Teach. 2018;40(4):387–94.

Natanasabapathy P, Maathuis-Smith S. Philosophy of being and becoming: a transformative learning approach using threshold concepts. Educ Philos Theory. 2019;51(4):369–79.

Neve H. Learning to become a primary care professional: insights from threshold concept theory. Educ Prim Care. 2019;30(1):5–8.

Neve H, Hanks S. When I say . . . capability. Med Educ. 2016;50(6):610–1.

Neve H, Wearn A, Collett T. What are threshold concepts and how can they inform medical education? Med Teach. 2016;38(8):850–3.

Neve H, Lloyd H, Collett T. Understanding students' experiences of professionalism learning: a 'threshold' approach. Teach High Educ. 2017;22(1):92–108.

Neve H, Gilbert K, Lloyd H. PBL as learning vehicle, threshold concept or capability? Audio-diary research in medical education. In: Savin-Baden M, Tombs G, editors. Threshold concepts and problem-based learning. Rotterdam, The Netherlands: Sense Publishers; 2018. p. 49-64

Neve H, Hothersall E, Rodriguez V. Exploring threshold concepts in population health. Clin Teach 2019. Published online 4 Sep 2019. https://doi.org/10.1111/tct.13087

Nicola-Richmond KM, Pépin G, Larkin H. Transformation from student to occupational therapist: using the Delphi technique to identify the threshold concepts of occupational therapy. Aust Occup Ther J. 2016;63(2):95–104.

Novak JD, Canas AJ. The theory underlying concept maps and how to construct them. Technical report IHMC CmapTools 2006-01 [Internet]. Florida Institute for Human and Machine Cognition; 2006. Available from: http://cmap.ihmc.us/Publications/ResearchPapers/TheoryUnderlyingConceptMaps.pdf.

Perkins D. Constructivism and troublesome knowledge. In: Meyer J, Land R, editors. Overcoming barriers to student understanding: threshold concepts and troublesome knowledge. London/New York: Routledge; 2006. p. 33–47.

Perkins D. Beyond understanding. In: Land R, JHF M, Smith J, editors. Threshold concepts within the disciplines, Educational futures: rethinking theory and practice. Rotterdam/Taipei: Sense Publishers; 2008. p. 3–20.

Pinnock R, Anakin M, Jouart M. Clinical reasoning as a threshold skill. Med Teach. 2019:1–7.

Rattray J. Affective dimensions of liminality. In: Land R, JHF M, Flanagan MT, editors. Threshold concepts in practice, Educational futures rethinking theory and practice. Rotterdam/Boston/Taipei: Sense Publishers; 2016. p. 67–76.

Reimann N. Learning about assessment: the impact of two courses for higher education staff. Int J Acad Dev. 2018;23(2):86–97.

Rodger S, Turpin M. Using threshold concepts to transform entry level curricula. Res Dev High Educ High Educ Edge [Internet]. 2011 July [cited 2016 Jul 20];34. Available from: http://www.herdsa.org.au/publications/conference-proceedings/research-and-development-higher-education-higher-education-56.

Ross PM, Taylor C, Hughes C, Kofod M, Whitaker N, Lutze-Mann L, et al. Threshold concepts: challenging the way we think, teach and, learn in biology. In: JHF M, Land R, Baillie C, editors. Threshold concepts and transformational learning, Educational futures: rethinking theory and practice. Boston: Sense Publishers; 2010. p. 165–78.

Rowbottom DP. Demystifying threshold concepts. J Philos Educ. 2007;41(2):263–70.

Ryan T. Medical student reflections of newborn medicine: looking back for threshold concepts. 2014. In: From personal practice to communities of practice [Internet]. Dublin:Ireland: NAIRTL; p. 28–9. Available from: http://www.nairtl.ie/documents/BookofAbstracts_ONLINE.pdf.

Savin-Baden M. Second life PBL: liminality, liquidity and lurking, keynote speech. In: Republic Polytechnic, Singapore; 2007.

Savin-Baden M. Liquid learning and troublesome spaces: journeys from the threshold. In: Land R, JHF M, Smith J, editors. Threshold concepts within the disciplines, Educational futures: rethinking theory and practice. Rotterdam/Taipei: Sense Publishers; 2008. p. 75–88.

Schuwirth LWT, Van der Vleuten CPM. Programmatic assessment: from assessment of learning to assessment for learning. Med Teach. 2011;33(6):478–85.

Shopkow L. What decoding the disciplines can offer threshold concepts. In: JHF M, Land R, Baillie C, editors. Threshold concepts and transformational learning, Educational futures: rethinking theory and practice. Boston: Sense Publishers; 2010. p. 317–31.

Sibbett C, Thompson W. Nettlesome knowledge, liminality and the taboo in cancer and art therapy experiences: implications for learning and teaching. In: Land R, JHF M, Smith J, editors. Threshold concepts within the disciplines, Educational futures: rethinking theory and practice. Rotterdam/Taipei: Sense Publishers; 2008. p. 227–42.

Smith JA, Blackburn S, Nestel D. Crossing the thresholds: challenges in the commencement of consultant cardiothoracic surgical practice. Heart Lung Circ. 2015;24:e15.

Smith JA, Blackburn S, Nestel D. Challenges in the commencement of consultant surgical practice: a study of threshold concepts in junior cardiothoracic surgeons. Int J Pract-Based Learn Health Soc Care. 2018;6(1):78–95.

Spillane S. The failure of whiteness in art education: a personal narrative informed by critical race theory. J Soc Theory Art Educ [Internet]. 2015 Aug 26;35(1). Available from: https://scholarscompass.vcu.edu/jstae/vol35/iss1/6.

Springfield E(L)A, Rodger S, Gustafsson L. Threshold concepts and authentic assessment: learning to think like an occupational therapist. Pract Evid Scholarsh Teach Learn High Educ. 2017;12(2):125–56.

Taylor C. Threshold concepts, troublesome knowledge and ways of thinking and practising – can we tell the difference in biology? In: Land R, JHF M, Smith J, editors. Threshold concepts within the disciplines, Educational futures: rethinking theory and practice. Rotterdam/Taipei: Sense Publishers; 2008. p. 185–96.

Taylor C, Meyer J. The testable hypothesis as a threshold concept for biology students. In: JHF M, Land R, Baillie C, editors. Threshold concepts and transformational learning, Educational futures: rethinking theory and practice. Boston: Sense Publishers; 2010. p. 179–92.

Taylor C, Liu D, Pye M, Tzioumis V, Meyer J. Using threshold concepts to design a first year biology curriculum. Proc Aust Conf Sci Math Educ Former UniServe Sci Conf [Internet]. 29 Aug 2012 [cited 2018 Apr 26]. Available from: https://openjournals.library.sydney.edu.au/index.php/IISME/article/view/6018.

Taylor, CE. Concepts in biology: do they fit the definition? In: Meyer J, Land R, editors. Overcoming barriers to student understanding: threshold concepts and troublesome knowledge. London/New York: Routledge; 2006. p. 87–99.

Timmermans JA. Changing our minds: the developmental potential of threshold concepts. In: Threshold Concepts and Transformational Learning. Meyer JHF, Land R, Baillie C, editors. Rotterdam: Sense Publishers; 2010. p. 3–19.

Timmermans JA, Meyer JHF. A framework for working with university teachers to create and embed 'integrated threshold concept knowledge' (ITCK) in their practice. Int J Acad Dev. 2017;17:1–15.

Treloar A, Stone T, McMillan M. Learning about mental health nursing: linking threshold concepts to practice, learning about mental health nursing: linking threshold concepts to practice. J Probl-Based Learn J Probl-Based Learn. 2018;5(1):21–8.

Vaughan K. Vocational thresholds: developing expertise without certainty in general practice medicine. J Prim Health Care. 2016;8(2):99.

Vosniadou S, Ioannides C. From conceptual development to science education: a psychological point of view. Int J Sci Educ. 1998;20(10):1213–30.

Vygotsky LS. Mind in society: development of higher psychological processes. Boston: Harvard University Press; 1978.

Wearn A, O'Callaghan A, Barrow M. Becoming a different doctor: identifying threshold concepts: when doctors in training spend six months with a hospital palliative care team. In: Land R, JHF M, Flanagan MT, editors. Threshold concepts in practice, Educational futures rethinking theory and practice. Rotterdam/Boston/Taipei: Sense Publishers; 2016. p. 223–38.

Wilkinson L. The problem with threshold concepts [Internet]. Sense & Reference. 2014 [cited 2018 Apr 26]. Available from: https://senseandreference.wordpress.com/2014/06/19/the-problem-with-threshold-concepts/.

Wilkinson I. Nurturing and complexity – threshold concepts in geriatric medicine. Int J Pract-Based Learn Health Soc Care. 2018;6(1):64–77.

Zimmerman BJ. A social cognitive view of self-regulated academic learning. J Educ Psychol. 1989;81(3):329–39.

Social Semiotics: Theorizing Meaning Making

21

Jeff Bezemer

Contents

Introduction 386
Sign Making 387
Doing Clinical Work 388
    Interpretation 388
    Expression 391
Reviewing Clinical Work 396
Projecting Clinical Work 397
Conclusion 399
Cross-References 400
References 400

Abstract

This chapter outlines a theoretical framework to account for practices of meaning making in health care and sets out an agenda for clinical educational research. It shows how meaning making pervades all aspects of clinical work and how it can be explored and made explicit within a framework derived from social semiotics. The chapter illustrates how the framework produces accounts of the ways in which clinicians make sense of and interact with the world, in situations where they give, review, and imagine care. It explores how clinicians interpret, and communicate through, human bodies, tools, and technologies, giving meaning to, and expressing meaning through, distinct material forms. In so doing, the chapter begins to render visible the semiotic skills that clinicians develop to prepare for, provide, and evaluate clinical care.

J. Bezemer (✉)
Institute of Education, University College London, London, UK
e-mail: j.bezemer@ucl.ac.uk

© Springer Nature Singapore Pte Ltd. 2023
D. Nestel et al. (eds.), *Clinical Education for the Health Professions*,
https://doi.org/10.1007/978-981-15-3344-0_26

Keywords

Social semiotics · Clinical education · Sign making · Communication · Multimodality

Introduction

Clinicians make signs all the time. They look for, interpret, and/or produce such varied formations as the yellowness of a human skin, the depth of a surgical stitch, the extent of a hand movement, the pitch contour, syntax and lexical items of spoken utterances, the waveform on a patient monitor, and the contrasts of entities rendered visible on a CT scan. This chapter explores how clinicians (learn to) recognize these forms as meaningful entities, i.e., as *signs*.

The chapter makes three contributions. First, it develops an encompassing model for understanding practices of meaning making that have hitherto been dealt with by separate branches of semiotics. Medical semiotics has been claimed to be one of the oldest branches of semiotics (Sebeok 1985); it explores how clinicians and patients interpret and communicate about the patient body. Social semiotics (Hodge and Kress 1988) developed from critical linguistics and has to date engaged little with clinical work. Where it has, its focus was on communication and learning, rather than on meaning making more broadly (cf. Bezemer et al. 2012). The framework outlined in this chapter aims to encompass meaning making across all clinical work, providing theoretical means of recognizing, documenting, and explaining how clinicians interpret the world around them, express themselves, and communicate with others.

Second, the chapter advances social semiotics by developing its foundational concepts to fit the distinct and multifaceted character of meaning making in the clinical world. Traditional semiotics has brought forth conceptual models of the basic "building block" for making meaning, the sign, and classifications of different types of signs (de Saussure 1916; Peirce 1931). *Social* semiotics has advanced semiotic theory through empirical research and refocused attention on the sign maker in the material world and the social mechanisms that shape meaning making. It has explored principles of and resources for meaning making in public media, such as magazines, films, and social media, and in traditional pedagogic spaces, such as textbooks and classrooms (van Leeuwen 2005). The chapter will show that clinical education raises new questions for social semiotics, e.g., about the body as a resource and target for meaning making.

Third, the chapter draws from original qualitative data sets from research on clinical practice and clinical education in hospitals in the UK, along with examples from previously published research. They cover different types of texts and activities that involve a range of different technologies. Main data sources include video recordings of clinical work in the operating theatre (Bezemer 2015) and in situ simulations of resuscitation events in a pediatric intensive care unit. These materials were explored through detailed transcription, annotation, and micro-analysis (Bezemer et al. 2017).

Looking across these data sets, the chapter explores two kinds of semiotic work: interpretation and expression. The focal setting for exploring these phenomena is the clinical environment, where clinical work "gets done." Following this, the chapter considers types of activities and texts aimed at reviewing and projecting clinical work, respectively. The chapter opens with an outline of basic theoretical premises of sign making and concludes with a discussion of implications of the framework for learning and clinical education.

Sign Making

The sign is the basic unit of meaning making. Eco (1976), following Peirce, defines it as "everything that, on the grounds of a previously established social convention, can be taken as something standing for something else" (p. 16). The model of the sign adopted in this chapter originates from de Saussure (1916) and has been adapted by Kress (2010) to refer to conjunctions of meaning and a material form. *Social* semiotics is concerned with the ways in which people recognize (selections of) forms and invest them with meaning. Inscriptions, sounds, vibrations, shapes, shades, and movements are all examples of forms ("signifiers") that can come to stand for something ("signifieds") to somebody.

Social semiotics draws on four basic premises about sign making. The first premise is that sign makers draw on *regularities* and *conventions* developed from social histories. Over time, some forms have come to be associated with particular meanings among a social network, e.g., medical students, radiologists, theatre nurses, and patients with Parkinson disease. The regularities are the result of social interactions. At the same time, they enable members of the network to communicate: they are generative, allowing people to guess, with some degree of plausibility, what others mean by, e.g., a gesture or word, or how they might interpret "natural" forms such as the yellowness of a patient's skin. Social semiotics sets out to identify such regularities in sign making that a given network has developed over time in response to their social needs.

The second premise is that sign makers recognize *configurations* of and *relations* between different forms. For example, clinicians attach meaning to a collection of noticeable forms on a patient body. Makers and readers of a textbook make connections between (selections of) graphic elements that appear on the page: orthographic elements, diagrammatic elements, photographic elements, and so on. Parties to face-to-face encounters also make connections between forms of various kinds: a co-occurring string of sounds and hand movement may be recognized as a speech-gesture-whole, carrying meaning that is greater than and different to the sum of its individual parts. Social semiotics aims to identify the principles underpinning these combinatory operations.

The third premise is that sign making is always *particular* to a sign maker and a situation. That means that even if a network of sign makers can draw on a long history of social interaction and strongly developed shared understandings, their sign making is never entirely predictable. Shared understandings may have been made explicit in grammars, dictionaries, textbooks, and so on, yet these "code books" do not account for the situated semiotic work of an individual sign maker. Sign makers use regularities in sign making as resources, rather than as prescriptions, in response to dynamic, unpredictable, emergent situations. The signs that people make, even when orienting to what appears to be the "same" form, will vary depending on their prior professional/life experiences. Social semiotics sets out to identify how sign makers through each new semiotic act transform meaning potentials of forms, thus expanding possibilities for interpretation and expression (Kress 2010). The notion of *transformation* acknowledges that sign makers do not "copy," or "acquire," somehow straightforwardly "internalizing" or "absorbing" signs made by others (Bezemer and Kress 2016).

The fourth premise is that *semiotic effort* is gradual: the work that sign makers put into interpretation and expression varies. Their commitment is not evenly spread; some signifiers are given more attention than others. Engaging with Twitter, for example, "reading" might mean anything from scrolling down five tweets per second to identifying tweets that might contain relevant information to skim-reading a text of 180 words and scrutinizing a CT scan of an atypical case that was posted. Equally, a clinician in conversation with a patient making a drawing to locate a disease will focus their efforts on those elements that they want to highlight and deem of particular relevance to the communication. Social semiotics aims to identify the principles of selection and distribution of effort. This includes a concern with the means that designers have at their disposal to shape the semiotic efforts of others.

Doing Clinical Work

Interpretation

To anyone entering a clinical environment, there is a wealth of "stuff" to attend to and interpret. As sign makers, clinicians and patients engage selectively with that environment; they recognize some forms and subject some of them to interpretation. By selectively recognizing and giving meaning to forms, they build a subjective reality, their "Umwelt" (von Uexküll 1936/1992).

Sign makers might recognize forms in any materiality. Clinicians are particularly likely to recognize forms on artifacts (artifactual forms) and bodies (corporeal forms). Artifactual forms are, for example, forms recognized on buildings, tools, documents, and other relatively durable structures designed by other human agents, who may or may not be co-present. Corporeal forms are forms recognized on or in the bodies of other human actors who are co-present, physically or virtually.

Sign makers can attribute social functions to forms they recognize. First, artifactual and corporeal forms may be interpreted as having been produced to communicate, i.e., in deliberate acts of expression by another semiotic agent who is addressing others, for example, using speech, gesture, or image. Second, they may be interpreted as having been produced to accomplish practical tasks. For example, clothing, tools, and body movements may be taken to have been produced for this purpose.

Any form can be subjected to interpretation, i.e., be made into a sign, including forms produced for practical purposes. For example, scrubs can be read as a sign of health and safety regulations and a body movement as a sign of what someone is going to do next and perhaps even as signs of what the interpreter is expected to do to facilitate the completion of the task. For example, an ICU nurse might establish when and how to assist an anesthetic trainee preparing for intubation on the basis of interpretation of the anesthetist's bodily actions. A consultant anesthetist might establish when to provide what instructions or when to take over from the trainee on the same basis. A team leader might interpret repeated attempts to intubate as signs of trouble and propose to the member giving chest compressions to stop for a moment. Thus the communicative and practical functions of forms are not always separable, all the more so when teams work on the tacit agreement that a particular body movement should be taken as instruction, as is often the case in clinical settings.

A special class of corporeal forms that clinicians attend to is what they call "signs and symptoms." In Western medicine, "symptoms" refer to signs made by the patient, i.e., certain sensations experienced by the patient are described by them as "dizziness," or "nausea." "Signs" are signs made by a clinician, who observes forms directly, such as skin color, or, indirectly, using tools such as a thermometer. These forms are often thought of as "natural signs" that have not been produced for communicative (or indeed practical) purposes. Alternatively, living organisms may be treated as semiotic agents that communicate with each other, their host (the patient), and their environment (e.g., the clinician). In that perspective, the patient body becomes "an inextricably complex *text*" (Sebeok 1985, p. 2, my emphasis).

Social semiotics is particularly interested in how clinicians and patients develop semiotic resources to *read* and communicate about this "body text" in their respective social networks. The underlying disposition of clinicians that shapes this "body text reading" might be described as a "professional vision" (Goodwin 1994) or, more specifically, as the "clinical gaze" (Foucault 1963/2003). Of interest are "the terms [. . .] that physicists [. . .] have worked out to transpose sign processes of their fields of phenomena into the human language and that can be interpreted as translations (Jakobson 1971)" (von Uexküll 1986, p. 209). These meaning making practices underpin all clinical action and all expression in response to engagement with a patient body. It includes practices of seeing, touching, and hearing through which the clinician comes to recognize forms as instances ("tokens") of categories ("types") developed and shared within the clinical community and an expressive repertoire that enables them to represent and communicate about these forms.

Technologies assist health professionals by mediating sensory experiences, e.g., a stethoscope amplifying sound or a laparoscopic monitor magnifying the view of the camera. Other technologies, such as the patient monitor, help *translate* sensory experiences. They have taken over some of the sensory and semiotic work from

Fig. 1 Medical Fellow (left) with Foundation Doctor (right)

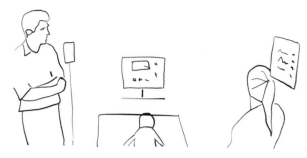

clinicians, automatically rendering measurements ("sensations") into numerical values (e.g., thermometer, or pulse reader) or graphic representations (e.g., imaging). New technologies are taking over more and different kinds of semiotic work. For example, computer vision supports the detection of breast cancer, thus shaping a judgment that was traditionally made by radiologists. These changes are having profound effects and warrant further social semiotic research.

Interpretation is shaped by many social factors, including training, experience, and role. Clinicians recognize different forms and attach different meanings to forms they recognize, whether on a patient, a colleague, or an artifact such as a CT scan (efforts to minimize these differences are discussed in the following section). The same applies to processes of selection for interpretation from a wider field. Take the Medical Fellow (a post at resident level) in Fig. 1. When he arrived by the patient's bedside, he looked for the Foundation Doctor (doctor within first 2 years of graduation from medical school) who paged him. When she started presenting the case ("Hi, this Katie, she's just come from theatre..."), she changed her gaze in accordance with the information she provides about the patient. When she said that Katie is hypotensive and tachycardic, she looked at the patient monitor, thus drawing attention to the evidence of that claim. When she referred to a nurse who was preparing bolus, she looked over to her. All the while, the junior doctor followed her gaze. The Foundation Doctor's gaze thus shaped the Medical Fellow's engagement with this clinical environment. Some minutes later, the Consultant (attending physician) arrived, called in by the Medical Fellow. Unlike him, she scanned the environment as she arrived, displaying orientation to the patient, infusion pump, patient monitor, and some members of the team, respectively. Their differing approaches to the environment are illustrated in Figs. 1 and 2.

These patterns have been explored in more detail using eye tracking technology. For example, Law et al. (2018) found that members of resuscitation teams direct 35% of their fixations on the patient and 26% on peripheral displays. In another study, inexperienced anesthetists were found to focus more on the patient monitor when a critical incident happened during induction, while spending less time engaging with manual tasks; the experienced anesthetist's time spent looking at the monitor did not change, and they spent more time on manual tasks (Schulz et al. 2011).

21 Social Semiotics: Theorizing Meaning Making

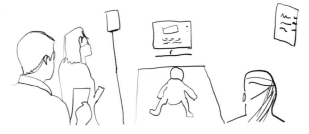

Fig. 2 Medical Fellow (left), Consultant (middle) and Foundation Doctor (right)

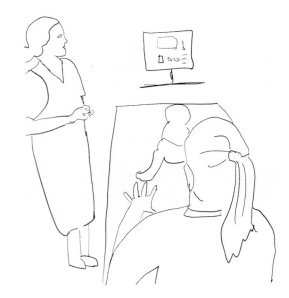

Fig. 3 Gesture in the ICU

Expression

Modes

Some of the artifactual and corporeal forms produced for communicative purposes are modal. Modes are conventionalized means of communicating meaning that are organized around a particular set of material resources (artifactual or corporeal) and means of and tools for manipulating these resources. Speech, writing, gesture, and image are examples of modes. Modes serve as semiotic resources for sign makers who, with each communicative act, transform them; it is the sign maker that "fixes" meaning, not the modes.

Modes typically co-occur. For instance, in the ICU, when staff call in colleagues, as in Figs. 1 and 2, much of what is communicated involves speech. Writing is used by the scribe to record how the event unfolds. The patient monitor translates vital signs in several different modes of communication: numbers, diagrams, writing, and sound tunes. Gesture also plays a role, as in the case depicted in Fig. 3.

The figure shows the Foundation Doctor making a "squeezing" hand movement, thus simulating the movements involved in "bagging" for ventilation, a common manual operation in this setting. The gesture indexes the object that the operation is typically performed on: the breathing apparatus. And the gesture stands for a command. By reaching out her left arm, she "places" the gesture in the direction of the nurse: she addresses her. Timing – the gesture is made just after the crash call – and the proximity of the nurse relative to the object to be pulled out provide further contextual grounding for the interpretation of the gesture.

Modes are typically combined to make signs with simultaneously produced forms. For instance, a surgical educator might identify a specific object in a field through pointing while describing it to a medical student in medical terms (e.g., "That's the liver"). In this case, a gesture is combined with a spoken utterance; they are co-produced, and semiotically interrelated. Without either one or the other, the joint identification of a relevant form in a complex, "messy" field would have been difficult to achieve.

A choice of modes is generally motivated by an assessment of the distinct semiotic potential of modes. For example, the Foundation Doctor's choice of gesture, as opposed to speech, might be explained by a combination of the following factors: (1) talk was already going on between the Consultant and the Medical Fellow; (2) what had to be communicated was expressible in gesture; and (3) given their relative position, the gesture could be performed within sight of the nurse.

As well as communicative modes that are also used in everyday life, such as speech, gesture, and image, clinicians have developed modes that are organized around certain operations on the patient body. To them, the patient body is more than an object on or in which forms are read. It is also a moldable object through which they can communicate with others: through intervention they leave traces, which might be read by colleagues, trainees, and the patient. Learning to read these traces is a major part of the clinical experience. For example, a medical student learns to recognize the possibilities for manipulating stitching material and human tissue (using tools), while at the same time learning what the resulting forms stand for in the medical world. Some stitching may signify a "rough and ready" job; other stitching signifies strength, care, insight in suturing material, and so on. Aesthetics come into this, as evidenced by the frequent use of evaluative adjectives, such as "nice." Knowing that their work will be read, assessed even, gives communicative potential to the act of stitching: it becomes a means for the trainee to communicate with the assessor. Clinicians frequently encounter traces of interventional work from colleagues on and in the bodies of patients, which they subject to interpretation. In other areas, such as reconstructive and plastic surgery, the work is also visible to and judged by the patient.

As with all modes, the moldable body can be classified in terms of the material "stuff"; it is made up of different types of human tissue, prosthetic material, and their basic properties. These properties might include, durability, elasticity, weight, and so on. They have an effect on possibilities for manipulation and thus on possibilities for sign making: they put limits on the forms that can be obtained in a given materiality, *and* they provide dimensions for variation. Material variation produces potential for expression. As sign makers gain experience in fashioning new forms out of certain material resources, they expand their possibilities for expression. Through interaction in social networks, people working with the same material resources will develop understandings of variations in form and of the ways in which other members of the network have exploited these possibilities for making meaning. In other words, the capacity to manipulate material resources comes with a recognition of certain regularities in meaning-form connections. It is for this reason that surgery is often described as an art and craft and compared to, e.g., the work of tailors, potters, and so on (cf. Schlegel and Kneebone 2018).

Directing Others

Each mode offers distinct possibilities to educators, team leaders, and others to guide engagement and interaction within the clinical environment. For instance, the attention of a clinician can be shaped through spatial arrangement of equipment, tools, technologies, and people in a room and through the arrangement of graphic elements on a patient monitor, a page from a textbook, or packaging. What the designers want their addressees to differentiate between can be given different colors; what needs to be highlighted can be given a more central place or a bigger space than other elements; and so on. New 3D-image techniques and technologies projecting predesigned visual maps onto patient bodies take guidance through graphics to a new level, helping interventional clinicians safely navigate anatomical structures.

In the absence of such advanced technologies, gaze and gesture can be used to direct someone's attention. Figure 3 already showed how a Foundation Doctor guides through gaze. Pointing gestures are frequently made when clinicians jointly inspect parts of a patient's body, directly, or aided by optical technologies. Distinct possibilities for shaping engagement are also offered by *contiguous gesture*, which can be used by a supervisor to, e.g., position the hand of a trainee, as for example when a retractor needs re-placing (Mondada 2014). Speech, too, provides means to draw attention and provide guidance.

Each of these modes offers distinct possibilities for shaping engagement. Take the command in operating theatres. In speech, a surgeon can choose an (elliptic) imperative ("Scalpel!"), an interrogative ("Can I have the scalpel please?"), or a declarative ("I need a scalpel"). Each grammatical form projects a different social relation, form of politeness, and/or sense of urgency. We might compare this to commands in gesture. How might a surgeon make a command by holding up their hand, and what might be the effects? A hand gesture always involves a stroke, its main movement. After the stroke, the hand is sometimes held in position for some time before the hand is withdrawn again (Kendon 2004). The speed of the stroke, the place where it is held in position, subsequent "grabbing" movements of the tips of fingers, and so on, all offer means of projecting social relations, forms of politeness, and a sense of urgency. By combining these forms with facial expressions, the possibilities for expression are multiplied: a hand held up while turning one's gaze in the direction of the addressee and displaying a smile means differently relative to the same gesture produced without a smile. We could extend this to the patient monitor interface: how do its graphics and sound tunes vary, and how has this variation been used to design different types of commands for action? That is another question for further semiotic research.

Developing Shared Understandings

Crucially, in a clinical environment, modes provide means for *expressing* understandings of the patient's condition. This includes possibilities for communicating sensory experiences. As clinicians inspect, palpate, and auscultate, they make meaning; they attach meaning to corporeal forms. Speech, writing, drawing, and other modes of communication are available to articulate the meanings made, enabling them to develop joint accounts of the patient and *calibrate* (Goodwin 2018) their understandings.

A number of different factors prompt deliberate efforts at developing shared understandings through communication: first, asymmetries in knowledge about a patient. For example, when the Consultant in Fig. 2 arrived on the scene, the Medical Fellow told her that the patient has just come back a few hours ago from having had TGA (transposition of the great arteries) surgery. The Foundation Doctor then adds that she's lost saturation. The Consultant, looking at the patient monitor, then remarked that she is hypotensive and started a recount of their joint observations ("So she's two hours post-op..."). Second, clinicians experiencing semiotic challenges in, e.g., interpreting corporeal forms. For example, in one laparoscopic cholecystectomy, the operating surgeon started the following dialogue with two experienced colleagues who were co-present:

SURG1: Look at that
SURG2: It's, it's weird. I would go into that space
SURG1: That might be the artery and that might be the duct. Can you see this anatomy
SURG2: Just twisted
SURG3: Yeah, it's really weird, it's twisting round each other
SURG1: Yeah. and what that's doing is it's, torting the Hartmann's pouch over

Speech, along with gesture, is used here to express uncertainty and hypotheses about what-is-what in this patient and how it compares to "normal" anatomy and about what might be the best next action.

Third, asymmetries in experience prompt calibration efforts. The example in Fig. 4 features a surgical trainee who is operating under the supervision of a consultant. The trainee is separating tissue that attaches the colon to the abdominal wall. The Consultant explains that "this bit is best done with your left hand closed [...] So that left hand kind of closed into the space and then like sweeping movements leftwards." A few minutes later, he takes over and demonstrates that movement. This is where the teaching episode in Fig. 4 begins.

The supervisor, now operating, demonstrates a movement, drawing attention to it by making the movement seamlessly yet slowly. He uses speech to connect the

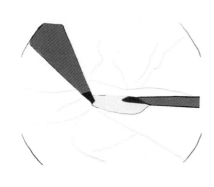

"So once we get into that position this is the movement that I was saying. [...] Now can I just get a bit of more traction higher up there. So Simon what I need is counter-traction. This is something Dave that you must get me to do when I'm giving back to you in a minute. To actually just get me moving upwards and opposite you the entire time. So you can hold that one there. You can see that that little flat bit of tissue now becomes a cul-de-sac. And that cul-de-sac is kind of what I'm always aiming to do. Because then I can put that left hand instrument in closed. And with the right hand just kind of thin it out."

Fig. 4 Surgical demonstration

movement to the description he had provided of it a little earlier; and to instruct the assistant what he needs to do to ensure that the movement produces the desired effect; and to instruct the trainee to mimic those instructions when he is back in the operating role. At one point, the supervisor also repositions the instrument held by the assistant. He then draws attention to what he describes as "that little flat bit of tissue" and to the shape it is adopting as a result of their concerted action – a shape he describes metaphorically as a "cul-de-sac." He then describes the movements he subsequently makes with his two instruments. The line drawing in Fig. 4 captures the point at which these are described as "thin[ning] it out."

In this fragment, the forms that the supervisor makes serve both practical and communicative functions. His manual movements, mediated by the instruments, not only serve to proceed with the dissection, they are also gestures that represent, iconically, the hand movements that this trainee is required to learn. These manipulations are shown *and* described. Speech is also used to describe changes in the stuff that is being manipulated, highlighting the body as medium.

Achieving shared understandings is limited by the expressive potential of the modes of communication available. This is felt sharply by patients trying to articulate the pain they feel, for example. Yet even with the semiotic resources that clinicians have developed over time to suit their needs many challenges remain. Not all forms that surgeons want to draw attention to have generic names, and so the surgeon in Fig. 4 relies heavily on pointing gestures to identify what area he refers to when talking about "that little flat bit of tissue." As well as limitations of naming parts of a human body, modes are limited in their potential to represent body movements and other kinds of processes, and individual sign makers have limited access to the specialist resources of surgeons. This has implications for what can be taught in what mode. It also highlights the need for educators to learn to be creative semiotically.

Reviewing Clinical Work

Clinical work is frequently reviewed by those who were party to that environment and external observers. Typically, this happens when reviewers are spatially and/or temporally detached from the clinical event under review. Different types of reviewing events can be characterized in terms of who reviews what for whom, how, and why. In the UK, examples of common types of reviewing events include the debriefing, workplace-based assessment, and the Schwartz Round.

Like doing clinical work, reviewing it is mediated by modes of communication. For instance, a clinical event may be recorded in written notes or numbers representing judgments along pre-defined categories ("rating"). It may also be automatically recorded, e.g., as video or digital data from equipment, sensors, and so on; all these recordings can be subjected to interpretation. Reviewers express their interpretations and build joint accounts of (recollections or recordings of) events using speech, gesture, and so on and may produce an official report, typically in writing. Reviewing, then, is an instance of "resemiotization" (Iedema 2003), in which meanings are made and re-made ("translated") according to specific needs and semiotic structures and possibilities for expression. This comes with a shift in focus from developing (shared) understandings of the patient to developing (shared) understandings of the clinician.

For example, Pelletier and Kneebone (2016) shows what participants in simulation-based training courses in the UK selected for expression and evaluation in their debriefings and how these accounts were then sampled and re-categorized by the course facilitators, e.g., as instances of strong "nontechnical skills" and other pre-defined categories derived from human factors. As they translated the participants' accounts, the facilitators introduced hierarchical and causal relations between the actions and events described by the participants, replacing, e.g., cohesive devices such as "and" with, e.g., "so," thus reshaping the account to suit the institutional aims of the training course.

Iedema et al. (2015) explored how clinicians gave meaning to video recordings of their own practices in an Australian hospital ward. Prompted to reflect on infection control, one junior doctor in their study noticed that "I put the dirty crepe bandage on his clean bed" (nurse) and that "I scratch my face when I'm in there" (p. 158). Collaboratively teams noticed cross-contamination risks when transferring a patient from the ward to an isolation room and designed solutions to mitigate these risks. As in the case reported by Pelletier, these reviewing practices were framed as opportunities for learning through reflection. One important difference between the two examples is that the reviewing event described by Iedema et al. was not only retrospective; it also was also prospective in that the participants jointly discussed how to redesign their own clinical environment to further minimize risk of infection control.

Schwartz Rounds are explicitly framed as a forum for reflection, rather than an improvement or problem solving exercise (Point of Care Foundation n.d.). They have been introduced in the USA, UK, and elsewhere to create a space for healthcare staff to talk about the emotional impact of their work. Here, clinical experiences are retold as personal stories, rather than joint accounts. Originally aimed at staff, Schwartz Rounds are now being opened up to medical students (Gishen et al. 2016). On top of these institutionally supported, structured forums, clinicians and students review their experiences in numerous other as yet little researched discursive spaces, e.g., in mentor- and student-led, curricular and extra-curricular, and regular and one-off meetings, and online and offline, local and global, open and closed, and inclusive and exclusive spaces. Each of these will afford distinct types of modes of communication for reviewing (speech, writing, dance, painting) and possibilities for participation, reflection, expression, interaction, and learning.

Other review types are embedded in a formal assessment structure. For example, in the UK workplace-based assessments are part of a framework set up by professional bodies responsible for postgraduate medical training. Junior doctors are required to organize for their involvement in different types of clinical events to be reviewed by their supervisors. They are then expected to jointly record the outcomes of the review in writing on an online pro forma. For instance, the pro forma used in surgery (ICSP 2018) asks the assessor to comment on "strengths," "development needs," and "recommended actions." The trainee is asked to address "trainee reflections on this activity," "what did I learn from this experience," "what did I do well," "what do I need to improve or change? How will I change it?" In practice, both sections are usually completed by the junior doctor and validated by the assessor some period of time after the event. The written comments found on these forms do not "replicate" the reviewing event; they are translations of selected observations expressed during the reviewing event. The selections and translations are shaped by the pre-defined categories on the form and by what can be expressed in writing and in anticipation of future use of the forms, which become part of a portfolio that is considered annually by an assessment panel. Research of this meaning making process, and the "gains and losses" involved in this type of reviewing, is under way (Tahim et al. 2019).

Projecting Clinical Work

Another area of semiotic work for and by clinicians is the making of texts that *project* clinical work. They include guidelines, protocols, learning resources, and reference books, such as anatomy atlases. While the reviewing practices discussed in the previous section are (primarily) retrospective, these are prospective. As with doing and reviewing clinical work, projecting it involves efforts by one party to shape engagement and understandings of others using a range of different modes of communication.

Take, for example, current guidance for health professionals on communication (Royal College of Physicians 2017). Like so many guides, it describes and visually represents a model for handovers which is comprised of four discrete elements that have a fixed ordering: situation, background, assessment, and recommendation. As with the categories that the facilitators imposed in Pelletier's study, and the rubrics

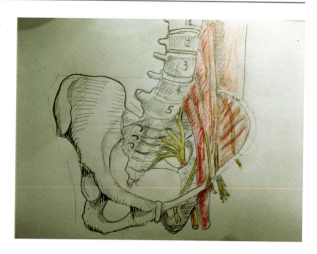

Fig. 5 Drawing by surgeon. (Copyright Tom Quick)

on the WBA pro forma, they are pre-defined and get reproduced through reviewing and projecting.

Elsewhere, clinicians produce their own texts to prepare for clinical work. For example, Fig. 5 is a drawing by a peripheral nerve surgeon that was used in communication with a pelvic surgeon, highlighting the sciatic nerve in the pelvis he was planning to operate on.

Questions that social semiotics raises in this area relate to, e.g., representational processes of selection (what is included and what is excluded?), arrangement (how do representational forms cohere?), foregrounding (what is highlighted, what is backgrounded?), and social positioning (what relation between drawer and reader does it project?) (Bezemer and Kress 2016). Consider, for instance, two learning resources designed for medical students preparing for the OSCE skin suturing station (discussed in Bezemer 2017). One is a set of revision notes; the other one is a short video published on YouTube (https://youtu.be/bE8SEOXjTpo). The "notes" consist mainly of writing, with some still images. The video consists of a much wider range of means of representation, including speech, gesture, and animation. (Note that the popularity of YouTube and other video sharing platforms among clinical learners is testimony to the potential of *video* for demonstration).

The two multimodal configurations project skin suturing differently. The written notes offer generalized, abstract instructions – "rules of thumb" – which students can apply in the actual, concrete situations they will be confronted with. For students who revised using the notes, the semiotic work involved is largely that of deduction: they are to follow a set of general rules to deal with the concrete, unique instance given in the OSCE. The video, unlike the notes, is organized around a concrete situation, showing an actual (simulated) body part (and, occasionally, patient), an actual suture and skin pad, etc., from which generalizations are sometimes inferred and articulated in writing superimposed and in animations added in the post production, edited stage. For students watching, the semiotic work demanded is largely that of induction, i.e., to analyze and infer from the concrete, unique instance shown a set of general rules that they can follow. While in principle both writing and moving image can be used to design the two learning environments, the level of "concreteness" achieved in the video would be difficult to match in the written notes; and the level of abstraction in the writing would be difficult to achieve in the video.

In each case, the modes used shape the representation of the suturing procedure. For instance, by default, the video shows all movements involved in suturing continuously. In writing, choices always need to be made about what movements to select and which ones to leave out. Movements that appear simultaneously on the video are to be presented sequentially, one after another, in writing. Each of these epistemological "losses" may at the same time count as pedagogic gains: a "reduced" account may be perfectly fitting to certain trainees, relative to their knowledge and skills.

Given the mediating effects of modes, no two learning resources or activities provide the same potential for learning, even if they were designed to "cover" the "same" body of knowledge. In the contemporary world, clinical trainees are rarely restricted to only one site. Instead they move between –and learn – across many different sites, each uniquely configured: workplace, simulation center, online platforms, etc. Social semiotics provides means for exploring what is "unique" in each and how they are used by educators and trainees to facilitate learning.

Experimental research is used to explore the effects that multimodality can have on learning. For instance, in one study, medical students were given learning materials on chest drains. One group was given a handout made up of traditional written text and diagrammatic representations, while another group was given a handout that included comical drawings (Junhasavasdikul et al. 2017). The latter appeared to have made greater progress in the 2-week period between the pre- and post-test. Similar questions can be asked about the effect of relative new text genres, such as (serious) *games* (see Gorbanev et al. 2018 for a review), and the potential of new technologies, such as touch screens and virtual reality, and AI, for creating multimodal, interactive, and personalized learning environments, which simultaneously project *and* review (simulated) clinical work.

Conclusion

At present, the domains for meaning making outlined above are not given equal recognition in curricula for clinical trainees. One area that *is* acknowledged in the medical curriculum as a matter of meaning making is diagnosis. Hence, clinical educators have taught medical students' principles of meaning making through the interpretation of art, on the assumption that the capacities for meaning making thus developed would be transferrable to diagnosis (Tredinnick-Rowe 2017).

The materials discussed in this chapter show that practices of meaning making pervade all clinical work, not only diagnosis. The quality and safety of clinical work is contingent on novice clinicians learning across all domains of sign making sketched above. This includes communication, an area that has been introduced into clinical curricula in recent decades in the Western world. Social semiotics draws attention to the multimodal character of communication, whether in consultations with patients, handovers to colleagues, or in the context of complex, dynamic team work. Drawing and gesture are widely used modes of communication in clinical work and clinical education, but hardly ever taught or reviewed. The meaning potential of the moldable patient body gets attention in some specialties and is made explicit in some cases, e.g., in a textbook for plastic surgery, and yet overall, remains "under the radar." Research is needed to further map and explicate these domains of meaning making in clinical work.

Doing clinical work, and indeed reviewing and projecting it, relies on semiosis. To advance practices in any and all of these domains, clinicians need to develop skills in signification and communication, i.e., they need to expand their semiotic repertoire. By expanding the expressive repertoires of clinical educators, possibilities for teaching increase. Effective clinical educators are effective, multimodal communicators. Underdeveloped semiotic repertoires can have real effects on what does and what does not get recognized and therefore becomes available for valuation, evaluation, and learning. Thus, there is a need for refinement and diversification of (meta-)semiotic resources, including specialist vocabulary and visual methods, to enable better communication about the semiotic work of clinicians. This is how social semiotics can be put to practical use.

Cross-References

▶ Arts and Humanities in Health Professional Education
▶ Debriefing Practices in Simulation-Based Education
▶ Learning and Teaching in Clinical Settings: Expert Commentary from an Interprofessional Perspective
▶ Supporting the Development of Patient-Centred Communication Skills
▶ Team-Based Learning (TBL): Theory, Planning, Practice, and Implementation

References

Bezemer J. Partnerships in research: doing linguistic ethnography with and for practitioners. In: Snell J, Shaw S, Copland F, editors. Linguistic ethnography: interdisciplinary explorations. Basingstoke: Palgrave Macmillan; 2015. p. 207–24.
Bezemer J. Visual research in clinical education. Med Educ. 2017;51(1):105–13.
Bezemer J, Kress G. Multimodality, learning and communication: a social semiotic frame. London: Routledge; 2016.
Bezemer J, Kress G, Cope A, Kneebone R. Learning in the operating theatre: a social semiotic perspective. In: Cook V, Daly C, Newman M, editors. Work-based learning in clinical settings: insights from socio-cultural perspectives. Abingdon: Radcliffe; 2012. p. 125–41.

Bezemer J, Cope A, Korkiakangas T, Kress G, Murtagh G, Weldon S-M, Kneebone R. Micro analysis of video from the operating room: an under-used approach to patient safety research. BMJ Qual Saf. 2017;26(7):583–7.

de Saussure F. Cours de linguistique générale. Paris: Payot; 1916.

Eco U. A Theory of Semiotics. Bloomington: Indiana University Press; 1976.

Foucault M. The birth of the clinic. London: Routledge; 1963/2003.

Gishen F, Whitman S, Gill D, Barker R, Walker S. Schwartz Centre rounds: a new initiative in the undergraduate curriculum—what do medical students think? BMC Med Educ. 2016;16:246.

Goodwin C. Professional vision. Am Anthropol. 1994;96(3):606–33.

Goodwin C. Co-operative action. Cambridge: CUP; 2018.

Gorbanev I, Agudelo-Londoño S, González R, Cortes A, Pomares A, Delgadillo V, et al. A systematic review of serious games in medical education: quality of evidence and pedagogical strategy. Med Educ Online. 2018;23(1):1–9.

Hodge R, Kress G. Social semiotics. Cambridge: Polity Press; 1988.

Iedema R. Multimodality, resemiotization: extending the analysis of discourse as multi-semiotic practice. Vis Commun. 2003;1(2):29–57.

Iedema R, Hor S, Wyer M, Gilbert G, Jorm C, Hooker C, O'Sullivan M. An innovative approach to strengthening health professionals' infection control and limiting hospital-acquired infection: video-reflexive ethnography. BMJ Innov. 2015;1(4):157–62.

ISCP. Workplace based assessment. 2018. Retrieved 22 Aug 19, 2018, from https://www.iscp.ac.uk/curriculum/surgical/assessment_wbas.aspx.

Jakobson R. Language in relation to other communication systems. Collected Writings Vol. 2. The Hague: Mouton; 1971.

Junhasavasdikul D, Sukhato K, Srisangkaew S, Theera-Ampornpunt N, Anothaisintawee T, Dellow A. Cartoon versus traditional self-study handouts for medical students: CARTOON randomized controlled trial. Med Teach. 2017;39(8):836–43.

Kendon A. Gesture. Visible action as utterance. Cambridge: CUP; 2004.

Kress G. Multimodality. A social semiotic theory of communication. London: Routledge; 2010.

Law BHY, Cheung P, Wagner M, et al. Analysis of neonatal resuscitation using eye tracking: a pilot study. Arch Dis Child Fetal Neonatal Ed. 2018;103:F82–4.

Mansbridge C. Skin suturing. Retrieved 1 Feb 2016 from: OSCEstop.com.

Mondada L. Instructions in the operating room: how the surgeon directs their assistant's hands. Discourse Stud. 2014;16(2):131–61.

Peirce C. Collected papers of Charles Sanders Peirce. Cambridge: Harvard University Press; 1931–1958.

Pelletier C, Kneebone R. Learning safely from error? Reconsidering the ethics of simulation-based medical education through ethnography. Ethnogr Educ. 2016;11(3):267–82.

Point of Care Foundation. Schwartz rounds information pack for larger organisations. n.d. Document retrieved from https://s16682.pcdn.co/wp-content/uploads/2018/11/Attach-1.-New-Information-pack-big-2.pdf

RCP. Improving teams in healthcare. Resource 3: team communication. London: Royal College of Physicians; 2017.

Schlegel C, Kneebone R. Taking a broader view: Exploring the materiality of medicine through cross-disciplinary learning. BMJ Simulation and Technology Enhanced Learning, Bmjstel; 2018.

Schulz CM, Schneider E, Fritz L, Vockeroth J, Hapfelmeier A, Brandt T, et al. Visual attention of anaesthetists during simulated critical incidents. Br J Anaesth. 2011;106(6):807–13.

Sebeok T. Vital signs. Am J Semiot. 1985;3(3):1–27.

Tahim A, Gill D, Bezemer J. How do postgraduate surgeons-in-training learn through the use of workplace-based assessment? Short communication, Association for Medical Education in Europe annual scientific meeting, August 2019, Vienna. 2019

Tredinnick-Rowe J. The (re)-introduction of semiotics into medical education: on the works of Thure von Uexküll. Med Humanit. 2017;43:1–8.

van Leeuwen T. Introducing social semiotics. London: Routledge; 2005.

Von Uexküll T. Medicine and semiotics. Semiotica. 1986;61(3):201–18.

Von Uexküll J. A stroll through the worlds of animals and men. A picture book of invisible worlds. Semiotica. 1992;89(4):319–91.. (Originally published in English in 1957, originally published in German in 1934)

Communities of Practice and Medical Education

22

Claire Condron and Walter Eppich

The positive development of a society in the absence of creative, independently thinking, critical individuals is as inconceivable as the development of an individual in the absence of the stimulus of the community.
Albert Einstein

Contents

Introduction 404
Application of Theory 407
CoP in Healthcare 407
CoP in Health Professions Education 409
CoP in Simulation 410
Critiques of CoP 411
Conclusion 411
Cross-References 412
References 412

Abstract

Learning is fundamentally a social process, which depends highly on context. Effective education requires learning that is embedded in authentic practice, wherein learners engage in increasingly more complex tasks within social communities. The development of professional identity is a dynamic negotiated process realized through interactional relationships that foster clear understanding

---

C. Condron (✉)
RSCI University of Medicine and Health Sciences, Dublin, Ireland
e-mail: ccondron@rcsi.ie

W. Eppich
RCSI SIM Centre for Simulation Education and Research, RCSI University of Medicine and Health Sciences, Dublin, Ireland
e-mail: WEppich@rcsi.ie

© Springer Nature Singapore Pte Ltd. 2023
D. Nestel et al. (eds.), *Clinical Education for the Health Professions*,
https://doi.org/10.1007/978-981-15-3344-0_28

of professional standards, ethical values, ideology, and conduct. Communities of practice provide a rich framework for approaching cross-discipline learning that champions innovation and understanding at boundaries of workplace interprofessional interactions. Intentional collaboration in landscapes of practice enables interdisciplinary CoPs to work as teams to prepare learners for successful interprofessional collaboration in practice. The concept of CoP has given impetus to the diversified field of research and theory of "practice-based studies."

Keywords

Communities of practice · Landscapes of practice · Professional identity · Situated learning · Sociocultural learning theory · Legitimate peripheral participation

Introduction

Health professions education continues to evolve rapidly. In the last decade, curriculum revisions around the world have accelerated transitions from predominantly didactic, discipline-based formats to highly interactive, case-based, patient-centered, integrated, and centrally administered programs. However, because of this frequent and rapid change, educators risk designing formal and informal workplace curricula untethered to relevant theory, and learning suffers. Theoretical underpinnings and conceptual frameworks should guide the choices made by health professions educators from curriculum design, implementation, and program evaluation (Bordage 2009). In this chapter, we discuss the origination of the CoP theory, its evolution, and its application to medical education. We provide examples of CoP in training and aim to broaden the discussion to provide insights on how learning in and across communities prepare learners for practice.

Educators' conceptualizations about learning processes shape how we design, innovate, and implement education. The ways of thinking about learning have evolved since the late 1980s, with a disruption of traditional notions of knowledge as packages of ideas developed by some and ingested by others. More than individual information gathering, learning is situated in complex social contexts. If we consider representative metaphors of learning, "learning-as-acquisition" focuses on purposeful accumulation of knowledge, skills, and attitudes, whereas "learning-as-participation" emphasizes full participation in a social practice (Sfard 1998). Thus, concepts of knowledge acquisition have been complemented by learning-in-context models of social participation and experiential engagement in relevant environments. From simulation settings to authentic workplace experiences, we view learning as not only an individual cognitive process but also a social and participative activity (Gherardi 2000, p. 251). One such theoretical framework foregrounds the participatory nature of learning: communities of practice (CoP). Lave and Wenger (1991) first described the term community of practice (CoP) as the relationships between people and the activities they perform, which are a prerequisite for learning (Lave and Wenger 1991, p. 98). These authors understood the workplace community as a living curriculum in which novices and experts interact, providing for *"situated learning."* Therefore, learning processes are inextricably linked to participation in that CoP with its situated and specific embedded knowledge. For newcomers to a community, participation is at first legitimately peripheral but evolves gradually through engagement and complexity to full participation in the sociocultural practices of the community. For example, consider the junior medical student observing on a first clinical placement progressing to the senior student entrusted with some clinical duties under direct proactive supervision. The student graduates to internship and manages patients with indirect, reactive supervision. The senior house officer works unsupervised, and the resident on the team provides supervision to more junior learners (Cate 2018).

Situated learning theory posits that learning is fundamentally a social process and must be situated within authentic activity, context, and culture (Lave and Wenger 1991; Schatzki 2012). Knowledge and meaning are socially constructed resulting from social processes and relationship, dependent on shared thinking, priority cultural and historical context (Handley et al. 2006). Vygotsky described consciousness as a phenomenon that unifies attention, intention, memory, reasoning, and speech. His sociocultural theory asserts that cognition is developed through social interaction and introduces the idea of instructional scaffolding to support the learner's development and provide structures to get to the next level (Raymond 2000). Sociocultural learning theory is a lens through which to view participative education; it involves adopting distinct practices and language and adhering to cultural norms and constraints (Kahlke et al. 2019). For example, activity theory bridges the gap between the individual subject and the social reality in the activity system with the concept of object-oriented, collective, and culturally mediated human activity (Leont'ev 1981; Yrjö et al. 1999). Activity theorists argue that consciousness is not a set of discrete disembodied cognitive acts such as decision-making, classification, or remembering rather consciousness is central to a depiction of activity and is located in everyday practice: *you are what you do* (Nardi 1996). Collective systems participate in goal-directed action based on motives shared by the activity system members (Leont'ev 1981). Engeström integrated the elements of Vgotsky's and Leont'ev's frameworks and introduced the idea of community rules and outcomes. Activity theory therefore includes the notion that an activity is carried out within a social context or specifically in a community (Engeström 1993).

Based on situated learning theory, individual learning should be considered emergent alongside the identity formation and development, and participation in the community provides opportunities to practice as well as a sense of belonging and commitment. CoPs are formed by people who engage in a process of collective learning in a shared domain of endeavor. Thus, CoP views learning as occurring in practice and involves an investment of identity in these social contexts (Pyrko et al. 2019; Carlsen 2006; Gherardi et al. 1998; Swan et al. 2002). Usually, a CoP represents an informal peer group characterized by identity and participation in authentic activities, discussion, and learning. A shared domain of interest, namely a practice they wish to improve, motivates community members to participate and connects them with each other, helping them to develop shared identity (Li et al. 2009; Wenger et al. 2002). Through regular interaction, participants in a CoP become better at the practice in which they are all engaged and motivated to improve (Wenger 1998).

Identity formation is central to CoP and captures the developing knowledgeability and stature achieved through validation by other community members (Wenger-Trayner and Wenger-Trayner 2015). Professional identity reflects the ways of being and relating in professional contexts and develops through a dynamic process of identification by which individuals classify their place in the world as both individuals and members of collectives. Professional identity develops through the processes of social construction, the influence of role models, and the common narrative or shared stories woven through experiences, which are critical to understand and further nurture the CoP (Goldie 2012). In CoPs, "practice" refers to a history of learning in a social context, where learning drives practice, and a sense of community forms organically around it (Wenger 1998). Further, professional identity develops in interactional relationships during which individuals may be influenced more by the categorizations of others than her/his own cognitions and emotions (Ashmore et al. 2004). The conceptualization of identity as a sole, distinct, fixed entity has moved to a dynamic conception of multiple identities (Shotter and Gergen 1994) situated in social relationships (Eisenberg 2001; Gergen 1991). This integrative developmental process involves establishing core values, moral principles, and self-awareness mediated through discourse (Lave and Wenger 1991). These professional identities are "constructed and co-constructed through talk" (Monrouxe 2010), and as such, health professionals shape their professional identifies through verbal interactions in a working community, learning to talk to and about patients. Socialization involves learning to speak like other community members (Lingard et al. 2003). Learners model their behaviors after experienced practitioners in learning to deal with and convey uncertainty, using modal auxiliaries (e.g., can, could, may, might must, shall) and adverbs (e.g., perhaps, maybe) when presenting patient cases (Lingard et al. 2003; Eppich et al. 2016).

In an interview, Wenger-Trayner elaborated on the original CoP concept and articulated the notion of landscapes of practice (LoP) (Omidvar and Kislov 2014), which describe how different yet related CoPs interact, depend on, and are accountable to one another's practice-based knowing, rather than relying exclusively on their own, local situated practices. The landscape of practice encompasses all the communities of practice, and learners can move between these (Hodson 2020). Stalmeijer and Varpio (2021) used the CoP and LoP frameworks to challenge traditional notions of intra- versus inter-professional education, i.e., doctors teaching doctors and nurses teaching nurses. Specifically, the authors proposes that health professionals may claim membership to multiple communities in healthcare; members in a physician CoP cross boundaries in the healthcare LoP and derive learning from interactions across professional boundaries. The capacity to navigate knowledge acquisition and identity formation across the landscape is considered "knowledgeability," recognizing a person's relationship to multiple communities within a broader LoP in complex social systems (Brown and Peck 2018. Health professions educators might promote boundary-crossing across CoP through deliberate approaches captured by "collaborative intentionality" (Morris and Eppich 2021).

CoP thus encompasses ideas that shifts the debate from cognitive theories of learning and knowledge to social theories of learning (Gherardi 2009). CoP and LoP provide processes through which individual learning advances organizational learning. The learning becomes embedded in an organization's institutional memory through the creation of structures and artefacts. These structures and artefacts, or reifications, include common ways of speaking, standard operating procedures, policies, and organizational customs.

Application of Theory

CoP has influenced theory in many domains, finding practical applications in many and varied contexts, which in turn has spurred the continuous expansion and theory development (Omidvar and Kislov 2014). The concept of CoP has influenced a diverse field of research involving "practice-based studies" (Gherardi 2009). Different generations of CoP theory share the notion of learning as a participatory social process and as a rationale to create conditions in which learners develop specific skills as well as theoretical and practical knowledge. Knowledge management within organizations supports the organization's learning processes and initiatives like participation in CoP, which have tangible benefits that foster innovation (Chindgren-Wagner 2010).

Researchers and practitioners in many different settings such as federal government (Chindgren-Wagner 2010), business (Wenger and Snyder 2000), education (Truscott and Stevens 2020), and professional associations have considered CoP as a beneficial approach to knowing and learning. CoP enables a perspective on knowing and learning that shapes learning systems at scale, from local communities and individual organizations to cities and regions, and across the world (Wenger-Trayner and Wenger-Trayner 2015). In a significant departure from the original concept that depicted CoPs as developing organically, Wenger expanded the original concept of CoP by proposing that CoPs improve the collection and dissemination of knowledge within organizations. He suggested that explicitly engineered or cultivated CoPs allow organizations to manage knowledge workers and enhance competitiveness (Wenger et al. 2002). However, others report that successful CoPs are characterized by authentic connection and arise organically, features that are incompatible with top-down implementation (Amin and Roberts 2008).

CoP in Healthcare

CoPs are increasingly being adopted in healthcare as quality improvement initiatives (Li et al. 2009). Fung-Kee-Fung et al. proposed a CoP model as a process for disseminating and implementing clinical guidelines for cancer screening and treatment and for providing a supportive infrastructure for quality improvements in cancer surgery in large-scale healthcare collaborations. This research designed an evaluation framework based on the knowledge conversion methods of organizational memory, social capital, innovation, and knowledge transfer (Fung-Kee-Fung et al. 2014). Kothari et al. describe using a CoP framework to facilitate health systems change to improve the care of seniors. These authors report that the CoP functioned as an incubator that brought together best practices, research, experiences, a reflective learning cycle, and passionate champions. However, the efforts of CoPs to stimulate practice changes were met with broader resistance (Kothari et al. 2015).

Organizational communities of practice (OCoPs) are more formalized, purposeful, and bounded forms of CoPs and characteristically operate alongside the conventional team structures (Kirkman et al. 2013). Kitto et al. (2018) explained how an engineered CoP created tension with the natural CoPs from their training programs with which surgeons identified; this tension contributed to inactive or marginal participation by some surgeons. These authors identified wide variation in the understanding of and participation in the CoP by surgeons. They noted that structural, economic, and cultural factors influenced participation in the CoP. Furthermore, an operational tension existed between the twin purposes of the CoP as a regionalization/rationalization activity in Ontario based on the volume-outcome hypothesis and as an educational intervention to enhance and maintain the members' surgical competence.

Unfortunately, CoPs co-opted by governing bodies do not necessarily capture the power and potential of situated learning (Kitto et al. 2018). To address this gap, Braithwaite et al. set out to understand how groups of professionals work together. This research used rigorous methodologies to evaluate the effectiveness of CoP and social–professional networks to optimize these interactions in order to improve organizational effectiveness and service delivery (Braithwaite et al. 2009b). The authors drew two main conclusions: (a) clinicians work best when they are empowered to mobilize their expertise, and (b) clinicians flourish in groupings of their own interests and preference. They prefer being invited, empowered, and nurtured rather than directed, micro-managed, and controlled through a hierarchy (Braithwaite et al. 2009a). Thus, a CoP cannot simply be created by regulatory agencies; rather they need to be supported in a way to evolve naturally. CoPs have a culture built on personal relationships, professional networking, shared knowledge, and common skills. With voluntary participation, CoPs provide contributors with opportunities to experience autonomy, mastery, and purpose beyond their routine work (Pink 2009).

We have much to learn about establishing and supporting CoPs to maximize their potential to improve healthcare (Ranmuthugala et al. 2011). Waring et al. (2013) examined knowledge brokering for patient safety initiatives and challenged the idea of using CoP to drive knowledge sharing in hospitals. Rather these authors suggested people whose roles operate at the boundaries of CoP and legitimately straddle several CoPs such as clinical managers are best suited as knowledge brokers (Waring et al. 2013), which aligns with the notion of LoP introduced earlier. Indeed, boundary spanning underpins knowledge translation processes. Evans and

Scarbourgh proposed the idea of "blurring" as a method of boundary spanning across healthcare CoPs. Blurring refers to knowledge translation happening as a continuous and incremental process situated within routine, daily practices where overlapping relations between working communities transform professional expertise into knowledge that transcends specialist domains. With patient safety as the driver, professional groups implicitly pursued the mutual adaptation of good practices. Clinicians and organizations more easily adapt relevant learnings because they better understand environmental considerations of overlapping work settings indicative of LoP (Evans and Scarbrough 2014). Considered discretely, each individual action of knowledge translation is minor but considered together across the spectrum, blurring has the potential for large-scale translation of knowledge and impact on practice, across complex boundaries (Carlile 2004).

CoP in Health Professions Education

Increasing evidence shows that undergraduate medical education inadequately prepares students for the tasks of internship particularly with respect to key professional competencies and skills (Monrouxe 2010; Hawkins et al. 2021). The traditional focus of medical education has been on knowledge acquisition; however, educators now recognize the performance-based component of clinical competency (Anderson et al. 2001). Modern team-based healthcare faces high complexity and needs workers who can work, negotiate, and create in groups, thus collaborative educational experiences are more essential than ever. Learning arises through shared participative practices in authentic work and includes both processes of becoming a HCP and belonging to the health care team (Morris 2018). Pressures from overladen curricula in medical education can demote boundary-crossing and knowledge-sharing experiences.

Stensaker and Fumasoli (2017) associated the increasing complexity, fragmentation, and managerialism of modern medical curricula with a reduction in collegiality, and advised academics to build initiatives that foster a collaborative working environment. The literature recognizes the impact of collaborative, situated learning within CoPs for academic development at an institutional level (Southwell and Morgan 2009; Viskovic 2006) and at a more individual, organic level (Monk and McKay 2017; Warhurst 2006). Gibbs (2013) argued that effective curriculum development must align with "the health and vigour of the community of teaching practice." Collaborative modes of working that enable a sense of shared responsibility provides the emotional and social support to enable change (Anakin et al. 2017). Online CoPs offering collegiality helps to counter the isolation of casual academic teaching (Dean and Forray 2018). Models of organizational change have supplemented underlying assumptions about how individuals change. Identity becomes fragile and fractured, and new boundaries are re-created to feel safe (Wenger-Trayner and Wenger-Trayner 2015). Participation in a CoP has a positive impact on academics sense of community and their knowledgeability in relation to new teaching approaches in a blended curriculum (Brown and Peck 2018).

Wenger-Trayner and Wenger-Trayner (2015) urge educators to support meaningful cross-border learning such that learners can succeed across the range of communities in which they work and learn. The LoP framework supports the interprofessional education required by the twenty-first century healthcare professionals delivering the complexities of modern patient care (de Nooijer et al. 2021). Gillespie and Dornan (2021) warn, however, that we must do more than encouraging interprofessional education; we must also nurture interprofessional practice of patient care to realize its full potential. Along these lines, Morris and Eppich (2021) outline strategies to foster collaborative intentionality and promote boundary crossing in both education and practice: (a) identifying explicit interprofessional clinical learning moments such as interdisciplinary ward rounds, (b) fostering workplace team inclusiveness to promote team learning behaviors, (c) formalizing cross-professional educational structures, and (d) embedding boundary-crossing behaviors in simulation-based education (SBE).

CoP in Simulation

Simulation bridges classroom and workplace. Through the lens of situated learning theory, we may consider simulation experience as a form of legitimate peripheral participation, in which learners safely practice the skills they need to provide safe care to patients in the real world (Bradley and Postlethwaite 2003). Learning occurs within and across the boundaries between the different systems in which learners operate. Since learning is fundamentally a social process that foregrounds the critical role of context, learning is suboptimal if individual cognitive processing remains the sole focus. Cleland's research examining the socio-cultural influences during surgical simulation bootcamps demonstrated that participants viewed the course as a vehicle not just for learning skills but for gaining "insider information" on how best to progress in surgical training. In addition, the faculty members use the surgical bootcamp to welcome trainees into the world of surgery. This important work demonstrated that social and cultural processes are as important to participants as individual, cognitive and acquisitive learning. These insights about education and an entry into a CoP should inform planning for similar educational activities and offer new perspective on SBE research (Cleland et al. 2016).

Simulation educators belong both to a CoP of educators and to a healthcare professional CoP; they move between these communities, and they have opportunities for brokering or advocating for changes of practice (Tamás et al. 2020). Those working as clinicians and simulation educators facilitate the transfer of newly acquired skills for the other members of their CoP (Tamás et al. 2020). Virtual CoPs can develop on social media platforms, encouraging educators to engage online for their own benefit and professional development of healthcare simulation educators (Thoma et al. 2018). Hovancsek et al. describe a 3-year international project with 17 contributors from eight different countries employing web-based courses for faculty development in nursing simulation education and outline the benefits and rewards and challenges and barriers of this CoP approach (Hovancsek et al. 2009). Unfortunately, simulation innovation and research arising from local CoP may not be disseminated to the wider simulation community due to a lack of collaboration between different stakeholders, departments, and hospital simulation centers. Peddle et al. recommend that the CoPs should develop networking opportunities to form research collaborative that can improve the publication and dissemination of activities and innovations from simulation in different settings (Peddle et al. 2020).

Sociocultural learning theory in general and CoP in particular view knowing and learning as emerging in complex nonlinear systems in which human actors and the material environment produce and shape each other (Hager 2011). Such socio-material approaches to simulation-based education value the complexity of professional learning (Fenwick and Dahlgren 2015). Also, social situations shape learning, and anxiety and emotion play a significant role. Understanding the relationships between motivation, engagement, identity, responsibility, and preparedness for practice will provide educators with theory-informed guidance to develop simulation-based education.

Critiques of CoP

As a theoretical framework, CoP has been highly influential and frequently applied. However, there is also danger of CoP becoming all things to all people, who interpret and use CoP differently to satisfy their particular yet diverse needs or expectations. From its origins, the social and situated dimension of learning embedded within conceptualizations of CoP evolved differently in different communities of researchers. While studies in the management literature shifted its emphasis to identifying, cultivating, and managing the dimension of community, online communities stressed the social competences necessary to make up for a missing interactive dimension with technology (Gherardi 2009). Thus, the CoP approach has been critiqued for its conservatism, managerialism, and limited analysis of power relations in learning situations, and for its romantic notions of "community," and its vague analyses of practice and participation (Hughes et al. 2007). In some workplaces, poor working practices and unethical values and beliefs such as sexism or racism can be learned or further entrenched and reinforced (Hodkinson and Hodkinson 2004). Hay argues that, *"students have no 'space' to create knowledge within the community of practice until they reach a certain station in relationship to the center of the community"* (Hay 1996). The hidden curriculum of medical education manifests in CoP where relationships between learner and educator are key. Research on relationships as a central construct is absent in the CoP literature, and more work is needed to understand how relationships and the hidden curricula impact access to participating and learning in CoPs (Jarecke 2010).

Conclusion

Health professions education requires an approach that deconstructs issues of power and hegemony which can permeate the clinical environment (Wear 1997) and CoP provide a theoretical lens to begin this process. Identity formation in health professions is a complex exercise as the roles and responsibilities of physicians, nurses, physician associates, and allied healthcare professionals continually develop and grow. Educators and clinicians alike must attend to the quality of CoP and LoP that shape both interactions and learning (Davies 2006). By fully exploiting their potential, educators should leverage the theoretical frameworks of situated learning and CoP and incorporate the concepts of LoP to foster a strong interprofessional healthcare team approach to health professions education, which will ultimately benefit patient care (Stalmeijer and Varpio 2021). Safe healthcare practice requires a lifelong commitment to learning and reflective practice, and CoPs have a role in improving healthcare performance. Further research is required to understand the factors at play, which hinder or influence success when cultivating CoPs to benefit organizational knowledge management (Ranmuthugala et al. 2011).

Cross-References

▶ Competencies of Health Professions Educators of the Future
▶ Developing Professional Identity in Health Professional Students
▶ Focus on Selection Methods: Evidence and Practice
▶ Focus on Theory: Emotions and Learning
▶ Future of Health Professions Education Curricula

References

Amin A, Roberts J. Knowing in action: beyond communities of practice. Res Policy. 2008;37(2): 353–69.

Anakin M, Spronken-Smith R, Healey M, Vajoczki S. Int J Acad Dev. 2017;23(1):1–13. https://doi.org/10.1080/1360144X.2017.1385464.

Anderson RC, Fagan MJ, Sebastian J. Teaching students the art and science of physical diagnosis. Am J Med. 2001;110(5):419–23.

Ashmore RD, Deaux K, McLaughlin-Volpe T. An organizing framework for collective identity: articulation and significance of multidimensionality. Psychol Bull. 2004;130(1):80–114. https://doi.org/10.1037/0033-2909.130.1.80. PMID: 14717651

Bordage G. Conceptual frameworks to illuminate and magnify. Med Educ. 2009;43(4):312–9.

Bradley P, Postlethwaite K. Simulation in clinical learning. Med Educ. 2003;37(1):1–5.

Braithwaite J, Runciman WB, Merry A. Towards safer, better healthcare: harnessing the natural properties of complex sociotechnical systems. Qual Saf Health Care. 2009a;18:37–41. https://doi.org/10.1136/qshc.2007.023317.

Braithwaite J, Westbrook JI, Ranmuthugala G, et al. The development, design, testing, refinement, simulation and application of an evaluation framework for communities of practice and social-professional networks. BMC Health Serv Res. 2009b;9:162. https://doi.org/10.1186/1472-6963-9-162.

Brown M, Peck C. Expanding the landscape: developing knowledgeability through communities of practice. Int J Acad Dev. 2018;23(3):232–43. https://doi.org/10.1080/1360144X.2018.1473252.

Carlile PR. Transferring, translating, and transforming: an integrative framework for managing knowledge across boundaries. Organ Sci. 2004;15(5):555–568. http://www.jstor.org/stable/30034757.

Carlsen A. Organizational becoming as dialogic imagination of practice: the case of the indomitable gauls. Organ Sci. 2006;17(1):132–49.

Cate OT. A primer on entrustable professional activities. Korean J Med Educ. 2018;30(1):1–10. https://doi.org/10.3946/kjme.2018.76.

Chindgren-Wagner TM. Climate of innovation in government communities of practice: focusing on 400 knowledge gains and relationships. In: Paper presented at PMI® Research Conference: Defining 401 the Future of Project Management. Washington: Project Management Institute; 2010.

Cleland J, Walker KG, Gale M, Nicol LG. Simulation-based education: understanding the socio-cultural complexity of a surgical training 'boot camp'. Med Educ. 2016;50(8):829–41. https://doi.org/10.1111/medu.13064.

Davies J. The importance of the community of practice in identity development. Int J Allied Health Sci Pract. 2006;4(3) https://nsuworks.nova.edu/cgi/viewcontent.cgi?article=1111&context=ijahsp. Accessed 31 May 2021.

de Nooijer J, Dolmans DHJM, Stalmeijer RE. Applying landscapes of practice principles to the design of interprofessional education, teaching and learning in medicine; 2021. https://doi.org/10.1080/10401334.2021.1904937.

Dean KL, Forray JM. Collegiality and collaboration in an era of competition. J Manag Educ. 2018;42(1):3–7. https://doi.org/10.1177/1052562917743014.

Eisenberg EM. Building a mystery: toward a new theory of communication and identity. J Commun. 2001;51(3):534–52. https://doi.org/10.1111/j.1460-2466.2001.tb02895.x.

Engeström, Y. Developmental studies of work as a testbench of activity theory: the case of primary care medical practice. In: Chaiklin S, Lave J (eds) Understanding practice: perspectives on activity and context (Learning in Doing: Social, Cognitive and Computational Perspectives, pp. 64–103). Cambridge: Cambridge University Press; 1993. https://doi.org/10.1017/CBO9780511625510.004.

Eppich W, Rethans JJ, Pim WT, Dornan T. Learning to work together through talk: continuing professional development in medicine. In: Billett S, et al., editors. Supporting learning across working life, Professional and practice-based learning, vol. 16. Cham: Springer International Publishing Switzerland; 2016. pp. 47–73. https://doi.org/10.1007/978-3-319-29019-5_3.

Evans S, Scarbrough H. Supporting knowledge translation through collaborative translational research initiatives: 'Bridging' versus 'blurring' boundary-spanning approaches in the UK CLAHRC initiative. Soc Sci Med. 2014;106:119–27. https://doi.org/10.1016/j.socscimed.2014.01.025.

Fenwick T, Dahlgren MA. Towards socio-material approaches in simulation-based education: lessons from complexity theory. Med Educ. 2015 Apr;49(4):359–67. https://doi.org/10.1111/medu.12638.

Fung-Kee-Fung M, Boushey RP, Morash R. Exploring a "community of practice" methodology as a regional platform for large-scale collaboration in cancer surgery-the Ottawa approach. Curr Oncol 2014;21(1):13–8. https://doi.org/10.3747/co.21.1662.

Gergen KJ. The saturated self: dilemmas of identity in contemporary life. London: Basic Books; 1991.

Gherardi S. Practice-based theorizing on learning and knowing in organizations. Organization. 2000;7(2):211–23. https://journals.sagepub.com/doi/abs/10.1177/135050840072001

Gherardi S, Nicolini D, Odella F. Toward a social understanding of how people learn in organizations: the notion of situated curriculum. Manag Learn. 1998;29(3):273–97.

Gherardi S. Community of practice or practices of a community? In: The SAGE handbook of management learning, education and development; 2009. Chapter 27 (pp. 514–530). https://doi.org/10.4135/9780857021038.n27.

Gibbs G. Reflections on the changing nature of educational development. Int J Acad Dev. 2013;18(1):4–14. https://doi.org/10.1080/1360144X.2013.75169.

Gillespie H, Dornan T. The wolf shall dwell with the lamb: the power dynamics of interprofessional education. Med Educ. 2021;55:883–885. https://doi.org/10.1111/medu.14568.

Goldie J. The formation of professional identity in medical students: considerations for educators. Med Teach. 2012;34(9):e641–8. https://doi.org/10.3109/0142159X.2012.687476.

Hager P. Theories of workplace learning chapter 2. In: M Malloch, L Cairns, K Evans (Eds) The SAGE handbook of workplace learning. SAGE Publications Ltd; 2011, pp 17–31. https://doi.org/10.4135/9781446200940.n2.

Hay K. Legitimate perihperal participation, instructionism and constructivism: whose situation is it anyway?. In: H McLellan (ed). Situated learning perspectives. New Jersey: Educational Technology Publications; 1996, pp 89–99.

Handley K, Sturdy A, Fincham R, Clark T. Within and beyond communities of practice: making sense of learning through participation, identity and practice*. J Manag Stud. 2006;43(3):641–53.

Hawkins N, Younan H-C, Fyfe M, Parekh R, McKeown A. Exploring why medical students still feel underprepared for clinical practice: a qualitative analysis of an authentic on-call simulation. BMC Med Educ. 2021;21(1):165.

Hodkinson H, Hodkinson P. Rethinking the concept of community of practice in relation to schoolteachers' workplace learning. Int J Train Dev. 2004;8:21–31. https://doi.org/10.1111/j.1360-3736.2004.00193.x.

Hodson N. Landscapes of practice in medical education. Medical Education. 2020;54(6):504–9.

Hovancsek M, Jeffries PM, Escudero E, Foulds BJ, Husebø SE, Iwamoto Y, Kelly M, Petrini M, Wang A. Creating simulation communities of practice, nursing education perspective. Nurs Educ Perspect. 2009;30(2):121–5.

Hughes J, Jewson N, Unwin L. Communities of practice critical perspectives. Routledge; 2007. (London and New York) Chapter 1 (pp. 1–16).

Jarecke J, Taylor EW. Exposing medical Education's hidden curriculum through an exploration of teacher-learner relationships. In: Adult Education Research Conference. 2010. https://newprairiepress.org/aerc/2010/papers/34 Accessed 31 May 2021.

Kahlke R, Bates J, Nimmon L. When I say … sociocultural learning theory. Med Educ. 2019;53:117–118. https://doi.org/10.1111/medu.13626.

Kitto SC, Grant RE, Peller J, et al. What's in a name? Tensions between formal and informal communities of practice among regional subspecialty cancer surgeons. Adv Health Sci Educ. 2018;23:95–113. https://doi.org/10.1007/s10459-017-9776-z.

Kirkman BL, Cordery JL, Mathieu J, Rosen B, Kukenberger M. Global organizational communities of practice: the effects of nationality diversity, psychological safety, and media richness on community performance. Hum Relat. 2013;66(3):333–62.

Kothari A, Boyko JA, Conklin J, Stolee P, Sibbald SL. Communities of practice for supporting health systems change: a missed opportunity. Health Res Policy Syst. 2015;25(13):33. https://doi.org/10.1186/s12961-015-0023-x. Erratum in: Health Res Policy Syst 2015;13:65. PMID: 26208500.

Lave J, Wenger E. Learning in doing: social, cognitive, and computational perspectives. In: Situated learning: legitimate peripheral participation. Cambridge: Cambridge University Press; 1991. https://doi.org/10.1017/CBO9780511815355.

Leont'ev AN. Problems of the development of the mind. (Kopylova, M., Trans.). Moscow Progress Publishers. (Original work published 1959); 1981.

Li LC, Grimshaw JM, Nielsen C, et al. Use of communities of practice in business and health care sectors: a systematic review. Implement Sci. 2009;4:27. https://doi.org/10.1186/1748-5908-4-27.

Lingard L, Garwood K, Schryer CF, Spafford MM. A certain art of uncertainty: case presentation and the development of professional identity. Soc Sci Med. 2003;56(3):603–16. https://doi.org/10.1016/s0277-9536(02)00057-6.

Monk S, McKay L. Developing identity and agency as an early career academic: lessons from Alice. Int J Acad Dev. 2017;22(3):223–30. https://doi.org/10.1080/1360144X.2017.130653.

Monrouxe LV. Identity, identification and medical education: why should we care? Med Educ. 2010;44(1):40–9.

Morris CS. On Communities of Practice in Medical Education. Acad Med. 2018;93(12):1752. https://doi.org/10.1097/ACM.0000000000002462.

Morris M, Eppich WJ. Changing workplace-based education norms through 'collaborative intentionality'. Med Educ. 2021 Aug;55(8):885–887. https://doi.org/10.1111/medu.14564.

Nardi BA. Context and consciousness: activity theory and human-computer interaction. Cambridge, MA. The MIT Press; 1996.

Omidvar O, Kislov R. The evolution of the communities of practice approach: toward knowledgeability in a landscape of practice. An interview with Etienne Wenger-Trayner. J Manag Inq. 2014;23(3):266–75. https://doi.org/10.1177/1056492613505908.

Peddle M, Livesay K, Marshall S. Preliminary report of a simulation community of practice needs analysis. Adv Simul. 2020;5:11. https://doi.org/10.1186/s41077-020-00130-4.

Pink DH. Drive: the surprising truth about what motivates us. New York: Riverhead Books; 2009.

Pyrko I, Dörfler V, Eden C. Communities of practice in landscapes of practice. Manag Learn. 2019;50(4):482–99. https://doi.org/10.1177/1350507619860854.

Ranmuthugala G, Georgiou A, Braithwaite J, Cunningham FC, Westbrook JI, Plumb JJ. How and why are communities of practice established in the healthcare sector? A systematic review of the literature. BMC Health Serv Res. 2011;11(1):273. https://doi.org/10.1186/1472-6963-11-273.

Raymond E. Cognitive characteristics. In: Learners with mild disabilities. Needham Heights, MA: Allyn & Bacon, A Pearson Education Company; 2000, pp 169–201.

Schatzki TR. Foreword. In: Hager P, Lee A, Reich A, editors. Practice, learning and change: practice-theory perspectives on professional learning. Dordrecht: Springer; 2012.

Sfard A. On two metaphors for learning and the dangers of choosing just one. Educ Res. 1998;27(2):4–13. https://doi.org/10.3102/0013189X027002004.

Shotter J, Gergen KJ. Social construction: knowledge, self, others, and continuing the conversation. Ann Int Commun Assoc. 1994;17(1):3–33. https://doi.org/10.1080/23808985.1994.11678873.

Southwell D, Morgan W. Leadership and the impact of academic staff development and leadership development on student learning outcomes in higher education : a review of the literature : a report for the Australian learning and teaching council (ALTC) / Queensland University of Technology. Brisbane: Dept. of Teaching and Learning Support Services; 2009

Stalmeijer, RE, Varpio, L. The wolf you feed: challenging intraprofessional workplace-based education norms. Med Educ. 2021;55:894–902. https://doi.org/10.1111/medu.14520.

Stensaker B, Fumasoli T. Multi-level strategies in universities: coordination, contestation or creolisation? Higher Educ Q. 2017;71(3):263–73. Special Issue: European flagship universities: autonomy and change

Swan J, Scarbrough H, Robertson M. The construction of "communities of practice" in the management of innovation. Manag Learn. 2002;33(4):477–96.

Symon B, Spurr J, Brazil V. Simulcast: a case study in the establishment of a virtual community of simulation practice. Adv Simul. 2020;5:5. https://doi.org/10.1186/s41077-020-00122-4.

Tamás, É. Södersved Källestedt M-L, Hult H, Carlzon L, Karlgren K, Berndtzon M, Hultin M, Masiello I, Allvin R. Simulation educators in clinical work: the manager's perspective. J Health Organ Manage. 2020;34(2):181–91.

Thoma B, Brazil V, Spurr J, Palaganas J, Eppich W, Grant V, Cheng A. Establishing a virtual Community of Practice in simulation: the value of social media. Simul Healthc. 2018;13(2): 124–30. https://doi.org/10.1097/SIH.0000000000000284.

Truscott D, Stevens BK. Developing teacher identities as in situ teacher educators through communities of practice. New Educ. 2020;16(4):333–51. https://doi.org/10.1080/1547688X.2020. 1779890.

Viskovic A. Becoming a tertiary teacher: learning in communities of practice. High Educ Res Dev. 2006;25(4):323–39. https://doi.org/10.1080/07294360600947285.

Warhurst RP. "We really felt part of something": participatory learning among peers within a university teaching-development community of practice. Int J Acad Dev. 2006;11(2):111–22. https://doi.org/10.1080/13601440600924462.

Waring J, Currie G, Crompton A. An exploratory study of knowledge brokering in hospital settings: facilitating knowledge sharing and learning for patient safety? Soc Sci Med. 2013;98:79–86.

Wear D. Privilege in the Medical Academy: A Feminist Examines Gender, Race, and Power (Athene Series) (1997) 1st Edition Teachers College Print ISBN-10: 0807762881.

Wenger E. Communities of practice: learning, meaning, and identity. Roy Pea, John Seely Brown, Jan Hawkins (Eds). Cambridge University Press; 1998. https://doi.org/10.1017/CBO9780511803932

Wenger EC, Snyder WM. Communities of practice: the organizational frontier. Harv Bus Rev. 2000;78(1):139–46.

Wenger E, McDermott RA, Snyder W. Cultivating communities of practice: a guide to managing knowledge. Boston: Harvard Business School Press; 2002.

Wenger-Trayner E, & Wenger-Trayner B (2015) Learning in a landscape of practice: A framework. In E. Wenger-Trayner, M. Fenton-O'Creevy, S. Hutchinson, C. Kubiak, & B. Wenger-Trayner (Eds.), Learning in landscapes of practice: Boundaries, identity, and knowledgeability in practice-based learning (pp. 13–29). New York, NY: Routledge.

Yrjö E, Reijo M, Raija-Leena P. Perspectives on activity theory. Cambridge: Cambridge University Press; 1999.

Activity Theory in Health Professions Education Research and Practice

23

Richard L. Conn, Gerard J. Gormley, Sarah O'Hare, and Anu Kajamaa

Contents

Introduction 418
An Overview of Activity Theory 420
    Origins 420
    Activity Systems 421
    Contradictions 425
    Expansive Learning 426
Using AT in Health Professions Education Research and Practice Development 428
    AT as a Theoretical Framework 429
    Data Collection 429
    Analysis 430
    AT as a Driver of Change: The Change Laboratory Method 431
Future Directions: AT in Educational Development 434
    Activity Theory as a Sense-Making Tool 435
    Activity Theory and In Situ Simulation: SimLab 435
Conclusion 436
Cross-References 437
References 437

Abstract

This chapter describes activity theory (AT) and its emerging role within health professions education (HPE). We outline AT's historical roots, before exploring its concepts and theoretical models in detail. We then describe its practical applications in HPE, in both analysis and intervention, before concluding with a discussion of its rich future possibilities.

R. L. Conn (✉) · G. J. Gormley · S. O'Hare
Centre for Medical Education, Queen's University Belfast, Belfast, UK
e-mail: r.conn@qub.ac.uk; g.gormley@qub.ac.uk; sohare23@qub.ac.uk

A. Kajamaa
Faculty of Education, University of Oulu, Oulu, Finland
e-mail: anu.kajamaa@oulu.fi

© Springer Nature Singapore Pte Ltd. 2023
D. Nestel et al. (eds.), *Clinical Education for the Health Professions*,
https://doi.org/10.1007/978-981-15-3344-0_30

Keywords

Health professions · Health professions education · Learning clinical education · Learning in practice · Interprofessional health education · Evidence-based educational methods · Quality improvement · Sociocultural theory · Activity theory · Cultural-historical activity theory

Introduction

To say that healthcare is complex has practically become a cliché. But what underlies healthcare complexity? And what are its implications for practitioners, educators, and researchers? Healthcare complexity can be considered on multiple levels.

First, and most intuitively, healthcare is clinically complex. Patients present in varied ways with unique, often coexisting, healthcare needs – and increasingly so, given the well-recognized issues of aging populations, multimorbidity, and polypharmacy (Whitty et al. 2020). Patient expectations are changing, with increasing demand for care that is person-centered, individualized, and co-constructed (Richards et al. 2015). Modern healthcare routinely requires professionals to act on provisional, incomplete clinical information in circumstances where diagnosis, treatment, and outcome are far from clear (Tonelli and Upshur 2019). And all the while, practitioners must deal not only with patients on an individual basis, but with the conflicting demands posed by caring for multiple patients in the context of limited resources, and cultural and political drivers around how to use those resources (Leung et al. 2012).

Second, healthcare is technically complex. Advances in diagnosis, investigation, and treatment, whilst promising technological efficiency and improved clinical outcomes, pose significant challenges for staff on the front line. Practitioners are required to employ specialized technologies, make use of increasingly sophisticated systems, and keep up with date with an ever-growing body of research and best practice guidelines (Plsek and Greenhalgh 2001).

Finally – and crucially – healthcare is socially complex (Greig et al. 2012; Kajamaa et al. 2019). Care is increasingly delivered by multilevel, multidisciplinary teams, whose successful function hinges not only on individual competence but on effective interactions between members (Lingard et al. 2004; Noble and Billett 2017). Clinical teams are not stable entities, but fluid, dynamic collaborations whose formation is shaped by factors such as evolving patient needs, increasing sub-specialization, and recent working hours restrictions;(Cristancho et al. 2019) in these circumstances, care is increasingly sophisticated, but its delivery is increasingly fragmented (Stange 2009).

Together, these interwoven layers of complexity underpin many of the major problems facing modern healthcare. They confound translation of innovations into practice (Davis et al. 2003), lead novice practitioners to feel routinely underprepared to begin work (Monrouxe et al. 2018), and contribute to widespread medical error

(Makary and Daniel 2016), creating a pressing need for practice changes in healthcare organizations.

These issues also represent urgent challenges for Health Professions Education (HPE), whose role is to support students and practitioners to prepare for and navigate the demands placed on them by their work. The Case Study below exemplifies one such issue – the educational problem of successfully implementing "best practice" in complex and diverse social contexts and physical environments.

In the face of these challenges, the Finnish educationalist Yrjö Engeström – the leading contemporary exponent of *cultural-historical activity theory* (CHAT; alternatively and here referred to as activity theory, AT) – argues that healthcare must move beyond traditional dominant ways of thinking (Engeström 2018). Drawing on decades of study in specific healthcare contexts, Engestrom concludes that expertise must be viewed as a collective, rather than an individual, attribute, defined by the ability to work within inherently unstable conditions. On this basis, educators need new theoretical tools to help understand how human activity and learning are shaped over time by complex social, cultural, and contextual factors – and to help them intervene within this activity.

AT provides such tools. It offers a valuable lens for understanding practitioners' work in local organizational contexts, as well as methods to bring about change within those contexts, that may support educators in both research and practice. In contrast to individualistic models, AT, as a sociocultural theory, situates learners as subject to social and historical discourse, and cognition as distributed across people and artifacts making up a community (Bleakley 2006). In AT, the human mind and the external milieu are seen as inseparable, and activity systems (and, further, networks of interdependent activity systems across different work-based contexts) form the basic unit of analysis (Bleakley 2006).

Activity theory has already begun to impact HPE research, having been applied to support both analysis and intervention in diverse areas of study. Yet AT has potential to impact HPE further – both within research, but also by directly shaping clinical and educational practice, supporting and driving innovation and change, helping practitioners to think critically about their work, and promoting greater alignment between education and healthcare.

In this chapter, our aim is to describe – in a way that is accessible to both researchers and practitioners – the development, use, and practical applications of AT in the field of HPE. We first outline AT's historical and theoretical roots, before exploring in detail its concepts and theoretical models. We then describe how these models can be used in HPE research, both within analysis and intervention, with reference to specific detailed examples from literature. To support understanding, we twice return to the Case Study introduced after this introduction, using it to exemplify AT's theoretical constructs and, later, to illustrate its practical applicability. Finally, we conclude with a discussion of AT's future possibilities in the field of healthcare and HPE.

> **Case Study: Part 1 – Preparing for Primary Care Emergencies**
>
> Max is an academic general practitioner who works in a large inner city general practice. The practice is moving into a newly built community healthcare building. They will share this space with other general practices, physiotherapy clinics, social workers, and mental health practitioners. Max is keen to consider how best they will set up arrangements to manage medical emergencies in this new setting. Given the physical layout of the building, and co-occupying with other healthcare providers, simply transferring their previous systems may not adequately prepare them for managing such emergencies.
>
> Whilst such emergencies are infrequent in community healthcare settings, he recognizes they are increasing and require an immediate and coordinated response to help provide the best outcome for patients. In order to address this issue, Max is keen to conduct an in situ simulation, i.e., using a simulation manikin and techniques – to "mock up" a medical emergency in this new environment. During this process, he is keen to consider how staff respond to this emergency, but more importantly how they can enhance their systems in order to improve their readiness if such an emergency were to happen in the future. Given Max's academic background he is keen to use this opportunity to conduct research into this topic. He has read about activity theory as a theoretical framework that can provide the analytical tools to understand complex activities in real-world clinical practice. Importantly it may have the potential to inform and guide in situ simulation to facilitate organizational change.

An Overview of Activity Theory

Origins

It hardly seems appropriate to attempt to define AT without considering its cultural-historical evolution. The theoretical foundations for AT were laid in the 1920s revolutionary Russia, driven by Marxist ideology and the work of Vygotsky, Leontiev, and Luria, the so-called "founding troika" of "cultural-historical" theory (Blunden 2011). They drew, in particular, on Marx and Engels' concept of *dialectical materialism* (Jordan 1967). *Dialectics* refers to the idea that progress occurs through the clash and resolution of contradictory ideas. *Materialism* is a philosophical stance concerning the primacy of material conditions – taken to include intangible external factors such as social interaction, language, and culture – over internally held ideas. In other words, human consciousness is shaped by real world conditions, rather than being a product of the mind's perceptions, as was held within then prevailing idealist philosophy (Marx and Engels 1967). Dialectical materialism therefore holds that human activity, driven by real-world conditions (especially, in

Marxist theory, factors such as social class, labor relations, and economic factors), produces contradictions, from which progress (e.g., reformed social structures) arises. Building on this idea – and in contrast to the then prevalent separation of mind and body espoused by Cartesian dualism (Kenny 1968), Vygotsky asserted the fundamental role of history, culture, and social interaction in shaping activity, therein forming the basis of what is now referred to as sociocultural theory (Wertsch et al. 1995). Importantly, Vygotsky also asserted that humans do not experience history and culture directly, but through interactions with people and physical objects. This process was termed *mediation*, occurring through interaction with *tools* or *artifacts*, either physical or psychological (Engeström et al. 1999; Vygotsky 1978). Most important amongst psychological tools is language (*semiotic mediation*), which acts as a "go-between" linking the outside world and individuals' construction of meaning (Vygotsky 1978).

Together, these ideas led to an understanding of human activity as "artifact-mediated and object-oriented action."(Vygotsky 1978; Kerosuo et al. 2010) In other words, activity (or work) is directed towards a purpose (its *object*) driven by real-world needs, and this purpose is achieved through multiple interactions with physical tools, dialogue, and documents. This conception is considered to represent *first-generation activity theory*, which concerns the triangular relationship between the *subject* (the person doing the activity) and the object, as mediated by artifacts.

Activity Systems

Vygotsky's work primarily concerned individuals in their social, historical, and cultural context. Following Vygotsky's death, however, Leontiev shifted AT's emphasis from individual to collective activity, driven by a common object (Leontiev 1981). Carrying these ideas forward, Engeström represented the structure of human activity as a dynamic model of an *activity system*, which represents *second generation activity theory* (Fig. 1). The topmost triangle contains subject, object, and mediating *instruments* (equivalent to tools and artifacts), the elements that comprise first generation activity theory (Engeström 2018). Underneath lie the "less visible social mediators," added by Engeström, of *rules*, *community*, and *division of labor*. The bidirectional arrows between all elements indicate their interrelated nature and point to the fact that activity systems must be understood holistically, and not simply as the sum of individual elements. The activity system, referred to as second-generation AT, is a key focus of activity theoretical research (Engeström et al. 1999; Engeström 2015).

More recently, Engeström and colleagues have further developed AT by incorporating the idea that, particularly within complex organizations, multiple, adjacent activity systems interact within a wider system. Thus, in what is referred to as *third-generation activity theory*, the "constellation of at least two interacting activity systems is frequently used as an extended unit of analysis" (Fig. 2) (Engeström 2015). The idea that two or more activity systems can be considered as interlinked, forming a network, is key to the concept of expansive learning, discussed in detail later in this chapter.

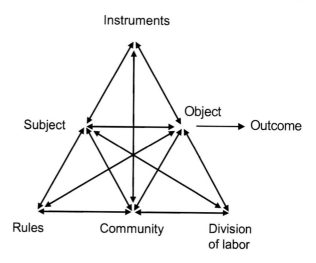

Fig. 1 The structure of human activity as a dynamic model of an activity system Engeström et al. 1999

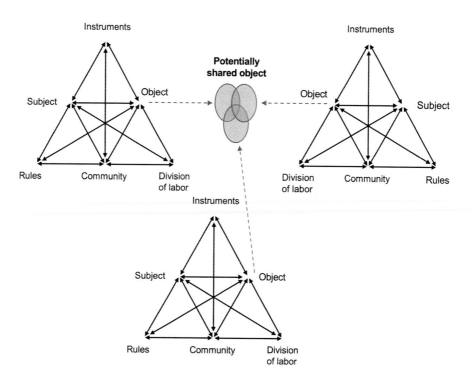

Fig. 2 Human activity as a dynamic model of interlinked activity systems Engeström 2018

While elements of activity systems are interrelated, it remains useful to define each in turn.

Subject

Following Engeström's ideas (Engeström 2015), the subject – or, more typically, group of subjects – is the agent (i.e., an individual who takes an active role in producing change) of the activity in question. Who is considered a subject depends on the nature of the activity under consideration and the analytic focus; in complex work environments, practitioners are typically subjects within many activity systems simultaneously. For example, the subject of a "surgical care" activity system might be a multidisciplinary team conducting a procedure (e.g., surgeons, anesthetists, and theatre nurse specialists) or, alternatively, if considering how residents learn to perform surgery, the subject might be the surgeons specifically. Similarly, an anesthetist serving many care processes taking place in parallel theaters can be considered a subject within multiple activity systems. Subjects' actions are always directed toward an *object*, which includes a collective motive for the activity. The concept of object, in view of its central importance in AT, is discussed in detail below.

Outcome

The outcome of activity is the tangible "product" that results from the collective activity. In a healthcare context, this might involve a treatment plan or the curing of a disease. Actions, in pursuit of the object, are mediated by tools and artifacts, known collectively as instruments.

Instruments

Instruments comprise physical tools (e.g., stethoscope, drug chart), language (e.g., medical terminology), and cognitive instruments, including analytical models and concepts (e.g., heuristics such as "rule out worst-case scenario" diagnostic reasoning). When using an activity theoretical approach to make sense of complex activity, it is essential to move beyond understanding of instruments as inert, physical items, and to recognize their role as social mediators. A stethoscope, for example, is not just an instrument for auscultating a patient's chest; it is also a badge signifying that its holder is a legitimate member of the healthcare community. Instruments therefore have the capacity not just to facilitate activity, but to shape it. A medical student with a stethoscope slung around her neck may be afforded opportunities to participate in activities of physicians that she would not otherwise. While clearly instruments do not possess intrinsic agency, their ability to enable, legitimize, condition, influence, impede, or inhibit activity means that they can be considered agentic (MacLeod and Ajjawi 2020). Within AT, instruments provide a way to understand the activity and its mediational nature, to give it meaning, and to develop it, but must always be considered in relation to the context in which they are used (Engeström 2015; Cole and Engeström 1993).

As human activity, and healthcare activity in particular, becomes more complex, it frequently calls for not just single tools, but multilevel instrumentality (Engestrom 2007). In particular, sophisticated new instruments have been created as a consequence of the revolution in information and communication technologies, which, as alluded to in the introduction, have profoundly impacted healthcare. The introduction of new technologies may precipitate qualitative transformations of entire activity systems. Implementing an electronic prescribing system, for example, may impact when and where doctors prescribe, how they access support from others, and the pattern of errors that occur (Puaar and Franklin 2018). These transformations are not reducible to the new technology but relate to resultant issues of responsibility and collaboration (Engeström 2004; Engeström et al. 2010) – an increasingly relevant consideration with the advent of artificial intelligence (AI) aiming to augment or replace practitioners' decision-making (Hodges 2021).

Rules

Rules, as the name implies, refer to regulations or procedures governing a particular activity. Rules may be formal and codified, such as a hospital's policy on staff sickness, but are very often informal, tacit, and socially defined, such as the prevalent cultural norm that healthcare professionals should work through minor illnesses to avoid letting colleagues down.

Division of Labor

Division of labor refers to the social structures, networks, and hierarchies that determine responsibility for particular actions within an activity system. Again, these may be enacted formally – senior doctors are given overall responsibility for patients within their care – or informally – consultants frequently delegate prescription writing responsibility to junior doctors rather than doing it themselves (Lewis et al. 2018).

Community

Community refers to the "actors" involved in the activity system that form its social context. Healthcare (and all human) activity always takes place within a community governed by a certain division of labor and by certain rules. How the community is defined and bounded depends on the historical development of the activity system (Engeström et al. 2010).

Object

Many discussions of AT deal with the concept of the object (Engeström et al. 2003; Miettinen 2005), reflecting its position as "perhaps the most challenging theoretical construct of AT," but one that holds central importance (Engeström 2018). Activity is always collective and driven by a shared object-related motive (Leontiev 1978). On this basis, individual actions can be said to be *goal-oriented*, whereas overall activity is *object-oriented*. In healthcare contexts, patient care can be considered the common, overarching object. In practice, however, the object is constructed within a given healthcare activity. For example, in considering doctor-patient encounters, Engeström describes individual patients as "raw material" from which the object ("a collaboratively constructed understanding of the patient's life situation and care plan") is formed (Engeström 2018).

The object holds the community together and gives it a long-term purpose (Engeström et al. 2003). On the other hand, the object is conceptualized differently (and often subconsciously) by different participants, making it *multivoiced* (Engeström 2018). Moreover, the object of activity may be constructed between adjacent activity systems with differing but overlapping purposes, referred to as a *potentially shared object*. That the object of activity is constantly molded, shaped, and negotiated by the activity systems that reproduce it means that object-orientated actions are often unpredictable and surprizing (Engeström and Blackler 2005). It is this dynamic, evolving quality of the object that underlies activity systems' potential for change; over time, activity systems and their elements reorientate themselves towards a new understanding of the object, whether as a natural consequence of activity, or due to conscious intervention by researchers and practitioners (Engeström 2004, 2015). This process, called *expansion of the object*, is the basis of the theory of *expansive learning*, discussed later.

Contradictions

Activity systems change in response to *contradictions*. Stemming from the previously discussed concept of *dialectics* – that progress occurs from the clash of opposing ideas – contradictions are inevitably occurring points of tension within and between activity systems, whose resolution leads activity systems to reformulate. Indeed, the activity system model is designed to explore tension-laden relationships between elements of singular activity systems, and between multiple interacting activity systems.

Contradictions "are not the same as problems or conflicts" that occur between practitioners on the ground (Engeström 2018). Instead, contradictions are systemic, structural tensions that manifest at different levels. Contradictions often surface as discursive manifestations such as dilemmas, conflicts, and double binds. Once healthcare practitioners begin to consider the concept of contradictions, they can begin to identify them within their own practice. For example, the increasingly recognized interdependence of patients' physical health, mental health, and wellbeing challenges the traditional biomedical separation between body and mind (with even the descriptors used in this sentence a testament to this tension). Or, in another example, primary care practitioners are all too aware of the contradiction between the need to see patients quickly (e.g., in short ten-minute appointment slots) while attempting to feel that their needs, both medical and interpersonal, are met through high-quality care.

Contradictions can be classified as *primary, secondary, tertiary,* and *quaternary* and their location may be denoted within the activity system model (Fig. 2) (Engeström 2015). Primary contradictions occur *within* single elements of activity systems and arise, Engeström argues, from the Marxist idea of "use value" and "exchange value" (Engeström 2018). Use value refers to an item's intrinsic usefulness in mediating activity, whereas exchange value refers to what an item is worth when traded (i.e., its market value). For example, healthcare professionals have skills that are used in service of patients yet, as employees of healthcare organizations, are also exchanged for financial reward, an arrangement that invariably gives rise to primary contradictions. In another example, medications (which can be considered instruments) have a use value in their potential to relieve symptoms and illness, but also a monetary exchange value. Again, this may create contradictions for practitioners responsible for making treatment decisions. *Secondary contradictions* are those that occur *between elements* of a *single activity system*. For example, professional guidance suggests that doctors should not act beyond their limitations (rules), but a colleague may have made clear that they do not wish to be awoken with queries during a night shift (community). *Tertiary contradictions* are those which occur *between an activity system* and its *future, redeveloped form*, and may manifest as inertia or resistance to change. For example, switching from a paper-based to a computerized hospital discharge system might be met with opposition, with knock-on effects on division of labor, community, rules, etc. For progress to occur (toward a new, shared object), tertiary contradictions must be overcome. Finally, *quaternary contradictions* occur *between activity systems*; typically, such contradictions arise from the potential for a shared object. For example, both healthcare education and practice aspire to the outcome of excellent patient care, but their specific objects – educating students within practice and delivering a safe, time-efficient clinical service, respectively, – frequently conflict. This particular example represents one of HPE's signature challenges (Larsen et al. 2019), which has been the subject of previous activity-theoretical study (Gillespie et al. 2021).

While a potential source of turmoil, contradictions enable organizational development because they build and accumulate over time, stimulating practitioners to look for new, stable ways of working in which they seek to establish shared objects of activity. Put more formally, the collective analysis and resolution of contradictions enables organizational transformation through renegotiation and reorganization of collaborative relations and practices, and through actions such as the construction of new tools (Engeström 2015). This process, involving expansion of the object, constitutes *expansive learning* (Engeström 2018).

Expansive Learning

Educators more familiar with more dominant theoretical perspectives in HPE, such as cognitivism, might come to question AT's role in understanding practitioners' learning and development. First generation AT, based on Vygotsky's work, is deeply concerned with individuals' development of meaning. In contrast to other individualistic, cognitively-focused models, however, Vygotsky's (sociocultural) framing held learning to be an essentially participatory process (Sfard 1998), in which learners, through material and social interactions, progress towards their developmental potential, termed a *zone of proximal development*. Moreover, Vygotsky characterized learning as a process of development of identify and self; in activity theoretical terms, people not only construct knowledge, but they also create their historical realities in object-oriented activity (Engeström et al. 1999; Vygotsky 1978). In sharing common roots in sociocultural theory, AT is linked to other educational theories, such as Communities of Practice (Johnston and Dornan 2015), which characterize learning as a socially mediated process.

Activity theory's shift in focus, from individual to collective, called for a further paradigm shift in what constitutes education and learning. In his most recent book, Engeström argues for a new vision of expertise that is collective, heterogeneous, boundary-spanning, and transformative. That this kind of expertise is needed may resonate with healthcare professionals and educators familiar with the challenges presented by the ever-changing landscape of practice, including those described in the introduction to this chapter. This framing forms the basis for expansive learning. Expansive learning refers to the development of new professional knowledge and new forms of work activity, by systematically questioning, reflecting on, and expanding the object of activity. By its nature, expansive learning views cognition as distributed and emphasizes organizational development over individual identity formation. The formal expansive learning cycle is described later, in relation to the Change Laboratory method, which is designed to systematically facilitate and structure the process.

Just as "every way of seeing is a way of not seeing,' (Burke 1935), health profession educators may contend that AT's emphasis on large-scale change, with activity systems as the unit of study, might detract from understanding how learners develop within object-oriented activity, particularly the novice practitioners with whom HPE is often concerned. Exploring how HPE can best embrace collective understandings of performance, and the issue of how individual practitioners learn and form identities within an activity theoretical framework, may represent areas of interest for HPE researchers moving forward.

> **Case Study – Part 2: Using AT to Make Sense of Complex Activity**
>
> Max is preparing to perform an in situ simulation in the new community healthcare building. In doing so, many of his colleagues comment *"are you preparing an emergency trolley?"* For Max, his intentions are much more than "just" preparing an emergency trolley. He is keen to step back and consider the wider perspective of how best to prepare for medical emergencies that may occur in the building. Increasingly he is drawing upon AT in his understanding of this complex activity.
>
> For Max, the overall purpose of his activity is to bring about change that enhances readiness to provide best care to an acutely unwell individual (i.e., *object*) in the vicinity of the healthcare facility. In doing so he wants to bring a multi-disciplinary team (i.e., *subject*) of healthcare professionals (including doctors, nurses, physiotherapists, social workers) who will be key individuals in responding to an emergency. In terms of preparedness, he also wants to consider the various *instruments* for managing an acutely unwell patient. Whilst emergency equipment such as airways and emergency drugs are of critical importance – he also wants to consider the physical layout of the building.

(continued)

> **Case Study – Part 2: Using AT to Make Sense of Complex Activity** (continued)
>
> Of course there is a wider *community* of individuals within the healthcare facility who also need to be considered – including the administrative personnel and other clients (patients) who may be in the facility at the time. Importantly there are explicit *rules* that apply across clinical settings governing the treatment of a patient who is experiencing an emergency (e.g., resuscitation guidelines). However, there are also local rules, whether explicit (such as local protocols around using emergency medications) or tacit, existing within the minds of Max and his colleagues, whether discussed or left unspoken. Within these local rules lies potential for development. Are there policies on who will update and maintain the emergency equipment? Are there procedures to ensure new staff are orientated to the emergency process?
>
> Finally, Max also turns his attention to "who will do what" in an emergency situation (i.e., *division of labor*). Whilst it is important to consider the practical tasks of managing an emergency (e.g., placement of a defibrillator on a patient) – it will be important to consider the many other tasks and who has responsibility for them; for example, ensuring that other patients in the facility are not distressed by the situation. Who updates and maintains the emergency trolley? Should it always be "the doctor" who manages the emergency? What if they were unavailable at the time?
>
> As Max prepares to plan a "mock up" simulation – he anticipates there will be contradictions between and within these various elements. Through this in situ simulation, he is keen to bring these contradictions to the surface – but more importantly, to bring about a positive change through renegotiation and reorganization of all of these aspects of a complex care scenario.

Using AT in Health Professions Education Research and Practice Development

That AT is well suited to researching and understanding problematic topics within HPE is reflected in an increasing body of literature, introducing AT to HPE audiences, describing its relevance to specific problems, and applying it directly within empirical study. Specific instances include book chapters (Johnston and Dornan 2015), a recent themed issue in a leading HPE journal (Dornan et al. 2021) and methodological articles within wide-ranging domains such as simulation (Gormley et al. 2020; Battista 2017), cultural complexity (Frambach et al. 2014), and interprofessional collaboration (Varpio and Teunissen 2021). Empirical articles have applied AT to analyze and address educational problems on topics such as prescribing (Kajamaa et al. 2019), patient safety (de Feijter et al. 2011), clinical examination (Ajjawi et al. 2015; Wearn et al. 2008), organizational development (Kerosuo et al. 2010), and student learning goals (Larsen et al. 2017). Having set out

AT's theoretical constructs, this section now explores practical considerations for using AT within HPE research, with reference to specific examples.

AT as a Theoretical Framework

AT can usefully inform all stages of research, including study design, data collection, and analysis. AT can be applied flexibly; there is no single approach to its use. In some cases, for example, it may be that AT can be used on a "post hoc" basis, applied to existing or routinely collected data, to enable deeper understanding. Nevertheless, it is important that researchers remain conscious that activity theoretical research has particular underpinning assumptions. For example, it gives primacy to social and cultural influences; it focuses on object-oriented activity rather than purely abstract or theoretical considerations; and it is concerned with systemic relationships rather than elements in isolation. It is essential that researchers reflect on the affordances created by these assumptions, questioning and ensuring alignment between them and their research questions, methodology, and methods.

In doing so, researchers may decide, for example, that AT might be a less appropriate theoretical lens to study the cognitive aspects of medical students' self-directed learning but, conversely, that AT may be appropriate for studying how their learning goals are enacted within specific healthcare contexts. In all cases, it is good practice for researchers to make decisions reflexively and to describe them in relation to the theoretical orientation of their work.

Data Collection

Taking the activity system as the basic unit of analysis has implications for how researchers might choose to collect data in activity theoretical studies. While quantitative data may contribute, the desire to explicate and explain social relationships, culture, and historical development means that qualitative data is the mainstay of AT research. In seeking to explicate these aspects of activity, multiple forms of data collection (perhaps in combination) may be considered, depending on the specific nature of the study. Researchers should reflect on how particular forms of data might shed light on the various elements that have comprised activity. For example, qualitative interviews might explore participants' experiences of workplace social relations, hierarchies, and informal rules of practice. Ethnographers might seek to identify significant instruments and, through observation and discussion with practitioners, understand their practical and cultural significance. Alternatively, documentary analysis may help trace the historical development of activity and the rules which govern it.

In examining how participation in simulation supported students' learning, Battista drew upon video recorded scenarios, transcripts of speech, and instructional design documents (Battista 2017). Videos enabled the researcher to produce narrative accounts of participants' activities; transcripts gave insight into social exchanges and participants' verbalized goals; and documents revealed tools, rules, and participant roles within scenarios. Together, these modes of data collection, chosen to align with an activity theoretical approach to analysis, enabled the researcher to explain how simulation-based scenarios might support students' learning by scaffolding object-orientated activity, and how tools, artifacts, and social interactions might mediate this.

Analysis

Activity theory is also and perhaps most commonly, applied as an analytic framework, in both exploratory and interventional research studies. Researchers may choose to describe and analyze activity systems in their entirety or, alternatively, use AT concepts to inform their analysis. In the former approach, researchers frequently "populate" the activity system model (as presented in Figs. 1 and 2) (Gormley et al. 2020). By defining individual elements – subject, rules, community, etc. – contradictions may be identified, particularly in subjects' conceptions of the object of activity. A recent study applied this approach to analyze an educational intervention (Gillespie et al. 2021), enabling the authors to address a key issue within HPE: the aforementioned contradiction between the object of the educational activity system (teaching and assuring students' competence) and the clinical activity system (providing safe and efficient patient care). This contradiction explained on-the-ground problems, such as clinicians' unwillingness to engage students in practice because it was seen to take too much time and pose a risk to patient safety. Carrying this forward, the researchers were able to show how their intervention – introduction of medical student "pre-prescribing" (authentic prescribing for real patients with sign-off by qualified doctors) – led to an expansion of the object, as clinicians and students reshaped their activity toward the shared purpose of caring for patients. In this instance, post-hoc application of AT added significantly to the transferability of the work, highlighting an important contradiction and a potential solution that will resonate with educators in other settings.

Rather than formally depicting full activity systems, Kajaama et al., aiming to understand doctors-in-training' experiences of the error-prone antibiotic prescribing process, drew on the concept of contradictions to focus their analysis (Kajamaa et al. 2019). They first used existing literature (e.g., national policy documents) and stakeholder input to develop a process map, reflecting the rules and procedures underpinning antibiotic prescribing. They then analyzed narrative interviews with doctors-in-training about their prescribing practice. This enabled the researchers to identify "disturbances" (contradictions) between the idealized process map and doctors' authentic prescribing experiences, such as when junior doctors struggled to reconcile conflicting advice given by ward-based consultants and microbiologists. In these cases, doctors were often more preoccupied with short-term goals (such as getting a prescription written) than the espoused object of achieving safe and effective treatment. This approach, emphasizing contradictions, enabled the authors to point to priority areas where interventions would be likely to have most impact.

Similarly, within a wider activity system analysis, Larsen et al. used the concept of *knotworking* – the way in which subjects form temporary, fluid teams centered around a specific purpose (Engeström 2018) – to explain how stakeholders came together to realize students' learning goals (Larsen et al. 2017). The authors argued that learning goals could act as tools, leading students, supervisors, and patients to come together in support of students' learning, but that "the knot was just as likely to unravel as tighten," as competing forces conspired to prevent these interactions. In this instance, the knotworking metaphor, drawn from AT, enabled the authors to explain and powerfully illustrate the dynamic, elusive, and context-dependent nature of students' learning.

AT as a Driver of Change: The Change Laboratory Method

AT differs from some other sociocultural theories in that it aspires to facilitate practical change, not just abstract understanding, and provides methodological tools in support of this aspiration. Engeström, whose approach to AT is now largely concerned with harnessing its creative potential to facilitate social change and forward movement, argues that change is inherently local, with "decontextualized prescriptions typically [leading] to solutions alien to the local activity system's developmental dynamics [leading them to be] rejected or unpredictably altered" (Engeström 2018). In other words, stakeholders within activity systems are best placed to conceptualize, develop, and bring about transformation.

To facilitate this sort of transformation, Change Laboratory (CL; often referred to as Change Lab) is a research-assisted intervention method, which draws theoretically from AT (Vygotsky 1978; Leontiev 1978) and, especially, from expansive learning (Kerosuo et al. 2010; Engeström 2015; Engeström et al. 1996; Virkkunen and Newnham 2013; Skipper et al. 2016; Morris et al. 2021). Change Laboratory is commonly used as an intervention in the context of research, although the CL approach need not be the subject of formal study. As described above, expansive learning is a collective process, aimed at overcoming tensions, leading to the formation of a new, expanded, and (at least partially) shared object between the participants of the activity (Engeström 2015). The purpose of CL is to facilitate an expansive learning cycle (Fig. 3) (Kerosuo et al. 2010; Engeström et al. 1996; Virkkunen and Newnham 2013).

The CL method is participatory and aims to enable stakeholders to understand the systemic nature of their daily activities and, through discussion (Haapasaari et al. 2016), to develop and implement new models and work practices (Engestrom 2007; Engeström et al. 2010). While not prescriptive, well-established procedures exist to support researchers in facilitating CL (Engeström et al. 1996; Virkkunen and Newnham 2013). Facilitators initially collect "mirror data" – data that enables participants to hold up a mirror to their own practices – by, for example, conducting observations. The CL intervention itself typically involves 6–10 sessions in which researchers and key stakeholders convene, facilitating a series of actions:

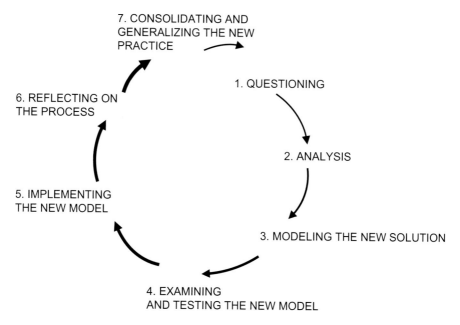

Fig. 3 Sequence of learning actions in an expansive learning cycle. (Adapted from Engeström and Sannino (2010) see also Engeström 1987/2015 (2015))

questioning, analyzing, modeling a solution, examining the model, and implementing (Engeström et al. 1999; Engeström and Sannino 2010).

Exemplifying the use of CL approach in healthcare practice, Diniz et al. set out to counteract disrespectful care of women during childbirth – including inappropriate obstetric interventions and impersonal treatment – in an academic maternity hospital in Brazil (Diniz et al. 2021). Using CL principles within a process of action research, and supported by mirror data collected through observation, interviews, focus groups, and historical and documentary analysis, they convened discussion sessions with clinicians and managers. Within these sessions, contradictions were identified, leading participants to suggest, model, and implement solutions. Specifically, the CL approach enabled identification of a key contradiction between mothers' wishes for person-centered care and clinicians' desire for residents to practise procedures. Principles of AT helped researchers explain cultural and historical issues underpinning this contradiction, such as culturally embedded hierarchical tensions between doctors and nurses and between men and women, and anachronistic beliefs that procedures could be performed without informed consent. As a result, changes were introduced, resulting in a friendlier environment, improved patient privacy, and fewer unnecessary procedures, although the authors did note that "changes that do not challenge hierarchies are easier to implement." This highlights that, while CL provides a powerful forum to explicate and redefine power relations, the methodology alone cannot bring about change without stakeholders' engagement and agreement.

Case Study – Part 3: Using AT to Bring About Practical Change

Following discussion with all of the stakeholders in the health center, Max organizes a series of meetings to consider how best they could prepare for managing emergencies in this new building. In the first meeting, Max prepares an in situ simulation of an emergency (a patient who had collapsed because of a cardiac event). Max was able to co-ordinate key stakeholders to meet over lunch time (when no real patients were in the health center). They include GPs from each of the separate clinics sharing the building, pharmacists, social workers, and members of the nursing and administrative teams. He briefs everyone about the simulation and then asks them to "go about their normal routines." Meanwhile, Max sets up a CPR manikin in the waiting room to recreate a collapsed patient scenario, and briefs a medical student to act as a distressed relative. An "emergency" is declared and the various healthcare workers respond to this simulated emergency. As the simulation unfolds, Max video records the event with his smartphone. Once the simulation has finished, all of the healthcare workers meet in the common room to have lunch and discuss the simulation. Following a debrief, Max explores with the group the "best practice" cardiac arrest guidelines. He then asks the group to review the video footage of how the cardiac arrest simulation was managed. Though the arrest was managed appropriately, it becomes evident that the overall response had areas that could be improved. The video footage provides an insightful "mirror" to what happened and reveals a number of contradictions. For example, not all of the staff knew where emergency equipment, such as the cardiac defibrillator, was located. Surprisingly, the pharmacists did not leave their desk to help with the emergency – given that the "unwritten rule" was that it was always doctors who managed emergencies. However, the GPs who responded to the emergency felt they would have really benefitted from the assistance of a pharmacist, particularly with administering medication to the collapsed patient. It also becomes evident that, although an emergency ambulance was called for promptly, no one had thought to look out for the paramedics and direct them to the scene, despite the vast size of the building. Max reflects with the group on a number of these issues. He also draws their attention to AT and discusses how that these "issues" can be considered to represent "tensions" between the various elements of activity. Following this meeting, participants are given notebooks to record tensions brought to their awareness as a result of the simulation. Moreover, they are asked to consider potential solutions to overcome these tensions.

At a follow up meeting a few weeks later, all of the healthcare workers meet again and have a round table discussion. They consider, collectively, the tensions identified and solutions to improve their overall preparedness for dealing with an acutely unwell patient. Through dynamic discussions, facilitated by Max, imagined meaningful changes surface and are considered.

(continued)

Case Study – Part 3: Using AT to Bring About Practical Change (continued)

Following this meeting the various stakeholders go about making changes that were collectively agreed upon. For example, they develop an emergency trolley that houses all essential clinical equipment. Importantly this trolley is located in a central area and with appropriate signage. Induction policies are modified to ensure that all new staff are oriented to where the emergency trolley is located. Equally, all current members of staff are oriented to the trolley and the new arrangements. Located in the emergency trolley are "prompt cards" that provide guidance on the important steps in managing various emergencies. Importantly, based on the previous simulation, a card is included that highlights the need for an individual (e.g., a member of the administration team) to wait at the front door, to beckon the paramedics and take them to the collapsed patient. Policies are also put in place that if a pharmacist is present in the building, that they also should be called to help in an emergency situation.

The third and final meeting is also held over a lunch time a few weeks later. At this meeting a further simulation is mocked up, this time involving a patient having a seizure. The response to this acutely unwell patient is again filmed by Max. Following debriefing, the various healthcare workers reflect on how much improved the response was: everyone knew where the emergency equipment was located; the pharmacists provided invaluable advice in helping to treat the patient; and an administration team member waited for the paramedics and brought them to the scene. The team express their thanks for Max's input in enhancing their organizational response to dealing with a medical emergency in the building. The team describe feeling much more confident and continue to suggest further modifications to enhance their response. It is agreed by the team that these changes would be made and a further simulation carried out to test them. Max is delighted and volunteers to conduct the further simulation in a few weeks' time. He also reflects that this would make the basis of an interesting research project.

Future Directions: AT in Educational Development

We would like to stress that AT involves many important concepts relevant to HPE beyond those described in this chapter; we encourage interested readers to read more deeply (with suggestions for useful resources given below).

We also encourage readers not to view AT as a finished product: like activity systems themselves, AT is changing, evolving, and expanding. Its use within HPE should serve to extend, not just apply, its concepts and methods. We conclude this chapter by reflecting specifically on how AT can be used within educational practice,

23 Activity Theory in Health Professions Education Research and Practice

not just research, and with specific reference to the emerging field of in-situ simulation.

Activity Theory as a Sense-Making Tool

While AT's development and main applications have been in a research context, we suggest that its ability to support practitioners to make sense of complex situations means that it can be used more widely. In applying AT principles, for instance, practitioners may begin to reflect more deeply on how contradictions arise within their own workplaces and, indeed, how solutions may be found. For example, a health professions educator, frustrated that students appear more interested in passing exams than interacting with real patients, might begin to perceive a primary contradiction: students focus on assessments because they must be passed in exchange for the right to practice as a doctor (Reid et al. 2021). This does not imply that change will be easy, but it may at least influence the educator's understanding that solutions might lie at the level of the educational system rather than in addressing students' motivation.

Activity Theory and In Situ Simulation: SimLab

Just as AT can be used to help make sense of complexity, we also suggest that it has the potential to augment, inform, and energize change efforts (even without adopting a formal CL approach), including service reconfiguration, quality improvement, and – of particular relevance to HPE – educational development.

In an example, which informs the case studies within this chapter, the authors have gained experience in using AT alongside in situ simulation to improve organizational responses to medical emergencies (Gormley et al. 2020). Medical emergencies, such as cardiac arrest or acute anaphylaxis, are time-dependent and difficult to manage well. Aside from the complex nature of the clinical presentation, healthcare professionals rely on a wide range of complex technical tools (e.g., defibrillators; emergency medications), which they must be able to access and use immediately. Furthermore, they must be able to coordinate their actions within a team to achieve optimal outcomes. Yet, due to the relatively rarity of events and fluid nature of healthcare teams, the clinical environment and the other team members may be unfamiliar to them.

Simulation, because of its ability to afford learning opportunities that are not readily available in real clinical environments, is regularly used to improve preparation for emergencies. Typically, however, simulation occurs in dedicated facilities remote from real clinical environments (e.g., simulation centers). To address this, there has been increasing interest in situ simulation, in which scenarios are conducted in authentic clinical workplaces. While this adds contextual richness, individual learning has remained in situ simulation's main emphasis. Our work hypothesizes that AT, as a systemic framework, can extend the use of in situ simulation, enabling it to drive organizational transformation alongside practitioner development. Recordings of initial simulations can provide powerful mirror data for subjects to reflect on their responses in relation to best practice (e.g., resuscitation guidelines). The principles of AT, through facilitated discussions, can enable subjects to consider issues, beyond individual performance, that might not otherwise come to light. By identifying contradictions, participants can scope, agree, and implement solutions within the workplace. A simulation-based approach provides an opportunity for solutions to then be tested, refined, and consolidated. We argue that this "SimLab'" approach exemplifies how educators can use AT to "expand the object" of conventional education, bringing it into closer alignment with the needs of real world clinical practice.

Conclusion

In the face of increasing healthcare complexity and the challenges this poses, both clinical and educational, it seems appropriate that HPE is beginning to embrace new "ways of knowing." This article outlines the increasingly recognized theoretical framework of AT, describing its roots, conceptual constructs, and applications within HPE. Given its focus on practices, multiple actors, and disturbances, which when collectively identified and analyzed are potential drivers for change and development, AT is particularly well suited for studying healthcare practice and education. Further still, under Engeström, AT has been iteratively developed and refined through extensive empirical study in healthcare contexts. While initially challenging at a conceptual level, AT offers huge potential as an approach to make sense of complex issues and as the basis of established methodological procedures that support both analysis and intervention.

Given healthcare's challenges, it is perhaps AT's explicit concern with implementation and change that appeals most. Unlike some other theoretical constructs, AT does not aspire to exist only in the abstract, unconcerned with the needs of practice. As Engeström puts it: "In the face of the pervasive and often dramatic changes in workplaces, avoidance [of putting theory to use in organizational development] amounts to hiding one's head in the sand" (Engeström 2018). Instead, he argues that AT should be used to drive healthcare reform: "disturbances and conflicts in everyday medical work . . . challenge the medical social system to understand and manage complexity, identify the dynamics of contradictions and utilize them in emancipatory transformations" (Engeström and Pyörälä 2021). This approach, in which development is not simply continual forward progress but "partially destructive rejection of the old" (Engeström 2018), may be challenging for healthcare and HPE to embrace (Dornan et al. 2021). It requires practitioners to continually question existing ways of doing things, accepting that learning is a lifelong process. It threatens prevailing structures, hierarchies, and power relationships. It undermines the continued dominance of the translational model in HPE, in which teachers teach, students learn, and improved clinical outcomes are taken for granted (Teodorczuk et al. 2017). Yet, by the same token, AT offers the potential for reforms that are sorely needed. It enables social boundaries between clinicians, students, and patients to be reassessed and redrawn, leading to healthcare that is more inclusive and more equitable. It promotes a conceptualization of expertise that takes account of healthcare's inherently collaborative and unstable nature. And it gives rise to the possibility that practitioners themselves are best placed to lead transformations within their local contexts. We encourage readers to reflect on how they might use AT to bring about change in their place of work.

Cross-References

▶ Embedding a Simulation-Based Education Program in a Teaching Hospital
▶ Focus on Theory: Emotions and Learning
▶ Social Semiotics: Theorizing Meaning Making

References

Ajjawi R, Rees C, Monrouxe LV. Learning clinical skills during bedside teaching encounters in general practice: a video-observational study with insights from activity theory. J Work Learn. 2015;27(4):298–314. https://doi.org/10.1108/JWL-05-2014-0035.

Battista A. An activity theory perspective of how scenario-based simulations support learning: a descriptive analysis. Adv Simul. 2017;2(1):1–14. https://doi.org/10.1186/s41077-017-0055-0.

Bleakley A. Broadening conceptions of learning in medical education: the message from teamworking. Med Educ. 2006;40(2):150–7. https://doi.org/10.1111/j.1365-2929.2005.02371.x.

Blunden A. An interdisciplinary theory of activity. Leiden: Brill; 2011.

Burke K. Permanence and change. New York: New Republic; 1935.

Cole M, Engeström Y. A cultural-historical approach to distributed cognition. In: Salomon G, editor. Distributed cognitions, psychological and educational considerations. Cambridge: Cambridge University Press; 1993.

Cristancho S, Field E, Lingard L. What is the state of complexity science in medical education research? Med Educ. 2019;53(1):95–104. https://doi.org/10.1111/medu.13651.

Davis D, Evans M, Jadad A, et al. Learning in practice journey from evidence to effect. BMJ. 2003;327:33–5.

de Feijter JM, de Grave WS, Dornan T, Koopmans RP, Scherpbier AJJA. Students' perceptions of patient safety during the transition from undergraduate to postgraduate training: an activity theory analysis. Adv Heal Sci Educ. 2011;16(3):347–58. https://doi.org/10.1007/s10459-010-9266-z.

Diniz CSG, de Bussadori JC, Lemes LB, Moisés ECD, de Prado CA, McCourt C. A change laboratory for maternity care in Brazil: pilot implementation of mother baby friendly birthing initiative. Med Teach. 2021;43(1):19–26. https://doi.org/10.1080/0142159X.2020.1791319.

Dornan T, Kearney GP, Pyörälä E. Destabilising institutions to make healthcare more equitable: clinicians, educators, and researchers co-producing change. Med Teach. 2021;43(1):4–6. https://doi.org/10.1080/0142159X.2020.1795102.

Engeström Y. The new generation of expertise: seven thesis. In: Rainbird H, Fuller A, Munro A, editors. Workplace learning in context. London: Routledge; 2004.

Engestrom Y. Enriching the theory of expansive learning: lessons from journeys toward coconfiguration. Mind Cult Act. 2007;14(1–2):23–39. https://doi.org/10.1080/10749030701307689.

Engeström Y. Learning by expanding – an activity-theoretical approach to developmental research. 2nd ed. New York: Cambridge University Press; 2015.

Engeström Y. Expertise in transition: expansive learning in medical work. New York: Cambridge University Press; 2018.

Engeström Y, Blackler F. On the life of the object. Organization. 2005;12(3):307–30. https://doi.org/10.1177/1350508405051268.

Engeström Y, Pyörälä E. Using activity theory to transform medical work and learning. Med Teach. 2021;43(1):7–13. https://doi.org/10.1080/0142159X.2020.1795105.

Engeström Y, Sannino A. Studies of expansive learning: foundations, findings and future challenges. Educ Res Rev. 2010;5(1):1–24. https://doi.org/10.1016/j.edurev.2009.12.002.

Engeström Y, Virkkunen J, Helle M, Pihlaja J, Poikela R. The change laboratory as a tool for transforming work. Lifelong Learn Eur. 1996;1(2):10–7.

Engeström Y, Miettinen R, Punamaki R-L, editors. Perspectives on activity theory. Cambridge: Cambridge University Press; 1999.

Engeström Y, Engeström R, Kerosuo H. The discursive construction of collaborative care. Appl Linguist. 2003;24(3):286–315. https://doi.org/10.1093/applin/24.3.286.

Engeström Y, Kajamaa A, Kerosuo H, Laurila P. Process enhancement versus community building: transcending the dichotomy through expansive learning. In: Yamazumi K, editor. Activity theory and fostering learning: developmental interventions in education and work. Kansai University Press; 2010.

Frambach JM, Driessen EW, van der Vleuten CPM. Using activity theory to study cultural complexity in medical education. Perspect Med Educ. 2014;3(3):190–203. https://doi.org/10.1007/s40037-014-0114-3.

Gillespie H, McCrystal E, Reid H, Conn R, Kennedy N, Dornan T. The pen is mightier than the sword. Reinstating patient care as the object of prescribing education. Med Teach. 2021;43(1):50–7. https://doi.org/10.1080/0142159X.2020.1795103.

Gormley GJ, Kajamaa A, Conn RL, Hare SO. Making the invisible visible: a place for utilizing activity theory within in situ simulation to drive healthcare organizational development? Adv Simul. 2020;5(29):1–9.

Greig G, Entwistle VA, Beech N. Addressing complex healthcare problems in diverse settings: insights from activity theory. Soc Sci Med. 2012;74(3):305–12. https://doi.org/10.1016/j.socscimed.2011.02.006.

Haapasaari A, Engeström Y, Kerosuo H. The emergence of learners' transformative agency in a change laboratory intervention. J Educ Work. 2016;29(2):232–62. https://doi.org/10.1080/13639080.2014.900168.

Hodges BD. Performance-based assessment in the 21st century: when the examiner is a machine. Perspect Med Educ. 2021;10:3–5. https://doi.org/10.1007/s40037-020-00647-4.

Johnston J, Dornan T. Activity theory: mediating research in medical education. In: Researching medical education. Wiley; 2015. p. 93–103. https://doi.org/10.1002/9781118838983.ch9.

Jordan ZA. The evolution of dialectical materialism. London: Macmillan; 1967.

Kajamaa A, Mattick K, Parker H, Hilli A, Rees C. Trainee doctors' experiences of common problems in the antibiotic prescribing process: an activity theory analysis of narrative data from UK hospitals. BMJ Open. 2019;9(6). https://doi.org/10.1136/bmjopen-2018-028733.

Kenny A. Descartes: a study of his philosophy. New York: Random House; 1968.

Kerosuo H, Kajamaa A, Engeström Y. Promoting innovation and learning through change laboratory: an example from Finnish health care. Cent Eur J Public Policy. 2010;4(1):110–31.

Larsen DP, Wesevich A, Lichtenfeld J, Artino AR, Brydges R, Varpio L. Tying knots: an activity theory analysis of student learning goals in clinical education. Med Edu. 2017;51(7):687–98. https://doi.org/10.1111/medu.13295.

Larsen DP, Nimmon L, Varpio L. Cultural historical activity theory: the role of tools and tensions in medical education. Acad Med. 2019;94:1255.

Leontiev AN. Activity, consciousness and personality. Englewood Cliffs: Prentice-Hall; 1978.

Leontiev AN. Problems of the development of the mind. Moscow: Progress Publishers; 1981.

Leung A, Luu S, Regehr G, Murnaghan ML, Gallinger S, Moulton CA. "First, do no harm": balancing competing priorities in surgical practice. Acad Med. 2012;87(10):1368–74. https://doi.org/10.1097/ACM.0b013e3182677587.

Lewis PJ, Seston E, Tully MP. Foundation year one and year two doctors' prescribing errors: a comparison of their causes. Postgrad Med J. 2018;94(1117):634–40. https://doi.org/10.1136/postgradmedj-2018-135816.

Lingard L, Espin S, Whyte S, et al. Communication failures in the operating room: an observational classification of recurrent types and effects. Qual Saf Heal Care. 2004;13(5):330–4. https://doi.org/10.1136/qshc.2003.008425.

MacLeod A, Ajjawi R. Thinking sociomaterially: why matter matters in medical education. Acad Med. 2020;95(6):851–5. https://doi.org/10.1097/ACM.0000000000003143.

Makary MA, Daniel M. Medical error – the third leading cause of death in the US. BMJ. 2016;353: i2139. https://doi.org/10.1136/bmj.i2139.

Marx K, Engels F. Capital: a critique of political economy. New York: International Publishers; 1967.

Miettinen R. Object of activity and individual motivation. Mind Cult Act. 2005;12(1):52–69. https://doi.org/10.1207/s15327884mca1201_5.

Monrouxe LV, Bullock A, Gormley G, et al. New graduate doctors' preparedness for practice: a multistakeholder, multicentre narrative study. BMJ Open. 2018;8(8). https://doi.org/10.1136/bmjopen-2018-023146.

Morris C, Reid AM, Ledger A, Teodorczuk A. Expansive learning in medical education: putting change laboratory to work. Med Teach. 2021;43(1):38–43. https://doi.org/10.1080/0142159X.2020.1796948.

Noble C, Billett S. Learning to prescribe through co-working: junior doctors, pharmacists and consultants. Med Educ. 2017;51(4):442–51. https://doi.org/10.1111/medu.13227.

Plsek PE, Greenhalgh T. The challenge of complexity in health care. BMJ. 2001;323(7313):625–8. https://doi.org/10.1136/bmj.323.7313.625.

Puaar SJ, Franklin BD. Impact of an inpatient electronic prescribing system on prescribing error causation: a qualitative evaluation in an English hospital. BMJ Qual Saf. 2018;27(7):529–38. https://doi.org/10.1136/bmjqs-2017-006631.

Reid H, Gormley GJ, Dornan T, Johnston JL. Harnessing insights from an activity system–OSCEs past and present expanding future assessments. Med Teach. 2021;43(1):44–9. https://doi.org/10.1080/0142159X.2020.1795100.

Richards T, Coulter A, Wicks P. Time to deliver patient centred care. BMJ. 2015;350:1–2. https://doi.org/10.1136/bmj.h530.

Sfard A. On two metaphors for learning and the dangers of choosing just one. Educ Res. 1998;27(2):4. https://doi.org/10.2307/1176193.

Skipper M, Musaeus P, Nøhr SB. The paediatric change laboratory: optimising postgraduate learning in the outpatient clinic. BMC Med Educ. 2016;16(1):1–12. https://doi.org/10.1186/s12909-016-0563-y.

Stange KC. The problem of fragmentation and the need for integrative solutions. Ann Fam Med. 2009;7(2):100–3. https://doi.org/10.1370/afm.971.

Teodorczuk A, Yardley S, Patel R, Rogers GD, Billett S, Worley P. Medical education research should extend further into clinical practice. Med Educ. 2017;1098–100. https://doi.org/10.1111/medu.13459.

Tonelli MR, Upshur REG. A philosophical approach to addressing uncertainty in medical education. Acad Med. 2019;94(4):507–11. https://doi.org/10.1097/ACM.0000000000002512.

Varpio L, Teunissen P. Leadership in interprofessional healthcare teams: empowering knotworking with followership. Med Teach. 2021;43(1):32–7. https://doi.org/10.1080/0142159X.2020.1791318.

Virkkunen J, Newnham D. The change laboratory – a tool for collaborative development of work and education. Rotterdam: Sense Publishers; 2013.

Vygotsky L. Mind in society: the development of higher psychological processes. Cambridge, MA: Harvard University Press; 1978.

Wearn AM, Rees CE, Bradley P, Vnuk AK. Understanding student concerns about peer physical examination using an activity theory framework. Med Educ. 2008;42(12):1218–26. https://doi.org/10.1111/j.1365-2923.2008.03175.x.

Wertsch JV, del Rio P, Alvarez A, editors. Sociocultural studies of mind. Cambridge: Cambridge University Press; 1995.

Whitty CJM, MacEwen C, Goddard A, et al. Rising to the challenge of multimorbidity. BMJ. 2020;368:1–2. https://doi.org/10.1136/bmj.l6964.

Suggested Further Reading

In-depth Discussion of Expansive Learning

Engeström Y. Expertise in transition: expansive learning in medical work. New York: Cambridge University Press; 2018.

Overviews of AT and Its Use in HPE

Engeström Y, Pyörälä E. Using activity theory to transform medical work and learning. Med Teach. 2021;43(1):7–13.

Dornan T, Kearney GP, Pyörälä E. Destabilising institutions to make healthcare more equitable: clinicians, educators, and researchers co-producing change. Med Teach. 2021;43(1):4–6.

Change Laboratory and Organisational Development

Morris C, Reid AM, Ledger A, Teodorczuk A. Expansive learning in medical education: putting change laboratory to work. Med Teach. 2021;43(1):38–43.

Kerosuo H, Kajamaa A, Engeström Y. Promoting innovation and learning through change laboratory: an example from Finnish Health care. Cent Eur J Public Policy. 2010;4(1):110 31.

Gormley GJ, Kajamaa A, Conn RL, Hare SO. Making the invisible visible : a place for utilizing activity theory within in situ simulation to drive healthcare organizational development? Adv Simul. 2020;5(29):1–9.

Reflective Practice in Health Professions Education

24

Jennifer M. Weller-Newton and Michele Drummond-Young

Contents

Introduction	442
Overview of Reflective Practice Theories	443
Meaning Perspectives	443
Dimensions of Reflection	444
Types of Reflection	444
Professional Practice and Donald Schön	446
Frameworks and Models to Guide Reflection	448
Pedagogical Approaches for Developing Reflectivity	452
Being Creative with Reflective Approaches	452
Reflective Learning Groups	452
Using Creativity	453
Digital Media	454
Scaffolding across the Years	455
Case Study 1	457
Case Study 2	458
Conclusion	459
Cross-References	459
References	459

J. M. Weller-Newton (✉)
Department of Rural Health, Melbourne University, Melbourne, VIC, Australia

School of Nursing, McMaster University, Hamilton, ON, Canada

Nursing and Midwifery, Monash University, Melbourne, VIC, Australia
e-mail: jennifer.wellernewton@unimelb.edu.au

M. Drummond-Young
School of Nursing, McMaster University, Hamilton, ON, Canada
e-mail: drummond@mcmaster.ca

© Springer Nature Singapore Pte Ltd. 2023
D. Nestel et al. (eds.), *Clinical Education for the Health Professions*,
https://doi.org/10.1007/978-981-15-3344-0_32

> **Abstract**

In health professions, reflection is a central tenet that assists practitioners in development of their professional knowledge and practice. Indeed, for many health professions, critical reflectivity has become a core competency within registration standards. This chapter presents the theory that underpins reflective practice beginning with a historical overview. John Dewey's seminal work *How We Think* (1933) paved the way for the current thinking on reflective practice. In presenting the theoretical underpinnings of reflective practice, pedagogical examples are provided. Discussion on the tensions between reflective practice as a pedagogy, service learning, where the reflective learning activity is given lip-service by students, versus clinical practice is provided. We explore how reflective practice in theory can become reflective practice in action. The exciting opportunities that current technologies afford in being creative with reflective practice are presented along with suggested pedagogical activities in scaffolding reflective practice.

> **Keywords**

Critical reflection · Dewey · Gibbs · Mezirow · Professional practice · Reflectivity · Reflective models · Schön

Introduction

The concept of reflection stems from educational and philosophical theories. John Dewey's seminal text *How We Think* laid the foundation among educationalists to reconsider approaches to learning. Dewey theorized that education should focus on individual growth, active learning experiences, and the social aspects of learning (Dewey 1934). He challenged us to consider reflection as a persistent form of thinking that is derived from experience. He defined reflective thought as:

> Active, persistent, and careful consideration of any belief or supposed form of knowledge in the light of the grounds that support it, and the further conclusion to which it tends, (Dewy 1997, p. 6)

Reflective thinking, Dewey suggests, is formed through five phases. The first phase is centered on an idea that comes to mind when initially confronted by a puzzling problem. The problem has become puzzling as it is seen as a whole, instead as small or distinct entities. A hypothesis is then formed when the problem is reconsidered in terms of what can be done with it or how it can be used or tentatively tested. Through reasoning, linking information, ideas, and previous experiences one can expand on suggestions. In the final phase the hypothesis is tested to ascertain how well one has thought through the problem situation. However, one may not always be right, and Dewey suggests failure is instructive as it sheds new light to a problem Dewey (1933, pp. 110–114) and so directs us to further reflective thinking.

Dewey's work underpinned teaching and learning on reflective practice for over 40 years before alternate theories proliferated in the late 1970s and into the 1980s. These latter theories are explored in the next section followed by the uptake of reflective practice in health professions education. Importantly as we review the theories, we need to recognize that reflection and the process of reflective practice are inextricably associated with learning and professional development in health professions. This is because the process of reflection on professional practice facilitates both practitioners and students to identify their learning needs. Reflection on personal beliefs and attitudes allows assimilation into one's discipline's culture (Mann et al. 2007). Through the divergent thinking that is undertaken, reflection enables professional growth and improved practice that can inform new understanding about self and the situated practice (Sadlon 2018).

Overview of Reflective Practice Theories

An early prominent theory is that of Jack Mezirow. For Mezirow (1990) the central function of reflection is validating what is known. Unlike Dewey, Mezirow claims that thoughtful action does not necessarily imply reflection. He defines reflection as "examination of the justification of one's beliefs, primarily to guide action and to reassess the efficacy of the strategies and procedures used in problem-solving" (Mezirow 1990, p. xvi). His 1970 theory on transformative learning originated from researching factors related to the success, or failure, of women's re-entry to community college programs. The researchers concluded that the subjects had undergone personal or perspective transformation. In his theory, Mezirow describes a ten-phase transformational process that was influenced by three educational philosophers: Kuhn's (1962) paradigm, Freire's (1970) conscientization, and Habermas's (1971–1984) domains of learning (Mezirow 1978, 1991, 2000). These phases included disorienting dilemma, meaning schemes, meaning perspectives, perspective transformation, frame of reference, levels of learning processes, habits of mind, and critical reflection (Kuhn 1962; Freire 1970; Habermas 1971, 1984). Over the decades, Mezirow refined this theory resulting in the construction of three distinct types of meaning perspectives.

Meaning Perspectives

A "meaning perspective is the structure of assumptions that constitute the frame of reference for interpreting the meaning of an experience" (Mezirow 1990, p. xvi). How we shape a particular interpretation of an experience is what Mezirow calls a "meaning scheme" which is a configuration of concepts, belief, judgments, and feelings (Mezirow 1994, p. 223). Learning within meaning schemes involves, for example, students building on what they already know, moving from a simple understanding of a situation (comforting a grieving parent) to one that is complex and nuanced. In more complex situations students may be challenged in their thinking and become aware of preconceived values and prejudices. Through critical self-reflection, students' learning can become transformed when they learn new insights about themselves. The three meaning perspectives are as follows: *epistemic*, related to knowledge and how a person uses it; *sociolinguistic*, language and how it is used in social settings; and *psychological*, the way people view themselves.

Dimensions of Reflection

Experiences that trigger reflection tend to arise when our assumptions become problematic: where we find a disconnect between our frames of reference, assumptions, and our environment (Mezirow 1994). Mezirow (1990) classifies our actions as the result of what we have learned in the formal and informal sense. In his model of reflection, Mezirow (1990) differentiates between *reflective action* and *non-reflective action*. *Non-reflective action* consists of two dimensions: habitual automatic action occurring without thought or rote action and thoughtful action which involves consciously drawing on what one knows to guide one's action (p. 6). This occurs without reflection. The reflective branch of his model encompasses thoughtful action with reflection and reflection on prior action. All reflection encompasses content and process dimensions. Only premise reflection is considered to embrace critical reflection and critical self-reflection. This asks why our frameworks and assumptions exist and whether they are congruent with our environments (Mezirow 1990, pp. 13–18).

Habitual action might occur when carrying out a psychomotor skill like changing a wound dressing. Thoughtful action occurs when drawing from what is known to guide one's response, for example, making decisions about how to redress a wound that has become infected. This along with habitual action is not reflecting. Although it solves a problem (applying an appropriate dressing), it does not challenge prior frames of reference or assumptions, rather decision-making is informed by shifting to another paradigm of prior knowledge. Reflective action is thoughtful but also incorporates a pause to critically challenge assumptions. This can occur in the moment or can involve looking back on an incident. This type of reflection primarily involves examination of the justification for one's beliefs to guide behavior or to assess how effective our task-oriented problem-solving strategies and process were. Mezirow (1981) describes seven hierarchical levels of reflection (see Table 1) which can assist us in understanding our assumptions and how we might respond to a given situation. He refers to the first four levels of reflectivity as "consciousness" and the last three as "critical consciousness." These latter three levels are when we become aware of the reasons that we might have made judgments or assumptions about people or the situation.

Types of Reflection

Thus, as illustrated in Table 1 critical self-reflection is central to transformative learning. According to Mezirow (1991), there are three distinct domains of

24 Reflective Practice in Health Professions Education

Table 1 Mezirow's levels of reflectivity

Level of reflectivity	Description of reflectivity
Reflectivity	Having an awareness of specific perceptions, meanings, or behavior
Affective	The individual's awareness of feelings about what is being perceived, thought, or acted on
Discriminant	Assessing the efficacy of perceptions, thoughts, and behavior; being able to identify reasons why you might respond in a particular way; and the impacts that relationships have on your actions
Judgmental	An awareness of value judgments made on perceptions, thoughts, and behavior
Conceptual	Assessing the adequacy of the concepts involved in clinical decision-making and the identification of the need for further learning; i.e., being able to critique your own actions and questioning the adequacy of and morality of concepts that you have encountered in the situation
Psychic	Recognition of the habit of making precipitant judgments on limited information, i.e., recognizing your own prejudices by acknowledging we often judge others on limited information
Theoretical	An awareness that one set of perspectives, e.g., taken for granted practice or culture, may explain personal experience less satisfactory than another perspective. This is about changing your underlying assumptions resulting in transformation

Table 2 Mezirow's domains of reflection

Type of reflection	Key elements
Content	Examines the acquisition of skills and knowledge from one's prior learning. Through pausing and thinking back, critiquing if what is learnt is congruent with current circumstance. Outcome of this level of reflection involves a transformation of meaning schemes (Mezirow 1995)
Process	Entails considering one's actions origins and related factors, checking problem-solving methodology being used. Has one understood the problem, is one's response congruent with societal norms. Also, may transform meaning schemes (Mezirow 1995)
Premise	Entails learning through meaning transformation through critically examining one's prior interpretations and assumptions to form new meaning as a result of asking "why." This transformation is profound (Mezirow 1995)

reflection: content, process, and premise (see Table 2). These are used to interpret and give meaning to our experiences (Mezirow 1991, p. 104).

In 2000, in a revised version of his transformative learning, Mezirow argued that a meaning perspective is a frame of reference comprising habits of mind and subsequent points of view. Habits of mind were expanded to include a variety of dimensions: sociolinguistic, moral ethical, epistemic, philosophical, psychological, and aesthetic (Mezirow 2000). Mezirow (1998) suggested that "learning to think for oneself involves becoming critically reflective of assumptions and participating in discourse to validate beliefs, intensions, values and feelings" (p. 197). Mezirow's transformative learning theory has been widely used in education. However, the proliferation of reflection and reflectivity particularly in health professional disciplines and education has been greatly influenced by the work of Donald Schön.

Professional Practice and Donald Schön

In our everyday professional practice, our knowing, Schön (1983) argues, is embedded in our actions. Professional education, Schön proposes, gives rise to systematic technical-rational forms of knowledge which are incongruent with the forms of professional knowledge and the changing characteristics of professional practice settings. The knowledge used in professional practice is broad, deep, multifaceted, and not easily articulated and is acquired overtime through developing a repertoire of expectations, images, and techniques. This practice knowing, Schön (1991) suggests, becomes increasingly tacit, spontaneous, and autonomic. When professional practitioners are confronted with complex situations, Schön contends that these are often insolvable through the technical-rational problem-solving approach of science. He suggests, in the "swampy world" of practice, one needs to refocus problems in terms or context that can be understood. Schön believes this can be done through a reflective conversation, where one draws upon their experience to understand, frame, and suggest actions to resolve the situation. Thus, reflective practice is an essential component of professional practice.

Schön (1983, 1987, 1991) articulates three forms of reflection: *reflection-in-action*, *reflection-on-action*, and *reflection-for-action*. *Reflection-in-action* involves becoming conscious of the tacit knowledge incorporated in the routines of practice and subjecting that knowledge to critical examination. Schön argues that reflection-in-action is central to the art by which professionals handle and resolve their difficulties and concerns about practice while actually in practice. It entails thinking about what one is doing in the midst of performing that action. *Reflection-on-action* is systematic and deliberate thinking back over one's action. It is a way that one can come to know their "tacit" knowledge. Tacit knowing can be hard to capture and articulate. Often what we know, we cannot verbalize, as Schön suggests, our knowing is ordinarily tacit and implicit in one's actions. *Reflection-for-action* is the desired outcome of reflection in and on action. It is anticipatory in nature – drawing upon past experiences in preparing for a future situation (Schön 1991).

Inextricably linked with Schön's (1983, 1987, 1991) concept of reflection is the notion of single- and double-loop learning. Argyris and Schön (1974) and Argyris (1976) contend that we all have theories-in-use, which are governed by the values one holds and the behavioral strategies that one uses. These theories-in-use are often dissonant with one's espoused theories, the ones we claim allegiance to. For example, as a health practitioner, one might claim that one's practice is underpinned by person-centered care; yet in the reality and business of everyday work, the concept of person-centered care becomes just a task list of activities to achieve during the shift, with little regard to the needs of the individual patient.

24 Reflective Practice in Health Professions Education

Table 3 Boud et al.'s (1985) phases of reflection

Phase	Key aspects
Preparation for the experience	Personal – What the individual brings to, wants from the experience The experience – The context, the constraints, and opportunities afforded by the experience The learning strategies – what strategies the individual will use (Boud 1992)
Returning to the experience	Description of the experience; recollecting the salient events, should be devoid of judgments to avoid clouding recollections Acknowledging feelings, both positive and negative
Attending to feelings	Feelings need to be discharged through either oral or written expression as they can affect the experience
Re-evaluating the experience	Association – Relating new information and ideas to relevant pre-existing knowledge Integration – Seeks to find relationships between current or observed experience and pre-existing knowledge to determine usefulness and meaningfulness Validation – Testing for internal consistency between new appreciations and existing knowledge and beliefs Appropriate – new information which has become integrated is accepted and becomes one's own, i.e., becomes part of one's value system (Boud et al. 1985; Boud and Walker 1991)

A further educational theory on reflection that became popular at the same time was the work of Boud et al. (1985). They originally proposed three phases to the reflective process, though in response to criticism Boud (1992) later included a further phase. These phases are outlined in Table 3. In reviewing these early prominent theorists' concepts of reflection, a common theme emerges, reflection is more than just thinking. It is about challenging one's previously underlying values, beliefs, and assumptions.

Reflection can be a useful learning tool for developing knowledge from practice because it can enable practitioners to identify their learning needs. Reflecting on personal beliefs and attitudes allows their integration into the professional culture (Mann et al. 2007). The combination of these elements is what makes reflective practice so distinct. As the process of reflection enables continuous professional growth and improved clinical practice amongst those who use it, through the distinct form of divergent thinking that is undertaken. This can lead to new understandings about self and the situated practice (Sadlon 2018). Within healthcare professions, the practice of reflective practice has been applied to many aspects of work in nursing and midwifery, such as clinical supervision, practice development, and education, and has also been utilized in social work, occupational therapy, and medicine (Taylor 2010).

However, as Dewey (1933, p. 35) writes: "While we cannot learn or be taught to think, we do have to learn how to think well, especially how to acquire the general habit of reflecting." Boud et al. (1985) consider reflection to be an intellectual and affective activity used to explore experiences to form new appreciations and understandings. As more professional disciplines and educationalists recognized the value and importance of reflection, several frameworks and models to assist individuals to engage in reflective practice have been developed. Several of these frameworks and models are presented in the next section.

Frameworks and Models to Guide Reflection

During the latter half of the twentieth century, a range of frameworks and models emerged. While Dewey (1933) offered five phases of reflective thinking, later educational theorists and even health practitioners recognized that key to reflection is articulating essential questions. A simple model proposed by Gibbs (1988) orientates the individual through a sequence of questions (see Fig. 1). Each stage of the model poses a series of questions that encourage the individual to make sense

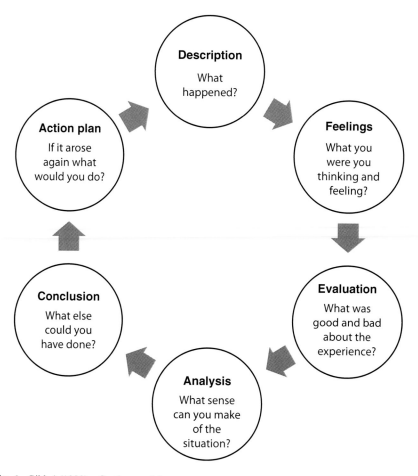

Fig. 1 Gibbs' (1988) reflective model

of the situation and consider their emotions and alternative actions if a similar situation was to occur. Gibbs' model has been widely used as an educational framework, e.g., for structured debriefing; however criticisms of this model includes its applicability to professional practice, the introversion on self, the lack of context in which learning is taken place, along with the lack of criticality (Timmins 2008).

A more complex guide to structured reflection was developed in 1995 by Chris Johns. His model of structured reflection (MSR) was advanced through the analysis of guided reflection relationships with nurses. Johns (1995) offered the model to be used as a "heuristic tool." The intention of the model is to provide a framework for reflection "whilst enabling the practitioner to transcend the model to reflect, in response to the unfolding situations that present in everyday practice" (p. 226). His model offers more depth through "looking in" at emotions, e.g., how was I feeling in this situation and what made me feel that way and how did the person or persons feel, to "looking out" at what external factors that may have led to the action or decision.

Johns has since refined and enhanced his original MSR as he explored epistemological and ontological approaches of reflection. He notes that the theories of Gibbs (1988), Boud et al. (1985), and Mezirow (1981) frame their reflective approach as a linear or cyclic progression that reflects a Western technological approach to learning. Seeking to balance this rational approach to reflection, Johns studied the more esoteric influences of Buddhism and Native American lore (Johns 2013). He does not subscribe to the distinction between reflection and critical reflection and contends that "all reflection has the capacity to move into a consideration of the nature and consequence of power and hegemony within everyday practice" (p. 40). Johns' (2017) 17th iteration of his MSR model is outlined in Table 4, although a thorough reading of the reference (*Becoming a Reflective Practitioner* fifth edition) is recommended.

While the cues in Johns' MSR are arranged in a sequential order, he stresses that they do not have to be used sequentially, as they "reflect a dynamic movement

Table 4 Model for structured reflection edition 17 (Johns 2017, p. 38)

Phase	Cues (questions to help you break down your experience and reflect on the processes and outcomes)
Preparatory	Bringing the mind home
Descriptive	Write a description of an experience
Reflective	What in particular seems significant to pay attention to? Why did I respond as I did? Was I effective in terms of consequences for others and myself? What factors influenced my response?
Anticipatory	Given the situation again, what are my options for responding more effectively? What are the potential consequences of responding differently? How do those influencing factors need to shift so I can respond differently?
Insight	What tentative insights do I draw? How does extant theory/ideas inform and deepen my insights? How does exploring with guides and peers challenge my insights? How do I feel now about the situation?

towards gaining insight" (p. 37). With increased use, the cues become embodied and shape practitioners' mindful attention.

Taylor developed her REFLECT model (Taylor 2010, p. 62), as she was concerned that reflective practice fails to acknowledge the ways in which reflective accounts construct the world of practice. Cognizant of Schön's concern that successful reflection requires coaching Taylor's model is a mnemonic represented as **R**eadiness, **E**xercising thought, **F**ollowing systematic processes, **L**eaving oneself open to answers, **E**nfolding insights, **C**hanging awareness, and **T**enacity in maintaining reflection. Her model has the image of a globe at the center which reflects the world of practice, encompassing the contextual features within the work setting. The band REFLECT flows around the globe in a systematic manner, encapsulating the processes of the world of practice. This flow of reflective processes, Taylor (2010) suggests, is dependent on the clinical issues within the work context, and internal and external constraints, that could be occurring at any given point of time. In an attempt to simplify reflection, Taylor considers that there are three main types of reflection: *technical* which is focused on thinking about issues relating to clinical procedures. These issues will require rational thinking for specific, manageable problems. Underlying concepts include scientific reasoning, critical thinking, and problem-solving. *Practical* reflection is focused on interactions and role relationships to improve communication. *Emancipatory* reflection enables the recognition of sociocultural constraints, questioning the status quo that might be impacting on one's practice and developing critical knowledge. It is worth noting that these three levels of reflection are not dissimilar to van Manen's (1977) levels of reflection: technical, practical, and critical. This third level he suggests entails reflecting on the sociopolitical influences that systematically and ideologically influence practice. Taylor provides a detailed set of questions/cues for each type of reflection, which enable the practitioner to determine if their reflection is across all three levels or whether they are wanting to focus on a particular aspect of their practice. A thorough reading of Taylor's REFLECT model (*Reflective Practice for Healthcare Professionals*, third ed.) is recommended.

Two further models are briefly considered next, both of which have been developed in the 2010s. The first is by Bassot, who has drawn upon several approaches (e.g., Gibbs and Johns) to create the Integrated Reflective Cycle (Bassot 2013, 2016). While highlighting the strengths of the theoretical models that precede it, Bassot has incorporated questions around the cycle to facilitate one's thinking. In doing so, she purports that questioning professional practice is "an excellent way of delving deeper into not only what you did, but why. . ." (p. 111) – an issue which is central to critical reflective practice. Bassot's (2013) Integrated Reflective Cycle is presented in Fig. 2.

A relatively new reflection model that seeks to promote transformative learning at both the personal and societal level is the Bass Model of Holistic Reflection (Bass et al. 2017). This model incorporates six inter-dependent phases: (1) self-awareness (inner); (2) description (external/internal); (3) reflection (thoughts and feelings, internal); (4) influences – knowing external; (5) evaluation (analysis) conclusions external; and (6) learning (synthesis) action internal/external. These phases are embedded within a circular design reflecting the iterative rather than linear nature

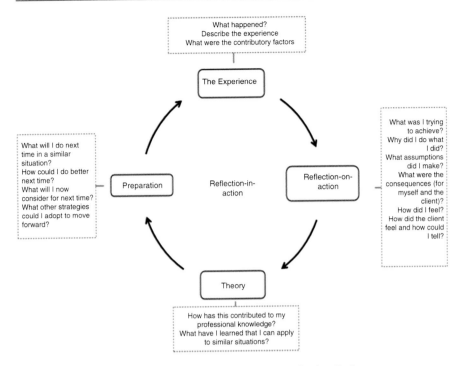

Fig. 2 Adapted from Bassot's (2013, p. 110) the Integrated Reflective Cycle

of reflection. Each phase is integrated to promote critical reflection at a deep personal level, contributing to the development of holistic reflective practice throughout the continuum of the learning cycle (Sweet and Bass 2019). The model makes explicit the forms of knowing used to make sense of practice, empirical (the know that of science), personal, moral, and aesthetics (the know-how of practice) along with emancipatory knowing as outlined by Habermas (1979). While initially designed for midwifery practice, the integrative, holistic nature of this model sits well in it being utilized by other disciplines. In particular, its application within curricula design maybe useful, which will be discussed in the chapter's section on scaffolding reflection across the years of a degree program.

This section has highlighted just a few models and frameworks available to guide reflection. Johns (2013) offers the advice that practitioners "should be guided to review all models for their value, rather than accepting the authority of any model on face value. Rather like the skilled craftsman, one needs to choose the tool that is most helpful" (p. 48). Importantly, reflection should not be understated, it is a complex and holistic activity that engages the mind in all stages or cues (Johns 2017). It is not necessarily a linear process, but an iterative process of weaving through the different stages. It could be a cycle or spiral, as befits the aspect of practice or the incident that triggered the reflection. Given that reflection requires the development of skill in acquiring this habit of mind, the next section explores some of the pedagogical approaches used in facilitating health professional practitioners' reflectivity.

Pedagogical Approaches for Developing Reflectivity

Reflection, as argued in this chapter, is a cognitively demanding and complex skill that is not acquired overnight and that requires carefully planned pedagogical strategies (Braine 2009). Most reflective activities in health professional education are in the form of reflective portfolios or journaling (Epp 2008; Mann et al. 2007). These reflective activities, in entry to practice programs, are frequently incorporated in their placement experiences, requiring students to explore their clinical or learning experience through writing about what occurred. However, practicum experience does not necessarily provide opportunities for students to develop their reflection skills (Nagle 2009). This is possibly due to the complex nature of the healthcare workplace which can impede on students understanding of their practice (Newton 2011) where they are unfamiliar with the requirements of the work environment.

Journal writing is not new. Diary or journal writing as a means of self-expression and reflection, historically, is an old form of writing (Lukinsky 1990). Writing reflections in a journal can create space in one's busy life (Johns 2013). However, there are emergent concerns whether written journals are the most effective way to develop students' reflective abilities (Newton and Butler 2019). Some students collate piles of reflective accounts, a number of which could be fictitious (Braine 2009; Newton 2004), while others find it difficult to engage with tasks such as journaling or reflective writing if there is no assessment attached to them (Braine 2009; Newton 2004). While reflective journals can be useful for promoting learning and reflection, there are other approaches to facilitate student learning (Chirema 2007). One needs to acknowledge how the advancement of technology is impacting on the current generation of students, who may not value nor find meaning in written tasks (Sandars and Homer 2008; Sandars and Murray 2009). Yet, as Boud (2010) suggests, one should not lose sight of the original focus of reflection, which is constructing personal knowledge. Reflection "is a means to engage in making sense of an experience in situations that are rich and complex..." (2010, p. 29). Hence, Boud contends, reflection needs to be located in the context of practice; otherwise it does not take into consideration the complexity of the workplace. So, what pedagogical strategies can be used to promote the development of reflection in practice? In the last decade, there has been an increase in the use of alternative pedagogies (other than journaling or portfolios) to support reflection, and several approaches are presented in the next section. Johns (2013, 2017) directs us to the importance of curiosity in opening one's mind to enable creativity in supporting reflectivity.

Being Creative with Reflective Approaches

Reflective Learning Groups

Reflective learning groups have been successfully used with final year nursing students (Newton 2011). Premised in the principles of action learning, an important element of reflective learning groups is the expectation that the students will identify their own action points at the end of each learning group. These actions need to be revisited in subsequent learning groups to encourage a sense of personal empowerment and in doing so foster reflexivity (Fook 2010). Reflectivity can become a tool for students to use as part of their repertoire of personal professional skills, enabling them to reflect about a problem in its practice context, to resolve it and then be able to move on to something else. Reflective learning groups allow for consideration of multiple perspectives of practice issues not available to individuals engaging in personal reflection (Duffy 2008). Through a reflective learning group, students' values and understandings can be shared, debated, challenged, and changed (Field 2004). Harrison et al. (2019) adapted this type of reflective activity in a project that explored the use of Clinician-Peer Exchange Groups (C-PEGs) with final year medical students on clinical placement. The C-PEGs provided peer-only, face-to-face forums for students to share learning with their peers in groups of five. Topics for discussion were comparatively open-ended topics. The C-PEGs were scheduled throughout the students' placement, and the nature of the C-PEGs created a safe learning environment for the students to share content that mattered to them. The scheduling of these sessions assisted the students to engage in a reflective process in a genuine and open way. Participation in these types of reflective learning groups supports Boud's (2010) argument that reflection needs to be contextualized, embodied, and co-produced, contextualized in terms of taking into account the actual people involved and the practice setting; embodied in the context of emotional engagement, that is, participants must choose to undertake reflection; and co-produced in that differences of power and position within the group are accommodated.

Using Creativity

Challenged with encouraging final year nursing students to reflect on their learning in preparation for transition to becoming a graduate nurse, a reflective assignment was introduced which encouraged students to use any form of creative arts media for their reflection (Newton and Plummer 2009). The students were required as a component of their assignment to submit a 300-word accompaniment that explained the meaning underpinning their creative work. The students' creativity was expressed in many differing media – photographic displays, paintings, sculptures, tapestries, board games, songs, and quilts. The reflective assignment became an eagerly anticipated activity to do, with students seeking to commence working on their creative work prior to the semester commencing (Newton and Plummer 2009). Such an approach highlights that creative art can be a way of communicating beyond words (Horsfall and Welsby 2007) by enabling the articulation of the unknown or previously expressible (Higgs and Titchen 2007). Using poetry or combining words with art enables the creative spirit to be nurtured by unlocking the right side of the brain, opening up space for reflection and imagination (Johns 2017).

Digital Media

Improving engagement in reflection can also be achieved through using digital media such as podcasts, video storytelling, and weblogs (Coulson and Harvey 2013). In health professional education, digital storytelling has been effectively utilized to develop increased insight into students' experiences and enhanced depth of understanding of both the clinical context or environment and the patient as a person within the healthcare process. Digital storytelling incorporates the use of photos, videos, animation, sound, text, music, and voice narrative in which students explore an issue or share an experience (Price et al. 2015). In this group activity, the process of creating the digital story encourages reflection on behaviors, scenarios, values, or experiences and helps link theoretical concepts to personal experiences. Reflection is promoted across the two phases of the digital storytelling process: students engage in reflection as they choose suitable photos, images, or dialogue to tell their story and reflect again as they share their story with others and receive comments and feedback. Through the preparation and engagement in the digital storytelling, it offers students new insights and assists with their application of content to practice facilitating their reflective learning by enhancing students' ability to notice things (Price et al. 2015). This sharing of experiences exposes learners to other ideas, worldviews, and perspectives, thereby augmenting both their own and their peers' reflections (Sandars and Murray 2009; Price et al. 2015).

Digital storytelling gathers pedagogical acceptance video, and the use of Vlogs (video blogs) is emerging as another approach to enhance the development of reflection across a range of disciplines, including both education and healthcare. The range of applications of video to enhance student reflection and also of practitioners is vast and includes video-supported reflection on action or clinical skill (e.g., in simulation debriefing), as an avenue for creating safety (e.g., real-time clinical practice). Though each of these activities varies slightly in design, they generally share a common purpose: to enhance clinical skills through reflection on actions; to increase understanding of actions, behaviors, and experiences (i.e., to enhance self-awareness, safety); and to improve students and practitioners' theoretical knowledge and decision-making (Al Sabei and Lasater 2016; Coffey 2014; Iedema 2011). As debriefing is a structured process of facilitated reflection on a clinical or simulated scenario, it enables students or practitioners to explore their cognitive, affective, and psychomotor skills in order to identify strengths and weaknesses, link theory to practice, and enhance their future performance (Al Sabei and Lasater 2016; Cant and Cooper 2011). The general quality and amount of student reflection is enhanced through this form of reflection (Royle and Hargiss 2015) as students gain insight into their actions and their learning (Bowden et al. 2012; Yoo et al. 2009).

Newton and Butler (2019) piloted the use of reflective videos to capture entry to practice nursing students' learning from their community practicum. Students were provided with guidelines to promote their critical reflections about what they had learnt. A specific web-based interface (Moodle site) was created to facilitate the students to upload their videos and engage in a discussion forum. While only a small group of students participated, the analysis of the video content revealed that the students' videos offered significant learnings from their community placements, with a greater insight and critical reflectivity compared with the analysis of a prior cohort's written community placement portfolios (Newton and Butler 2019). Indeed, reflecting through video enabled the students to articulate their previously held values and reshaped their perspectives of their discipline practice. As technology advances, digital and creative pedagogical strategies that engage students and practitioners in reflection need to become mainstream. Central to such developments is the need for the health professional educator to not only be well-grounded in reflective practice to facilitate innovative pedagogical approaches but also to understand the importance of scaffolding reflection across the curriculum. The next section presents a reflective framework for scaffolding along with a case study of how scaffolding of reflection has been incorporated into a nursing program.

Scaffolding across the Years

If we recall the section on frameworks and models for reflective practice, there was some degree in variation in the simplicity and complexity of these frameworks. Choosing which one to use can be aligned to the notion of scaffolding an individual's development of their reflectivity ability. Scaffolding should not be mistaken with just "teaching" or "support" (Wilson and Devereux 2014); rather it encompasses the stimulation of judicious and independent orientation to assist students in making sense within the context of their discipline. It is about building capacity and enabling individuals to go beyond their existing capacity. Thus, in the context of reflective practice, scaffolding is important in supporting the novice in the development of their self-awareness, critical thinking, reasoning, decision-making, and behavior to become independent and autonomous reflective practitioners.

Within the context of clinical placements, Bandaranaike et al. (2012) adapted a Work Skills Development Framework (WSD) into a Clinical Reflective Skills (CRS) framework that promotes students' engagement in reflective practice through a continuum of five autonomous levels within defined clinical skills facets. Table 5 provides an example of a skill development along the continuum of student autonomy. This structured two-dimensional facet facilitates students not only about "collecting experiences" of their clinical placement, e.g., for a portfolio or journal, but actively engages the student in processing their learning and changing their behaviors. As Bandaranaike et al. (2012) suggest, the CSR framework can be used as a reflective tool. It also can be used as an assessment tool across health professions in enabling the development of professional skills through reflective practice.

A Canadian school of nursing's BScN curriculum utilizes similar scaffolding principles to the WSD framework. Students are introduced to their curriculum which is designed to cultivate an ethos of reflection in an attempt to promote ongoing transformative learning as students evolve as nurses throughout the program (Barnett 2009; Cranton 2002; Mezirow 2000; Taylor 2017). Faculty who deliver the course model "thinking out loud" when engaging in discussion as they teach content, process, and metacognitive aspects of the course. Additionally, as students progress

Table 5 Example of Clinical Reflective Skills Development Framework (Snelling and Karanicolas 2012)

Level of student autonomy

Facet of skill development	Level 1 Student requires a high degree of structure/guidance	Level 2 Student works with some degree of structure/guidance	Level 3 Student works independently within provided guidance	Level 4 Student works in an innovative manner with minimal reliance on guidelines	Level 5 Student works with self-determined guidelines appropriate to the context
Initiative Student establishes professional role within their scope of practice	Requires a high degree of guidance to identify and adapt to professional role	Able to restate professional role requirements, but requires some guidance to identify and adapt to position	Able to establish professional role requirements, and identifies and adapts to the position with minimal oversight	Readily establishes professional role requirements and identifies and adapts to position in a variety of contexts.	Highly developed sense of professional role in all clinical contexts.

through the program, they are taught the concept of being part of "a community of practice" where they will discover ways of being within the practice setting (Dall'Alba 2009). This evolves through explicit engagement in reflective practice by noticing and interpreting disconnects between their frames of reference, assumptions, and the practice environment (Mezirow 1994; Tanner 2006). Process learning within the curriculum is scaffolded to engender knowledge-based dispositions to professional growth and lifelong learning (Manankil-Rankin et al. 2013). This approach to scaffolding reflection has been formalized by A Guide for Developing Reflective Practitioners whereby nursing students are required to submit clinical reflections each placement. Instructions and expectations of the reflective activities, along with several optional lines of questioning for the students, are outlined in their clinical manual. In the first and second year of the degree program, the students are directed to use Gibbs' model. However, on entering third year, students are required to try a framework other than Gibbs' model. There is also an expectation by third year of the use of literature to inform their analysis and develop a deeper understanding of the problematic aspects of the encounter. How students' reflection is scaffolded is illustrated in two cases.

The first case is where a third-year student chose to use John's MSR framework. The core question students are directed to consider are as follows: What information do I need access to in order to learn through this experience? This question is followed by a number of "reflective questions": What was I trying to achieve? Why did I intervene as I did? What were the consequences of my actions for –

24 Reflective Practice in Health Professions Education

myself? – the patient/family – the people I work with? How did I feel about this experience when it was happening?

Case Study 1

Kim wanted to do a Mental Status Assessment (MSA) in a timely manner on a patient watching television. The student was new to this long-term placement and mental health patient and was rejected by them. Kim felt demoralized. The patient's staff nurse completed the assessment. Kim wrote...

> Dziopa and Ahern (2009) identify that mental health patient's benefit from less clinical interventions from nurses especially when first meeting them. They identified these alternative approaches as having someone to watch television with or having someone to go on a walk with (Dziopa and Ahern 2009). If I would have engaged with the patient initially in a non-clinical way, such as sitting with the patient to watch television or play cards, this may have helped to foster a trusting bond between the patient and me by allowing the patient to be seen as a whole person and not just a mental health patient who had to have a MSA in a timely manner. Patients on this ward stay for a long time, it is their home and they deserve to be treated like people first.

This excerpt demonstrates insight Kim gained as they accessed literature to help inform their understanding of the encounter. The faculty educator validated and supported the student's struggle and insight by responding: "It sounds as if you have experienced a valuable insight when you explored the effect your initial approach had on the patient, staff nurse and you." Further exploration of the lessons learned was encouraged by faculty questions such as, "Do you think this insight could be adapted to other practice setting? Why? How?"

In moving into fourth year, students enter the practice setting with a preceptor model of supervision. Each student has their own staff preceptor in the setting and is assigned to a faculty member for indirect supervision. Students meet with their assigned faculty member for 1 hour every second week. The faculty's primary concern for students is the pending transition from student to practicing novice nurse. It is the role of faculty to guide the student through the integrated phenomenon of descriptive, dialogic, and critical reflection. Critical reflection and analysis are employed as a means of gaining insights to transform their practice and self, examine issues from several perspectives, and understand how many problems, which surface at the point of care, have their grounding in a sociopolitical and economic dynamic that serves the status quo. At this stage students are encouraged to find a reflective framework that resonates with them. Moreover, they are no longer prescribed a reflective focus; instead students are encouraged to look up and out from their point of practice and critique the culture...to focus on why things are the way they are? Who benefits? And where they choose to situate themselves. The more complex or emotionally charged encounters require more tutor dialogue and probing to engage in analysis. The student relies on multiple communities to dig deeper to promote their transformation toward an accountable and self-regulated member of their community of practice (Manankil-Rankin et al. 2013).

Case Study 2

Leslie was working in a trauma unit caring for a young adult who had been repeatedly run over by a truck. Staff blamed the patient for his ill fate. Later that day the patient's sister came to visit. She shared with Leslie that her brother had been raped by a family friend at the age of 13 and that is why he is a drug abuser and out on the street. Leslie was taken aback by the news and sought to better understand the young man's predicament. This process is captured in an excerpt from Leslie's reflection below:

> A study by Medrano, Hatch, Zule, & Desmond found a correlation between childhood sexual abuse and substance abuse into adulthood (2002). Many of the participants in the study attribute their continuous drug use to the fact that the drugs decrease the psychological stress that they experience as a result of abuse during adolescence (Medrano et al. 2002). This information has shocked me into realizing how prejudiced I was. I blamed the patient for his accident and even resented that he was taking up an expensive hospital bed in the ICU. This lesson is something that I can carry forward in my clinical practice, since I will now remind myself of this correlation whenever I have a patient who is a drug user. I will not be so quick to blame their drug use and situation solely on their choices and will instead consider underlying factors that may be present. The acknowledgement of my previous bias in this situation has made me more aware of the potential for other biases that I may have. As in this situation, other biases may result in an immediate reaction to future patients that may also be inappropriate.

Here, Leslie choose to search for information as an entry into the issue of stigmatization. During their biweekly meeting, the faculty educator validated the student's struggle and explored how difficult it must have been for them to experience that critical insight. The student was also asked to explore what their former beliefs were about homeless substance using people and where that might have originated from. They were asked to consider whether what nurses believe might affect how they practice. The faculty educator then spent some time discussing how this situation was an excellent example of sociocultural inequities and how vulnerable people are failed by the healthcare system and fall through our social safety nets.

These two case studies demonstrate that with appropriate reflective scaffolding, achieved here through expectation of the use of more complex reflective models and supportive questioning, one can encourage individuals to gain insights into their previously held beliefs and values, enhancing their criticality and leading to transformational learning and change in practice. However, such learning entails a degree of reciprocity between the learner's critical thinking, their agency, and metacognition to develop and apply their reflective learning (Coulson and Harvey 2013). Learning to reflect is not a linear process. It requires the judicious blend of facilitation between learner and educator, to develop the learner's capacity for reflective thinking, enable the learner to make sense of the experience through synthesis and analysis of the experience, make connections with theory and practice, and identify how this learning can be drawn upon in future practice. Importantly though for some health professional educators, to engage in timely reflective scaffolding, it may require negotiating a zone of proximal development around reflective practice themselves before they are able to scaffold the novice practitioner's capacity for reflection (Coulson and Harvey 2013).

Conclusion

This chapter has highlighted theories of reflection along with several reflective frameworks that have been used within education and adapted for use in health professional education. Johns (2013) recounts a scenario where his partner introduced him as bit of "guru in reflective practice" to a local district nurse. Johns shares that the nurse indicated that "she hated reflective practice, that she had had it shoved down her throat" (p. 25). He goes onto write, "I could imagine her experience of being taught reflection in an instrumental way using a model of reflection by unreflective teachers. I know this because I see it everywhere," Johns (2013, p. 25). This chapter has illustrated the pedagogy of reflective practice requires health professional educators to not only be engaged, creative, and innovative but most importantly to be reflective practitioners themselves. It is through our own reflective practice that we learn and challenge ourselves to enhance our practice as a clinician and educator.

Cross-References

▶ Interprofessional Education (IPE): Trends and Context
▶ Medical Education: Trends and Context
▶ Obstetric and Midwifery Education: Context and Trends
▶ Transformative Learning in Clinical Education: Using Theory to Inform Practice

References

Al Sabei SD, Lasater K. Simulation debriefing for clinical judgment development: a concept analysis. Nurse Educ Today. 2016;45:42–7.

Argyris C. Theories of action that inhibit individual learning. Amer Pysch. 1976;31:638–54.

Argyris C, Schön D. Theory in practice: increasing professional effectiveness. San Francisco: Jossey Bass; 1974.

Bandaranaike S, Snelling C, Karanicolas S, Willison J. Opening minds and mouths wider: developing a model for student reflective practice within clinical placements. 9th international conference on cooperative & work-integrated education; June 20–22. Istanbul: University of Bahcesehir University; 2012.

Barnett R. Knowing and becoming in the higher education curriculum. Stud High Educ. 2009;34 (4):429–40.

Bass J, Fenwick J, Sidebotham M. Development of a model of holistic reflection to facilitate transformative learning in student midwives. Women Birth. 2017;30(3):227–35.

Bassot B. The reflective practice guide: an interdisciplinary approach to critical reflection. New York: Rutledge, Taylor and Francis Group; 2013.

Bassot B. The reflective journal. 2nd ed. London: Macmillan Education; 2016.

Boud D. The use of self-assessment schedules in negotiated learning, Studies in Higher Educ, 1992;17(2):185–200.

Boud D. Published in proceedings of the 35th adult education research conference, 20–22 May. Knoxville: College of Education, University of Tennessee, 1994; 1992. p. 49–54.

Boud D. Relocating reflection in the context of practice. In: Bradbury H, Frost N, Kilminster S, Zukas M, editors. Beyond reflective practice. Abingdon/Oxon: Routledge; 2010.

Boud D, Walker J. Experience and learning: reflection at work. Melbourne: Deakin University; 1991.

Boud D, Keogh R, Walker D. Reflection, turning experience into learning. London: Kogan Page; 1985.

Bowden T, Rowlands A, Buckwell M, Abbott S. Web-based video and feedback in the teaching of cardiopulmonary resuscitation. Nurse Educ Today. 2012;32(4):443–7.

Braine ME. Exploring new nurse teachers' perception and understanding of reflection. Nurse Educ Prac. 2009;9(4):262–70.

Cant RP, Cooper SJ. The benefits of debriefing as formative feedback in nurse education. Aust J Adv Nsg. 2011;29(1):37–47.

Chirema KD. The use of reflective journals in the promotion of reflection and learning in post-registration nursing students. Nurse Educ Today. 2007;27(3):192–202.

Coffey AM. Using video to develop skills in reflection in teacher education students. Aust J Teach Educ. 2014;39(9)

Coulson D, Harvey M. Scaffolding student reflection for experience-based learning: a framework. Teach High Educ. 2013;18(4):401–13.

Cranton P. Teaching for Transformation. New Directions for Adult Continuing Educ. 2002;93:63–72.

Dall'Alba G. Learning professional ways of being: ambiguities of becoming. Educ Phil Theory. 2009;41(1):34–45.

Dewey J. How we think. Revised edition. Boston: DC Health; 1933.

Dewey J. The supreme intellectual obligation. Science; New Series. 1934;2046(79):240–3.

Dewy J. How we think, vol. 6. Mineola/New York: Dover Publications Inc.; 1997.

Duffy P. Engaging the YouTube Google-Eyed generation: strategies for using web 2.0. Teaching and learning. Electron. J. e-Learn. 2008;6(2):119–30.

Dziopa F, Ahern K. Three different ways mental health nurses develop quality therapeutic relationships. Issues Ment Health Nurs. 2009;30(1):14–22.

Epp S. The value of reflective journaling in undergraduate nursing education: a literature review. Intern J Nsg Stud. 2008;45(9):1379–88.

Field D. Moving from novice to expert – the value of learning in clinical practice: a literature review. Nurse Educ Today. 2004;24(7):560–5.

Fook J. Beyond reflective practice: reworking the 'critical' in critical reflection. In Bradbury H, Frost N, Kilminster S, Zukas M. editors. Beyond Reflective Practice: Abingdon Oxon: Routledge; 2010.

Freire P. Pedagogy of the oppressed. New York: Herter and Herter; 1970.

Gibbs G. Learning by doing: a guide to teaching and learning methods. London: Great Britain Further Education Unit; 1988.

Habermas J. Knowledge of human interests. Boston: Beacon; 1971.

Habermas J. Communication and the evolution of society. Cambridge: Polity Press; 1979.

Habermas J. The theory of communicative action. 1: reason and the rationalization of society (trans: McCarthy T). Boston: Beacon; 1984.

Harrison J, Molloy E, Bearman M, Ting CY, Leech M. Clinician peer exchange groups (C-PEGs): augmenting medical students' learning on clinical placement. In: Billett S, Newton J, Rogers G,

24 Reflective Practice in Health Professions Education

Noble C, editors. Augmenting health and social care students' clinical learning experiences. Professional and practice-based learning. Dordrecht: Springer; 2019. p. 25.

Higgs J, Titchen A. Journey of meaning making through transformation, illumination shared action and liberation. In: Higgs J, Titchen A, Horsfall D, Bridges D, editors. Creative spaces for qualitative researching: living research. Sydney: Hampden Press; 2007. p. 301–10.

Horsfall D, Welsby J. If someone actually asked us, you'd find we have a lot to say. In: Higgs J, Titchen A, Horsfall D, Armstrong H, editors. Being critical and creative in qualitative research. Sydney: Hampden Press; 2007.

Iedema R. Creating safety by strengthening clinicians' capacity for reflexivity. BMJ Qual Saf. 2011;20:i83–i6.

Johns C. Framing learning through reflection within Carper's fundamental ways of knowing in nursing. J Adv Nsg. 1995;22:226–34.

Johns C. Becoming a reflective practitioner. 4th ed. West Sussex: Wiley; 2013.

Johns C. Becoming a reflective practitioner. 5th ed. United Kingdom: Wiley, Incorporated; 2017.

Kuhn T. The structure of scientific revolutions. Chicago: University of Chicago Press; 1962.

Lukinsky J. Reflective withdrawal through journal writing. In: Mezirow J, editor. Fostering critical reflection in adulthood. Oxford: Jossey-Bass Publishers; 1990. p. 213–34.

Manankil-Rankin L, Noesgaard C, Drummond-Young M, Matthew-Maich N, Diamond A, Sheremet D, McGraw MJ. A Guide for developing reflective practitioners. Hamilton: McMaster University; 2013. p. 3–30.

Mann K, Gordon J, MacLeod A. Reflection and reflective practice in health professions education: a systematic review. Adv Health Sci Educ. 2007;14:595.

Medrano MA, Hatch JP, Zule WA, Desmond DP. Psychological distress in childhood trauma survivors who abuse drugs. Amer J Drug and Alcohol Abuse. 2002;28(1):1–13.

Mezirow J. Education for perspective transformation: Women's re-entry programs in community colleges. New York: Teacher's College, Columbia University; 1978.

Mezirow J. A critical theory of adult learning and education. Adult Educ Quart. 1981;32(3):3–24.

Mezirow J. Fostering critical reflection in adulthood. San Francisco: Jossey-Bass; 1990.

Mezirow J. Transformative Dimensions of Adult Learning. San Francisco: Jossey-Bass; 1991.

Mezirow J. Understanding transformation theory. Adult Educ Quart. 1994;44(4):222–32. 6 pp 13–18.

Mezirow J. Transformation theory of adult learning. In: Welton MR, editor. In defense of the lifeworld. New York: State University of New York Press; 1995. p. 39–70.

Mezirow J. On critical reflection. Adult Educ Q. 1998;48(3):185–98.

Mezirow J. Learning as transformation: critical perspectives on a theory in progress. The Jossey-Bass Higher and Adult Education Series; 2000.

Nagle JF. Becoming a reflective practitioner in the age of accountability. The Educ Forum. 2009;73:76–86.

Newton JM. Learning to reflect – a journey. Reflec Prac. 2004;5(2):155–66.

Newton JM. Reflective learning groups for student nurses. In: Billett S, Henderson A, editors. Promoting professional learning: Integrating experiences in university and practice settings. Dordrecht: Springer; 2011. ISBN: 978-90-481-3936-1.

Newton JM, Butler A. Facilitating students' reflections on community practice: a new approach. In: Billett S, Newton J, Rogers G, Noble C, editors. Using post-practicum interventions to augment healthcare students' clinical learning experiences: outcomes and processes. Dordrecht: Springer; 2019.

Newton JM, Plummer V. Using creativity to encourage reflection in undergraduate education. Reflective Pract. 2009;10(1):67–76.

Price DM, Strodtman L, Brough E, Lonn S, Luo A. Digital storytelling: an innovative technological approach to nursing education. Nurse Educ. 2015;40:66–70.

Royle C, Hargiss K. Comparison of baccalaureate nursing Students' experience of video-assisted debriefing versus Oral debriefing following high-Fidelity human simulation. Int J Strateg Inf Technol Appl. 2015;6:2. https://doi.org/10.4018/IJSITA.2015040103.

Sadlon PP. The process of reflection: a principle-based concept analysis. Nsg Forum. 2018:1–5.

Sandars J, Homer M. Reflective learning and the net generation. Med Teach. 2008;30(9):877–9.

Sandars J, Murray C. Digital storytelling for reflection in undergraduate medical education: a pilot study. Educ Primary Care. 2009;20(6):441–4.

Schön D. The reflective practitioner: how practitioners think in action. New York: Basic Books; 1983.

Schön D. Educating the reflective practitioner. London: Jossey-Bass; 1987.

Schön D. The reflective practitioner. 2nd ed. San Francisco: Jossey Bass; 1991.

Snelling C, Karanicolas S. In Bandaranaike S, Snelling C, Karanicolas S, Willison J. Opening Minds and Mouths Wider: Developing a model for student reflective practice within clinical placements. In Proceedings of the 9th International Conference on Cooperative & Work-Integrated Education 2012;1–16.

Sweet L, Bass J. The continuity of care experience and reflective writing: enhancing post-practicum learning for midwifery students. In: Billet S, Newton J, Rogers R, Noble C, editors. Using post-practicum interventions to augment healthcare students' clinical learning experiences: outcomes and processes. Dordrecht: Springer; 2019.

Tanner CA. Thinking like a nurse: a research-based model of clinical judgment in nursing. J Nurs Educ. 2006;45(6):204–112.

Taylor BJ. Reflective practice for healthcare professionals: a practical guide. 3rd. ed. Berkshire: Open University Press; 2010.

Taylor EW. Critical reflection and transformative learning: a critical review. PAACE J Lifelong Learn. 2017;26:77–95.

Timmins F. Making Sense of Nursing Portfolios: A Guide for Students, McGraw-Hill Education, 2008.

Van Manen M. Linking ways of knowing with ways of being practical. Curric Inquiry. 1977;6(2): 205–28.

Wilson K, Devereux L. Scaffolding theory: high challenge, high support in academic language and learning (ALL) contexts. J Acad Lang Learn. 2014;8(3):A91–A100.

Yoo MS, Son YJ, Kim YS, Park JH. Video-based self-assessment: implementation and evaluation in an undergraduate nursing course. Nurse Educ Today. 2009;29(6):585–9.

Transformative Learning in Clinical Education: Using Theory to Inform Practice

25

Anna Jones

Contents

Introduction 464
What Is Transformative Learning? 464
Transformative Learning in a Clinical Context 468
Identifying and Evaluating Transformation 472
Vignette 472
Implications and Recommendations 476
Conclusion 477
Cross-References 477
References 477

Abstract

Transformative learning is a way of understanding learning when the central focus is profound change in both thinking and behavior. Although Mezirow is key to transformative learning, the work has been developed and used in a range of contexts. In clinical education the notion of transformative learning is increasingly being used as a framework to understand the ways in which clinicians learn in ways that promote fundamentally new ways of thinking. As a tool for curriculum design and teaching development, transformative learning provides a means by which educators can plan for learning. The key elements of transformative learning are disequilibrium or a "disorienting dilemma" that is a trigger to prompt critical reflection. The final stage is a change in both thinking and action. These stages can then be expanded into a much more fine-grained process. This

---

A. Jones (✉)
School of Medical Education, King's College London, London, UK
e-mail: anna.jones@kcl.ac.uk

© Springer Nature Singapore Pte Ltd. 2023
D. Nestel et al. (eds.), *Clinical Education for the Health Professions*,
https://doi.org/10.1007/978-981-15-3344-0_33

chapter provides the theoretical background to transformative learning before examining its use in clinical education. This is illustrated through a vignette. While transformative learning requires effort and persistence on the part of both learner and educator, the possibilities for creating learning environments that enable a flexibility of thought, interdisciplinary collaborations, and an openness to new ways of working are essential in a rapidly changing healthcare system.

Keywords

Transformative learning · Transformation · Change · Reflection · Critical thinking

Introduction

The notion of learning as a transformation is a powerful one and the journey that learners take from student to clinician can be profound. Many clinicians are conscious of the change they underwent from students entering a clinical degree to the professionals they have become. This change encompasses a large volume of knowledge, an understanding of clinical reasoning and decision-making, communication skills, a professional role, and often an accompanying change in identity. These transformation points often occur at entry into a clinical program, first clinical encounters and following graduation. The learners' journey has been documented from various perspectives, focusing on cognitive skills and social transformation (Abela 2009; Buchman 2012; Greenhill and Poncelet 2013; Walters et al. 2011). Beyond this, there are possibilities for transformation of experienced clinicians as they develop their view of knowledge, skills, leadership, and professional roles and identity. This chapter looks in detail at the idea of transformative learning, considering its theoretical underpinnings and application in clinical education. While the term is used frequently, in this chapter I examine the ways of defining transformative learning, its key elements, and how a clear understanding of transformative learning can provide a framework for designing for learning. Transformational learning is not a quick fix but requires understanding of the stages and careful planning on the part of the educator.

What Is Transformative Learning?

Transformative learning is the concept that some learning can lead to a fundamental change in one's worldview and ways of acting. It is more than just an acquisition of knowledge and skills, but requires fundamental change in the learner. Transformative learning draws upon the work of Friere (1970), although it is Mezirow (1991, 1997, 2000) who is most often cited as the author of the concept.

Mezirow's concept of transformative learning posits that people acquire a set of understandings about the world – a frame of reference or "meaning scheme" through which all experiences are filtered. Transformative learning then is the process by which this frame of reference can be confirmed or altered through critical reflection. In essence, it is a form of learning in which "disorienting dilemmas" challenge learners' thinking, causing them to change in both outlook and action. Using critical thinking and reflection, the learner questions their assumptions and beliefs. The three key phases of transformative learning are (a) a disorienting dilemma, (b) critical reflection, and (c) reflective discourse (Mezirow 1991: 78).

A disorienting dilemma is a situation in which the learner is faced with ideas or circumstances that do not match with their existing beliefs and frame of reference. In such cases, for transformative learning to occur, the learners begin to challenge their existing worldview and assumptions through critical reflection. According to Mezirow, this is an intellectual, rational, and social act. Critical reflection leading to transformative learning is grounded in reason and can be both triggered and facilitated by reflective discourse, in other words through dialogue with others. Central to transformative learning is cognitive struggle. Because the change is profound, a learner cannot transform without wrestling with ideas and the effort can be considerable and sustained.

Mezirow argues that transformative learning is a linear and strictly cognitive process defined by an initial trigger event and a clear conclusion, comprising change in both thinking and practice. He suggests that the stages in perspective change are psychological – understanding of the self; convictional – changing belief systems; and behavioral – changing actions. When broken down in a more fine-grained manner, this is a ten-phase process, ultimately based on dialogue with others (Taylor 2013).

These phases are:

1. The disorienting dilemma
2. Self-examination
3. Sense of alienation
4. Relating discontent to others
5. Explaining options of new behavior
6. Building confidence in new ways
7. Planning a course of action
8. Knowledge to implement plans
9. Experimenting with new roles
10. Reintegration of new thinking and action

Thus, the process requires serious thought, social learning, a period of uncertainty, and then experimentation, and finally a stage in which new ways of thinking and acting become an integrated part of one's worldview. Social learning encompasses learning with others, engaging with scholarship, wrestling with ideas collaboratively, putting ideas and questions into words, and problem solving with others. Experimentation encompasses trying out new ideas in conversation with peers and teachers, trying out new practices, and engaging with new ideas in more formal assessment tasks.

A more expansive understanding of transformative learning comes from Jarvis (2012), who suggests that **all** learning is transformative. The starting point of learning is a disjuncture, which is a problem that causes instability and a loss of equilibrium (as with Mezirow's disorienting dilemma). This disjuncture is puzzling, and so cannot be ignored, prompting questioning and critical thinking, which will in turn lead to a new model of thinking. While this is similar to Mezirow's conception of transformation, for Jarvis, learning is cognitive, emotional, and social, and encompasses the whole person (Illeris 2017). Jarvis sees learning not as an individual act but always as a relationship between the person and their social context. As Illeris points out, seeing all learning as transformative contrasts with Piaget's view that there are two forms of learning. The first is assimilative learning which is a process of adding to preexisting learning. The second is accommodative learning, which is a process of reconstruction of an existing mental model when it no longer fits with one's experience of the world (Illeris 2017).

While Mezirow (1991, 1997, 2000) developed a way of seeing transformation at a more individual, less political level, transformation can also be seen at a societal level. Friere (1970) argued that education can never be neutral: it either maintains the status quo and normalizes inequality, or works to enable liberation and the fight to transform society. According to Friere, education is always political. Where Mezirow's focus is on the transformation of the individual, Friere considers transformation as leading toward social change. Within a community of learners, critical reflection can identify oppressive social structures and can empower learners to act to promote change. Friere argues that it is through *praxis* – the interaction between reflection and action – that change can come about. From this view, transformative learning requires an interrogation of power and social structures; hence, the learner becomes willing and empowered to critique existing structures and to work toward social change. Transformation should be "epiphanic" or in other words a process of realization or revelation and should be more than just a new, more nuanced or sophisticated understanding. Rather, transformative learning requires a fundamental questioning and rethinking of central assumptions (Brookfield 2003: 142). It is that moment in which one says "ah, I never thought like that before, I see the world differently now." As such, transformative learning is a "reordering of social relations and practices" (p. 142). It requires us to think critically about power and oppression and to challenge these.

It appears then that there may be several ways of understanding transformative learning, and an ongoing question is its definition (Brookfield 2003; Dirkx 2012; Hoggan 2016; Newman 2012; Taylor and Cranton 2013). In some of the literature, transformative learning has been used to describe almost any instance of learning and hence has become almost meaningless (Hoggan 2016). In many cases, according to Newman (2012), transformation is actually conflated with learning: rather than a more fundamental change in thinking and behavior, the simple acquisition of new skills and knowledge is seen to be transformative. Moreover, Newman argues that transformation can be difficult to define because in some cases the acquisition of a new skill, albeit not requiring a fundamental change of beliefs and assumption, can be transformative because it gives the learner new opportunities and so can be said to be transformative. However, this may be pushing the point a little too far. Certainly, learning a new skill can open up transformative opportunities. Yet this is different from transformative learning. A new skill may provide opportunities that then enable a profound change in thinking. It may enable the learner to enter a particular career path which then promotes transformation through interaction with others prompting further learning, challenging one's original set of assumptions and identity. Yet the acquisition of the skill itself may not have been transformative, but rather the transformative aspect was the social setting which it enabled the learner to participate in and the challenges to the learners' original assumptions that this setting provoked. For example, learning to take a history will not make you a doctor, but is part of a set of skills and ways of thinking that may enable you to become one, and so to enter a world that is transformative. It may, if taught well, be a trigger to allow the learner to think critically about how she communicates, how she understands the patient, how she structures information, and how she reasons like a clinician. Learning to take a history could also prompt a learner to think about the different ways people communicate, the different psychosocial contexts that shape this, and the different ways that patients respond to clinicians and the power dynamics therein.

Different types of transformation can be identified (Taylor and Cranton 2013): psychocritical, which is the form proposed by Mezirow (1991, 1997, 2000) and which refers to the process of becoming aware of the assumptions and expectations that inform our worldview; psychodevelopmental, requiring a change in one's sense of self (Kegan 2000); psychoanalytic, requiring an expansions of one's consciousness (Dirkx 2012); and finally social emancipatory, referring to outcomes that involve a change in one's view of oneself as active in and empowered to promote social change (Friere 1970). Thus, in unpacking the notion of transformation, it is possible to view it as promoting quite different – yet always profound – change.

In aiming for increased clarity and precision around the notion of transformative learning, Hoggan (2016) argues that given the range of approaches to transformation, the term transformative learning should refer to the broad range of approaches such as those outlined above, whereas perspective transformation should refer more specifically to Mezirow's theory of transformation. He argues that this would increase clarity since it would be easier to identify the type of transformation and avoid the lack of precision around the terms. However, the term transformative learning is still current in the literature and still refers to a broad range of activity (Briese 2018; Kear 2013; Renigere 2014).

In order to achieve transformation, learners must reflect not only on their current practices but also on the paradigmatic assumptions that inform them. One possible critique of Mezirow is that his stages tend to imply a linear progression and a very rational approach to transformation. However, transformation through reflection can be recursive rather than linear and can involve periods of fear, doubt, and chaos. At each stage there can be blocks that prevent critical reflection and hence transformation from occurring (Larrivee 2000). A profound change in worldview can require emotional as well as intellectual struggle. So too can a change in one's sense of self as a result of this change in thinking and action. A new awareness of the world, a new conceptual framework, and a changed understanding, epistemology, and even ontology can not only be personally disorientating but can disrupt one's relationships with those around – albeit possibly only temporarily. In fact, the very term "disorientating dilemma" suggests an emotional element, since neither term is emotionally neutral. Beliefs, attitudes, and assumptions that have formed over time to make sense of the world only change with some effort, and this type of learning requires risk taking, openness to change, a willingness to be vulnerable, and the preparedness to have one's attitudes and assumptions challenged.

Transformative Learning in a Clinical Context

Transformative learning is an important aspect of clinical education because it enables a change in thinking and practice. Hence, in order to develop as a professional, both in the preregistration stage and for established clinicians, there are times when profound change is essential. For example, coping with very stressful situation, understanding professional behavior, learning to respond to feedback and reflect, clinical reasoning, ethical decision-making, taking on leadership roles, understanding the patient point of view, and becoming an effective educator may all require a different way of thinking that challenges existing assumptions and beliefs. As part of becoming a clinician, learners experience dramatic changes in professional perspectives which need to be built into teaching (King 2004). The process of transformative learning in a clinical context requires a safe and inclusive learning space, critical reflection, the opportunity to engage in critical conversations, and a learning environment that enables working with others in such a way that will foster challenge and reframing of thinking. It requires not only the right environment but also both the cognitive ability and disposition on the part of the learner to reframe thinking. In other words, the learner must be in an environment that is supportive and challenging, that encourages, models, and rewards reflection and rewards willingness on the part of learners to challenge their own worldview. In a clinical context, this can enable a way of thinking that promotes change, critical thought, and an openness to consider new ideas. All these are vital in a rapidly changing clinical and social environment. Transformative learning has the capacity to enable clinicians to broaden their worldview, think more flexibly, and draw on other fields of knowledge. However, it is not a quick or easy approach and requires careful planning on the part of educators and effort on the part of learners.

While transformative learning can occur in any environment, in an academic or clinical learning environment this can be carefully facilitated. Through careful design, learners can be presented with challenging new ideas that require serious intellectual engagement. This in turn may require learners to view the world through a whole new lens and take on new epistemological perspectives. Through thinking, writing, and conversation with other learners, they can start to consider these challenges by being encouraged to think critically. Transformation is often collaborative as learners rehearse new ideas, bouncing them off other learners as well as their teachers. Mezirow suggests that transformation learning requires dialogue with others and is a social process, while also requiring individual reading, thinking, and engaging with ideas (Mezirow 2000).

Given the level of challenge involved in transformative learning, it is essential not only to facilitate the social nature of learning and the reflective discourse with both teachers and peers but also to ensure that this is a safe environment in which one can trust and be trusted. Reflective dialogue requires time for relationships to be established, and it requires teachers who are able to create, foster, and maintain this environment. Brookfield (1990) argues that the capacity for critical thinking is developed though a cycle of concrete experiences, reflection, abstraction, and application. Yet a major deterrent to critical thinking is a lack of time to think deeply, to come to grips with abstract concepts, and to reflect. If the focus of teaching is a large volume of facts which learners must memorize for examination, Brookfield argues that they will not be able to develop the intellectual skills to think critically. Moreover, in the absence of a trusting learning environment, it is difficult to enable students to be challenged intellectually. Without critical thinking, it is unlikely that transformative learning can occur since it requires critical reflection.

In order to be reflective (and thus open to transformation), the learner needs to have time for solitary reflection, to be a perpetual problem-solver, and to question the status quo in ways that are invitational rather than confrontational (Larrivee 2000). Writing about critical reflection, Larrivee argues that the stages to transformation are firstly exploration, comprising questioning, challenging, and a desire for change; secondly struggle, comprising inner conflict, surrender, uncertainty, and chaos; and finally perpetual shift, comprising reconciling, personal discovery, and new practice. However, this is a dynamic process. Thus, she acknowledges the emotional element of transformation. She also acknowledges the very real possibility that at each stage there is the possibility for blocks and that transformation is not a given. The implications for teaching are that there must be time and space for reflection and problem solving as well as for challenge. Ultimately the end point is new practice, and without this, the transformation is incomplete.

Although transformation can be deliberate, serendipitous, or gradual, in order to enable it, educators must explicitly plan and design for it if this is what they wish to achieve. In her study into the use of problem based learning, Donnelly (2016) identified that the specific stages required were: activating or trigger events that prompted thinking, the identification and articulation of current assumptions, critical reflection, critical discourse and opportunities to test and apply new knowledge and perspectives, and this loosely follows Mezirow's stages. In this study, learners were exposed to disorienting dilemmas, given the opportunity to identify and articulate their own assumptions, explain their reasoning and thought processes. They were then encouraged to engage in critical reflection by considering their own assumptions and how these shaped their thinking. Critical discourse with other learners and the tutor took place as learners were encouraged to consider other ways of thinking. Finally, learners were given the opportunity to try out new ideas in practice. Donnelly suggests it is essential for the tutor to "strike a careful balance between support and challenge" (p. 14) and that trust is key to successful transformational learning.

In the context of medical school, educators play a vital role in encouraging self-reflection, but the extent of this can vary depending on the learning context

(Greenhill et al. 2018). The study by Greenhill et al. explored the development of self-awareness, patient centeredness, systems thinking, self-care, clinical skepticism, and understanding diversity in medical students. They found that medical students who experienced transformation were the ones who were active in engaging in very challenging learning opportunities and cultivated strong collaborative relationships with their peers and clinical educators. These participants developed a deep sense of the kind of doctor they wished to become, which was also reflected in their values and behavior with patients and changing role in the community. The students who experienced transformation reported experiencing a disorienting dilemma that facilitated a reconsideration and critical assessment of their previous assumptions. Greenhill et al. point out that the changes in ways of knowing is developed within the context of and directed by the medical curriculum. Those with the opportunity for the development of ongoing relationships and some stability and extended challenge reported more transformation. The medical students who were in long-term placements or well-supported rural placements were those who transformed in more fundamental ways. And so, while each learner will respond differently, their scope for transformation and the sort of transformation that occurs will be shaped by (and either enhanced or limited by) the curriculum and the experiences which the learners have (both formal and informal) as part of their medical education. Their findings point out that it is the context in which learning occurs which is critical in enabling transformative learning.

One technique for teaching for transformation outlined in the literature is through a carefully planned technique of giving learners a values-based survey focused on complex issues such as euthanasia, genetic research, and other difficult questions with no clear "correct" answer (Christie et al. 2015). The survey is done individually, but the anonymized results are discussed with the group and the rationale for the answers is considered. In the discussion, no one is required to reveal their own position, but the assumptions underlying each position are explored and alternatives are considered. In this way, learners can become aware of the prescriptive assumptions they hold, are presented with alternative viewpoints and evidence, and have the opportunity to examine their own perspectives in a safe environment.

In nursing, McAllister (2011) developed the STAR framework to promote transformative learning. This framework has three elements: sensitize (to human issues), take action (linking knowledge to action), promote reflection (through challenging assumptions and encouraging new perspectives). The sensitizing aspect is the disorienting dilemma and can be achieved through exposing nursing students to the patients' experiences through film, first-person testimonials, music, poetry, YouTube, media, and so on. The take action element enables students to make the connection between what they know and what they do and to understand the rationale for their actions and underlying assumptions. She suggests that it is essential to include and challenge this connection between actions and assumptions in order to prompt critical thinking. Further, students can be encouraged to consider their beliefs and assumptions through a think aloud technique (Offredy 2002). Reflection can then be encouraged by asking students the "why" questions, which again can promote a disorienting dilemma – and, if discussed carefully, can prompt reflection. The aim is that reflection on the dilemma (and the underlying assumptions) can enable transformation.

Teaching techniques designed for quick improvement of a skill or a general overview of facts will only result in superficial or temporary change (Gravett 2004). Using teaching development as a setting, Gravatt suggests instead that education theories should be explored, discussed, and challenged, using action research to promote a more reflective, analytical, and critical approach to teaching practice. She begins by asking learners to describe their assumptions about teaching and learning. She then enables learners to explore alternative approaches to teaching and to critically assess these alternatives.

In a study on a program designed to change residents' views on professionalism, Foshee et al. (2017) conclude that a 4-week program was more effective than a single seminar or lecture as it provided more scope for engagement and critical thought. However, they did acknowledge that developing empathy was difficult in a 4-week block, and might require a more extended program. Their work used transformative learning as a conceptual framework for evaluation, and their program aimed to develop professionalism. However, while they did report some changes, as the authors acknowledged, even in a program spread over 4 weeks, engendering fundamental change was not easy.

In time-pressured clinical environments, where teaching can be opportunistic and brief, where contact between teachers and learners can be fleeting, and where the stakes are high and patient safety is of paramount importance, taking the risks required to promote transformation may appear to be daunting. The cognitive load (Sweller 1988) and the time and effort required are significant, and so transformative learning is unlikely to occur in a quick one-off seminar or workshop. This, however, is not to undervalue these sessions, as they can teach vital skills and/or promote an interest in more fundamental change. Embarking on a program of transformative change requires time and planning. Paradoxically, a culture requiring continual innovation has meant that real transformation has been devalued. As we are increasingly required to constantly provide evidence of innovation, profound change has become more difficult because it requires more than a quick and easily reportable teaching session or identifiable criteria. A target-and-competency-driven culture also has put real reflection required in jeopardy, since what is required is serious critical thought, engagement with ideas, disciplined consideration, and mature creativity.

The high-profile Bawa-Garba case (Cook 2019) in the United Kingdom has raised the issue of the uses to which reflection (a central element of transformative learning) can be put. In this case a junior doctor and a nurse were found guilty of manslaughter following the death of a 6-year-old child. There has been ongoing debate about the case, in part because of the concerns regarding personal negligence versus systemic failure and in part because of the possible use of the doctors' reflective notes as evidence. While the court, in the case, stated that reflections were irrelevant to the facts to be determined, the Medical Protection Society acknowledged, that it "may well have been the case" that the reflections influenced the trial (Dyer and Cohen 2018: 572).

As a consequence (of this, and of other cases), there may be a reluctance on the part of doctors to reflect in ways that can be subsequently used for other purposes, particularly legal ones. There are also concerns that written reflections can jeopardize promotion and employment if used in the wrong way. This may limit transformative learning in some contexts, because it may stifle the ability to critically reflect and consider new ways of thinking and behaving.

Faculty development and engagement with formal clinical education programs can enable transformative learning. This is particularly the case when these programs can engage learners to think critically, to challenge their assumptions, to start to think differently, and to begin to put this all into practice in their own teaching. However, none of these are a given. As outlined earlier, if the program is carefully designed to enable space for disorienting dilemmas, critical reflection, and social learning, then transformation is possible.

Identifying and Evaluating Transformation

One issue for research into and reporting of transformative learning is the complexity of capturing, identifying, and evaluating transformation. Identifying and evaluating changes in perspectives and actions can be very difficult given that these changes often occur over an extended period and can be gradual or multilayered. There are a number of techniques in the research literature which aim to capture transformation, ranging from levels of change (Kirkpatrick 1994) to theory of change (Clark and Taplin 2012). These include qualitative research (Cranton and Hoggan 2012), questionnaires (Kember et al. 2000), learning activity surveys (King 2009), and transformative learning surveys (Stuckey et al. 2013). Yet context is so important, and perspective transformation can happen on so many levels (Romano 2017). Capturing real change in actions is perhaps even more difficult, particularly if these changes happen gradually and over time. Theory of change is one approach to evaluation that can capture transformation at a holistic level (Markless et al. 2019). For educators wishing to report their learning as transformation, identifying an evaluation technique that will capture the rich detail of the change is essential.

Vignette

The following vignette, based on an interview with a London clinician, is used to illustrate transformative learning.

Sara is one of the senior leadership team in a large medical school. She is an experienced clinician – a consultant – and highly regarded in her own field. She works in a London teaching hospital and has been involved in the medical

(continued)

school for many years in teaching, leadership, and strategic planning roles. Both her clinical and education roles are demanding, but she talks with enthusiasm about each and takes her responsibilities very seriously. She is interested in and concerned for the welfare of the students but conscious that her responsibility is to educate future doctors who are safe, knowledgeable, and compassionate. She is currently enrolled in a formal qualification in clinical education in the same institution where she is teaching. This course is a large, well-regarded master's in clinical education program, and she has now been studying part-time for nearly 3 years.

She commenced an education qualification somewhat reluctantly, encouraged by colleagues who persuaded her that it would be helpful for her career in medical education, and so she was driven by pragmatic considerations. During the first part of the program she spoke to her tutor and somewhat ruefully explained that she really felt that she had no idea what was going on. "I read the papers but I'm not sure I understand... I really do try, even though work is busy, I'm on call and dealing with all the dramas in the medical school. I thought education would be easy, I thought it would be common sense."

By the end of the course however, her views were different. She said: "This course has completely changed my way of thinking." She remarked, "it has made me aware that there is more than one truth and that has completely changed my way of thinking, both as an educator but also a clinician.

It has been really hard. REALLY hard. Like space exploration. I feel like I have been able to see other worlds. But it has been a real struggle. I come from a field that is really data driven. We don't take anything seriously unless there is 'gold standard' data. We dismiss papers unless they have the right kind of data. But now I have learnt that there are other ways of thinking. I am now able to see that we don't have to prove a hypothesis. And in some cases that just won't be possible anyway.

I have changed the way I think – before I would have thought the word 'ontology' was just jargon, but I think about these things now. I think about the idea of truth, about theory, about what it means to be a good educator and what sorts of evidence we can use and what questions we need to ask. I'm not certain I am a better educator, but I think more about it and about the decisions I make. I think perhaps it has made me irritating though, as I ask lots of questions now. Which probably annoys the people who don't.

But it has not only changed the way I think, but the way I do things. And not only as an educator – it has really changed me as a clinician. Now, with my patients I no longer impose the doctor's view. I don't just push my own point. Or I try to be aware that this will be understood in different ways depending on the patient. I'm much more aware that for each patient, things are going to be different, that there will be more than one truth – even in the same setting. And I think it has made me a better team worker. I'm more interested in different

(continued)

ways of seeing things, different skill sets. I can read the nursing literature or take a dietitian seriously. But I suppose the problem is that in my old life I used to be the unknowing unknower. I am now able to see other ways of thinking. Or at least be aware that they are there. And to see that it is worth asking the questions and to be aware that finding the truths might be a journey. But now I'm the knowing unknower and so I can't just blissfully be a bad communicator. I might still be a bad communicator. It is just that I now know that I might be bad.

I was talking to a colleague just recently. A patient had been really upset about a difficult conversation. And now I understand that people respond differently, there is not necessarily a single right way of doing things. I am not sure I am always a better communicator. But I understand when people don't respond the way I expected. And I can reflect on my practice in a critical way.

I am probably even more irritating now than I was before. I ask difficult questions. It is really nice because people now see me as the person with the educational expertise. I am one of the few people who can understand and do qualitative research. But I'm also annoying because I ask annoying questions, I challenge things.

But not everyone on the programme changed the way I have changed. Some people sail through the certificate and don't really think much differently. It is a piece of paper, they have done it and left. And there are people around here who have done other master's programmes and have not changed at all. So, I guess it really struck something for me, and I worked at it. It struck a chord. But this has certainly not been the same for everyone."

When musing about what it was about the course itself that had prompted this change, Sara suggested that it was because it was difficult and really pushed her to think. As she said: "the programme tutors don't let us off lightly, they make us think, read those impenetrable papers, question. When I first started, I thought what *IS* this? It was so different. But because it was over a period of time, it slowly began to sink in. I don't think I really started to get it until at least the second module. Maybe the third. And the way the modules are run, we discuss the ideas with each other and with the tutor. We keep coming back to the big ideas. We have to try and put our ideas into words. And then we have to try and write them in the essays. And although the tutors push us quite hard, they are supportive. There is a nice atmosphere in class and I enjoyed the camaraderie and support from others in class. It is a mixed class – there are a range of clinical professions there, so you get used to listening to other views. And I suppose, if someone puts a challenge there for me, I will take it. So, in the course, the tutors said 'well, think about it'. . . . So I did."

Key changes that can be identified were that she had changed her thinking in very fundamental ways, expanding beyond a set of assumptions based on the idea of a single and discoverable truth identified by hypothesis testing. While she does not dismiss this in the case of some medical research, she now argues that in the clinical and educational context, there are other ways of seeking understanding and the possibility of more than one truth. She is able to see the value of both intellectual paradigms and to see the importance of context. This axiomatic change in perspective has altered her fundamental ways of seeing the world. This change has influenced both her work as an educator and her work as a clinician. As she pointed out, it has changed the way she communicates with colleagues and with patients. It has changed what she believes "counts" as knowledge, and it has changed her thinking about the validity of different points of view. As such it has changed both her thinking and her behavior.

The aspects of the program that encouraged transformation were that it presented material that challenged Sara's original worldview and did so in a rigorous intellectual way. The program was over an extended period, so Sara had the opportunity to develop her thinking and her confidence and to revisit ideas. She had the opportunity to work with others and so was able to discuss the ideas with her peers and with the tutor. She had the opportunity to actively engage with the ideas and experiment with new ways of thinking both through rehearsing them in class and then wrestling with them in a more coherent way in the assessment. And although the environment was intellectually challenging, she found it psychologically safe and felt supported by both the tutors and by her fellow learners.

As the vignette has identified, transformation can be fundamental, and it can change the way in which someone sees the world and the way they practice, both in the context of the educational experience but also as clinicians. And yet this transformation is hard won. As Sara pointed out, it was difficult – the time commitment, and the intellectual and emotional challenge. And moreover, although she now sees herself as a better educator and a better clinician, this is not without its costs. She is perhaps less brashly confident – or at least more thoughtful and reflective because she sees the complexities as well as the certainties. She is now more likely to question herself because she is now a "knowing unknower." Her transformation has brought her benefits. Her enthusiasm in discussing the program and her changing worldview is palpable. She has valued skills and knowledge. She now challenges herself and subjects herself to a scrutiny that she perhaps did not do beforehand. Moreover, she now asks the "irritating" questions and challenges the assumptions of others which while valuable can potentially put her in difficult situations. Although she is senior, both clinically and in the medical school, these environments are very hierarchical, and challenges can be viewed as insubordination by more senior colleagues if not handled diplomatically.

As Sara pointed out, not everyone doing the course changed, or changed to the extent that she has done. As she suggests, it was not just the fact of doing the course but that something about it resonated with her. A transformative learning program will not necessarily change every participant (Greenhill et al. 2018). For Sara there were elements of the program itself that are key to transformative learning – the level of challenge, exposure to new ideas, continuity, support, and social contact. But there were also aspects of Sara herself that enabled transformation – her willingness to change, her ability to put in the time and effort and to persist, her emotional strength in facing the uncertainty of change, and her intellectual flexibility to adapt to a different way of thinking and to be able to integrate this with her earlier views so that she can now see the value of hypothesis-driven knowledge where this is appropriate and interpretive knowledge in other contexts.

Transformative learning is not a "quick fix," and not all valuable learning will be transformative. If transformative learning is understood to be a fundamental change in both one's worldview **and** behavior, then this is a profound change. All learning engenders change of some sort – new knowledge, new skills, and these in turn can prompt fundamental changes, for example, a promotion, new career path, and so on. Yet this is different from an axiomatic change in worldview. In Sara's case, understanding learning theory may not necessarily have changed how she thinks. Being knowledgeable about different models of debriefing in simulation need not necessarily be transformative, nor is using problem-based learning, or being able to unpack clinical reasoning in order to teach it better. Transformation is more than just new knowledge or skills, but is a fundamental change in worldview and an associated change in practice.

Implications and Recommendations

In summary, teaching for transformative learning appears to require a number of elements:

- Material that is challenging and has intellectual depth and rigor
- The ability to digest and revisit the material over time
- Social contact and collaboration with other learners
- Engagement and experimentation with the material
- A safe space for dialogue
- Support from teachers who are committed
- Awareness that time and effort are required

This is not to devalue other forms of teaching. Short courses can teach vital skills or can be the first steps toward more fundamental change. Transformation is not necessary (or even desirable) in all educational settings, and learning new skills and knowledge is of intrinsic value. Transformative learning requires planning and commitment from educators and learners. Educators who are aiming for transformative learning need to carefully integrate this into the curriculum.

Writing of the value of transformative learning in transdisciplinary research in the biosciences, Pennington et al. (2013) outline the process by which a group of scientists were forced to transform in the context of an unexpected infectious disease outbreak. A series of unexplained deaths which was determined to be an exotic viral hemorrhagic fever drew on a team of clinicians, pathologists, public health professionals, epidemiologists, and molecular biologists. This team was, by necessity, pulled together quickly and without preparation to work on the problem. Pennington et al. argue that this team of professionals and researchers were confronted with a disorienting dilemma they needed to face to solve the problem. In order to develop a shared vision and conceptual framework, the scientists had to find some way to engage with a range of different bodies of knowledge. As part of a multidisciplinary team, they were faced with an array of new information that did not fit their existing mental models – new assumptions, data, terminology, analytical methods, tools, technology, and ways of thinking. It was only through communication and critical reflection that the individual members of the team were able to revise their thinking to create a new and more integrative model to address the disease outbreak. The authors suggest that this process required a period of uncertainty and ambiguity, before a new conceptual framework could be formulated and the problem addressed. Yet this new framework enabled them to develop new research questions, new research paths, and use new techniques, thus expanding their own repertoire as they expanded outside their own disciplinary foundations.

Conclusion

Transformative learning is a central part of learning for clinicians, as it is a way of thinking about learning that can enable fundamental change. It is a way of conceptualizing teaching and learning that views as central profound change in both thought and action. Because critical reflection is central to the process of transformation, the new perspective or worldview that learners arrive at will be more inclusive, in that it accommodates or acknowledges other points of view. It will be more discriminatory in that it is grounded in an ability to think critically, integrative in that it draws upon, utilizes, and engages with wider range of knowledge. Finally, it will be more permeable in that it will be a perspective that is flexible, open, and available to new information. Transformative learning is one means by which clinical professions can develop and change. Through drawing upon new ideas, information, and ways of thinking, it can often enable a way of thinking that is open to other possibilities.

Cross-References

▶ Simulation as Clinical Replacement: Contemporary Approaches in Healthcare Professional Education

References

Abela J. Adult learning theories and medical education: a review. Malta Med J. 2009;21:11–8.

Briese PM. Application of Mezirow's transformative learning theory to simulation in nursing education. Leadership connection conference, September 15–18, 2018. Indianapolis; 2018.

Brookfield S. The skillful teacher: on technique, trust and responsiveness in the classroom. San Francisco: Jossey-Bass; 1990.

Brookfield S. Putting the critical back into critical pedagogy. J Transform Educ. 2003;1(2):141–9.

Buchman S. Transformative teachers. Can Fam Physician. 2012;58:1.

Christie M, Carey M, Robertson A, Grainger P. Putting transformative learning theory into practice. Aust J Adult Learn. 2015;55(1):9–30.

Clark H, Taplin D. Theory of change basics: a primer on theory of change. New York: Actknowledge; 2012.

Cook J. The Bawa-Garba case: a timeline. GP Online [Internet]. 8th June 2019.

Cranton P, Hoggan C. Promoting transformative learning through reading fiction. J Transform Educ. 2012;13(1):6–25.

Dirkx J. Self-formation and transformative learning: a response to 'calling transformative learning into question: some mutinous thoughts' by Michael Newman. Adult Educ Q. 2012;62(4):399–405.

Donnelly R. Application of Mezirow's transformative pedagogy to blended problem-based learning. Dublin: Dublin Institute of Technology ARROW@DIT; 2016. p. 1–21.

Dyer C, Cohen D. How should doctors use e-portfolios in the wake of the Bawa-Garba case? BMJ. 2018;360:572.

Foshee C, Mehdi A, Bierer B, Traboulsi EI, Isaacson JH, Spencer A, et al. A professionalism curricular model to promote transformative learning among residents. J Grad Med Educ. 2017;9:351–6.

Friere P. Pedagogy of the oppressed. New York: Continuum; 1970.

Gravett S. Action research and transformative learning in teaching development. Educ Action Res. 2004;12(2):259–72.

Greenhill J, Poncelet AN. Transformative learning through longitudinal integrated clerkships. Med Educ. 2013;47:336–9.

Greenhill J, Richards JN, Mahoney S, Campbell N, Walters L. Transformative learning in medical education: context matters, a South Australian Longitudinal Study. J Transform Educ. 2018;16(1):58–75.

Hoggan C. Transformative learning as a metatheory: definition, criteria and typology. Adult Educ Q. 2016;66(1):57–75.

Illeris K. Peter Jarvis and the understanding of adult learning. Int J Lifelong Educ. 2017;36(1–2):35–44.

Jarvis P. Teaching, learning and education in late modernity. London: Routledge; 2012.

Kear T. Transformative learning during nursing education: a model of interconnectivity. Nurse Educ Today. 2013;33:1083–7.

Kegan R. What 'form' transforms?: a constructive-developmental perspective on transformational learning. In: Mezirow J, editor. Learning as transformation: critical perspectives of a theory-in-progress. San Francisco: Jossey-Bass; 2000. p. 35–70.

Kember D, Leung DYP, Jones A, Loke AY, McKay J, Sinclair K, et al. Development of a questionnaire to measure the level of reflective thinking. Assess Eval High Educ. 2000;25(4):381–95.

King K. Both sides now: examining Transformative learning and professional development of educators. Innov High Educ. 2004;29(2):155–74.

King K. The handbook of the evolving research of transformative learning based on the learning activities survey. Charlotte: Information Age Publishing IAP; 2009.

Kirkpatrick DL. Evaluating training programmes: the four levels. San Francisco: Berrett-Koehler; 1994.

Larrivee B. Transforming teaching practice: becoming the critically reflective teacher. Reflective Pract. 2000;1(3):293–307.

Markless S, Jones A, Reedy G. Using theory-based evaluation: an approach to dealing with complexity. AERA conference, 5–9 April. Toronto; 2019.

McAllister M. STAR: a transformative learning framework for nurse educators. J Transform Educ. 2011;9(1):42–58.

Mezirow J. Transformative dimensions of adult learning. San Francisco: Jossey-Bass; 1991.

Mezirow J. Transformative learning: theory to practice. New Dir Adult Contin Educ. 1997;74:5–12.

Mezirow J. Learning as transformation: critical perspectives on a theory in practice. San Francisco: Jossey-Bass; 2000.

Newman M. Calling transformative learning into question: some mutinous thoughts. Adult Educ Q. 2012;62(1):36–55.

Offredy M. Decision-making in primary care: outcomes from a study using patient scenarios. J Adv Nurs. 2002;40(5):532–41.

Pennington D, Simpson G, McConnell M, Fair J, Baker R. Transdisciplinary research, transformative learning and transformative science. Bioscience. 2013;63(7):564–73.

Renigere R. Transformative learning in the discipline of nursing. Am J Educ Research. 2014;2(12):1207–10.

Romano A. The challenge of the assessment of process and outcomes of transformative learning. Educ Reflective Pract. 2017;1:184–219.

Stuckey HL, Taylor E, Cranton P. Developing a survey of transformative learning outcomes and processes based on theoretical principles. J Transform Educ. 2013;11(4):211–28.

Sweller J. Cognitive load during problem solving: effects on learning. Cogn Sci. 1988;12(2):257–85.

Taylor D. Adult learning theories: implications for learning and teaching in medical education. AMEE Guide No 83. Med Teach. 2013;83:e1561–e72.

Taylor E, Cranton P. A theory in progress? Issues in Transformative learning theory. Eur J Res Educ Learn Adults. 2013;4(1):33–47.

Walters L, Prideaux D, Worley P, Greenhill J. Demonstrating the value of longitudinal integrated placements to general practice preceptors. Med Educ. 2011;45:455–63.

Self-Regulated Learning: Focus on Theory

26

Susan Irvine and Ian J. Irvine

Contents

Introduction	482
Conceptual Framework of SRL	483
Phase 1: Cognitive Forethought, Planning, and Activation	483
Phase 2: Cognitive Monitoring	485
Phase 3: Cognitive Control	485
Phase 4: Cognitive Reaction and Reflection	485
Regulation of Motivation and Affect	486
Phase 1: Motivational Forethought, Planning, and Activation	486
Phase 2: Motivational Monitoring	487
Phase 3: Motivational Control	487
Phase 4: Motivational Reaction and Reflection	487
Regulation of Behavior	488
Phase 1: Behavioral Forethought, Planning, and Activation	488
Phase 2: Behavioral Monitoring	488
Phase 3: Behavioral Control	488
Phase 4: Behavioral Reaction and Reflection	488
Regulation of Context	489
Phase 1: Contextual Forethought, Planning, and Activation	489
Phase 2: Contextual Monitoring	489
Phase 3: Contextual Control	489
Phase 4: Contextual Reaction and Reflection	489
Self-Regulated Learning in the Clinical Context	490
Future Directions for Health Professional Education and Research	493
Education	493
Research	494

S. Irvine (✉)
Victoria University, Melbourne, VIC, Australia
e-mail: susan.irvine@vu.edu.au

I. J. Irvine
University of Newcastle, Newcastle, NSW, Australia
e-mail: ian.irvine@uon.edu.au

© Springer Nature Singapore Pte Ltd. 2023
D. Nestel et al. (eds.), *Clinical Education for the Health Professions*,
https://doi.org/10.1007/978-981-15-3344-0_34

Conclusion 495
Cross-References 495
References 495

Abstract

This chapter uses Pintrich's theory of self-regulated learning (SRL) and explores the associated interplay between areas of self-regulation, cognition, motivation/affect, behavior, context, and its application to student learning in the clinical setting. This theoretical approach provides explanations for the vast differences in how a learner regulates learning and accounts for differences in performance outcomes.

The theory of SRL is generally applied to the classroom setting; however, health professional education often consists of clinical placement. Therefore, the theory of SRL is used to demonstrate how a student self-regulates their learning in the clinical context. The need for educators to remediate student performance with SRL instructional support is discussed.

Finally, this chapter outlines future directions for education and research. Included in future directions is the need to link research methodologies to assess the effectiveness of student's SRL in the clinical environment. Research needs to identify how the theory of SRL is best modified to learning environments outside the classroom.

Keywords

Theoretical framework · Self-regulated learning · Clinical environment · Cognition · Metacognition · Motivation · Learning strategies · Affective behaviors · Instructional support

Introduction

In the past student's failure to learn was attributed to lack of intelligence (Dierking 1991). Educators struggled to explain the vast differences in learner's approaches to learning and study; why some learners seem highly motivated, retain information, and others seemed disinterested and struggled to understand. Self-regulated learning (SRL) developed from a need to include other constructs that impact learning, such as motivation, affect, and metacognitive strategies (Biggs and Moore 1993).

The following vignette exemplifies how the way in which the ineffective use of motivation and SRL strategies may cause a student to struggle with learning:

A final year OSCE is due in two weeks, Lisa has not set study goals, including a study schedule, and she cannot see the value of OSCE exams. Her self-talk tells her she must do her best to please her parents for paying her university fees. Lisa attributes previous failures to a lack of ability and intelligence, and because of this, she is too embarrassed to ask for help from her educator or peers. Exams make Lisa very anxious, and she has little confidence in passing the exam.

The theory of SRL assumes that learners like Lisa can improve their performance using adaptive motivation and learning strategies. This approach is consistent with the underpinning philosophical approach to health professional education in fostering independent, lifelong learners (Artino et al. 2012; Kuiper and Pesut 2004).

This chapter begins by outlining the conceptual framework of SRL as developed by Pintrich (2004). The next section examines the interplay between Pintrich's model of SRL within the clinical context. Finally, future directions for education and research are explored.

Conceptual Framework of SRL

This section details a social cognitive model of SRL as developed by Pintrich (2004). Within this model, the structure of learning involves an interactive process of four phases. The four phases include forethought, planning and activation phase, a monitoring phase, a control phase, and finally a reaction and reflection phase. Each phase interacts with areas of regulation. The areas of regulation include the dynamic interaction between cognition, motivation/affect, behavior, and context (Pintrich 2000). The following definition of SRL highlights this interaction:

> Self-regulated learning is an active, constructive process whereby learners set goals for their learning and then attempt to monitor, regulate, and control their cognition, motivation, and behavior, guided and constrained by their goals and the contextual features in the environment (Pintrich 2000, p. 453).

These areas for regulation and the phases are outlined in Table 1. The items located at the bottom of the table align with the areas of regulation and are used in a self-report instrument called the motivational strategy for learning questionnaire (MSLQ) developed by Pintrich and colleagues to measure areas involved in self-regulation (Pintrich et al. 1991).

Phase 1: Cognitive Forethought, Planning, and Activation

The forethought, planning, and activation phase involves the processes that precede efforts to learn and involves goal setting, activation of prior knowledge, and activation of metacognition (Pintrich 2004). Goal setting is used to guide cognition and monitoring of a task. Goal difficulty, or the level of task adeptness required, influences the effort used by learners to attain a goal (Pintrich 2000). Learners who are more self-regulatory or metacognitive will retrieve relevant information before performing a task or activate prior knowledge in a planned manner by using strategies such as self-questioning activities or self-prompts (Pintrich 2004).

Cognitive regulation involves the activation of metacognitive knowledge and strategies that enhance learning. For example, knowing that rehearsal as a strategy is useful for memorizing information, a learner studying for a drug calculation test may

Table 1 Phases and areas for self – regulated learning

Areas for regulation				
Phases and relevant scales	Cognition	Motivation/affect	Behavior	Context
Phase 1				
Forethought, planning, and activation	Target goal setting	Goal orientation adoption	Time and effort planning	Perceptions of task
	Prior content knowledge activation	Efficacy judgments	Planning for self-observations of behavior	Perceptions of context
	Metacognitive knowledge activation	Perceptions of task difficulty		
		Task value activation		
		Interest activation		
Phase 2				
Monitoring	Metacognitive awareness and monitoring of cognition	Awareness and monitoring of motivation and affect	Awareness and monitoring of effort, time use, need for help	Monitoring changing task and context conditions
			Self-observation of behavior	
Phase 3				
Control	Selection and adaptation of cognitive strategies for learning, thinking	Selection and adaptation for strategies for managing, motivation, and affect	Increase/decrease effort	Change or renegotiate task
			Persist, give up	Change or leave context
			Help-seeking behavior	
Phase 4				
Reaction and reflection	Cognitive judgments	Affective reactions	Choice behavior	Evaluation of task
	Attributions	Attributions		Evaluation of context
Relevant MSLQ scales	Rehearsal	Intrinsic goals	Effort regulation	Peer learning
	Elaboration organization	Extrinsic goals	Help-seeking	Time/study environment

(continued)

26 Self-Regulated Learning: Focus on Theory

Table 1 (continued)

Areas for regulation				
Phases and relevant scales	Cognition	Motivation/affect	Behavior	Context
	Critical thinking	Task value	Time/study environment	
	Metacognition	Control beliefs		
		Self-efficacy		
		Test-anxiety		

Reprinted from "A conceptual framework for assessing motivation and self-regulated learning in college" Pintrich, P. 2004, *Educational psychology review*, p. 390. Copyright 2004 Springer Science + Business Media, Inc. Reprinted with permission Regulation of Cognition

activate the knowledge of the usefulness of rehearsal and use it to remember drug formulas.

Phase 2: Cognitive Monitoring

The cognitive monitoring phase involves the awareness and monitoring of various aspects of cognition and is referred to as metacognition (Flavell 1979). One type of metacognitive judgment or monitoring involves self-judgments of what the learner understands. Self-judgments occur as the learner monitors their approach to a task and by asking themselves questions. Metacognitive awareness enables the learner to control and regulate cognition (Zimmerman 2000).

Phase 3: Cognitive Control

Cognitive Control The cognitive control phase includes the types of cognitive and metacognitive activities in which learners engage to adjust their cognition. Attempts to control, regulate, and change cognition is associated with cognitive monitoring, which provides information about any gaps between a goal and the performance toward achieving that goal (Zimmerman 2000). One of the central aspects of the control and regulation of cognition is the actual selection and use of various cognitive strategies for memory, learning, and problem solving (Pintrich 2004).

Phase 4: Cognitive Reaction and Reflection

The processes of the cognitive reaction and reflection phase involve learners' judgments and evaluations of their performance. Self-regulators evaluate their performance in comparison to learners who avoid self-reflection and self-evaluation and are more likely to adjust their performance (Zimmerman 2002). Further, this approach is linked to deeper cognitive processing, better learning outcomes, and achievement as well as positive motivational beliefs and behaviors such as high self-efficacy and persistent effort (Schunk 2012).

Attributions are judgments about success and failures that powerfully influence learners' academic self-regulation (Schunk 2012). Dunn and associates examined learners' causal attributions and their influence on their self-regulation. Results indicated that ability, effort, and luck attributions for success influenced learners' self-regulated learning and that ability did not have the most significant influence (Dunn et al. 2012). Therefore, educators can alter a learner's negative attributional thinking by encouraging the learner to use adaptive attributions, such as attributing results to effort.

Table 1 details the phases as a linear or hierarchical model where earlier phases precede later phases; however, in performing a task, the phases may occur in a cyclic manner (Pintrich 2000), as outlined in the following example.

A learner plans how they will take a patient's blood pressure (Phase 1-goal setting). During the procedure, the student is monitoring their performance and realizes the blood pressure cuff is too large (Phase 2 – judgment and Phase 1 – replanning) and adjusts the size of the cuff to ensure an accurate reading (Phase 3 – implementing a different strategy) and monitors the accuracy of the size of the cuff and the blood pressure reading (Phase 2 – metacognitive awareness and monitoring of cognition). At the end of the task, the learner reflected on their overall performance and made a mental note (Phase 4 – cognitive judgment), next time, to assess the cuff size before performing the task.

Regulation of Motivation and Affect

Phase 1: Motivational Forethought, Planning, and Activation

In this phase, motivational forethought, planning and activation involve the learners' perception of self-efficacy as well as motivational beliefs, the value and interest they have of a task (Pintrich 2004). To continually improve and become proficient at a specific task, a learner needs a high level of motivation to continue to self-regulate (Kitsantas and Zimmerman 2002). Regulation of motivation and affect includes the attempt to regulate motivational beliefs, such as the reason for doing a task (goal orientation), learners' beliefs about the importance of the task (task value), how interested they are in the task (task interest), and judgments about the level of competence to perform a task (self-efficacy) (Pintrich 2000). Positive performance outcomes are directly related to a student's control of learning beliefs. If a learner believes in their efforts to learn, they are more likely to use effective learning strategies to achieve the desired result (Pintrich 2004).

Learners that are intrinsically, goal-orientated find learning to be challenging and rewarding, enquiring beyond the tasks set, and exploring more in-depth the material to understand underlying concepts and structures. Therefore, intrinsic motivation is often associated with deep learning, which is characterized by higher-order cognition such as analysis, synthesis, and evaluation (Entwistle 2013). Conversely, extrinsically motivated learners have behaviors that are focused on specific outcomes that are externally controlled, such as passing an examination or achieving a high grade. Extrinsic motivation is linked to surface learning and is characterized by lower-order cognition such as knowledge recall using strategies such as memorizing and rehearsal (Zimmerman et al. 2011).

Learners' beliefs about the value and importance of the task and their goal orientations determine why and how they engage in a task and the metacognitive strategies used when performing a task. Perceptions of task difficulty or the level of task proficiency determine the effort that learners expend to attain a goal (Schunk 2012).

Phase 2: Motivational Monitoring

During the monitoring phase, the learner attempts to regulate their self-efficacy, their interest in the task, or their level of anxiety. However, to do this, they must be aware of these motivations and monitor them, and this occurs in the monitoring phase. Even when performance is poor, they do not give up; instead, they amend their efforts using new strategies. Therefore, metacognitive strategy use does not contribute to learning and performance if learners cannot motivate themselves to use these strategies and persist in the face of difficulties, distractions, or problems (Sungur 2007).

Phase 3: Motivational Control

In the control phase, there are many strategies a learner can use to control motivation and affect. For example, a learner can control self-efficacy through positive self-talk such as *I can do this or don't give up, keep going* (Bandura 1977), or moderating anxiety by changing any factors that increase anxiety. Ultimately, it is the learner's ability to monitor their affective behaviors and control these behaviors by the selection of strategies to manage them and enhance learning and performance.

Phase 4: Motivational Reaction and Reflection

Reaction and reflection occur after learners have completed a task with several possible outcomes, for example, happiness at success or disappointment with failure. Learners' reflections on the reasons for their performance and the type of reactions will impact on the learners' motivational beliefs and expectancy for future success (Schunk and Pajares 2010). Attributions or learners' beliefs about learning, such as the value they attribute to a task, their goal orientations, and high self-efficacy are associated with higher levels of metacognitive strategy use and therefore improved performance in the future (Valle et al. 2003).

Regulation of Behavior

Phase 1: Behavioral Forethought, Planning, and Activation

Regulation of behavior is an aspect of self-regulation that involves the learner's attempts to control their behavior with the aim of performing well (Pintrich 2004). In the forethought, planning, and activation phase learners engage in time-management activities, planning, and managing their study environments effectively (Pintrich et al. 1991). These activities are part of behavioral control, and the extent to which they are used is based on the learner's decisions on how they allocate their effort, the amount of work they will undertake and the control they exhibit in their study environment to reduce interruptions (Pintrich et al. 1991).

Phase 2: Behavioral Monitoring

The monitoring phase of behavior is where the learner monitors their time management and the amount of effort; they give to a task (Pintrich 2000). For example, a learner may decide to allocate more time to a task when they realize the task is more difficult than they anticipated. Monitoring performance in this way will lead the learner to implement a strategy to control their effort by using strategies such as spending more time studying or setting up a study group.

Self-regulators monitor behaviors and engage in self-judgments in which they assess their performance and identify reasons for their performance. The ability to monitor and reflect is crucial because attributions of failure can cause a learner to react negatively, such as procrastinating, becoming anxious, giving up, and not persisting and trying to improve (Zimmerman 2000).

Phase 3: Behavioral Control

Control of behavior may involve strategies to control academic learning, time, and the study environment, effort, and level of persistence with a task. For example, a learner may use help-seeking as a strategy, rather than giving up. The learner's ability to seek help from educators and peers can be vital to successful performance (Pintrich 2000).

Phase 4: Behavioral Reaction and Reflection

In the reaction and reflection phase, the learner reflects and makes judgments on their behaviors. A learner may reflect on how procrastination impedes their academic achievement and decide to take a different approach to their study and make different behavioral decisions, such as greater persistence and effort (Pintrich 2004).

Regulation of Context

Phase 1: Contextual Forethought, Planning, and Activation

Context is the final area of regulation involving how learners regulate tasks and the environment. Unlike the other areas of regulation, context is mostly out of the control of the learner. This phase involves the perceptions about the nature of the activities and the norms within the classroom (Pintrich 2004). For example, learners may have perceptions of the tasks, learning environment, learning activities, and perceptions about working with peers. For learners to do well in the classroom, they need to reflect on these perceptions as well as monitoring the requirements of the tasks, the contextual features or rules of the classroom (Pintrich 2004). The classroom is a social system and can provide opportunities or constraints that influence behavior and impact learning. If learners are not aware of the advantages of working with peers, they are less likely to adjust their performance or behaviors to give them the best opportunity of succeeding.

Phase 2: Contextual Monitoring

Contextual monitoring requires an awareness of perceptions that the learner may have of the learning context, for example, the tasks, the degree of autonomy the educator assigns to the learner or the rules of the group in which they participate. In their own learning environment, learners are required to monitor for distractions such as noise and the use of social media to control the environment by removing these distractions to ensure the environment is conducive to learning (Zimmerman 2000).

Phase 3: Contextual Control

This phase involves the learner controlling tasks and their environment (Pintrich 2004). Learners are required to regulate context in both the classroom and in their own private study. A learner may have limited control of context, for example, classroom activities are often assigned by the educator, for instance, in a didactic learning environment the learner may not be given the opportunity to negotiate tasks. In contrast, a learner-centered learning environment the learner is afforded the opportunity to negotiate academic tasks. Assigning the learner greater autonomy and creating more opportunities for learners to negotiate tasks to regulate and control their learning will foster self-regulated, independent learners (Zimmerman 2002).

Phase 4: Contextual Reaction and Reflection

In the reaction and reflection phase, learners reflect and make assessments of the academic tasks in both the classroom and their private study environment

(Zimmerman 2002). Educators can allocate time for learners to reflect on what is working in the classroom, for example, reflecting on their judgments of the peer group activities to decide on what is working or not working. These judgments can be fed back into phase one when learners undertake other tasks.

Lisa's story is revisited to demonstrate how the areas of regulation may impact Lisa's performance. Items in brackets are examples that relate to theoretical constructs listed in Table 1:

> A final year OSCE is due in two weeks, Lisa has not set study goals (lack goal setting), including a study schedule (lack of planning and regulation of time and study), and she cannot see the value of OSCE exams (low task value). Her self-talk tells her to do her best to please her parents for paying her university fees (extrinsic goal). Lisa attributes previous failures to a lack of ability and intelligence (negative attributions). Because of this, she is too embarrassed to ask for help from her educator or peer (lack of help-seeking). Exams make Lisa very anxious (negative affect), and she has little confidence in passing the exam (low self-efficacy).

Lisa may not be aware of the impact of her negative motivation such as anxiety, low task value, and low self-efficacy on her performance. Behaviors portrayed in the vignette are indicators of a learner who is likely to fail, and without appropriate remedial action, Lisa is likely to continue with these negative motivations. Retraining negative motivations and beliefs about the causes of failure and success is crucial for future success (Dunn et al. 2012; Durning et al. 2011; Sandars 2013).

This section described Pintrich's theory of self-regulated learning and provided an explanation for individual differences in learners' performance. The next section will explore SRL in the clinical context of health professional education.

Self-Regulated Learning in the Clinical Context

So far, this chapter has focused on SRL theory within the broad context of learning, mainly within the classroom setting. Given self-regulated learning is shaped by the interaction between the individual and the context, the purpose of this section is to explore the interplay of SRL in the clinical context. SRL is known to be depended on the degree to which learners can adjust or regulate their behavior to the clinical context and the extent they show motivational and proactive positive behaviors (Berkhout et al. 2017; Woods et al. 2011).

The health profession education curriculum incorporates a clinical practicum at different stages of the course whereby learners integrate and apply knowledge in the real world. The context of the clinical practicum has greater challenges for the learner than the classroom setting. These challenges will be explored, highlighting the implications for learners' ability to self-regulate, and perform at the expected level. To illustrate this, we follow Lisa in the first two hours of her first acute care clinical placement.

Lisa passed her OSCE and progressed to her first acute clinical placement. Day 1 Lisa arrives at 0700, feeling anxious and hoping she will get along with her educator (anxiety). Lisa attends the handover; however, the staff use unfamiliar abbreviations leaving Lisa unsure what they mean in relation to the patients she is caring for. Following the handover at 0720, she is given a time planner to set up the care of her 2 patients where she lists the various tasks (planning). She asked if she could look up the medical terminology. However, her educator suggested she could do that later in the shift when the unit wasn't as busy. Lisa is enthusiastic about the opportunity of administering the 0800 medications under the supervisor of her educator for the first time (task value). Lisa would like the time to look up the medications to hopefully impress her educator (external motivation). However, there isn't time to do this because one of her patients' needs assistance with feeding. Lisa catches up with the educator to administer the medications to one of her patients, including an antihypertensive and a hypoglycemic agent. The educator asks Lisa what the patient's blood pressure (BP) and blood sugar level (BSL) readings were, to which Lisa replied, "I didn't have time to attend to them" (lack of integration of knowledge and planning). The educator becomes very frustrated with Lisa because she should know to take the patient's BP and BSL as a priority. 0900 Lisa finds the daughter of one her patients very upset about her mother's condition and would like to speak to the RN who is attending to a medical emergency and is unable to assist Lisa with the competing demands including the upset daughter. At the end of the shift, Lisa's educator provides feedback on the areas Lisa must develop to ensure future care is provided in a safe and timely manner. However, Lisa is upset and not feeling confident of performing well (self-efficacy) on the next shift.

The vignette demonstrates the complexities that a novice faces in negotiating and balancing competing goals within the complex clinical setting. Although the vignette focuses on nursing, the principles, and the following discussion could be applied to other health professions.

The clinical context as described in the case of Lisa is one in which it may be difficult to learn because it's hard knowing what is expected coupled with the unpredictability of the clinical environment and competing demands (Prince et al. 2005). Developing competency in the clinical setting is reliant upon the degree to which self-regulation can be enhanced or inhibited by circumstances and context faced by learners such as Lisa, and whether they are afforded a supportive setting. In fact, studies in the health professional literature report many barriers to learning in the clinical context, with learners feeling unsupported (Berkhout et al. 2017; Newton et al. 2012). Learners require a great deal of support from clinical staff to balance the tension between the demands of learning, maximizing learning opportunities, and maintaining good relationships with the clinical educator and members of the health care team (Berkhout et al. 2017). Otherwise, these tensions within the clinical context may impede metacognitive awareness or critical thinking, which is a purposeful, self-regulatory judgment that involves a person's capacity to reflect on and monitor their performance. If the clinical context is chaotic, it may contribute to learners experiencing negative affect such as anxiety, low self-efficacy, decreased effort, and a reluctance to ask for help (Pintrich 2004).

These contextual factors of the clinical setting have negative implications for the novice learner such as Lisa because the development of metacognitive (reflective) strategies to evaluate monitor and adjust performance is difficult. In addition, their decision-making skills may be slower due to a lack of automaticity resulting from a lack of experience and encoded patterns (Benner 1984). This was highlighted in the case of Lisa, where she lacked the ability to integrate theory with practice, to manage competing goals and to plan and prioritize care. The more experienced learner may have the capacity to prioritize care effectively, practice more independently, and not rely on the support of the clinical educator as much as a novice (Sagasser et al. 2012). Experienced learners are known to adjust and use different strategies to regulate learning and vary the strategies dependent on the clinical case (Sagasser et al. 2012), concurring with the theory of SRL that strategy use is situational and influenced by the context (Pintrich 2004).

The individual differences in learner's ability to effectively regulate motivation and use effective learning strategies highlight the importance of self-regulatory instructional support within the clinical context (Butler 2002). If Lisa is not aware of the advantages of positive motivation, she is unlikely to adjust her behaviors to give her the best opportunity of succeeding. Conversely, Lisa's educator would need to be aware of the theoretical underpinnings of self-regulated learning to identify maladaptive self-regulatory behaviors and provide remedial action to facilitate Lisa's success.

Learners require instructional support to reflect on their causal thinking and their emotional reactions to successes and failures, as well as how those cognitive and emotional patterns affect their future behaviors (Sandars 2013). Educators can support learners to adopt more positive attributional tendencies by discussing the learners' judgment about reasons for success or failure (Dunn et al. 2012). The educator can highlight the role that effort plays in success and support learners to regulate cognition by goal setting, planning care, monitoring the outcomes of the care, and adjust care as required. This implies coregulation (Garrison and Akyol 2015) where the educator must regulate their own cognition, motivations/affect, behaviors, and context as well as supporting and mentoring the learner's self-regulation. The degree to which coregulation can be enhanced or inhibited by circumstances and context faced by Lisa and the educator is dependent upon a supportive context. van Houten-Schat Maaike et al. (2018) conducted a systematic review to explore self-regulated learning in the clinical context and found a focus on instructional support conjures positive self-regulatory behaviors in the clinical context.

Self-regulated learning microanalysis is a procedure that involves asking a series of questions about specific regulatory processes as learners engage in a task (Cleary and Sandars 2011; Sandars 2013). The following vignette is an example of an educator using a microanalytical approach to determine the SRL strategies used by Lisa as she performs a procedural task.

> Prior to the task [forethought, planning, and activation), the educator asked Lisa about her performance goals (goal setting) and what she needs to do to perform the task [assessing for planning and activation of prior knowledge]. During the task, the educator observed Lisa performing the task and at a specific point stopped Lisa and asked, 'What is the main thing you are focusing on and why?' [assessing for metacognitive awareness, monitoring, and affect]. After the task, the educator asks Lisa two questions. 'How well do you think you went? Is there anything you would do differently next time? (assessing reaction and

reflection). The outcomes of the microanalytical approach enabled the educator to provide feedback and offer instructional support on SRL processes to enhance Lisa's performance. The educator encourages Lisa to ask herself the questions in future performances, so she progresses to a level of independence and self-regulation over the duration of the course (Kuiper and Pesut 2004).

Other types of instructional programs are reported in the literature, for example, Hall et al. 2004) found that two types of retraining programs significantly improved both high-achieving and low-achieving learners' attributional thinking. One type used cognitive strategies in which learners were taught to understand their thinking processes (metacognitive strategies) and the other understanding affective behaviors and reactions to successes and failures. A different example of instructional support using a computer-assisted instructional attributional training could be used in both the classroom and clinical context (Van der Hem-Stokroos et al. 2003). Retraining requires a safe and supportive learning environment (Van der Hem-Stokroos et al. 2003) and maybe supported by engaging learners in a discussion on how to learn in a clinical environment (Sandars 2010).

Future Directions for Health Professional Education and Research

Education

For decades the educational psychology literature has reported instructional support and remedial intervention to enhance SLR and learner performance with recent reports in the health professional education (Durning et al. 2011). However, this pedagogical approach needs to extend to all health professions and research to investigate specific training techniques for improving learners' self-regulatory strategy use and the effects of such training on learning outcomes in the clinical context.

Training low achievers to effectively utilize self-regulatory processes will improve their performance (Durning et al. 2011). For example, teaching learners to think about the process of performing a skill and self-monitoring during the performance, instead of focusing on the outcome has been shown to increase skill performance and motivation (Cleary and Sandars 2011). Developing learners as highly metacognitive and to become independent learners is an expectation of the health professionals once learners graduate (Kuiper and Pesut 2004). To achieve these practices, the novice learner must progress to a level of independence and self-regulation over the duration of the course (Kuiper and Pesut 2004). Hence, the need for instructional support and developing students as self-regulated learners (Durning et al. 2011; Ten Cate et al. 2004).

Further development of the curriculum requires a greater emphasis on assessment and detection of self-regulatory strategy use in the clinical context. According to Cleary and Sandars (2011), microanalysis has a strong potential as a structured assessment technique examining the self-regulatory processes underlying psychomotor skills and could make important contributions to identify and remediate strugglers in the clinical context.

Peer learning is known to be an effective self-regulatory strategy affording learners greater support and improving learner performance in the clinical environment (Irvine et al. 2017). There is increasing evidence that dyadic practice (learning in pairs) improves efficiency for a wide range of clinical skills without compromising learning. This is illustrated in a study comparing the effectiveness of simulation-based ultrasound training in dyads with that of training as an individual (Tolsgaard et al. 2015). However, peer learning in the health professional literature indicates this pedagogical approach is implemented mostly on an informal basis with few programs integrated into the curriculum (Irvine et al. 2017). When it is embedded into the curriculum it can have very positive effects on learners' self-efficacy (Mckenna et al. 2018).

Research

There are three tensions that arise from the definition of SRL in relation to "self," having implications for further research. Firstly, the concept; of "self" in the theory of SRL implies it is an individualistic motivation (Boekaerts 2002). It raises the question of how a learner develops as a "self" regulated learner when the "self" – goals may compete with the goals of the curriculum. For example, the educator creates the goals based on the goals of the curriculum and imposes those goals onto the learners. This raises the question, to what degree can the curriculum accommodate the individual goals of the learner? Secondly, tensions may occur within the context of group work or collaborative learning where the goal of the individual learner conflicts with the goals of the group (Ben-Eliyahu and Bernacki 2015).

Finally, theories of SRL, including Pintrich's framework, do not deal with the learner as a whole person (Boekaerts 2002). The theory focuses on academic goals ignoring cultural, social, and personal goals of the learner, which may create tensions between the learner and educator. For example, a learner wants to complete a classroom task on time but has a social goal that involves communicating a message to a friend in the classroom. The educator requests that the learner stop chatting and focus on the academic task. The learner has the option of maintaining the goal of the educator or pursing the personal goal and risk creating tensions between themselves and the educator. The learner in this situation could choose a regulatory strategy such as writing a note to the friend and then continuing with the task set by the educator. However, the educator may view as the learner self-managing the situation rather than the learner regulating the conflicting goals.

The impact of conflicts between learner's cultural, social, and personal goals and the goals of academic learning within the classroom and the clinical contextual, remains unknown. Further studies in health professional education are required to examine how learners manage these tensions and the impact on the learners' ability to self-regulate in different learning environments. Additional studies are required to gain a deeper understanding of how various aspects of the clinical context influences or inhibits learner's ability to self-regulate and what support provides adaptive self-regulatory behavior. The outcomes of such research may contribute to the theory of SRL.

van Houten-Schat Maaike et al. (2018) reported that studies on SRL in the health professional literature lack a theoretical framework (e.g., Zimmerman's, Pintrich) and the theory, when applied is mainly in a classroom setting. Given context is a strong influence of learners' performance, methodologies appropriate to the complex clinical setting require a move beyond reliance on self-report data (Pintrich 2004), to real-time studies such as think-aloud protocols (Greene et al. 2011; Irvine et al. 2005) and microanalysis (Cleary and Sandars 2011; Cleary et al. 2016). Insights into self-regulatory behaviors and causal attributes of learners in real-time in the simulated and clinical setting will inform learner feedback and provide the opportunity to implement remedial action where necessary.

Newly graduated health professionals are required to demonstrate the ability to problem-solve complex patient care issues. This requires higher-order strategies such as critical thinking and metacognition. Longitudinal studies are required to assess the development of SRL strategies throughout a course, and how these can be supported to create highly self-regulating, life-long learners.

Conclusion

This chapter used Pintrich's theory of SRL explored the phases and areas of regulation of cognition, motivation/affect, behavior, and context, relating the theory to health professional education, research, and practice. Learners would benefit if educators were aware of how learners regulate their learning, to determine the need for individual instructional support. Highlighted in the chapter are the implications for the novice and struggling learner if instructional support is not provided. The chapter identified the need to link research methodologies to the assessment of learner's SRL in the clinical environment. Finally, research to identify how the theory of SRL is best modified to learning environments outside the classroom context.

Cross-References

▶ Learning and Teaching in Clinical Settings: Expert Commentary from an Interprofessional Perspective

References

Artino AR Jr, Dong T, DeZee KJ, Gilliland WR, Waechter DM, Cruess D, Durning SJ. Achievement goal structures and self-regulated learning: relationships and changes in medical school. Acad Med. 2012;87(10):1375–81. https://doi.org/10.1097/ACM.0b013e3182676b55.
Bandura A. Self-efficacy: toward a unifying theory of behavioural change. Psychol Rev. 1977;84(2):191–215. https://doi.org/10.1037/0033295X.84.2.191.

Ben-Eliyahu A, Bernacki ML. Addressing complexities in self-regulated learning: a focus on contextual factors, contingencies, and dynamic relations. Metacogn Learn. 2015;10(1):1–13. https://doi.org/10.1007/s11409-015-9134-6.

Benner P. From novice to expert – excellence and power in clinical nursing practice. California: Addison-Wesley Publishing Company Nursing Division Melno Park; 1984.

Berkhout JJ, Helmich E, Teunissen PW, van der Vleuten CPM, Jaarsma ADC. How clinical medical students perceive others to influence their self-regulated learning. Med Educ. 2017;51(3):269–79. https://doi.org/10.1111/medu.13131.

Biggs J, Moore P. The process of learning. Sydney: Prentice Hall; 1993.

Boekaerts M. Bringing about change in the classroom: strengths and weaknesses of the self-regulated learning approach—EARLI presidential address, 2001. Learn Instr. 2002;12(6):589–604. https://doi.org/10.1016/S0959-4752(02)00010-5.

Butler D. Qualitative approaches to investigating self-regulated learning: contributions and challenges. Educ Psychol. 2002;37(1):59–63. https://doi.org/10.1207/S15326985EP3701_7.

Cleary T, Sandars J. Assessing self-regulatory processes during clinical skill performance: a pilot study. Med Teach. 2011;33:7. https://doi.org/10.3109/0142159X.2011.577464.

Cleary TJ, Durning SJ, Artino AR Jr. Microanalytic assessment of self-regulated learning during clinical reasoning tasks: recent developments and next steps. Acad Med. 2016;91(11):1516–21. https://doi.org/10.1097/ACM.0000000000001228.

Dierking L. Learning theory and learning styles: an overview. J Museum Educ. 1991;16(1):4–6. https://doi.org/10.1080/10598650.1991.11510159.

Dunn KE, Osborne C, Link HJ. Exploring the influence of students' attributions for success on their self-regulation in pathophysiology. J Nurs Educ. 2012;51(6):353–7. https://doi.org/10.3928/01484834-20120420-01.

Durning SJ, Cleary TJ, Sandars J, Hemmer P, Kokotailo P, Artino AR. Perspective: viewing "strugglers" through a different lens: how a self-regulated learning perspective can help medical educators with assessment and remediation. Acad Med. 2011;86(4):488–95. https://doi.org/10.1097/ACM.0b013e31820dc384.

Entwistle NJ. Styles of learning and teaching: an integrated outline of educational psychology for students, teachers and lecturers: Routledge; 2013. Available from. https://doi.org/10.4324/9781315067506.

Flavell JH. Metacognition and cognitive monitoring: a new area of cognitive-developmental inquiry. AmP. 1979;34(10):906–11.

Garrison RD, Akyol Z. Thinking collaboratively in educational environments: shared metacognition and co-regulation in communities of inquiry. In: Lock J, Redmond P, Danaher PA, editors. Educational developments, practices and effectiveness: global perspectives and contexts. London, UK: Palgrave Macmillan Limited; 2015. p. 39–52.

Greene JA, Costa L, Dellinger K. Analysis of self-regulated learning processing using statistical models for count data. Metacogn Learn. 2011;6(3):275–301. https://doi.org/10.1007/s11409-011-9078-4.

Hall NC, Hladkyi S, Perry RP, Ruthig JC. The role of attributional retraining and elaborative learning in college student's academic development. J Soc Psychol. 2004;144:591–612. https://doi.org/10.3200/SOCP.144.6.591-612.

Irvine IJ, Jeanneret N, Cantwell RH. A methodology for representing the regulation of the composing process. In: Forrest D, editor. Proceedings of the XV National Conference of Celebration of Voices. Melbourne: Australian Society for Music Education; 2005. p. 111–7.

Irvine S, Williams B, McKenna L. How are we assessing near-peer teaching in undergraduate health professional education? A systematic review. Nurse Educ Today. 2017;50:42–50. https://doi.org/10.1016/j.nedt.2016.12.004.

Kitsantas A, Zimmerman B. Comparing self-regulatory processes among novice, non-expert, and expert volleyball players: a microanalytic study. J Appl Sport Psychol. 2002;14(2):91–105. https://doi.org/10.1080/10413200252907761.

26 Self-Regulated Learning: Focus on Theory

Kuiper R, Pesut D. Promoting cognitive and metacognitive reflective reasoning skills in nursing practice: self-regulated learning theory. J Adv Nurs. 2004;45(4):381–91. https://doi.org/10.1046/j.13652648.2003.02921.x.

McKenna L, Irvine S, Williams B. 'I didn't expect teaching to be such a huge part of nursing': a follow-up qualitative exploration of new graduates' teaching activities. Nurse Educ Pract. 2018;32:9–13. https://doi.org/10.1016/j.nepr.2018.06.010.

Newton JM, Jolly BC, Ockerby CM, Cross WM. Student centredness in clinical learning: the influence of the clinical teacher. J Adv Nurs. 2012;68(10):2331–40. https://doi.org/10.1111/j.1365-2648.2012.05946.x.

Pintrich P. The role of goal orientation in self-regulated learning. In: Boekaerts M, Pintrich P, Zeidner M, editors. Handbook of self-regulation. San Diego: Academic Press; 2000. p. 451–502.

Pintrich PR. A conceptual framework for assessing motivation and self-regulated learning in college students. Educ Psychol Rev. 2004;16(4):385–407. https://doi.org/10.1007/s10648-004-0006-x.

Pintrich P, Smith D, Garcia T, McKeachie W. A manual for the use of the motivated strategies for learning questionnaire (MSLQ). Mitchigan: The University of Mitchigan; 1991.

Prince KJ, Boshuizen HP, Van Der Vleuten CP, Scherpbier AJ. Students' opinions about their preparation for clinical practice. Med Educ. 2005;39(7):704–12. https://doi.org/10.1111/j.1365-2929.2005.02207.x.

Sagasser M, Kramer A, van der Vleuten C. How do postgraduate GP trainees regulate their learning and what helps and hinders them? A qualitative study. BMC Med Educ. 2012;12(1):67. https://doi.org/10.1186/1472-6920-12-67.

Sandars J. Pause 2 learn: developing self-regulated learning. Med Educ. 2010;44(11):1122–3. https://doi.org/10.1111/j.1365-2923.2010.03824.x.

Sandars J. When I say . . . self-regulated learning. Med Educ. 2013;47(12):1162–3. https://doi.org/10.1111/medu.12244.

Schunk D. Attributions as motivators of self-regulated learning. In: Schunk DH, Zimmerman BJ, editors. Motivation and self-regulated learning: theory, research, and applications, vol. 2012. New York: Routledge; 2012. p. 245–66. Available from: http://search.proquest.com/docview/62678326?accountid=12528.

Schunk D, Pajares F. Self-efficacy beliefs. In: Peterson P, Baker E, McGaw BP, Baker E, Peterson P, Baker B, editors. International encyclopedia of education. 3rd ed. Oxford: Elsevier; 2010. p. 668–72.

Sungur S. Modeling the relationships among Students' motivational beliefs, metacognitive strategy use, and effort regulation. Scand J Educ Res. 2007;51(3):315–26. https://doi.org/10.1080/00313830701356166.

Ten Cate OL, Snell L, Mann K, Vermunt JD. Orienting teaching toward the learning process. Acad Med. 2004;79(3):219–28.

Tolsgaard MG, Madsen ME, Ringsted C, Oxlund BS, Oldenburg A, Sorensen JL, et al. The effect of dyad versus individual simulation-based ultrasound training on skills transfer. Med Educ. 2015;49(3):286–95. https://doi.org/10.1111/medu.12624.

Valle A, Cabanach RG, Nunez JC, Gonzalez-Pienda J, Rodriguez S, Pieniro I. Cognitive, motivational, and volitional dimension of learning. Res High Educ. 2003;44:557–80. https://doi.org/10.1023/A:1025443325499.

Van der Hem-Stokroos HH, Daelmans HE, Van der Vleuten CP, Haarman HT, Scherpbier AJ. A qualitative study of constructive clinical learning experiences. Med Teach. 2003;25(2):120–6. https://doi.org/10.1080/0142159031000092481.

van Houten-Schat MA, Berkhout JJ, van Dijk N, Endedijk MD, Jaarsma ADC, Diemers, AD. Self-regulated learning in the clinical context: a systematic review. Med Educ. 2018;52(10):1008–1015.

Woods NN, Mylopoulos M, Brydges R. Informal self-regulated learning on a surgical rotation: uncovering student experiences in context. Adv Health Sci EducTheory Pract. 2011;16(5):643–53. https://doi.org/10.1007/s10459-011-9285-4.

Zimmerman BJ. Chapter 2 – Attaining self-regulation: a social cognitive perspective. In: Boekaerts M, Pintrich PR, Zeidner M, editors. Handbook of self-regulation. San Diego: Academic Press; 2000. p. 13–39.

Zimmerman B. Becoming a self-regulated learner: an overview. Theory Pract. 2002;41(2):64–70. https://doi.org/10.2307/1477457.

Zimmerman B, Moylan A, Hudesman J, White N, Flugman B. Enhancing self-reflection and mathematics achievement of at-risk urban technical college students. Psychol Test Assess Model. 2011;53:108–27. Available from: http://www.psychologie-aktuell.com/fileadmin/down load/ptam/1-2011_20110328/07_Zimmermann.pdf

Critical Theory

27

Nancy McNaughton and Maria Athina (Tina) Martimianakis

Contents

Introduction	500
Critical Paradigm and Methodological Implications	501
Reflexivity	502
Location of the Authors	502
Critical Versus Constructivist and Positivist Paradigms	503
Relevance to Clinical Education	504
Part 1: An Exploration of Power	506
Power as Hegemony and Oppression	506
Power as Ideology	507
Power as Linguistic and Discursive Power	508
Theoretical Alignments	510
Summary of Part One	511
Part Two: Power, Critical Theories, and Clinical Education	511
Critical Theory Projects and Different Foci Within Clinical Education	511
Hidden Curriculum	511
Colonialism and Postcolonial-Oriented Projects	512
Marxist and Neo-Marxist Perspectives	513
Feminist and Gender Approaches	514
Anti-racist Approaches	515
Intersectional Approaches	515
Conclusion	516
Cross-References	516
Glossary	516
References	519

N. McNaughton (✉)
Wilson Centre for Research in Education, University of Toronto and University Health Network, Toronto, Canada
e-mail: n.mcnaughton@utoronto.ca

M. A. T. Martimianakis
Department of Paediatrics, Faculty of Medicine, University of Toronto, Toronto, Canada
e-mail: tina.martamianakis@utoronto.ca

© Springer Nature Singapore Pte Ltd. 2023
D. Nestel et al. (eds.), *Clinical Education for the Health Professions*,
https://doi.org/10.1007/978-981-15-3344-0_35

499

Abstract

The chapter describes and situates the critical research paradigm as valuable to the study of clinical medicine settings. In the introduction, the authors define critical theory, situate it historically, and describe its most salient features. The remainder of the chapter is organized into two parts. The first part outlines three different definitions of power accompanied by a discussion of their relevance within clinical education. The second part of the chapter examines specific critical theories with a discussion of their different applications within clinical education.

Keywords

Critical theory · Power · Hegemony · Ideology · Discourse · Hidden curriculum · Intersectionality · Marxist · Feminist · Postcolonial

Introduction

What is critical theory?

We find that question difficult to answer because: a) there are many critical theories, not just one; b) the critical tradition is always changing and evolving; and c) critical theory attempts to avoid too much specificity, as there is room for disagreement among critical theorists.
(Kincheloe and McLaren 2011)

Situating Critical Theory as an Approach Has Several Different Foci and Goals. Critical theory, sometimes called the Frankfurt School, began in Germany in the 1930s as an interdisciplinary, action-oriented approach to social analysis that attempted to integrate Marxian economic and social theory and Freudian psychoanalysis (Code 2000). Critical theory as a particular viewpoint grew in popularity through uptake in schools of literary studies, cultural studies, and social studies, as well as philosophy. At first glance it might seem that critical theorists are organized around a common political project, that of bringing awareness to the impact of power on the capacity of individuals to share equally in social, political, cultural, and economic life and that they also share the same history. It is now acknowledged that this unified political project of addressing inequities occurred over time, and around the world, in a haphazard way. The many perspectives that flourished from the Frankfurt School or that emerged independent of this group have a shared focus on power relations but with different histories and trajectories. Take, for example, feminist, antiracist, postcolonial, and Marxist perspectives, all of which focus on power relations as central however with different research foci and political projects.

In other words, the term critical theory now represents a category of theories with specific characteristics, rather than just one comprehensive framework. As identified in the quote above, not only are there many different critical theories, but also theorists who identify as critical often intentionally do not obligate themselves to one theory alone. Paradigmatically, critical research is inherently dynamic, changing, and evolving because it is irrevocably linked to contemporary social justice movements, which endeavor to transform society to be more equitable. We realize that this makes for a less than stable starting point to understand what critical theory is and why it is relevant within clinical education contexts. However, this ambiguity is a central feature of critical research. While there is not one "critical theory" to speak of, there are specific characteristics that distinguish critical inquiry from other research approaches. We will thus begin with an outline of the basic tenets that underpin the family of theories and methodologies that fall under the critical paradigm.

Critical Paradigm and Methodological Implications

Paradigms are described by Guba and Lincoln (1994) as "a basic set of beliefs that guide action." Informing this set of beliefs is a view about the nature of reality (ontology) and knowledge (epistemology). The relationship between these ideas and beliefs shapes how we see the world and act in it, as well as the questions we may ask and interpretations we may bring to our experiences (Denzin and Lincoln 1994). At the core of a critical research perspective is an understanding that truth is not a given but is responsive to different contextual, historical, and political conditions that may benefit some at the cost of others. Critical scholars share a restlessness to break free from assumptions about what is said to be "true" and a desire to try to see the world with fresh eyes. Methodologically, this allows critical researchers to focus on effects of power by deconstructing what we have come to think of as normal and naturally occurring. As a process, it draws attention to how we construct truths about ideas, people, and institutions. The goal of such research is to make visible the ways in which disadvantage, oppression, discrimination, and other negative effects of power are socially constructed and reproduced, either explicitly or implicitly. Research conducted through a critical lens may have any one of the several aims that exist along a continuum. One aim may be to give voice to those who are marginalized or to raise awareness of inequitable power arrangements. Another may be to effect change in the material conditions of a specific group. This kind of critical research is a form of advocacy and praxis which refers back to the work of Paulo Freire (1921–1997), a Brazilian philosopher and educator. He believed that education was a vehicle for change which could be harnessed for the goal of emancipation from oppression through an awakening of the critical consciousness. When critical consciousness is achieved, he believed that individuals are able to transform their world through social critique and political action (Freire 1970). Another aim may be to contribute to sociopolitical reform through policy or practice. Critical approaches address issues of discrimination and disadvantage, in whatever form they may take in a given context. The focus on power is thus a central tenet of critical inquiry with implications for how the researcher conceptualizes their role in the research process.

Reflexivity

Critical perspectives presume that researchers will always be active in the meaning-making process. In other words, there is no location from which to inquire about a topic or phenomenon in which the researcher is not involved. Who a researcher or educator is in the world, their gender, race, ethnicity, their religious affiliations, their socioeconomic status, their sexual orientation, their professional training, and other aspects of their identity, all inform their world view which in turn influences their approach to knowledge (epistemology) and what they believe can be known (ontology).

Insert our stories here.

Location of the Authors

Both authors are white cisgendered women, born and raised by working-class parents, who recently immigrated to Canada, and afforded the opportunities and privileges of their white settler heritage. They identify within a critical theory paradigm as a result of a number of intersecting personal and professional locations and experiences. Professionally, NM is located as a health professional education scholar who uses critical social science perspectives to inform questions about health professional socialization and intersections of power as they relate to equity, access, and constructions of knowledge legitimacy (McNaughton 2013). She has worked in the area of human simulation as an SP, a trainer, administrator, researcher, and educator for most of her educational life. This experience as well as other life experiences has led to her interest in exploring education as an embodied cultural and political undertaking that shapes and is shaped by emotion and affect. Her inquiry is informed by post-structuralist feminist writers on emotion, as well as Michel Foucault's (Foucault 1977) genealogical historical approach and principally Gilles Deleuze and Felix Guattari's writings that engage an alternative ontology which encompasses the idea of nomadology (Deleuze and Guattari 1987). Her project is critical in that it seeks to interrupt the taken-for-granted assumptions about the work and place of emotion in the field of health professions education while offering an alternative reading that includes acting, emotion, affect, medicine, and the place of women, patients, and simulated participants in health professional arenas. McNaughton, N. (2012) believes that the focus on SPs and how they are engaged is important for clinical education to consider because they act as vehicles for the transmission of medicine's prevailing ideas about patients, illness, and expected professional clinician behavior (Martimianakis and McNaughton 2015).

TM is a critical social scientist working in the Department of Paediatrics and the Wilson Centre at the University of Toronto, where she studies how culture, politics, and organizational practices impact health professional identity and socialization. Her research generates evidence that brings attention to the effects of marginalization and discrimination in medical training and practice (Lam et al. 2019). Theoretically, she is influenced by neo-Marxist, feminist, and Foucauldian scholars. She is particularly drawn to Foucault's notions of governmentality and subjectivity for its potential to show the power of discourses (institutionalized ideas and practices) (Martimianakis et al. 2015). Her research primarily focuses on elucidating the effects of discourses such as interdisciplinarity, collaboration, humanism, professionalism, and globalization on clinical working and learning spaces (Martimianakis and Hafferty 2013). Her work on identity explores how clinical learners and faculty come to appreciate what counts as expertise and the implications this has for how they approach patient care. Her approach has allowed her to understand and identify the ways in which expertise and knowledge are sidelined or stratified in specific contexts and how organizations inadvertently stifle the career potential of faculty and learners. For over 15 years, she has applied this theoretical lens to initiatives that target misalignments in educational vision and practice (Martimianakis et al. 2015).

In other words, critical researchers are expected to be reflexive about their standpoint and how it affects their knowledge-making process. Reflexivity is a marker of rigor and quality in critical research, as is an explicit appreciation of power relations, and a social justice orientation that contributes in some way to social transformation and egalitarianism. Participants are invited as partners in critical projects that aim to give voice to marginalization, oppression, and discrimination and to contribute to resolving those injustices. For example, standpoint theorists and approaches purposively select to work with groups designated as vulnerable (such as women, people of color, indigenous peoples, transgendered people, people with disabilities, and others) in order to articulate the material effects of power relations from their standpoint. The assumption is that knowledge about oppression can be more meaningfully derived from the perspectives of those who are oppressed. Critical participatory action researchers go one step further to incorporate actionable approaches for empowerment as an end goal of the research.

Critical Versus Constructivist and Positivist Paradigms

Critical theorists view social structures such as educational institutions, professional organizations, and professions themselves – along with the rules, practices, and positions of authority that maintain them – as shaped by political, cultural, economic, gender, and other social forces. These beliefs and ideas, namely, that social reality is dynamic, interconnected, and politically consequential, distinguish the critical paradigm from constructivist and positivist worldviews. Reality and knowledge about the social world are conceptualized theoretically not only as constructed through interactions but also importantly shaped by power relations that have historically privileged certain groups over others. Knowledge making is always perceived to be situated in a social, political, and historical context. For example, many critical scholars have shown that what we have come to associate as knowledge is the accumulation of interests, beliefs, and preferred methods of inquiry. It is often Eurocentric and Western voices that tend to dominate the academic world scene in publications and other scholarly engagements. This dominance is often a result of their location at, and access to, resource-rich research-intensive universities. Scholars at prestigious academic institutions are provided entitlements and networking opportunities that increase their reach through participation at international conferences. In medical education and other health academic contexts, the lead academic journals publish papers in English, thus providing an explicit advantage to English-speaking scholars. However, while we can generalize that power relations can constitute marginalization and discrimination around the world, we would never assume that this marginalization and discrimination would be experienced in the same way by people in different geographic locations and at different points in history.

Another idea that sets critical theories apart from constructivist and positivist theories is the belief that language does not merely describe but in fact interactively produces the truths upon which our institutions and organizations are based. In other words, the labels we use to identify objects and people have histories and cultural meanings that also dictate a particular way of relating back to those things to which we give a label. For example, when a person with an illness is described as a "patient" versus "a disease" versus a "client," or by their birth or chosen name, it engenders a particular relationship between a health-care provider and a person who needs care. Each label connotes a particular way of subjecting the person to a situated history of what counts as care, with immediate implications for how the person experiences the health-care system (i.e., paternalistically, as objectification, as an exchange of services, as relational).

As identified above, these features specific to critical theory approaches make them recognizable and defensible as a way of examining and exploring different clinical phenomena and topics. When we think about critical theories and clinical education, it is perhaps more useful for us to frame critical theory as a particular way of looking at the world, which directs our attention to issues of power and its effects. From this perspective, clinical education in all its varied practices can be conceptualized as an important vehicle for knowledge production, which powerfully influences how we come to appreciate and experience health and illness. Critical theorists working within clinical domains orient their inquiry toward making visible how the act of knowing and caring for the human body has the potential to support and reproduce truths that privilege some over others. While not all research conducted from a critical perspective is intended to directly inform change, critical theorists seek to identify and describe how marginalization, discrimination, and oppression occur in medical contexts and to generate evidence that can be used to make health-care education and practice more inclusive and equitable.

Relevance to Clinical Education

> Critical theory in education is concerned with the workings of power in and through pedagogical discourses, and....addresses the relations among schooling, education, culture, society, economy and governance. (Popkewitz and Fendler 1999)

Popkewitz and Fendler's description holds as true for the role of critical theory in health professions education as it does for education more broadly. The world of clinical education is dynamic, with a multiplicity of intersecting forces. Power relations inform knowledge claims or put another way who gets to decide whose knowledge is more important than another's knowledge. Pedagogical approaches, curriculum design decisions, and issues of professionalism and identity formation are shaped by these claims. For example, historically, and across the world, there are ongoing debates about what should be considered foundational clinical knowledge. Most schools around the world would consider basic and life sciences as integral to the future skills and knowledge of health-care practitioners. As a result, these subjects are often given more curricular time and possibly more human and technical resources than subjects that relate to the social dimensions of health. In the process, and often inadvertently, a tacit message is being delivered about which knowledge counts more in the training of health-care professionals as well as in the care of patients. Such educational decisions will have implications for how patients experience health-care encounters. It also contributes to how divisions of work take place in the clinical setting. Tasks that are not specific to the biological symptoms of a patient, such as their capacity to access food on a regular basis, may be seen as problems that should be resolved outside of the clinic and by individuals who are not health-care professionals.

Education takes place in milieus that are as socially and culturally constructed as they are scientifically informed. Many "ways of doing things" become taken for granted over time, and the rationales for various practices become invisible. Critical theory perspectives, thus, can be helpful in bringing to light what is often considered invisible or taken for granted in clinical education contexts, particularly around the ways that practices are organized and decisions made about what to teach, who to train, and how to educate about the body, health, illness, care, and treatment. Critical theory perspectives take what is accepted as status quo in relation to biomedical and psychosocial knowledge, health, disease, and care and question who benefits from specific arrangements. Pursuing this question may reveal unseen dimensions that can lead to welcome transformations in how we train clinical personnel to approach and treat patients and their families. Throughout the rest of the chapter, we will describe a selection of different critical theories and illustrate their relevance within clinical education contexts. Specifically, the remainder of the chapter is divided into two parts. In part one we will explore different definitions of power and the ways in which they can be understood and engaged with in critical theoretical projects. In part two we will examine the different relationships between power, critical theories, and clinical education, using specific projects to illustrate how a critical theory lens may help the reader understand the direct application and significance of critical scholarship in their day-to-day practices.

Part 1: An Exploration of Power

There are many definitions of power, with each bringing to bear different analytical considerations for clinical education. Three of these will be discussed below: power as hegemony, power as ideology, and power as discourse.

Power as Hegemony and Oppression

Hegemony can be traced back to the scholar Antonio Gramsci (1891–1937) and to Karl Marx (1818–1893) before him. It refers to the idea that a ruling class can manipulate the value system and mores of a society, so that their view becomes the dominant world view. Hegemony is a slight of hand that presents a social, political, and economic status quo as inevitable, natural, and beneficial to everyone rather than as an artificial social construct that benefits only the ruling class. Hegemonic power is invisible, described sometimes as pervasive and unnoticed as the air that we breathe. We are not aware of it affecting us, even though it impacts our daily lives. Socially we don't question the way things are organized around us. It is just the way it is. Medicine, for example, is taken for granted to be at the top of the health professions pyramid. Other health professions labelled as "allied" have developed and are identified within this group not by their own health professional knowledge and skills base but through there relation to whom they are allied. Medicine represents a taken-for-granted status quo with implications for access to resources, decision-making, and priority setting within institutions.

Another characteristic of hegemony is the idea that domination occurs not through force but by winning people's consent to be dominated through cultural institutions such as schools, the media, the family, and religion. An example of hegemony at work in the clinical realm is the notion that patients must come to a hospital or clinic to receive care. While this was not always the case, the formalization of the health professions into organized, regulated occupations with control over a body of expert knowledge has concentrated the delivery of care in specific settings. These have, in turn, implications related to who can access health-care resources and under what conditions. Another routine example is the scheduling of committee meetings at 7:30 AM or following work after 5:00 PM. The rationale for this practice is the notion that committee meetings should not interfere with clinical work. Thus, the time is set to privilege or convenience those conducting patient rounds or patient clinics. The question about who this arrangement may inconvenience is not really considered. Clinician parents needing to drop off or pick up children, or those whose schedules do not conform to institutional arrangements, are not thought about. Patients who are woken up early for rounds after a sleepless night or needing to fit in a doctor's appointment during working hours are also not considered. To interrupt the institutional organization for a particular group of individuals is difficult – if not impossible – given the inevitable logic of certain arrangements. It is this hidden logic, and our unquestioning acceptance of the arrangements, to which hegemony refers.

Power as Ideology

> We may be unconscious of some of this gap, but even when conscious we are silent or inarticulate about the dissonance and, in silence, do not assist our students to understand our challenges when attempting to live up to our profession's ideals. (Coulehan 2006)

An ideology is a set of ideals, principles, doctrines, or myths of a large group, such as an institution, profession, or nation, which explains how society should work and which offers a political and cultural blueprint for a certain social order. Communism, for example, is an ideology that constructs a particular classist vision of society as true, complete with roles, societal rules, and predictive outcomes. Importantly, power as ideology is political in nature. Ideologies are central to the constitution of both political subjectivities (what we hold to be true about ourselves as citizens) and social and political relations. Thus, there are different political ideologies, concerning different aspects of a society. For example, ideas about how the economy, education, health care, law, etc. should function inform our decision-making at social, institutional, and political levels.

It is important to consider ideological power in clinical education settings, because ideology can drive decisions and actions toward achieving a particular goal – often without consideration of possible unintended effects. Actions that are anchored in ideological appreciations of health care and illness may reproduce the status quo and can lead to actions that have material consequences. The most common ideological divide is around whether health care should be delivered through a universal access or private health-care model. Committing to one or the other approach will influence many facets in a country's political and economic organization, including the capacity for a specific government to introduce health-care reform that is ideologically misaligned with the dominant system; e.g., the introduction of Obama care in the United States was opposed even by individuals who would benefit from the reform, because it was perceived to challenge the ideology of free determination (see below the comments on neoliberalism). Another example, more specific to clinical training, relates to admission requirements for medical school. The medical professional is socialized over many years into a particular way of viewing their role and their patients. The process begins with decisions about who is considered eligible for medical school and continues through "...specialized language of the medicine disciplines [which have] defined, organized, contained and made seemingly immutable a group of attitudes, values and behaviours subsumed under the label 'professional' or 'professionalism'" (Wear and Kuczewski 2004). Much like a hegemonic system of power in which benefits are accrued by some at the expense of others, an ideology that holds professionalism as a particular set of traits and values attached to an ideal vision of an altruistic expert also privileges some individuals at the expense of others. For example, a dominant ideology in North America is neoliberalism. Neoliberalism refers to the ideology that the "market," and hence market-based solutions, is the most efficient and effective way to address public sector problems (Kearney et al. 2019). The prevailing common sense of neoliberalism suggests that as free persons, individuals are responsible for securing their well-being by making good choices, developing marketable skills, and competing to accumulate personal resources and property. It promotes the notion of self-determination and does not consider sociohistorical determinants in the career success of individuals. In a medical education context, power works through neoliberal ideology to enact new practices and rituals of accountability, orienting social relationships around individual responsibility and economic competitiveness (De Lissovoy and Cedillo 2016). This plays out not only in competitive entry requirements for medical schools and decision-making processes about who might make a suitable candidate but also in ideas about competence. For example, the eligible candidate for medical school in North America until recently was often white, male, Christian, of a particular class, and preferably with a strong science background. The gendered and racist dimensions of not considering why white, male Christian men only emerged as top candidates was not problematized. This was not necessarily consciously upheld during selection processes, but rather these characteristics came to construct an ideal picture of a physician – by virtue of who had ended up in medical schools. It has taken deliberate intervention through enacting policies and processes to develop diversity in medical schools. Power in neoliberalism also asserts itself by constructing an enclosed ideological universe, which is maintained through everyday rituals and practices (De Lissovoy and Cedillo, 2016). In this process of enclosure, a competitive and entrepreneurial determination of education is secured through the very structure of the experience of school. In other words competitive processes are set up and rewarded in ways that sustain the culture. Ideas about professionalism are operationalized within reform and accreditation documents as a complex array of competencies to be mastered as part of a larger medical enterprise.

Power as Linguistic and Discursive Power

> Discourses of power refers to…. "Practices and rules about what can and cannot be said, who can speak with the blessings of authority and who must listen, whose social constructions are valid and whose are erroneous and unimportant." (Adapted from Kinchloe and McLaren 2011)

Critical theorists for whom power is seen through a linguistic or discursive lens look largely to post-structuralist thinkers such as Michel Foucault (1926–1984), who wrote prolifically on a number of topics such as the birth of clinical medicine and medical education, public health, psychiatry, schools and examinations, the body, physical and laboratory examination, sexuality, and ethics. Indeed, some of his notions – including discourse, bio-power, and technologies of the self and the clinical gaze, just to name a few – have major importance for clinical education today (Hodges et al. 2014). Foucault coined the term bio-power to describe the processes by which populations are regulated and bodies disciplined. Think about the practices in our early school years of lining up for entry into school or raising a hand in class to answer a question or the process of handing test sheets into the teacher in an orderly fashion. Training is a form of disciplining bodies that takes place within institutions like prisons, schools, and the military as organized practices. The resulting behaviors become normalized and internalized, thereby creating greater control especially where large groups are involved. In societies where it is common practice to teach children to line up to enter their class, it is also common to see lines forming to access busses, to buy tickets, and to order food at a take-out restaurant to name a few. Lines will form in places where there is no explicit sign or instruction to form a line. This type of self-regulation has implications for how we come to perceive behaviors of others who do not naturally conform to line forming, including attributing rudeness, incivility, or unprofessionalism to individuals who try to cut in line (entering a queue at any position other than the end). A specific type of disciplining by medicalizing behaviors relates to Foucault's concept of bio-power. He was interested in examining the different ways in which knowledge was put to work through practices within institutional settings in order to regulate the conduct of others in relation to physical health without exerting direct force upon the person (Hall 2001). For example, when it became common practice to relate to people in terms of their life stage (infancy, childhood, adolescence, adulthood, middle age, old age), the medical fields also established milestones and healthy behaviors and practices for each life stage. The application of this medical thinking made certain previously acceptable social practices such as child labor, child marriages, or sexual relationships between adults and teenagers, which were common in previous eras, to be considered deviant practices in contemporary societies. This is a different way of conceptualizing power than either hegemony or ideology. It is seen as an effect of social relations, practices, rules, and positions of authority but not as a top-down application of power. Foucault's interest was to make visible the way power circulates and less about the ways it oppresses as a direct force from one person onto another. The focus is on the relationships between knowledge, power, the body, and the regulation of conduct according to a set of implicit truths that are institutionalized as discourses.

For example, the idea that collaboration is an essential good has been institutionalized in North American clinical contexts, making it very difficult for health professionals to act in ways that contrast to the idea of practice in health-care teams. Learning and delivering in teams has generated many activities, objects, and practices that did not exist prior to the institutionalization of the idea that collaboration in health care is a good thing. The relationships between knowledge, truth, and power were of a concern for Foucault because of the disciplining effect they had without the direct and top-down exercise of power. Disciplinary processes at an institutional level are most efficient and effective when "... individuals take up the task of self-regulation and self-disciplining, something that occurs as persons take up identities offered them through the discursive practices of social institutions and professions" (Jaye et al. 2006). The effect of these relationships is to produce a normalized set of practices that become invisible or taken for granted. Foucault's notion of bio-power and in particular how it applies to the regulation and self-regulation of professional behaviors offers us insight into the role of power within medical training (McNaughton and Snelgrove 2019).

For Foucault and other post-structuralist thinkers (such as Gilles Deleuze, Jacques Derrida, Julia Kristeva, Judith Butler), language does not simply describe but actually constructs our social world and the different ways in which we may participate. In this way it shapes our social relations and subjects us within different discourses. As we described earlier, the different ways in which a person with an illness is called a "patient," a "disease," a "client," or by their name create a particular relationship between health-care provider and person who needs care. It also subjects that person to speak in different ways with different effects. According to Foucault, a discourse is an organized system of thought made up of "practices that systematically form the objects of which they speak" (Foucault 1972). So, practices and rules about what can and cannot be said, who can speak with the blessings of authority and who must listen, and whose social constructions are valid and whose are erroneous and unimportant are all affected by discourses.

For example, a medical trainee's developing identity within the profession is tied to the manner in which he or she "performs" an understanding about their own skill and knowledge as well as their place in the professional hierarchy. The training process is a subjecting practice: the trainee is shaped into a particular kind of subject by the expectations of the professional community. A disciplinary discourse serves to regulate behaviors and attitudes to a normalizing process. For example, a medical student reporting a patient history to a staff person is expected to deliver the information in a particular order and know which information to include and exclude in order to be perceived as competent. Foucault's critical discourse explicates the various ways in which taken-for-granted rules about professional conduct get built into day-to-day processes and practices. The relevance for clinical educators is in the different ways that these taken-for-granted disciplinary practices become internalized and continue to reproduce professional norms of legitimacy.

The main difference between discursive power and power as an ideological force is the view that language is actively involved in creating our possible roles, practices, and knowledge claims. In this iteration of power, it is not an oppressive force but rather one that circulates among institutions, roles of authority, practices, and ways of saying and doing that like our other forms of power have material and symbolic effects.

Theoretical Alignments

The above three definitions of power align with theories that clinical educators may find helpful when designing curriculum, justifying pedagogical choices, or analyzing outcomes from their day-to-day educational practice. In all three of the definitions of power described, the emphasis is on the social, political, and historical forces that shape individual choices and behaviors. The individual is the product of processes that are self-regulating and normalizing in that they choose to conform to ideas about legitimacy – whether in order to get into a medical school or to fit in once they are accepted. There are overlapping ideas within these three perspectives on power. All three systems of power create a consenting subject who is willing to adopt practices that conform to a norm of legitimacy put forward by those in positions of power. The manner in which this occurs is different in all three; however their roots are the same; these refer us back to the Frankfurt School of the 1930s.

Summary of Part One

In the first part of the chapter, we have situated critical theory historically and described its salient features. As a theoretical perspective, critical theories share across the spectrum of different approaches an interest in exploring relations of power. Three definitions of power – hegemonic, ideological, and discursive – were described, with examples that highlight their different foci while acknowledging their overlapping principles.

Part Two: Power, Critical Theories, and Clinical Education

Critical Theory Projects and Different Foci Within Clinical Education

As we have noted above, there are many different ways to approach scholarship from a critical perspective in the clinical education domain. Depending on the area of interest and goals of the particular project, a critical theoretical approach can offer analytical tools to help explore and possibly uncover unseen underlying mechanisms. Clinical education encompasses a broad landscape of possible interests and projects: from student admissions to methods of learning and from curriculum design and assessment to professionalism, to name only a few. Below we provide examples of different projects and accompanying critical theoretical considerations.

Hidden Curriculum

> The hidden curriculum highlights the importance and impact of structural factors on the learning process. Focusing on this level and type of influence draws our attention to...commonly held "understandings", customs, rituals and taken-for-granted aspects of what goes on in the life-space we call medical education. This concept also challenges medical educators to acknowledge their training institutions as both cultural entities and moral communities, intimately involved in constructing definitions about what is "good" and "bad" medicine. (Hafferty 1998)

Hidden curriculum is an important critical concept that directs our attention to tacit influences that contribute to the socialization of learners into health professional practice. While the hidden curriculum can be both positive and negative, most scholars focus on making sense of the incongruence in what we purport to value in health professions training (as written into official curricular documents) and what is actually practiced by clinical faculty, learners, and practicing professionals . With roots in sociology and education, the concept draws our attention to the influence of organizational structure and culture on the execution of a school's stated mission and objectives for training. The hidden curriculum is theorized to affect the nature of learning through routine professional interactions and clinical practice. When using the concept of the hidden curriculum to conduct research, the aim is to identify inadvertent tacit influences within a health professions training program that socializes learners to the knowledge, behaviors, practices, and values that represent the culture and practice of health care in a particular context and to see whether these tacit messages reinforce the learning objectives of the formal curriculum, or work against them. In other words, identifying the potential to undermine the mission of the health professions school through routine and unproblematized practices in clinical workplaces is the object of hidden curriculum research. First introduced into medical education by Fred Hafferty in the early 1990's, (Hafferty 1994) the concept has been applied to issues ranging from admissions to accreditation, and includes topics such as professionalism lapses, the erosion of humanism and empathy, the erasure of identities through socialization, and other features of the learner and faculty experience that are incongruent with the aim of producing caring, competent health professionals who will address the needs of all patients and their families. Hidden curriculum scholarship has also made visible the role of education in creating a hierarchy of what counts as important knowledge and what constitutes good medical practice in a given context. Hidden curriculum projects within clinical medicine may include exploring the taken-for-granted power relations behind choices of what to include in the curriculum. Another project may be an examination of how the norms, values, expectations, and practices of medical schools work to reinforce gender stereotypes.

Colonialism and Postcolonial-Oriented Projects

> Post-colonialism is 'a cultural, intellectual, political, and literary movement of the twentieth and twenty-first centuries characterized by the representation and analysis of the historical experiences and subjectivities of the victims, individuals and nations, of colonial power. Post-colonialism is marked by its resistance to colonialism and by the attempt to understand the historical and other conditions of its emergence as well as its lasting consequences.' (Fidel Fajardo-Acosta 2005)

The main goal of postcolonial perspectives is to make visible ways in which we continue to reproduce and reinforce notions of "developed" and "underdeveloped" that privilege settler groups over indigenous groups when organizing and delivering medical education. For example, there are statistically fewer First Nations, Inuit and Metis people, and people of color in many Canadian medical schools. Postcolonial theories document how colonial relationships historically established through military and government intervention are perpetuated by practices, policies, and protocols in the day-to-day activities of Canadian society. Postcolonial theoretical perspective can contribute to "understanding how continuities from the past shape the present context of health and health care" (Browne et al. 2005).

One postcolonial project relevant to clinical education explored traditional approaches to health promotion. The authors worked with a group of aboriginal peoples on the west coast of Canada to develop a decolonizing approach in the context of an urban garden project. The authors argue that health promotion must be "linked to decolonization efforts, a process that centres on regaining political, cultural, economic and social self-determination as well as positive identities as individuals, families, communities and nations . . .. addressing the legacy of colonialism and drawing on knowledge and practices from pre-colonial times" (Mundel and Chapman 2010).

Theories that explore colonial and postcolonial relationships are important orientations for troubling the dominance of Eurocentric and other Western ways of thinking in the health professions. In addition, these perspectives focus an exploratory lens on the historical effects of colonialism and on the capacity of those colonized to access resources and to receive education that is organized and delivered in ways that respect their cultural orientation to health, illness, and overall way of life. In many parts of the world where European colonies took root (such as Canada, Australia, the United States, and countries of Latin American and Africa), indigenous medical students continue to experience forms of oppression. A critical theorist may call on postcolonial theories to better understand the various political and power relations that contribute to indigenous students' experiences of professional schools, such as medicine and nursing including issues of representation stereotyping, explicit racism, and devaluing of indigenous healing practices. They might also focus on ways in which biomedical approaches to health silence perspectives on alternative ways of caring for patients and healing illness and create health inequities where indigenous peoples fail to obtain the level and quality of care offered to those with more power in society. The loss of voice and self-determination is a major tenet in this line of research. This does not preclude also exploring intersections of power related to other sources of discrimination, including gender or class:

> It is important to note that postcolonial theory is not only relevant to practitioners and researchers working with Aboriginal populations. The forces of colonization have had global effects and many of us have direct and indirect experiences of colonization that we bring with us from other parts of the world. At some level, it could be argued that we have all internalized colonization and we are both the oppressor and the oppressed. (Postcolonial Theory for Beginners September 1 2010, in Aboriginal/Indigenous Research Methodology)

Marxist and Neo-Marxist Perspectives

Marxist theories explore the sociocultural and economic conditions that give rise to class distinctions. Class issues specifically orient the exploration to social divisions that are differentially constituted on the premise of material and symbolic wealth. They track the reproduction of class divisions through explicit and implicit mechanisms and bring attention to how people in lower socioeconomic groups experience life. Issues of access to health and education have been a central topic for critical scholars inspired by Marxist perspectives. Issues of class have been concerns across the health professions education literature. For example, there is work that documents the cost of preparing for and applying to medical school. This line of research shows that students from lower socioeconomic groups, who have the same potential as students from higher socioeconomic groups, may be disadvantaged by admission processes that are financially burdensome or that require additional educational preparation that is costly and out of reach to many students, such as having overseas volunteer experience. Other work has focused on showing how achieving training in a clinical field secures a higher status in society. The privilege associated with the practice of medicine (financial and cultural) makes these professions coveted and exclusionary.

Feminist and Gender Approaches

There is a plethora of theories that identify themselves as feminist, with some not focusing on gender per se but rather the mechanisms of privilege and exclusion that are premised on competition and other organizational attributes considered to derive from masculine orientations. All feminist theories consider the role of women and female-identifying people in society and contend that they have been excluded from full participation in society by virtue of their gender. Patriarchy is a form of power that is linked to feminist inquiry and that denotes the ways in which male dominance has historically taken root in different cultural contexts over time. Feminist writing is very closely linked to the feminist movement and is concerned with improving how women and female-identifying groups experience the world. For example, feminist standpoint theories emerged in the 1970s as a reaction to essentialist feminist movements and writing that conceptualized all women to be equally marginalized. In contrast, standpoint theorists drew out the specific ways in which some women and female-identifying groups are more marginalized than others. For example, black feminist writers distinguished themselves as giving voice to the particularities of the lives of black women, in a way that could only be captured by someone who is of that group. Theoretically, feminist standpoint theorists make three principal claims: (1) Knowledge is socially situated (therefore it has cultural and social dimensions that are contextually specific). (2) Marginalized groups are socially situated in ways that make it more possible for them to be aware of things and ask questions than it is for the non-marginalized (therefore it is best to learn about these experiences from a member of this group directly). (3) Research that focused on power relations should begin with the lives of the marginalized (in other words, to appreciate the exclusion of women requires that you study women, not to extrapolate from what we know of men and generalize to women). Feminist scholars working within a number of disciplines – such as Dorothy Smith (1987), Nancy Hartsock (1983), Bell hooks (1984), Sandra Harding (1986), Patricia Hill Collins (2000), Alison Jaggar and Bordo (1989), Arlie Hochschild (2003), and Donna Haraway (2006) – have advocated taking women's lived experiences, particularly experiences of (caring) work, as the beginning of scientific inquiry. Central to all these theories are feminist analyses and critiques of relations between material experience, power, and epistemology and of the effects of power relations on the production of knowledge. This is especially because, for thousands of years, what we have come to associate with knowledge that has been conceptualized and actualized by men.

Anti-racist Approaches

Anti-racist scholars focus on ways in which skin color can be deterministic in how a person experiences social, cultural, and economic life. Race is thus the pivotal point of departure for making visible the forces of marginalization and exclusion. Anti-racist scholars are particularly concerned with white privilege and dominance in all contexts and have documented the plight of visible minorities around the world. In health professional training, anti-racist scholarship has served to document the exclusion of learners and faculty on the basis of their race and to track the disadvantage in their careers associated with stigma and racialization. In addition, health research from an anti-racist perspective has exposed how race has been used in eugenics projects, implicating medicine in reproducing and maintaining social inequities. From unethical experimentation on black, aboriginal, and other visible minority groups to an inappropriate extrapolation of findings derived from a geographically similar population to all populations, the problematization of science and medical practice from an anti-racist lens has made visible ways in which medical education and care occupy a political space with sociocultural, economic, and health implications for patients and their families.

Intersectional Approaches

Intersectional theory asserts that people are often disadvantaged by multiple sources of oppression: their race, class, gender identity, sexual orientation, religion, and other identity markers. In other words, rather than seeing social identities and intersections of power as a single defining characteristic of an individual's status and capacity to act in society, intersectional approaches look at ways in which, for example, gender, class, race, ability, ethnicity, sexual identity, and immigration status operate to create complex configurations of opportunity and disadvantage. As in previous approaches, the goal is to identify and chart ways in which oppression, marginalization, and discrimination happen and to develop strategies for addressing inequities in society. In medical education, intersectionality perspectives are used to document the interacting factors that create social inequities for patients, learners, and faculty (Tsouroufli et al. 2011). Intersectional approaches offer a nuanced understanding of the complex factors that mediate the social relations of patients, learners, and faculty in health settings. For example, when we explore the career trajectories of female- and male-identifying learners or faculty, we may discover that female-identifying learners and faculty experience glass ceiling effects, with lower rates of promotion and lower earnings for similar tasks compared with male-identifying peers. An intersectional lens would allow the researcher to look more deeply into the categories of female and male and overlay analysis that draws out potential subgroup examples of privilege and marginalization. For example, one might find that in a particular context, black, male-identifying faculty experience lower rates of promotion than white, female-identifying faculty. Or, Muslim female trainees may experience higher rates of exclusion than other trainees identifying as a visible minority. Exploring students' experiences of their educational environment from multiple vantage points may be helpful for creating a deeper understanding about the forces that inform their professional identities or choice of specialty, as well as the barriers to success.

Conclusion

In this chapter, we have provided an overview of critical theory and various approaches to appreciating the effects of power that may be relevant for clinical educators to consider as they endeavor to prepare health professionals to meet the need of diverse people with different histories and access to health care. There are many different critical theories to choose from and a number of considerations with respect to how power figures in each. In the first part of the chapter, we situated critical theory historically and described its many features. As a theoretical perspective, critical theories share across the spectrum of different approaches an interest in exploring relations of power. Three definitions of power – hegemonic, ideological, and discursive – were described, with examples that highlight their different foci while acknowledging their overlapping principles.

We have defined critical theory as a valuable approach for bringing to light taken-for-granted and undervalued aspects of clinical education and explained a number of critical theories as they relate to clinical education contexts.

Cross-References

▶ Threshold Concepts and Troublesome Knowledge

Glossary

Advocacy Advocacy is the act of exercising one's power and privilege to support people or groups which experience marginalization, discrimination, oppression and other forms of compromised agency.

Agency Agency is theorized as the capacity to act in the world and exercise self-determination. Free choice can be limited by social structures. Critical theories are concerned with the limits on agency that are linked to intersecting power relations such as gender, class, religion, ability, race, ethnicity etc.

27 Critical Theory

Axiology Axiology(from Greek ἀξία, axia, "value, worth"; and -λογία, -logia) is the philosophical study of value. It is either the collective term for ethics and aesthetics, philosophical fields that depend crucially on notions of worth, or the foundation for these fields, and thus similar to value theory and meta-ethics.

Critical Discourse Practices and rules about what can and cannot be said, who can speak with the blessings of authority and who must listen, whose social constructions are valid and whose are erroneous and unimportant (Adapted from: Kincheloe and McLaren 2011)

Discrimination Prejudice or prejudicial outlook, action or treatment (i.e. racial discrimination); the act, practice or instance of discriminating categorically rather than individually (Merriam-Webster Dictionary)

Diversity Diversity is the range of human differences, including but not limited to race, ethnicity, gender, gender identity, sexual orientation, age, social class, physical ability or attributes, religious or ethical values system, national origin, and political beliefs.

Equity Derives from ideas of social justice and refers to access to fair and equal treatment under the law, regardless of race, social class or gender. "It represents a belief that there are some things which people should have, that there are basic needs that should be fulfilled, that burdens and rewards should not be spread too divergently across the community, and that policy should be directed with impartiality, fairness and justice towards these ends." (Falk, Jim, Hampton, Greg, Hodgkinson, Ann, Parker, Kevin and Rorris, Arthur, 1993, Social Equity and the Urban Environment, Report to the Commonwealth Environment Protection Agency, AGPS, Canberra, p.2.)

Equality The quality of being the same in quantity, measure, value or status (Princeton's WordNet)

Hegemony Preponderant influence or authority over others, domination of a state, group, persons. The social, cultural, ideological, or economic influence exerted by a dominant group, institution, country etc. (Merriam-Webster Dictionary)

Hidden curriculum The hidden curriculum is explored through the social norms and moral beliefs tacitly transmitted through the socialization process that structure classroom social relationships. (Giroux, 1983, 48 as found in Skelton, 177)

Inclusion The term "**inclusion**" has a number of different meanings, often relating to disabled or disaffected children. ...**Inclusion** is the continuous process of increasing the presence, participation and achievement of all learners in education establishments. www.orkney.gov.uk/Service-Directory/D/Defining-Inclusion.htm Inclusion means that all people, regardless of their abilities, disabilities, or health care needs, have the right to: Be respected and appreciated as valuable members of their communities. Inclusion, while closely related, is a separate concept from diversity. SHRM defines inclusion as "the achievement of a work environment in which all individuals are treated fairly and respectfully, have equal access to opportunities and resources, and can contribute fully to the organization's success.

Inequities Lack of fairness or justice (Merriam-Webster Dictionary)

Intersectionality The term intersectionality was coined by black feminist scholar Kimberlé Crenshaw in 1989 "Intersectionality" represents an analytic approach that attempts to identify how interlocking systems of power impact those who are most marginalized in society. Intersectionality considers that various forms of social stratification, such as class, race, sexual orientation, age, religion, creed, disability and gender, do not exist separately from each other but are woven together. While the theory began as an exploration of the oppression of women of color within society, today the analysis is potentially applied to all social categories, including social identities usually seen as dominant when considered independently."

Marginalization Marginalization has been defined as a complex process of relegating specific groups of people to the lower or outer edge of society. It effectively pushes these groups of people to the margin of society economically, politically, culturally and socially following the policy of exclusion. https://www.sociologyguide.com/civil-society/marginalization.php

Oppression A situation in which people are governed in an unfair and cruel way and prevented from having opportunities and freedom. (Merriam-Webster Dictionary)

Political Project An organized and focused campaign to raise awareness and interrupt the normative ideas that support the status quo. To produce material, ideological or political change.

Power The notion of power is a contested term; there is no one prevailing definition of power, just as there is no singular critical theory. Nevertheless, for scholarship to carry the label "critical," power will have to be foregrounded. Power is sometimes referred to as the capacity/ability to act or produce an effect, physical or mental might, the influence or exercise one's will over others, the possession of legal or political authority, the "ability of an individual or group to achieve their own goals or aims when others are trying to prevent them from realizing them" (Weber 1925b/1978:926). Critical scholars are concerned with applications of power that impact the capacity of individuals or groups to share equally in social, political, cultural and economic life.

Power Relations Power relations refers to the matrix of political, cultural, social and economic structures and relationships that influence who and what has power in a given content. "At the very heart of the power relationship, and constantly provoking it, are the recalcitrance of the will and the intransigence of freedom" (Foucault, The Subject and Power, p. 221, Afterward to H. L. Dreyfus and P. Rabinow, Michel Foucault: Beyond Structuralism and Hermeneutics, Chicago, University of Chicago Press, 1982)

Privilege Privilege is the socio-political and economic advantage enjoyed by or afforded to individuals or groups of people in society on the basis of their class, caste, gender, race, ethnicity, ability etc.

Reflexivity Thoughtful, conscious, self-awareness Examination of one's own assumptions and reasoning in the production of knowledgeAwareness of own

27 Critical Theory

social positioning, personal experiences, and socialization. Reflection on taken-for-granted aspects of daily life

Social Justice Justice in terms of the distribution of wealth, opportunities, health, wellbeing, opportunity and privileges within a society. Aim is to create a more egalitarian society.

References

Browne AJ, Smye VL, Varcoe C. The relevance of postcolonial theoretical perspectives to research in aboriginal health. Can J Nurs Res. 2005;37(4):16–37.

Code L. Encyclopedia of feminist theories. New York: Routledge; 2000.

Collins PH. Black feminist thought. New York: Routledge; 2000.

Coulehan J. You say self-interest, I say altruism. In: Wear D, Aultman J, editors. Professionalism in medicine: critical perspectives. New York: Springer; 2006.

De Lissovoy N, Cedillo S. Neoliberalism and power in education. In: Peters MA, editor. Encyclopedia of educational philosophy and theory. Singapore: Springer Science+Business Media Singapore; 2016. https://doi.org/10.1007/978-981-287-532-7_155-1.

Deleuze G, Guattari F. A thousand plateaus: capitalism and schizophrenia (trans: Massumi B). Minneapolis/London: University of Minnesota Press; 1987/2005.

Denzin NK, Lincoln YS, editors. Handbook of qualitative research. Thousand Oaks: SAGE; 1994. p. 279–314.

Fajardo-Acosta F. World literature web site (2001–2011). 2005. http://fajardo-acosta.com/worldlit. Accessed 01 Sept 2019.

Foucault M. The archeology of knowledge & the discourse on language (trans: Sheridan Smith AM). New York: Pantheon Books; 1972. p. 49.

Foucault M. In: Bouchard D, editor. Language, counter-memory, practice: selected essays and interviews. Ithaca: Cornell Press; 1977/1980.

Freire P. Pedagogy of the oppressed. New York: Bloomsbury; 1970.

Guba EG, Lincoln YS. Competing paradigms in qualitative research. In: Denzin NK, Lincoln YS, editors. Handbook of qualitative research. Thousand Oaks: SAGE; 1994. p. 105–17.

Hafferty F. The hidden curriculum, ethics teaching, and the structure of medical education. Acad Med. 1994;69(11):861–71. https://doi.org/10.1097/00001888-199,411,000-00001.

Hafferty F. Beyond curriculum reform: confronting medicine's hidden curriculum. Acad Med. 1998;73(4):403–7.

Hall S. Foucault: knowledge, power, and discourse. In: Wetherall M, Taylor S, Yates SJ, editors. Discourse theory and practice: a reader. London: SAGE; 2001. p. 72–81.

Haraway D. A Cyborg manifesto: science, technology, and socialist-feminism in the Late 20th century. In: Weiss J, Nolan J, Hunsinger J, Trifonas P, editors. The international handbook of virtual learning environments. Dordrecht: Springer; 2006. https://doi.org/10.1007/978-1-4020-3803-7_4.

Harding S. The science question in feminism. Ithaca/London: Cornell University Press; 1986.

Hartsock NCM. The feminist standpoint: developing the ground for a specifically feminist historical materialism. In: Harding S, Hintikka MB, editors. Discovering reality. Synthese library, vol. 161. Dordrecht: Springer; 1983. https://doi.org/10.1007/0-306-48017-4_15.

Hochschild AR. The managed heart: commercialization of human feeling. 11th ed. Berkeley: University of California Press; 2003.

Hodges B, Martimianakis MA, McNaughton N, Whitehead C. Meet Foucault. Med Educ. 2014;48:563–71. https://doi.org/10.1111/medu.12411.

hooks B. Feminist theory: from margin to center. London: Pluto Press; 1984.

Jaggar A, Bordo SR. Gender/body/knowledge: feminist reconstructions of being and knowing. New Brunswick: Rutgers University Press; 1989.

Jaye C, Egan T, Parker S. 'Do as I say, not as I do': medical education and Foucault's normalizing technologies of self. Anthropol Med. 2006;13(2):141–55. https://doi.org/10.1080/13648470 600738450.

Kearney G, Corman MK, Hart N, Johnston J, Gormley GJ. Why institutional ethnography? Why now? Institutional ethnography in health professions education. Perspect Med Educ. 2019:1–8. https://doi.org/10.1007/s40037-019-0499-0.

Kincheloe JL, McLaren P. Rethinking critical theory and qualitative research. In: Kincheloe JL, editor. Key works in critical pedagogy. Bold visions in educational research, vol. 32: Brill/Sense on-line Publishing; 2011. p. 285–326. ISBN: 9789460913969.

Lam J, Hanson M, Martimianakis MA. Exploring the socialization experiences of medical students for social science and humanities backgrounds. Acad Med. 2019;95(3):401–410.

Martimianakis MA, Hafferty F. The world as the new local clinic: a critical analysis of three discourses of global medical competency. Soc Sci Med. 2013;87:31–8.

Martimianakis T, McNaughton N. Discourse, governmentality, biopower and the hidden curriculum. In: Hafferty F, O'Donnell J, editors. The hidden curriculum and health professions education. Chicago: Chicago Press; 2015.

Martimianakis MA, Michalec B, Lam J, Cartmill C, Taylor JS, Hafferty FW. Humanism, the hidden curriculum, and educational reform: a scoping review and thematic analysis. Acad Med. 2015;90(11 Suppl):s5–s13.

McNaughton N. The role of emotion in the work of standardized patients: a critical theoretical analysis. Berlin: LAP Press; 2012. ISBN 978-3-659-26257-9

McNaughton N. Discourse(s) of emotion within medical education: the "ever present absence". Med Educ. 2013;47(1):71–9.

McNaughton N, Snelgrove R. The role of power in surgical education: a Foucauldian perspective. In: Nestel D, Dalrymple K, Paige J, Aggarwal R, editors. Advances in surgical education. Singapore: Springer Press; 2019.

Mundel E, Chapman GE. A decolonizing approach to health promotion in Canada: the case of the Urban Aboriginal Community Garden Project. Health Promot Int. 2010;25(2):166–73.

Popkewitz TS, Fendler L. Critical theories in education: changing terrains of knowledge and politics. New York: Routledge; 1999.

Postcolonial Theory for Beginners. 2010, September 1. In: Aboriginal/Indigenous, research methodology. https://fasdprevention.wordpress.com/2010/09/01/postcolonial-theory-for-beginners/. Accessed 01 Sept 2019.

Smith D. The everyday world as problematic. Boston: North Eastern University Press; 1987.

Stergiopoulos E, Fernando O, Martimianakis MA. Being on both sides: Medical students' experiences with disability and professional identity construction. Acad Med. 2018;93(10):1550–1559.

Tsouroufli M, Reese C, Monrouxe L, Sundaram V. Gender, identities and intersectionality in medical education research. Med Educ. 2011;45:213–6.

Wear D, Kuczewski M. The professionalism movement: can we pause? Am J Bioeth. 2004;4(2):1–10.

Focus on Theory: Emotions and Learning

28

Aubrey L. Samost-Williams and Rebecca D. Minehart

Contents

Introduction	522
What Is Emotion?	522
Neurocognitive Basis of Emotions	523
Theoretical Frameworks Connecting Emotion and Learning	524
Circumplex Model	525
Control Value Theory	527
Broaden and Build Theory	529
Emotional Intelligence	530
Implications and Strategies for Learning	532
Conclusions	533
Cross-References	533
References	534

Abstract

Many educators have lived powerful experiences that will stay with them long after the moments have passed; times they failed at something meaningful to them, the wonder of finally understanding and "cracking the code" of a very complex concept, and the curiosity of diving into a new learning topic. What

---

A. L. Samost-Williams
Department of Anesthesia, Critical Care and Pain Medicine, Massachusetts General Hospital, Boston, MA, USA

Harvard Medical School, Boston, MA, USA
e-mail: ASAMOST-WILLIAMS@PARTNERS.ORG

R. D. Minehart (✉)
Department of Anesthesia, Critical Care and Pain Medicine, Massachusetts General Hospital, Boston, MA, USA

Harvard Medical School, Boston, MA, USA

Center for Medical Simulation, Boston, MA, USA
e-mail: RMINEHART@mgh.harvard.edu

© Springer Nature Singapore Pte Ltd. 2023
D. Nestel et al. (eds.), *Clinical Education for the Health Professions*,
https://doi.org/10.1007/978-981-15-3344-0_36

makes these so impactful? This chapter explores how learning is impacted by emotional states, such that educators can consider these potent modifiers of learning. The chapter starts by defining emotion and understanding the neurocircuitry underlying the biological basis of emotion. Then, theoretical frameworks are explored for integrating the role of emotion with the learning process. Finally, the chapter considers what these theories mean for our educational approaches in healthcare.

Keywords

Cognitive reappraisal · Affective states · Motivation · Acceptance · Suppression · Affect labeling · Emotional intelligence

Introduction

Healthcare professionals receive education and deliver care under emotionally charged circumstances. How do these emotions shape learning? How can the links between emotions and learning be harnessed for improved educational outcomes? This chapter explores how learning is impacted by emotional states, such that educators can consider these potent modifiers of learning. The chapter covers prevailing definitions of emotion and reviews neurocircuitry underlying the biological basis of emotion. Theoretical frameworks for integrating the role of emotion with the learning process will be addressed, and considerations will be shared regarding educational approaches in healthcare.

What Is Emotion?

Emotion is incredibly complex to define; to some, it may seem overly simplistic to assign specific conditions or elements that make up a single emotion (Plutchik 2001). While the experience of an emotion is universal, operationalizing definitions of myriad emotions is a necessary and daunting task. This starting framework to define emotions will be explored next.

The classic categorization of emotions is first into affective traits and affective states. Affective traits are defined as an individual's tendency toward one type of behavior or response to a situation. Affective states are further subdivided into moods and emotions. Moods are affective changes that are longer, more diffuse, and less in response to external stimuli than emotions, which are far more situationally related (Hascher 2010). Emotions are defined as responses to situations categorized by multiple components, such as valence, arousal, and intensity (Hascher 2010; Fredrickson 2001). They impact cognition, motivation, expression, and even physiology with changes in heart rate, blood pressure, skin conductance, and more (Pekrun 2006). See Fig. 1 for this classification schema.

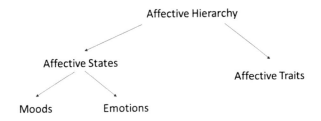

Fig. 1 Schematic representation of categorization of affective states and traits

Neurocognitive Basis of Emotions

The neurocognitive circuitry behind emotion consists of varied neurological pathways which are still under exploration. Broadly, emotions may arise from a stimulus that the brain processes, which then commands changes within the body, including physical manifestations, facial movements, body movements, and more (Barrett 2017). Therefore, consideration of the neurocircuitry will include a discussion of perception, then signal processing, and finally the execution of an emotion.

A major way humans identify emotions is by seeing and interpreting the facial expressions and body language of others they interact with. Visual stimuli, namely, the facial expression or body language demonstrated, travel from the retina along the optic nerve and eventually enter the visual cortices for processing. Compelling animal and human data suggest that certain critical sections of the brain (specifically the lateral portion of the inferior occipital gyrus, fusiform gyrus, and superior temporal gyrus) are largely involved in facial image processing (Adolphs 2002).

Two such structures, known as the amygdala (deep inside the brain) and the orbitofrontal cortex (right in front, behind the eyes), are believed to support further understanding of and interpretation of emotion from facial images. The amygdala is the classic neuroanatomic structure that many consider as a fundamental structure where emotions arise and undergo processing. While the amygdala has both cortical and subcortical connections, the subcortical connections have been shown to activate when research participants are shown subliminal images of faces, particularly showing fear. Both through cells on the brain's surface (cortical) and deeper within the brain (subcortical pathways), the amygdala plays a role in identifying emotions, including those particularly skewed toward a negative valence, such as fear, anger, and sadness. The orbitofrontal cortex shows a similar predilection for playing a role in negative emotion processing. There are some who theorize that these two structures may be important from an evolutionary perspective in helping with threat identification because of these notable negative predilections and their role in assisting humans in avoiding harm (Adolphs 2002).

The brain's "reward" system is a second structure to consider and is classically thought of as chemicals that signal other nerves in a specific area of the brain (the mesolimbic dopamine system). This system connects broadly to the rest of the brain, communicating with many areas (ventral tegmental area, nucleus accumbens, amygdala, and hippocampus). The mesolimbic dopamine system is most understood from studies with drug addiction where increased activation in this system leads to the feelings of euphoria and the classic "high" from drugs, but there is increasing evidence as well that lowered activity in this area can contribute to negative emotions too (Posner et al. 2005). It appears that this area is critical for processing the valence of emotion, whether positive or negative.

It is clear from research that the structures mentioned above are not the sole structures related to emotion recognition and processing. Patients with tumors or strokes in these areas can also show disrupted ability to identify different emotions in standardized pictures of faces. Functional MRI studies are emerging which suggest that emotional processing is the result of broad and diffuse neural networks (Barrett 2017; Posner et al. 2009). This evolution in understanding nicely mirrors the evolution in considering emotion from a psychological perspective, which is covered in the next section. As is true with any quest for understanding in science, a simple model over time has been adapted to add layers of complexity and nuance to better explain multifaceted and intricate phenomena.

The emerging theory of constructed emotion, based in neuropsychology, or the study of how brain structures, brain chemicals, and thinking interact (Barrett 2017), elucidates the shift toward considering the complexity and degeneracy in these neural pathways. This theory argues that each fear instance felt is slightly different from every other occurrence of that emotion, and this premise is the same for each instance of happiness or sadness, or any other unique emotion. Humans may make a slightly different grimace each time they are scared, and their heart rates rise to a slightly different elevated level. Therefore, it is argued that emotion is not something that can be easily categorized and then evaluated for what paths between brain cells appear to be involved, due to too much variability and degeneracy, which precludes prior approaches used in neuroscience. Rather, researchers should begin with understanding the connections in the brain, like the above-mentioned neural networks, and construct emotions from there.

Theoretical Frameworks Connecting Emotion and Learning

To start understanding the theoretical basis of role of emotions in learning, we must first start with pondering how emotion and learning might interact. There are four major routes through which emotions impact learning (Pekrun 1992): three are cognitive effects of emotion and the fourth involves motivation to learn.

The first cognitive impact is in the storage and retrieval of information, essentially a mood-dependent memory. There is reasonable empirical evidence that if a subject has learned something while in a particular emotional state, that subject will have easier recall of that material when in that emotional state. This appears to be a stronger effect when the mood and the material learned are congruent. There remains some debate regarding whether the valence of the emotional state or even the specific emotional state impacts this phenomenon.

The second impact on cognition is in the impact of emotion on cognitive strategies for problem solving. Small studies suggest that these impacts are at a subconscious level. It appears that positive mood states lead to more creative and big-picture thinking. This is postulated because positive moods typically occur when things are going well, there is little benefit to critically analyzing small details that may not benefit the larger situation. Conversely, negative moods tend to lead to more detail-oriented thinking with more analytical cognitive strategies. These are broad generalizations, and data do suggest that there are degrees of nuance that are not captured in the above rules of thumb.

The third cognitive impact of emotions is in syphoning off limited attentional and cognitive workload resources. The nature of cognitive workload (how much work it takes to "think through" something) and the workload resources available is hotly debated in the human factors literature. However, the idea here is that emotions like anxiety come with a cognitive component, namely, concerns, that can detract resources from being applied to a cognitive task, such as recall and problem solving on an exam. There is empirical data that suggest, but do not conclusively prove, that this is the mechanism underlying negative performance of students with test anxiety (Eysenck 1988).

Finally, emotions alter learning through motivation, both via intrinsic motivation and extrinsic motivation. There have been several different definitions of intrinsic and extrinsic motivation in the literature, but for this review intrinsic motivation can be thought of as motivation to perform a task for the sake of the task alone. Extrinsic motivation is motivation from the secondary gain of completing a task, be it recognition, pride, or even punishment at failure. Interest and joy are emotions linked to positive intrinsic motivation. The classic example of a negatively motivating emotion is boredom. Emotions are also linked to extrinsic motivation, most obviously fear of failure and pride in anticipated or retrospective success.

The four links between emotion and learning listed above were the starting point to researchers beginning to consider more complex frameworks for considering how emotions interact with each other and with learning. Building these frameworks and theories began to provide hypotheses that could be tested in a systematic fashion and start to advance this field of study in coherent paths forward.

Circumplex Model

The first framework that will be considered is the circumplex model that sought to link emotions to each other in a logical spectrum. Prior to the circumplex model being proposed, the prevailing theory among psychologists was that the human brain was wired to experience a finite number of discrete emotions, each acting independently of each other. For example, under this framework, sadness would be one independent affective scale ("degrees of sadness") and pleasure would be a separate and independent affective scale. However, this paradigm did not seem to fit psychological observations or even constructs of emotion. It appeared logical to most people that happiness and sadness were two ends of a wider spectrum and not two completely independent affective axes. More experimental data emerged showing that models of these affects as independent were statistically flawed.

Into this growing debate, James Russell introduced his new framework for conceptualizing emotions, known as the circumplex model of affect (Russell 1980). This framework proposed that emotions could be defined in two-dimensional space by the relation between two axes: valence and arousal. Valence ran from positive to negative, with the ends being marked by misery on one and pleasure on the other. Arousal ran from the extremes of full arousal to sleepiness. Other emotions populated the circumference of a circle defined by their respective positions along these two axes. See Fig. 2 for a pictorial representation of this two-dimensional circular spectrum.

The circumplex model of affect has several strengths because of its spectrum of affect. First, it better fits empirical data that suggest people are unable to describe discrete emotions, as this model presumes that all emotions sit on a spectrum without discrete borders, like a color wheel might blend smoothly from red to orange and so on before returning to red. This spectrum approach also helps explain the heterogeneity and degeneracy of the neurocircuitry involved in mood disorders and anxiety disorders. These two are highly intercorrelated at familial and genetic levels, and the circumplex model suggests that these affective states are also likely highly intercorrelated and merely differ by shades on a common spectrum (Posner et al. 2005). Overall, the circumplex model offers a more nuanced look at emotions and allows for finer and more blurred distinctions between the emotional states experienced in everyday life.

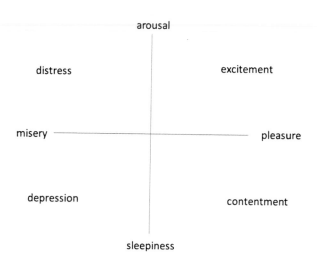

Fig. 2 The Circumplex Model of Affect. (Adapted from Russell 1980)

Control Value Theory

Russell's work in understanding the interconnectedness of affective states generated deeper understanding of the interrelatedness of these states and the nuances of the emotions. However, these definitions of emotions remained disconnected to learning. Over the intervening 20 years, researchers empirically evaluated individual emotion with regards to learning, but no central framework emerged for predicting and explaining the impacts of these emotions on learning. This glaring lack of clarity was highlighted as researchers found even conflicting evidence of the role of test anxiety. Test anxiety hurt attention, while simultaneously helping motivation (Eysenck 1988). A framework was necessary to explain these interactions.

As a response to heterogeneity in research designs and questions asked, one group began building a framework to cohesively understand the role of achievement emotions in learning. Achievement emotions are simply defined as emotions tied to the *outcome of* (outcome achievement emotions) or *act of doing* (activity achievement emotions) a particular activity (Pekrun 2006).

This theory posited that several key situational factors leading to any given outcomes would alter the emotions associated with that learning scenario for the student. The key axes considered were control and value, hence the control-value theory. "Control" was broken down into "self" versus "other." If the student had full control over the outcome of the scenario, then self-control was high. Self-control could be subdivided into high, medium, and low. "Other" was full external control over the outcome, with no control from the student. Value was the perceived positive or negative value of the student's object *focus* during this scenario. Object focuses could be outcomes, things like passing or failing a test, which were broken down into prospective outcome, retrospective outcome, or activity (i.e., the classic joy of learning itself). These categorizations were then charted into a framework to understand the overriding emotion that each scenario would evoke (Pekrun 2006). See Fig. 3 for a subset of emotions and their categorized scenarios adapted from this work.

This grid helps to link specific learning scenarios with their attendant emotions. Take, for example, the scenario of a student facing an important exam. They are worried that they might fail, but they realize that if they study, then they are likely to pass. This student will experience anticipatory relief as they study and prepare for that exam. Take a different student with the same high stakes exam but now they have a low ability to study effectively enough to pass this test. That student in the same scenario is going to experience hopelessness. The students experienced the same object focus (the test), the same value (negative consequence of failure), but different control levels (low versus high self-abilities) and therefore experienced different emotions as a result (Pekrun 2006).

Control-value theory has real world consequences. Consider the antiquated observation that male students performed better at math, which had been observed as early as the 1970s with little insight into why there might exist an achievement gap. When framed as a control-value theory problem, researchers might predict that boys would feel higher competence in math than girls while both rate math as highly

Object Focus	Value	Control	Emotion
Outcome (Prospective)	Positive	High	Anticipatory Joy
		Medium	Hope
		Low	Hopelessness
	Negative	High	Anticipatory Relief
		Medium	Anxiety
		Low	Hopelessness
Outcome (Retrospective)	Positive	Irrelevant	Joy
		Self	Pride
		Other	Gratitude
	Negative	Irrelevant	Sadness
		Self	Shame
		Other	Anger
Activity	Positive	High	Enjoyment
	Negative	High	Anger
	Either	Low	Frustration
	None	Either	Boredom

Fig. 3 Table of control-value combinations and their subsequent achievement emotions. (Adapted from Pekrun 2006)

important. This would lead boys to feel more joy and pride in their math skills while girls might report more negative emotions like anxiety, hopelessness, and shame. This was further demonstrated in an empirical study of elementary school students (Frenzel et al. 2007). Interestingly, the students in that study were performing identically well in mathematics at the time of the study. The ability of this theory to explain these empirically seen differences is powerful, but this theory's ability to broaden research in education and learning outside of a focus on anxiety has great potential. Research can move forward in mathematics education looking not only to minimize anxiety but also to maximize pride or joy, which are linked to later successes in future studies.

Additionally, control-value theory has consequences outside of closing the gender gap in mathematics education. This theory helps provide a framework for considering how educators can help learners shift from negative emotional scenarios to positive emotions. There are several levers that can be manipulated, including shifting goals, focusing on the joy of the activity itself instead of the consequences of an exam, for example. Educators can also help learners shift their views of their self-abilities, thus shifting their appraisal of control in certain situations (Pekrun et al. 2007). Shifting students from a low to a high control appraisal of their self-abilities can help them reframe problems from hopeless to neutral or even joyful.

Finally, these emotions tie back into cognition through the same four mechanisms as listed at the start of this section, linking emotion and learning. One can see here that if emotions were shifted from a more negative to a more positive valence regarding the material being learned, one might see increases in creative problem solving, decreases in cognitive workload and demands on attention, and an increase in intrinsic motivation (Pekrun et al. 2007). These shifts would greatly help students learn and engage with the material, simply from changing their emotional experience with the material.

Broaden and Build Theory

Researchers have also explored the role of emotions in impacting a person's overall cognitive abilities, leading to the broaden and build theory. This theory draws from ample evidence that negative emotions lead to stereotyped responses. For example, fear leads to a compulsion to escape the situation, while disgust leads to a desire to expel the source of that disgust. However, this theory further considered evidence that positive emotions did not lead to these single-purpose stereotypical responses. These observations formed the basis of the broaden and build theory, which posits that positive emotions lead to a broadening of thought-action repertoires, where thought-action pairs represent a host of possible responses to a particular action (Fredrickson 2001, 2004). Positive emotions such as interest foster exploration and discovery of new concepts, practices, skills, or worldviews. Joy can lead to play which allows for increased creativity and attainment of new skills. Positive emotions in general lead to increased social interactions and bonds. The broadening of the responses associated with positive emotions consequently leads to an increased acquired set of responses, skills, and social bonds that can be accessed in a threatening situation, therefore leading to an evolutionary advantage to the species (Fredrickson 2001). See Fig. 4 for a brief introduction to several positive emotions, their corresponding responses, and their consequent skills learned (Fredrickson 2013).

Emotion Label	Thought-Action Tendency	Resources Accrued
Joy	Play, get involved	Skills from experiential learning
Gratitude	Prosocial urge	Skills for promoting loyalty and social bonds
Interest	Explore and learn	Knowledge
Pride	Dream big	Achievement motivation
Inspiration	Strive towards your own big goals	Motivation for personal growth

Fig. 4 Select positive emotions and their associated thought-action tendencies and resources gained. (Adapted from Fredrickson 2013)

Broaden and build theory offers a framework, and associated empirical evidence, to understand how emotion might alter a learner's engagement with the material and therefore their success at learning. Fostering an environment of interest, joy, and pride can lead to student engagement, creativity, and a view of more success in future endeavors, all outcomes that would be ideal in learners. This has been borne out with studies in settings as diverse as learning a second language (MacIntyre and Gregerson 2012) and performing experiential learning exercises in psychology (Abe 2011).

Emotional Intelligence

The final theory we consider is the idea of emotional intelligence, an idea that has been interpreted and defined in different ways throughout its relatively young history. Emotional intelligence was first defined and conceptualized by Mayer and Salovey in 1990 but has been studied and adapted extensively since then. Broadly speaking, emotional intelligence is a person's ability to identify their own emotions and the emotions in the people around them, and then use those emotions to regulate their own thinking and actions (Brackett et al. 2013).

There have been two predominant schools of thought in research in emotional intelligence. The first framework, exemplified by the Mayer-Salovey Model, assumes that emotional intelligence is an intrinsic ability, likened to the concept of IQ being a cognitive ability. Given this assumption, emotional intelligence can be objectively measured, and people can demonstrate their emotional intelligence through assessments and performing tasks. In this model, emotional intelligence can be divided into three separate components: (1) recognition and expression of emotions, (2) emotional regulation, and (3) using those emotions to influence (Salovey and Mayer 1990). Figure 5 highlights the details of this framework. Mayer and Salovey went on later to subdivide recognition and expression of emotion

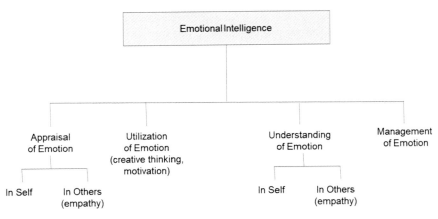

Fig. 5 Four-Branch Ability Model. (Adapted from Salovey and Mayer 1990; Brackett et al. 2013)

into two separate aspects of emotional intelligence (Mayer and Salovey 1997); hence their model is typically now referred to as the Four-Branch Ability Model.

The other framework that researchers have used to conceptualize emotional intelligence is called the mixed ability-trait model. This model assumes there is a component of emotional intelligence that is an ability that can be easily objectively measured but that there is another component that is based on intrinsic personality traits, such as optimism. Personality traits are much harder to objectively measure and analyze. The two popular models using this framework are the Bar-On Model and the Boyatzis-Goleman Model. Both of these, like the Four-Branch Ability Model, divide the larger concept of emotional intelligence into components or competencies, such as self-awareness, self-management, interpersonal skills, or intrapersonal skills (Brackett et al. 2013). There is significant debate between these two types of models, where the former is more objective but the latter might be more descriptive of the overarching phenomena; each has its adherents in the field.

What does emotional intelligence have to do with education? Emotional intelligence is an explicitly different concept from IQ, which one could easily conceptualize as being directly related to learning. However, as has been shown above, there are a tight links between learning and emotions, so one might hypothesize that higher emotional intelligence would lead to an ability to regulate some of these emotions more successfully and lead to better learning outcomes in a classroom setting. Studies bear out this hypothesis. For example, research from Portugal strongly correlated emotional intelligence correlated with tenth graders' grade point averages (Costa and Faria 2015). A recent meta-analysis demonstrated that even across cultures, higher emotional intelligence was significantly linked to higher academic achievement (Hanafi and Noor 2016). The same holds true in research looking at adults in the workplace. Having a higher emotional intelligence leads to better abilities to navigate learning and professional environments (Brackett et al. 2013). From these findings, it is easy to extrapolate the importance of emotional intelligence in health professions education at all levels from undergraduate through continuing and post-doctoral education, and decades into practice.

Implications and Strategies for Learning

Skillfully using emotional modulation is critical for simulation and other modalities, where learners may benefit from enhanced engagement, and may fall victim to the risk that comes with intense emotional (over)investment. In addition, learners may experience acute stress during educational activities, which may change their ability to perform higher-level cognitive processing (Arnsten 2009), a concept with which educators should be familiar. The circumplex model of learning situates an ideal learner state as being activated and slightly positive or negative in valence (Posner et al. 2005), neither too activated nor too far positive or negative, as learning may be grossly impacted as the theories above state. How is this achievable? This section will cover ways in which emotional states can be moderated as a prerequisite to learning.

As Vicki LeBlanc writes in her review of the effects of emotions on learning processes in healthcare education (LeBlanc et al. 2015), "Given that health care rarely occurs in emotionally neutral settings, it is important to understand how health professionals' emotional states affect their ability to interpret, make decisions about, and recall clinical information." Thus it follows that educators must include explicit instruction on how learners may modify their own emotional states to better care for patients, which they may readily practice during role-plays and other forms of simulated encounters. Some specific techniques which vary in their utility are *cognitive reappraisal* (or *reframing*), *acceptance*, *affect labeling*, *self-distraction*, and *suppression* (this last of which is not recommended but is widely performed).

Cognitive reappraisal is a cognitive strategy that involves effortful, deliberate reinterpretation of an event or situation to change one's emotional responses, both in the moment and for future experiences, leading to a different emotional experience when applied (Kalisch et al. 2006; Haga et al. 2009). It may also include distancing oneself from the emotional impacts (Torre and Lieberman 2018). Practical examples of the process of cognitive reappraisal have been published (Prehn 2012), and while this technique involves cognitive work, it is highly predictive of well-being (e.g., life satisfaction, absence of depression) as compared with other techniques such as suppression (Haga et al. 2009). Prehn's article lists common prompting questions to enhance the process of perspective generation, including, "If your friend/child were in a similar situation, what advice would you give?" (Prehn 2012).

Acceptance is welcome acknowledgment of one's situation and has strong links to mindfulness. People who practice acceptance have been shown to have less pain, stress, and anxiety in certain circumstances than those who do not (Wojnarowska et al. 2020). One practical example where acceptance may be a useful strategy for learners may center around learning to tolerate discomfort and anxiety that uncertainty brings, as uncertainty is nearly universal within health care.

Affect labeling has been called an "implicit emotion regulation" technique, where the act of assigning feelings to words may feel less effortful than some other explicit emotion regulation techniques (Torre and Lieberman 2018). In studies, affect labeling appears to have similar effects to cognitive reappraisal, although they are somewhat conceptually distinct techniques (Torre and Lieberman 2018), where affect labeling might manifest as, "I am feeling upset" or "He is looking upset." Affect labeling also distances oneself from the emotion, akin to mindfulness techniques (Torre and Lieberman 2018), and may be useful as an in-the-moment strategy.

Self-distraction is another self-directed emotion management strategy, whereby one intentionally refocuses on less emotional-laden parts of a circumstance, rather than reimagining or reinterpreting the circumstance. Self-distraction has been shown to be less successful at decreasing anticipatory anxiety than in reducing unwanted thoughts (Kalisch et al. 2006), and therefore potentially a less helpful emotion management technique overall.

Finally, *suppression*, as an emotion regulation technique, refers to deliberately inhibiting experienced emotions (LeBlanc et al. 2015). As this requires conscious effort and focus, where one is constantly seeking out to abolish specific emotions, it is unsurprisingly associated with worsened recall of information during times of high emotion (Richards and Gross 2006). Educators may choose to normalize suppression as a common technique for learners while simultaneously highlighting its shortcomings.

Conclusions

Emotions can be rich experiences for learners and can heighten excitement and solidify learning, or cause distress or dismay. Current theories of emotion may help educators anticipate and address bidirectional relationships between emotions and learning. Educators should seek to capitalize on a learner's intrinsic motivation for learning, enhance experience of self-control and joy, and teach emotion regulation techniques to enable learners to self-modulate emotions in learning and practice. Being deliberate with learners' emotions optimizes their potential in any educational setting.

Cross-References

▶ Cognitive Neuroscience Foundations of Surgical and Procedural Expertise: Focus on Theory
▶ Debriefing Practices in Simulation-based Education
▶ Well-Being in Health Profession Training

References

Abe JA. Positive emotions, emotional intelligence, and successful experiential learning. Personal Individ Differ. 2011;51:817–22. https://doi.org/10.1016/j.paid.2011.07.004.

Adolphs R. Neural systems for recognizing emotion. Curr Opin Neurobiol. 2002;12:169. https://doi.org/10.1016/S0959-4388(02)00301-X.

Arnsten AFT. Stress signalling pathways that impair prefrontal cortex structure and function. Nat Rev Neurosci. 2009 June;10(6):410–22. https://doi.org/10.1038/nrn2648.

Barrett LF. The theory of constructed emotion: an active inference account of interoception and categorization. Social cognitive and affective. Neurosciences. 2017;12:1–23. https://doi.org/10.1093/scan/nsw154.

Brackett MA, Bertoli M, Elbertson N, Bausseron E, Castillo R, Salovey P. Emotional intelligence: reconceptualizing the cognition-emotion link. In: Robinson MD, Watkins ER, Harmon-Jones E, editors. Handbook of cognition and emotion. New York: Guilford Press; 2013. p. 365–79.

Costa A, Faria L. The impact of emotional intelligence on academic achievement: a longitudinal study in Portuguese secondary school. Learn Individ Differ. 2015;37(1):38–47. https://doi.org/10.1016/j.lindif.2014.11.011.

Eysenck MW. Anxiety and attention. Anxiety Res. 1988;1(1):9–15. https://doi.org/10.1080/10615808808248216.

Fredrickson BL. The role of positive emotions in positive psychology: the broaden-and-build theory of positive emotions. Am Psychol. 2001;56(3):218–26.

Fredrickson BL. The broaden-and-build theory of positive emotions. Phil Trans R Soc Lond. 2004;359:1367–77. https://doi.org/10.1098/rstb.2004.1512.

Fredrickson BL. Positive emotions broaden and build. In: Devine P, Plant A, editors. Advances in experimental psychology, vol. 47. San Diego: Academic; 2013. p. 1–53.

Frenzel AC, Pekrun R, Goetz T. Girls and mathematics – a hopeless issue? A control-value approach to gender differences in emotions towards mathematics. J Psychol Educ. 2007;22 (4):497–514.

Haga SM, Kraft P, Corby EK. Emotion regulation: antecedents and well-being outcomes of cognitive reappraisal and expressive suppression in cross-cultural samples. J Happiness Stud. 2009;10:271. https://doi.org/10.1007/s10902-007-9080-3.

Hanafi Z, Noor F. Relationship between emotional intelligence and academic achievement in emerging adults: a systematic review. Int J Acad Res Bus Soc Sci. 2016;6(6):268–90. https://doi.org/10.6007/IJARBSS/v6-i6/2197.

Hascher T. Learning and emotion: perspectives for theory and research. Eur Educ Res J. 2010;9(1):13–28. https://doi.org/10.2304/eerj.2010.9.1.13.

Kalisch R, Wiech K, Herrmann K, Dolan RJ. Neural correlates of self-distraction from anxiety and a process model of cognitive emotion regulation. J Cogn Neurosci. 2006;18(8):1266–76.

LeBlanc VR, McConnell MM, Monteiro SD. Predictable chaos: a review of the effects of emotions on attention, memory and decision making. Adv Health Sci Educ. 2015;20:265. https://doi.org/10.1007/s10459-014-9516-6.

MacIntyre P, Gregerson T. Emotions that facilitate language learning: the positive-broadening power of the imagination. Stud Second Lang Learn Teach. 2012;2(2):193–213.

Mayer JD, Salovey P. What is emotional intelligence? In: Salovey P, Sluyter DJ, editors. Emotional development and emotional intelligence: educational implications. New York: Basic Books; 1997. p. 3–34.

Pekrun R. The impact of emotions on learning and achievement: towards a theory of cognitive/motivational mediators. Appl Psychol Int Rev. 1992;41(4):359–76.

Pekrun R. The control-value theory of achievement emotions: assumptions, corollaries, and implications for educational research and practice. Educ Psychol Rev. 2006;18:315–41. https://doi.org/10.1007/s10648-006-9029-9.

Pekrun R, Frenzel AC, Goetz T. The control-value theory of achievement emotions: an integrative approach to emotions in education. In: Schutz PA, Pekrun R, editors. Emotion in education. Amsterdam: Academic; 2007. p. 13–36.

Plutchik R. The nature of emotions: human emotions have deep evolutionary roots, a fact that may explain their complexity and provide tools for clinical practice. Am Sci. 2001;89(4):344–50. Retrieved from http://www.jstor.org/stable/27857503

Posner J, Russell JA, Peterson BS. The circumplex model of affect: an integrative approach to affective neuroscience, cognitive development, and psychopathology. Dev Psychopathol. 2005;17(3):715–34.

Posner J, Russel JA, Gerber A, Gorman D, Colibazzi T, Yu S, Wang Z, Zhu H, Peterson BS. The neurophysiological bases of emotion: an fMRI study of the affective circumplex using emotion-denoting words. Hum Brain Mapp. 2009;30(3):883–95. https://doi.org/10.1002/hbm.20553.

Prehn A. Create reframing mindsets through Framestorm. NeuroLeadership J. 2012;4:1–11.

Richards JM, Gross JJ. Personality and emotional memory: how regulating emotion impairs memory for emotional events. J Res Pers. 2006;40(5):631–51.

Russell JA. A circumplex model of affect. J Pers Soc Psychol. 1980;39(6):1161–78.

Salovey P, Mayer JD. Emotional intelligence. Imagin Cogn Pers. 1990;9:185–211. https://doi.org/10.2190/DUGG-P24E-52WK-6CDG.

Torre JB, Lieberman MD. Putting feelings into words: affect labeling as implicit emotion regulation. Emot Rev. 2018;10(2):116–24. https://doi.org/10.1177/1754073917742706.

Wojnarowska A, Kobylinska D, Lewczuk K. Acceptance as an emotion regulation strategy in experimental psychological research: what we know and how we can improve that knowledge. Front Psychol. 2020;11:242. https://doi.org/10.3389/fpsyg.2020.00242.

Ecological Systems Theory in Clinical Learning

29

Yang Yann Foo and Raymond Goy

Contents

Introduction	538
Ecological Systems Theory's Applicability for Clinical Education	539
Chapter Organization	540
Bronfenbrenner: His Life and Influences	540
Key Features of Ecological Systems Theory	542
Developmental Trajectory of Ecological Systems Theory	542
Phase 1: Emphasis on Contextual Influences on Development	542
Microsystem	543
Mesosystem	543
Exosystem	544
Macrosystem	544
Phase 2: Chronosystem and Emphasis on Process	544
Chronosystem	544
Emphasis on Process	545
Phase 3: Bioecological Theory, Proximal Processes, and the Process-Person-Context-Time Model	545
Ecological Systems Theory and Clinical Education	547
Health Professions Students	548
Clinical Learning	548
Transitions and Change	548
Working Trainees and Community of Practice (CoP)	549
Helping Trainees with Difficulties	550
Conclusion	551
Cross-References	551
References	551

Y. Y. Foo (✉)
Office of Education, Duke-NUS Medical School, Singapore, Singapore
e-mail: yangyann.foo@duke-nus.edu.sg

R. Goy
KKH Women and Children's Hospital, Singapore, Singapore
e-mail: raymond.goy.w.l@singhealth.com.sg

© Springer Nature Singapore Pte Ltd. 2023
D. Nestel et al. (eds.), *Clinical Education for the Health Professions*,
https://doi.org/10.1007/978-981-15-3344-0_37

Abstract

Ecological Systems Theory (EST) seeks to understand human development through examining the interactions between an individual's innate nature and the multiple influences from the environment. Its emphasis on understanding developmental issues from a nonlinear, multifactorial perspective suits the study of clinical education in an age where healthcare is a social system involving multiple factors that are inter-related in complex ways. In this chapter, we describe the potential uses of EST in understanding and exploring how contextual influences impact clinical learning, transitions and change, and helping trainees with difficulties.

Keywords

Urie Bronfenbrenner · Ecological Systems Theory · Bioecological Model · Process-Person-Context-Time Model · Contextual influences · Proximal processes

Introduction

Ecological Systems Theory (EST) was developed by Urie Bronfenbrenner (1917–2005), a Russian-born American developmental psychologist. As indicated by the subtitle of his seminal book published in 1979 – *The ecology of human development: experiments by nature and design*, Bronfenbrenner sought to understand human development by examining the complex interactions between the person's innate nature and the multiple influences from the environment (Bronfenbrenner 1979, 1986, 1988, 1989, 1999, 2001, 2005; Bronfenbrenner and Ceci 1993, 1994; Bronfenbrenner and Crouter 1983; Bronfenbrenner and Evans 2000; Bronfenbrenner and Morris 1998, 2006).

EST's strength lies in its unique ability to serve as a comprehensive framework that examines different sources of influences both immediate and remote, and of the importance of connections within and among systems (Hamilton and Luster 2005). Prior to Bronfenbrenner's theoretical expositions, the trend in developmental psychology (i.e., the study of human development) was to focus on the immediate and *unidirectional* influence of a parent on a child (Baumrind 1966). Remote and less obvious sources of influence were not considered, such as a parent's workplace demands on his or her ability to care for the child (Hayes et al. 2017), or how historical events such as the Great Depression in the 1930s affected breadwinners' ability to provide for their children during harsh economic times (Bronfenbrenner 1986). Bronfenbrenner's pioneering theory thus serves as a framework to consider holistically how a child's innate characteristics interact with multiple factors in the environment to influence his or her development.

As befitting its origins, EST has been widely used by developmental and educational scholars (Hayes et al. 2017; Riggins-Caspers et al. 2003; Small and Luster

1994; Zhang 2018). Notably, the theory is also deemed versatile and has been used in fields as diverse as natural disaster management (Boon et al. 2012), health promotion (McLeroy et al. 1988; Sallis et al. 2008), and public mental health research (Eriksson et al. 2018). However, EST is little known in the field of healthcare. Elements of the theory were only alluded to by D'Amour and Oandasan (2005) when they used concepts such as microsystem and mesosystem to explore why interprofessional *education* does not translate automatically into interprofessional *collaboration* in the healthcare setting.

Despite the initial lack of interest in EST, in more recent times, it seems to have gained the attention of some healthcare researchers. Bluteau et al. (2017) used it to study the impact of an online interprofessional education program they had developed. Using EST in the analysis of their data, Bluteau and associates were able to map the influence of both immediate (individual's interaction with the curriculum and institutional care settings) and remote (community and national care contexts) factors on their learners' interprofessional development. In 2019, Hamwey et al. suggested that EST "may be useful for exploring the multifactorial interactions that shape learners in health professions education," and could be used to "study the experiences of a learner who is performing poorly" (for a brief discussion, see section "Ecological Systems Theory and Clinical Education," p. 11).

Ecological Systems Theory's Applicability for Clinical Education

The incipient interest in EST is congruent with the paradigm shift observed in the healthcare systems. Thinking models such as knowledge pipeline that presupposed linear development from discoveries in the laboratory settings to clinical trials and clinical practice no longer predominate. Instead, healthcare is increasingly appreciated as being a complex social system involving multiple, inter-related factors interacting in complex ways (Braithwaite et al. 2018; Cristancho et al. 2019; Ellaway et al. 2017; Lipsitz 2012). Given its emphasis on understanding developmental issues from a nonlinear, multifactorial perspective, EST might serve as a useful theory for clinical educators in a variety of educational settings. For example, in the topic of career and specialty choices, what factors of influence would be considered as part of a student's or trainee's decision-making prior to the entry into health professions training? What would be the interplay between the environmental influences and the student/trainee, and how did these influences change as the learner transits from being a student to being a working trainee?

Using EST as a framework, clinical educators can think of how immediate factors of influences such as personal interest, work-life balance considerations, family, and peers would contribute more significantly to individual choices (Sanfey et al. 2006) for a health professions student. In some societies, parental and family expectations, and/or respect for a family member in the same profession, were important considerations (Saigal et al. 2007). At this stage of his or her development, the student could not have acquired experiential knowledge of more remote factors in order to make holistic decisions. The student might lack knowledge and insights into the remote, yet important, factors such as national policies, institutional and training resources, competitions for specialty jobs, specific specialty demands, and clinical space culture (Saigal et al. 2007).

A working trainee, on the other hand, would have developed a partial understanding of the healthcare system. Being older in age, the trainee could be more mature in his or her outlook, temperament, and emotions. He or she would have a better understanding of the demands of the profession; the degree of experience is dependent on situated learning and the clinical setting (Larsen et al. 2003). Motivation (or demotivation) to progress onto the next stage of the career could have been shaped by the previous encounters and experiences in the clinical learning environment and in the community of practice (Dornan et al. 2007).

As the succinct discussion above shows, EST could be used as a framework to understand the many factors that influence the way healthcare professionals make decisions about their career and specialty choices. More examples related to clinical education are found in the section "Ecological Systems Theory and Clinical Education."

Chapter Organization

As EST is relatively unknown in the health professions field, we aim to provide an introductory guide for clinical educators curious about the theory. This chapter is divided into three sections. Section "Bronfenbrenner: His Life and Influences" – offers information drawn from his life that accounts for key aspects of his intellectual development. Section "Key Features of Ecological Systems Theory" – looks at the developmental trajectory of the theory. Section "Ecological Systems Theory and Clinical Education" – provides examples of how the theory could be applied in clinical education for the health professions.

Bronfenbrenner: His Life and Influences

Bronfenbrenner received his Bachelor's Degree from Cornell University in 1938, where he majored in psychology. By 1942, he had completed his Master's Degree at Harvard University and received his Doctorate from the University of Michigan. He was then inducted into military service. After World War II ended, he took up position as assistant professor at the University of Michigan. In 1948, Cornell University gave him joint appointments in psychology (College of Arts and Sciences), as well as in child development and family relationships (College of Home Economics) (Hamilton and Luster 2005).

Although Bronfenbrenner forged his professional reputation in America, he was born in Moscow in 1917. At age 6, he emigrated to the United States with his parents as they were worried about raising a Jewish family in postrevolutionary Russia. Both his parents were instrumental in giving him an upbringing that shaped his future as a scholar. Under his mother's influence, Bronfenbrenner kept in touch with the

Russian language which in later life helped him access developmental psychology literature coming out of the Soviet Union. From his father, a pathologist who had also a degree in zoology, Bronfenbrenner came to understand ecology in the natural world where he saw how the physical environment influenced an organism such that the same plant looked different in two different locations. Through his father's work at an institution for the developmentally delayed, Bronfenbrenner also appreciated how feebleminded individuals could contribute to their community if they had the right kinds of support from the people around them (Hamilton and Luster 2005).

Besides his parents, two other individuals – both famous researchers in their own right – also featured prominently in Bronfenbrenner's intellectual formation: They were Lev Vygotsky and Kurt Lewin. It is useful to understand Vygotsky and Lewin's influence on Bronfenbrenner because readings on Bronfenbrenner would frequently also mention Vygotsky and Lewin.

Lev Vygotsky was a Soviet psychologist widely recognized for his social programs that sought to increase competence and halt dysfunctional development. He was also one of the first proponents of the sociocultural theory of learning. Although Vygotsky died in 1934, aged only 37, Bronfenbrenner, being fluent in Russian, came across Vygotsky's ideas through the scientific literature produced by Vygotsky's Moscow University colleagues and disciples such as Alexander Luria (Hamilton and Luster 2005).

In 1954, Bronfenbrenner met his Moscow University counterparts at an international meeting in Montreal, and together they set up an exchange program between the universities of Cornell and Moscow. Bronfenbrenner's visits to Russia culminated in the publication of a book (1970) entitled *Two worlds of childhood: US and USSR*. This work highlighted the impact of cultural differences on the development of American and Soviet children. By focusing on studying children in the settings where they lived, Bronfenbrenner became one of the first developmental psychologists not to rely on laboratory experiments to advance his field (Hamilton and Luster 2005). Prior to that, psychologists' predominant modus operandi were to study children in controlled environments. An example was noted psychologist Albert Bandura who used the Bobo Doll experiments to develop the social learning theory (Bandura et al. 1961).

Kurt Lewin was the other psychologist who had a strong influence on Bronfenbrenner. They met as colleagues when Bronfenbrenner was inducted into military service and assigned to the Office of Strategic Services. A pioneer of social, organizational, and applied psychology, Lewin's postulations that behavior is a function of the interaction between a person's characteristics and the environment strongly influenced Bronfenbrenner's conception of the ecology of human development (Hamilton and Luster 2005).

For his work with children and families, the American Psychological Association in 1996 gave Bronfenbrenner its first Award for Lifetime Contribution to Developmental Psychology in the Service of Science and Society. For his decades-long contributions to Cornell, the university honored him by establishing the Bronfenbrenner Life Course Center (Hamilton and Luster 2005).

Having explored the influences that shaped Bronfenbrenner's early intellectual development, we now turn our focus to EST's key features and the rationale underpinning the refinement of his theory over the different phases of his career.

Key Features of Ecological Systems Theory

Bronfenbrenner's key concepts have been presented in several different ways. While some sources present his nested theory as comprising four subsystems: *microsystem*, *mesosystem*, *exosystem*, and *macrosystem* (Bronfenbrenner 1979), others include a fifth called *chronosystem* (Bronfenbrenner 1986). Also, the prefix *"Bio"* is sometimes added to the term ecological (Bronfenbrenner 2005; Bronfenbrenner and Ceci 1994). To this potentially confusing mix is yet another of Bronfenbrenner's framework – the Process-Person-Context-Time (PPCT) model (Bronfenbrenner 2005; Bronfenbrenner and Evans 2000).

The numerous ways by which EST has been presented and applied can be confusing to clinical education scholars new to the theory. It is thus useful to discuss EST's key features according to the different phases of the theory's developmental trajectory (Bronfenbrenner 1979, 1986, 1988, 1989, 1999, 2001, 2005; Bronfenbrenner and Ceci 1993, 1994; Bronfenbrenner and Crouter 1983; Bronfenbrenner and Evans 2000; Bronfenbrenner and Morris 1998, 2006). This is to help clinical education scholars be cognizant of the different phases of EST's development so that they could state clearly which version of the theory they are using. This is critical as for any field to develop, research has to be theoretically driven and studies must be explicitly designed to test theories or call into question their key concepts for the purpose of supporting or expanding them (Tudge et al. 2009). Without stating clearly which version of a theory one is using, scholars familiar with a different version of the same theory will not be able to evaluate accurately one's study results. Thus, researchers should always state clearly which version of a theory they have used in their studies.

Developmental Trajectory of Ecological Systems Theory

Phase 1: Emphasis on Contextual Influences on Development

Bronfenbrenner developed and refined his theory over three phases starting from the 1970s to his death in 2005 (Tudge et al. 2009). In phase 1, which culminated in the publication of his 1979 monograph, he presented his theory as comprising four subsystems (Fig. 1) of contextual influences on development, nested one inside the other such as Russian dolls (Bronfenbrenner 1979).

The following explains how each subsystem contributes to the holistic understanding of child development. The examples are drawn from developmental psychology (i.e., the study of child development), the field for which Bronfenbrenner

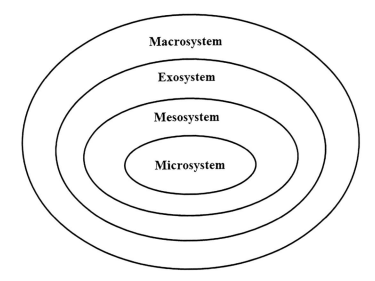

Fig. 1 Ecological systems theory's contextual influences on development (1979)

developed his theory. EST's application in clinical education will be discussed in section "Ecological Systems Theory and Clinical Education" (p. 11).

Microsystem

At the heart of the nested subsystems resides the microsystem. This is where the child comes into contact with his or her most *immediate* and *direct* sources of influence impacting his or her daily life (Bronfenbrenner 1979, 1986). One setting in which a child interacts with significant others is the family, namely his or her parents, sibling(s), and possibly extended family members such as grandparents. Another setting in which the child has immediate contact with others includes teachers and classmates in (pre)school (Hayes et al. 2017).

Mesosystem

The mesosystem consists of interactions between two or more settings in the microsystem (Bronfenbrenner 1979, 1986). The interactions in this subsystem also have a *direct* impact on the child. For example, if the child's parents and school teachers have incompatible educational goals and practices, the child's development might be adversely affected (Hamilton and Luster 2005). For instance, the child's parents might want him or her to engage in experiential learning activities which they consider meaningful. However, the child's teachers might teach in a way that requires him or her to do rote-learning, which the parents do not endorse (Foo 2018).

If not managed skillfully, in the interactional space of the mesosystem, the parents-child microsystem setting might clash with the teachers-child microsystem setting. The resulting tension might thus adversely affect the child's development.

Exosystem

The exosystem consists of *remote* settings in which a child does not actively participate. Nonetheless, events in the exosystem impact his or her development (Bronfenbrenner 1979, 1986). Take for instance a school board meeting (Hamilton and Luster 2005). While a child never attends such meetings, the decisions made by board members affect the teachers, who in turn will influence the child through the school setting within the microsystem.

Macrosystem

Remote influences within the macrosystem are of a sociocultural nature and include factors such as values, beliefs, and norms (Hamilton and Luster 2005). For instance, a mother does not engage private tutors for her son because she believes that he should be responsible for his own learning. However, many of his classmates who are doing well academically have tutors and are greatly outperforming her son. Given such prevailing societal norms, the mother might wonder if her parenting outlook would disadvantage her son and consider hiring tutors for him too (Foo 2018).

Phase 2: Chronosystem and Emphasis on Process

A self-reflective scholar, Bronfenbrenner continually developed his theory (Tudge et al. 2009). In the 1980s, he added another subsystem – the Chronosystem – to EST because historical data convinced him that time was a critical element in a person's development. Hence, from 1986, his theory has five instead of four levels of subsystems (Fig. 2).

Chronosystem

The impact of time on human development can be understood from two perspectives. First, it refers to the time-period influences. For instance, during the Great Depression in the 1930s, many fathers became unemployed, and this significantly diminished the resources families had for their children's nutritional and educational needs, thus adversely impacting their development (Bronfenbrenner 1986). Second, chronosystem refers to transitions taking place over time. For instance, as a preschool child grows older and begins attending primary school, his or her needs will change (Hayes et al. 2017). Thus, being aware of the changes wrought by time is important in deepening our understanding of a child's developmental needs.

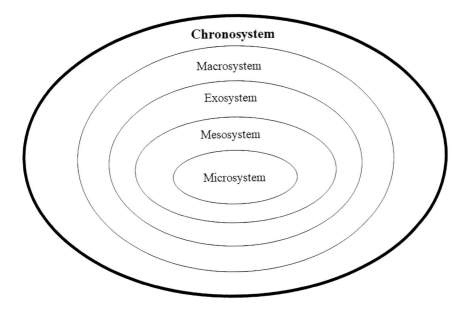

Fig. 2 Ecological systems theory's contextual influences on development (1986)

Emphasis on Process

As can be seen from the discussion of the various subsystems, Bronfenbrenner's theory offers a holistic, multifactorial framework with which to study human development. Not surprisingly, he came to be regarded as a theorist of context (Tudge et al. 2009). However, Bronfenbrenner was concerned that his early writings placed too much emphasis on contextual influences and not enough on the role played by the person in his or her own development (Tudge et al. 2009). To address the perceived imbalance, Bronfenbrenner began to focus on *process*, a concept that examines how the interaction between the person and his or her environment affects his development (Bronfenbrenner and Crouter 1983). The concept of process was further refined by Bronfenbrenner from the 1990s and came to be known as *proximal processes*, which is one of the four major concepts of Bronfenbrenner's mature theory; the other three concepts are person, context, and time (Bronfenbrenner 1999, 2005; Bronfenbrenner and Ceci 1993, 1994; Bronfenbrenner and Evans 2000; Bronfenbrenner and Morris 1998).

Phase 3: Bioecological Theory, Proximal Processes, and the Process-Person-Context-Time Model

Three elements mark phase 3 of the development of EST: the addition of the prefix "bio" to the word "ecological," the concept called "proximal processes," and the Process-Person-Context-Time (PPCT) model (Bronfenbrenner 2001, 2005;

Bronfenbrenner and Ceci 1994; Bronfenbrenner and Evans 2000; Bronfenbrenner and Morris 1998, 2006).

Bronfenbrenner added the prefix "bio" to the word "ecological" to emphasize the importance of the person and not merely focus on contextual factors shaping human development. The consequence of that was his creation of the concept called "proximal processes." If the nomenclature is reminiscent of the concept of "zone of proximal development," it is probably because Bronfenbrenner was influenced by the Soviet psychologist Lev Vygotsky, an early pioneer championing a sociocultural understanding of learning.

As posited by Bronfenbrenner, proximal processes are "the primary engines of development"; they help to explain how "human development takes place," which is "through ... (the) progressively more complex reciprocal interaction between an active, evolving biopsychological human organism and the persons, objects, and symbols in its immediate external environment," that is the microsystem (Bronfenbrenner and Morris 1998, p. 996). Some examples include a child playing with another child or in a group ("persons"), or reading a book ("objects" and "symbols"). These activities engender development as they allow individuals to "make sense of their world and understand their place in it" (Tudge et al. 2009, p. 200).

Proximal processes might be deemed the main engines of development by Bronfenbrenner, but as his PPCT model makes clear, to understand human development, what still matter are factors such as the person's characteristics, contextual influences, and time:

> The form, power, content, and direction of the proximal processes effecting development vary systematically as a joint function of the *characteristics* of the developing person; of the *environment* – both immediate and more remote – in which the processes are taking place ... over *time* through the life course and the historical period during which the person has lived. (Bronfenbrenner and Morris 1998, p. 996, italics added)

In the mature version of his theory, the "environment" refers to the four nested subsystems he created in his 1979 monograph. They include the microsystem, mesosystem, exosystem, and macrosystem. However, Bronfenbrenner further developed the concepts of person and time. He divided the concept "person's characteristics" into three types: demand, resource, and force (Bronfenbrenner 2001; Bronfenbrenner and Ceci 1994). Demand characteristics are characteristics such as age, gender, and physical appearance. Resource characteristics relate to mental and emotional resources such as intelligence, skills, experiences, and social class. Force characteristics refer to a person's temperament, motivation, and persistence. As with person's characteristics, time was also divided into microtime (what is occurring during some specific activity or interaction), meso-time (the extent to which activities and interactions occur with some consistency in the developing person's environment), and macrotime (aka the chronosystem; see pp. 8–9) (Bronfenbrenner and Morris 1998).

Section "Key Features of Ecological Systems Theory" presents the key features of Bronfenbrenner's EST by tracing its developmental trajectory. The following section will discuss how Phase 2 of EST might be applied in clinical education for the health professions.

Ecological Systems Theory and Clinical Education

This section aims to illustrate the relevance and applicability of EST in health professions clinical education. EST provides a useful framework for educators to examine how each individual learner interacts and responds to the changes in the learning and working environment. It can be used to explore, understand, and explain how these multiple and often inter-related influences shape the development of a health professional in a variety of educational situations.

These knowledges are important for several reasons. First, change (be it predictable or unpredictable) occurs daily in our healthcare system and can potentially result in upheavals in the educational mission. In the dynamic clinical environment, both learners and clinical teachers would have to respond appropriately in order to balance patient care and education (Teunissen 2015). The stakeholders' reactions to these changes can be shaped (knowingly or unknowingly) by their previous experiences nested within the EST's five systems. New knowledge and meaning are constantly derived from the current experience, following which reflection, learning, and exploration form the foundations of practice-based learning and resilience (Dennick 2016).

Second, learning and teaching in the clinical environment is complex and challenging (Gruppen et al. 2018). The quality of clinical learning is often varied, and dependent on multiple diverse factors, some of which are beyond the control of the learners and teachers. Mennin (2010) aptly characterized the nature of these factors as repetitive, variable in form, interdependent, and reflective. Hence, it is necessary for educators and curricular developers to recognize the existence of these influences and their impact on the formal curriculum. As part of the curriculum, the learner should be equipped with the knowledge and ability to recognize, acknowledge, and manage these influences in their daily lives. It is through the appreciation and reflection (Rahimi and Haghani 2017) of one's ecological system that self-regulated learning (Boekaerts 1997) can be practiced and integrated into daily practice.

Third, EST itself is a very versatile framework, with which we can apply to different educational contexts and situations (Bluteau et al. 2017; Ellaway et al. 2017; Hamwey et al. 2019). The following subsections will attempt to describe the applications of EST on the (1) development of a health professional student to a working trainee, and to a qualified healthcare provider, (2) challenges encountered by learners facing difficulties.

Health Professions Students

Clinical Learning

Situated learning forms the basis of clinical learning for health profession students (Artemeva et al. 2016). Learning takes place in a variety of clinical environments and is shaped by the students' interactions with their patients, their teachers, and other health professions (Brown et al. 1989). In order to safeguard the educational mission, learning resources (funding, time, and faculty) are provided for by the university or college. Hence, the students learn in a secure and managed micro-system, whereby they are generally shielded from the real-world demands of patient care. The educational and healthcare institutions communicate and plan training rotations on a regular basis (mesosystem).

Beyond the mesosystem, however, clinical learning can be uncertain and disruptive. For example, in understaffed or stretched health systems with high patient loads and/or with high expectations of clinical efficiency, contact time between the student and his clinical teacher can be significantly reduced (Al Kai et al. 2011). Pressures to achieve both clinical and educational outcomes can contribute to high levels of tension, stress, burnout, and emotional exhaustion in the clinical team (Gruppen et al. 2018). These challenges can in turn reduce the quality of learning and demotivate students.

Therefore, the EST can be used as a tool to analyze the student's needs in these uncertain situations, and identify potential disruptors in the clinical learning environment. Importantly, the framework allows for a more holistic examination of the influences (Nordquist et al. 2019) and also allows clinical teachers to communicate more effectively with the rest of the stakeholders (Table 1).

Transitions and Change

Transitions are common and necessary in training and career progression. Examples in health professions education include a student progressing through a training program, graduating to a working trainee, and becoming a certified health professional. Transitional change can be stressful if the educational and clinical support systems are not well established. Negative stress associated with poor transitions can lead to learning disengagement (Dewhurst 2010), learner demotivation (Williams et al. 2008), and exhaustion (physical, mental, and emotional) (Sturman et al. 2017).

Transitioning from a full-time student to a working trainee can be challenging. The learner will have to learn how to manage the responsibilities for complex patient care for the first time, yet simultaneously learning to cope with real-world demands and uncertainties. This transition stage has been characterized as a "steep learning curve," whereby the lack of appropriate guidance and support can result in poor engagement and learning (Sturman et al. 2017). Analysis of the EST's nested systems can inform of the likely positive and negative influences in the clinical and sociocultural context. Knowledge of these influences can aid us in the design and development of coping programs (Ellaway et al. 2017), such as structured

29 Ecological Systems Theory in Clinical Learning

Table 1 Applying EST framework to analyze the enablers and barriers in clinical learning for a student

	Enablers	Barriers
Individual	Motivation to engage and learn Optimal temperament and emotions	Poor motivation (individual and/or previous poor micro, meso, and exo experiences) Personality traits, inability to cope
Micro	Clear curricular and learning objectives Protected resources (university or college) Well-managed clinical environment for learning and teaching (hospital)	Unclear goals and objectives of the clinical attachment Poorly managed clinical environment Tensions in the clinical learning environment
Meso	Active communications between educational and healthcare institutions Good coordination between the educators and clinical teachers	Protected resources not actualized in the clinical setting Inadequate monitoring and reporting of educational issues
Exo	Appropriate and adequate case mix and load Good experience in the clinical learning environment	Patient presentations not matched to the curriculum Busy clinical teachers, distracted or unavailable Technological resources not supportive of learning
Macro	Clearly articulated hospital policies, including supervision policies Culture in the clinical workplace: welcoming, open, and fair Strong interprofessional collaborations	Poor clinical workplace organization and processes Patient refusal of consent or participation in education Inattention of learning goals and engagement by other professions
Chrono	Cumulative good experiences in the clinical workplace, department, and institution	Persistent poor experiences or ongoing conflicts with other staff in the clinical area

induction (O'Brien and Poncelet 2010), preparatory program (Teunissen and Westerman 2011), and job-shadowing initiatives (Hashim 2017).

Working Trainees and Community of Practice (CoP)

Working trainees are exposed to the challenges and demands of patient care. They work and learn in a clinical context that is dynamic and unpredictable. Learning is shaped by their engagement with the work practices, social norms, relationships, and sense of belonging within their local communities of practice. Wenger et al. (2002) proposed the model of integrative learning, in three elements: domain, practice, and community. "Domain" refers to the goals and shared interest of the group, "practice" refers to the professional activities of the group, and "community" refers to the meaningful relationships that unite the group. Table 2 illustrates some of the likely relationships between EST and the success in integration into the community of practice.

Table 2 Enablers and barriers in clinical training and integration into the CoP for working trainees

	Enablers	Barriers
Individual	Motivation to engage and learn within the CoP Stable emotional state and temperament to manage the demands Professionalism, interpersonal communications, empathy, and care as core attributes	Motivation affected by previous poor clinical or CoP experiences Other stressors: exams, jobs
Micro	Clear clinical learning and assessment goals Protected educational time and opportunities (programs and hospital) Stable and engaging CoP	Unclear CoP domain and practice goals Poorly controlled clinical environment (high noneducational clinical loads, manpower shortages)
Meso	Good communication between the program directors and clinical teachers on the curriculum, assessment, and progression criteria Clear articulation of supervision policies and empowerment of clinical responsibilities	Protected resources not actualized in the clinical setting (funding authority and hospital) Inadequate supervision, concerns with clinical risks by clinical teachers, and "blame" culture in managing patient complaints
Exo	Appropriate and adequate patient mix and load Good learning experience within the community (modeling, coaching, scaffolding, and mentoring)	Patient presentations not matched to learning goals Busy clinical teachers, distracted or unavailable for supervision Technological resources not supportive of patient care and learning
Macro	Clearly articulated hospital and clinical policies on patient care supervision Identification of purpose in the community of practice Strong CoP and interprofessional relationships	Poor educational support in the workplace Concerns with litigation of poor engagement with other professions
Chrono	Strong sense of belonging to the CoP built over time	Persistent conflicts and tensions within the CoP and hospital staff

Helping Trainees with Difficulties

Trainees with learning difficulties may encounter challenges in one or multiple EST systems. Given the interrelated nature of the influences, it is likely that barriers encountered in one system (for example, microsystem – understaffed clinical environment) could potentially influence other systems indirectly (exosystem – clinical teacher unavailable for guidance and supervision, macrosystem – breakdown in community). Some barriers that cut across several systems (such as poor team dynamics, conflicts, and system issues) could further compound the learning and well-being of a struggling learner (Houpy et al. 2017). Hamwey et al. (2019) provided an excellent example of the use of EST to analyze the experiences of a struggling learner. The framework reminds educators to refrain from adopting a narrow and presumptive view between learning and teaching shortcomings, and academic failures. Instead, they should take time to analyze, explore, and manage some of these barriers more holistically. Some of the examples elucidated by the authors included loss of financial resource and personal motivation in the learner (individual), unexpected changes in family, friends, and workplace relationships (micro), poorly managed microsystems of the learning environment (meso), persistent faculty issues (exo), and changes in hospital workplace norms, values, and culture (macro). Accurate and timely information is key to aid the struggling learner.

Conclusion

EST is a very versatile framework which can be applied to analyze different educational contexts and situations. Although its use is currently not fully explored in health professions education, its applicability extends beyond that of clinical education. Much promise lies in its use in understanding healthcare management issues and patient care challenges. Further research should be done to explore the influence of the systems on clinical workplace stress, clinician well-being, resilience and burnout, and patient compliance. In each of these situations, the EST can provide a useful common framework to unite the stakeholders.

Cross-References

▶ Communities of Practice and Medical Education
▶ Medical Education: Trends and Context
▶ Self-Regulated Learning: Focus on Theory

References

Al Kai HM, Al-Moamary MS, Elzubair M, Magzoub ME, AlMutairi A, Roberts C, et al. Exploring factors affecting undergraduate medical students' study strategies in the clinical years: a qualitative study. Adv Health Sci Educ. 2011;16(5):553–67.
Artemeva N, Rachul C, O'Brien B, Varpio L. Situated learning in medical education. Acad Med. 2016;92(1):134.
Bandura A, Ross D, Ross SA. Transmission of aggression through imitation of aggressive models. J Abnorm Soc Psychol. 1961;63(3):575.
Baumrind D. Prototypical descriptions of 3 parenting styles. Psychology. 1966;37:1966.
Bluteau P, Clouder L, Cureton D. Developing interprofessional education online: an ecological systems theory analysis. J Interprof Care. 2017;31(4):420–8.
Boekaerts M. Self-regulated learning: a new concept embraced by researchers, policy makers, educators, teachers, and students. Learn Instr. 1997;7(2):161–86.
Boon HJ, Cottrell A, King D, Stevenson RB, Millar J. Bronfenbrenner's bioecological theory for modelling community resilience to natural disasters. Nat Hazards. 2012;60(2):381.

Braithwaite J, Churruca K, Long JC, Ellis LA, Herkes J. When complexity science meets implementation science: a theoretical and empirical analysis of systems change. BMC Med. 2018;16 (1):63–14.

Bronfenbrenner U. Two worlds of childhood: US and USSR. New York: Basic Books; 1970.

Bronfenbrenner U. The ecology of human development: experiments by nature and design. Cambridge, MA: Harvard University Press; 1979.

Bronfenbrenner U. Ecology of the family as a context for human development: research perspectives. Dev Psychol. 1986;22(6):723–42.

Bronfenbrenner U. Interacting systems in human development. Research paradigms: present and future. In: Bolger N, Caspi A, Downey G, Moorehouse M, editors. Persons in contexts: developmental processes. Cambridge, UK: Cambridge University Press; 1988. p. 25–49.

Bronfenbrenner U. Ecological systems theory. In: Vasta R, editor. Annals of child development. Greench: JAI Press; 1989. p. 187–249.

Bronfenbrenner U. Environments in developmental perspective: theoretical and operational models. In: Friedman SL, Wachs TD, editors. Measuring environment across the life span: emerging methods and concepts. Washington, DC: American Psychological Association; 1999. p. 3–28.

Bronfenbrenner U. Human development: bioecological theory of. In: Smelser N, Baltes P, editors. International encyclopedia of the social and behavioral sciences. New York: Elsevier; 2001. p. 6963–70.

Bronfenbrenner U. Making human beings human: bioecological perspectives on human development. Thousand Oaks: Sage; 2005.

Bronfenbrenner U, Ceci SJ. Heredity, environment, and the question "how?": a first approximation. In: Plomin R, McClern GG, editors. Nature, nurture, and psychology. Washington, DC: American Psychological Association; 1993. p. 313–23.

Bronfenbrenner U, Ceci SJ. Nature-nurture reconceptualized in developmental perspective: a bioecological model. Psychol Rev. 1994;101(4):568–86.

Bronfenbrenner U, Crouter AC. Evolution of environmental models in developmental research. In: Mussen PH, editor. Handbook of child psychology: formerly Carmichael's Manual of child psychology. New York: Wiley; 1983.

Bronfenbrenner U, Evans GW. Developmental science in the 21st century: emerging questions, theoretical models, research designs and empirical findings. Soc Dev. 2000;9(1):115–25.

Bronfenbrenner U, Morris PA. The ecology of developmental processes. In: Damon W, Lerner R, editors. Handbook of child psychology, Theoretical models of human development, vol. 1. New York: Wiley; 1998. p. 993–1023.

Bronfenbrenner U, Morris PA. The bioecological model of human development. In: Damon W, Lerner R, editors. Handbook of child psychology: theoretical models of human development. New York: Wiley; 2006. p. 793–828.

Brown JS, Collins A, Duguid P. Situated cognition and the culture of learning. Educ Res. 1989;18 (1):32–42.

Cristancho S, Field E, Lingard L. What is the state of complexity science in medical education research? Med Educ. 2019;53(1):95–104.

D'Amour D, Oandasan I. Interprofessionality as the field of interprofessional practice and interprofessional education: an emerging concept. J Interprof Care. 2005;19(S1):8–20.

Dennick R. Constructivism: reflections on twenty five years teaching the constructivist approach in medical education. Int J Med Educ. 2016;7:200–5.

Dewhurst G. Time for change: teaching and learning on busy post-take ward rounds. Clin Med J R Coll Phys. 2010;10(3):231–4.

Dornan T, Boshuizen H, King N, Scherpbier A. Experience-based learning: a model linking the processes and outcomes of medical students' workplace learning. Med Educ. 2007;41(1):84–91.

Ellaway RH, Bates J, Teunissen PW. Ecological theories of systems and contextual change in medical education. Med Educ. 2017;51(12):1250–9.

29 Ecological Systems Theory in Clinical Learning

Eriksson M, Ghazinour M, Hammarström A. Different uses of bronfenbrenner's ecological theory in public mental health research: what is their value for guiding public mental health policy and practice? Soc Theory Health. 2018;16(4):414–33.

Foo YY. Parents' stories to live by in a competitive educational landscape. Singapore: Nanyang Technological University; 2018.

Gruppen L, Irby DM, Durning SJ, Maggio LA. Interventions designed to improve the learning environment in the health professions: a scoping review. MedEdPublish. 2018;7

Hamilton SF, Luster T. Bronfenbrenner, Urie. In: Fisher CB, Lerner RM, editors. Encyclopedia of applied developmental science. Thousand Oaks: Sage; 2005. p. 184–8.

Hamwey M, Allen L, Hay M, Varpio L. Bronfenbrenner's bioecological model of human development: applications for health professions education. Acad Med. 2019;94(10):1621.

Hashim A. Educational challenges faced by international medical graduates in the UK. Adv Med Educ Pract. 2017;8:441–5.

Hayes N, O'Toole L, Halpenny AM. Introducing Bronfenbrenner: a guide for practitioners and students in early years education. London/New York: Routledge; 2017.

Houpy JC, Lee WW, Woodruff JN, Pincavage AT. Medical student resilience and stressful clinical events during clinical training. Med Educ Online. 2017;22(1):1320187–8.

Larsen PD, McGill JS, Palmer SJ. Factors influencing career decisions: perspectives of nursing students in three types of programs. J Nurs Educ. 2003;42(4):168–73.

Lipsitz LA. Understanding health care as a complex system. JAMA. 2012;308(3):243.

McLeroy KR, Bibeau D, Steckler A, Glanz K. An ecological perspective on health promotion programs. Health Educ Q. 1988;15(4):351–77.

Mennin S. Complexity and health professions education. J Eval Clin Pract. 2010;16(4):835–7.

Nordquist J, Hall J, Caverzagie K, Snell L, Chan M-K, Thoma B, et al. The clinical learning environment. Med Teach. 2019;41(4):366–72.

O'Brien BC, Poncelet AN. Transition to clerkship courses: preparing students to enter the workplace. Acad Med. 2010;85(12):1862–9.

Rahimi M, Haghani F. Reflection in medical education: a review of concepts, models, principles and methods of teaching reflection in medical education. Res Med Educ. 2017;9(2):24–13.

Riggins-Caspers KM, Cadoret RJ, Knutson JF, Langbehn D. Biology-environment interaction and evocative biology-environment correlation: contributions of harsh discipline and parental psychopathology to problem adolescent behaviors. Behav Genet. 2003;33(3):205–20.

Saigal P, Takemura Y, Nishiue T, Fetters MD. Factors considered by medical students when formulating their specialty preferences in Japan: findings from a qualitative study. BMC Med Educ. 2007;7(1):31.

Sallis JF, Owen N, Fisher E. Ecological models of health behavior. In: Glanz K, Rimer BK, Viswanath K, editors. Health behavior and health education: theory, research, and practice. San Francisco: Jossey-Bass; 2008. p. 43–64.

Sanfey HA, Saalwachter-Schulman AR, Nyhof-Young JM, Eidelson B, Mann BD. Influences on medical student career choice: gender or generation? Arch Surg. 2006;141(11):1086–94.

Small SA, Luster T. Adolescent sexual activity: an ecological, risk-factor approach. J Marriage Fam. 1994;56(1):181–92.

Sturman N, Tan Z, Turner J. "A steep learning curve": junior doctor perspectives on the transition from medical student to the health-care workplace. BMC Med Educ. 2017;17(1):92–7.

Teunissen PW. Experience, trajectories, and reifications: an emerging framework of practice-based learning in healthcare workplaces. Adv Health Sci Educ. 2015;20(4):843–56.

Teunissen PW, Westerman M. Opportunity or threat: the ambiguity of the consequences of transitions in medical education. Med Educ. 2011;45(1):51–9.

Tudge JRH, Mokrova I, Hatfield BE, Karnik RB. Uses and misuses of bronfenbrenner's bioecological theory of human development. J Fam Theory Rev. 2009;1(4):198–210.

Wenger E, McDermott RA, Snyder W. Cultivating communities of practice: a guide to managing knowledge. Boston: Harvard Business School Press; 2002.

Williams KN, Ramani S, Fraser B, Orlander JD. Improving bedside teaching: findings from a focus group study of learners. Acad Med. 2008;83(3):257–64.

Zhang YL. Using Bronfenbrenner's ecological approach to understand academic advising with international community college students. J Int Stud. 2018;8(4):1764–82.

Philosophy for Healthcare Professions Education: A Tool for Thinking and Practice

30

Kirsten Dalrymple and Roberto di Napoli

Contents

The Substance of This Chapter 556
From Reflective Practice to Philosophy for Healthcare Professions Education 558
Changing Landscapes in Healthcare and Healthcare Education 559
Exemplifying Changing Paradigms in Healthcare Education 561
What Do We Mean by *Philosophy for Healthcare Professions Education*? Why Do We
Need It? 564
Toward a Philosophy for Healthcare Professions Education Approach: Two Case Studies ... 567
    Case Study One: Exploring Professional and Educational Values and Identity Through
    a Philosophical Approach to Practice 567
    Case Study Two: A Values-Based Philosophic Approach to Professionalism
    Development 568
Toward a Philosophy for Healthcare Professions Education: A Curricular Proposal 569
References 570

Abstract

This is a reflective chapter which focusses on the concept of Philosophy for Healthcare Professions Education. We consider this to be a heuristic device through which to engage, systemically and systematically, with ongoing changes in healthcare and healthcare education, with a view to furthering practice.

Philosophy for healthcare professions education implies adopting a personal philosophical attitude to dissect, critique, and synthesize healthcare practice in relation to specific contexts and wider norms, through educational encounters *with* and reflections *on* other disciplinary and professional fields (e.g., the social

---

K. Dalrymple (✉)
Department of Surgery and Cancer, Imperial College London, London, UK
e-mail: k.dalrymple@imperial.ac.uk

R. di Napoli
Centre for Innovation and Development for Education, St. George's University of London,
London, UK
e-mail: rdinapol@sgul.ac.uk

© Springer Nature Singapore Pte Ltd. 2023
D. Nestel et al. (eds.), *Clinical Education for the Health Professions*,
https://doi.org/10.1007/978-981-15-3344-0_21

sciences and humanities fields), and through contrasting theories and practices in healthcare professions. This means developing a critical stance that leads to a conscious and deep understanding of the nature, aims, and functioning of healthcare as both a theoretical and practical field. Achieving this requires a vigorous engagement with those current value systems and norms underpinning healthcare, through a focused reflection on foundational concepts of healthcare such as care, risk, quality, and responsibility afresh, to capture and contribute to the evolving nature of the field in both informed and agentic ways.

In the course of the chapter, we reflect on current changes in healthcare education, through several examples and two specific case studies, while unpacking the very notion of Philosophy for Healthcare Professions Education. In the last part, we bring our arguments and reflections together to propose Philosophy for Healthcare Professions Education as a conceptual tool for curricular changes in healthcare education.

Our arguments may be considered to be of a political nature, aiming toward a reacquisition of a sense of agency and professional judgment, on the part of healthcare professionals, at times of pervasive normativity.

We leave it to our readers to ascertain the possibilities and limitations of our proposal, in relation to their own professional and educational positioning within healthcare.

Keywords

Philosophy · Values · Professionalism · Knowledge · Curriculum · Professional judgment · Reflection · Agency

The Substance of This Chapter

This is a reflective piece generated by the educational experience of the two authors and their special interest in the nature and scope of philosophy in its relationship to the closely intertwined domains of healthcare and healthcare professions education. Neither author is a healthcare professional, but both have developed their careers through close contact with healthcare professionals, and healthcare professions students, especially in the United Kingdom (UK). Through these extended interactions, they have developed a general understanding of how the UK healthcare system works and how healthcare professions education is taught, its advancement, and its challenges in environments saturated by normativity (both institutional and disciplinary culture) as expressed in the protocols, policies, and initiatives issued by bodies such as the General Medical Council (GMC), higher education institutions, and professional and training bodies. In agreement with a recent editorial from the British Journal of General Practice (Shah et al. 2021), we register a sense of an identity crisis in healthcare professionals, uncomfortably situated between impersonal normativism (which facilitates risk-avoidance) and a personal contextualized and contingent approach (which, inherently, may divert practitioners from normativity toward risk-taking).

Against the background of a complex field filled with normativity, which can transform professional judgment into a rule-application exercise, we argue that both in healthcare and healthcare professions education it is time to return to rigorous and principled reflections on foundational concepts such as care, quality, risk, and responsibility, along with a renewed effort to encourage both students and practitioners to think cogently about the nature, values, and aims supporting their field of practice, through interdisciplinary encounters. These concepts, in our view, constitute the necessary lenses through which to reflect upon professional and educational practice today, to make it both deeply understood in its epistemological nature, and, importantly, in its links with sociocultural practices, and their underlying value systems. The aim of this chapter is to reinvigorate the debate about healthcare and its educational endeavors, by both illustrating work in progress and by making suggestions for empowering practitioners with the tools to critique norms and analyze practice as they occur in specific sociocultural contexts. We call this *philosophy for healthcare professions education* and see it as articulating on two interconnected levels.

First, we argue that philosophy for healthcare professions education implies adopting a personal philosophical attitude to dissect, critique, and synthesize healthcare practice in relation to specific contexts and wider norms, through educational encounters *with* and reflections *on* other disciplinary and professional fields (e.g., the social sciences and humanities fields, and through contrasting theories and practices in healthcare professions). In the first place, such expansive critical and reflective thinking with others would allow for a conscious and deep understanding of the nature, aims, and functioning of healthcare as a theoretical and practical field. Second and crucially, it means a vigorous engagement with current value systems and norms underpinning healthcare, through a focused reflection on foundational concepts of healthcare such as care, risk, quality, and responsibility afresh, to capture the evolving nature of the system and contribute to it actively and in informed ways. This would be achieved through discussions of ideas and insights which have been generated, over time, on those very concepts within healthcare, the humanities, and the social sciences.

To us, this approach to healthcare practice and professional education has the potential to transform the field into an evolving one *owned* by practitioners (in collaboration with patients), as they reflect on actions and experiences in a rigorous way, rather than obediently adopting superimposed rules and behaviors. We argue that it is time to look at the ethical foundations of healthcare and healthcare education afresh, through an engagement with its ethical basis and its epistemological premises, both systemically and systematically. We propose that philosophy for healthcare professions education, as both a theoretical framework and its application to practice and education, can revive the very meaning of healthcare professionalism, which, as we note, currently increasingly emphasizes the application of heterodirected norms and behaviors.

From Reflective Practice to Philosophy for Healthcare Professions Education

> To practise is to 'act within a tradition', but also to critique it and contribute to its evolution. It is the very continuing presence of contesting philosophical viewpoints that provides the oppositional tension, which is essential for critical thinking to perform this role. (De Cossart and Fish 2005, p. 78)

Reflective practice has grown over time in healthcare and healthcare professions education, increasingly, and leans toward an individualistic, introspective, and action-oriented approach (Finlay 2008; Hobbs 2007; Quinn 2000). Within healthcare, reflective practice tends to be technical in nature, with considerable differences between different professional subsets such as nursing and surgery, for instance (see ▶ Chap. 24, "Reflective Practice in Health Professions Education"). This kind of reflective practice, though useful to solve immediate practical problems, may do little to advance the discourse about the nature, scope, and aims of healthcare. Or, indeed, to nurture this in healthcare professions' learners and professionals who often are called to reflect on their practice in relation to superimposed norms and behaviors, without adopting an informed personal critical lens. Of course, we do not wish to underplay the role of normativity, and reflective practice underpinned by it; rather, we would like to promote the nourishing of an epistemologically informed and ethically bound reflective attitude in healthcare and healthcare education which can assist with the implementation of rules contextually and nourish professional judgment and development in focused and informed ways.

This, we argue, can reinvigorate the very soul of the overall healthcare profession by giving professionals the tools and know-how to engage with norms and regulations in an active way, which goes beyond implementation and adherence, toward a professional citizenship within the healthcare system. At times of confusion generated by continuous changes in the healthcare system, and in the face of new, emerging challenges, such as Covid, we believe it is time to go back to the foundations of healthcare and look at the current system from this angle. These challenges demand, in our view, new ways of thinking about healthcare professionalism, beyond a behavioral approach, to one that is critical in nature and is applied throughout a professional's career, from academic studies to lifelong learning based on different forms of professional development. To achieve this, we propose an interpretivist and practical approach, which we call *philosophy for healthcare professions education*.

We define philosophy for healthcare professions education as a professional attitude to look at practice through two lenses which are intimately linked to philosophical theory and practice: the lens of epistemology to fully understand the evolving nature and aims of the disciplines underpinning healthcare – and that of moral philosophy – to revive the overall discourse about the value system underpinning healthcare practice. This is an attitude not simply to reflect on and interpret in the abstract, but to link reflections to actions both for the patients' benefit and the nourishing of professional judgment, and growth. This requires an approach that goes beyond types of healthcare knowledge and practice of a biotechnical nature, toward a mindset that anchors technical knowledge within ethical foundations of and epistemological reflections on healthcare, and incorporates the professional and societal discourses in which the whole field is immersed. We argue that only by doing this can healthcare systems become fully educative in and for themselves, and for the end users who, in turn, need to appreciate what healthcare is and what it is for. We maintain that to achieve this aim it is important to take an interdisciplinary approach to healthcare education and practice, which, includes an understanding of the humanities, especially epistemology and moral philosophy, along with an ability to compare different practices in healthcare (dental, medical, social work, nursing, etc.).

As an attitude to practice, we argue that philosophy for healthcare professions education should accompany practitioners throughout their professional life span, from university studies to the time of exit from healthcare practice. Healthcare practice and healthcare education go hand in hand, as the one feeds upon the other in a continuous cycle. What we argue for is the adoption of a philosophical attitude *for* healthcare professions education that traverses the whole healthcare field and its educational efforts to develop the current and next generation of practitioners.

In this chapter, the reader will not find a discussion of the ideas of thinkers of all times about healthcare or education (which we call philosophy *of* healthcare professions education); rather, they will be encouraged to reflect on a proposal which we believe could help with the flourishing of healthcare and healthcare professions education field over time, within and beyond a system governed by normativity. The argument is tentative and open to application and discussion.

We start with an overview of macrolevel drivers in healthcare and healthcare professions education and the resulting approaches that have emerged on their overlapping landscapes. We then provide some conceptual distinctions before the chapter considers the importance of moral and epistemological thinking in healthcare and healthcare professions education as practice. We substantiate arguments with examples taken from our experience as healthcare professions educators fostering interdisciplinary encounters that nurture reflectivity on disciplinary knowledge and professional practice as well as moral reasoning. In the conclusion, we summarize our arguments by offering a synoptical framework for people to experiment within their educational efforts.

However, before we delve deeper into the concept of philosophy for healthcare and its practical applications, we start by offering a short summary of the changes which have affected healthcare and healthcare professions education in recent times – this provides the background against which our arguments are presented.

Changing Landscapes in Healthcare and Healthcare Education

To understand shifts in the healthcare education landscape, it is instructive to look first at healthcare itself. Healthcare has evolved considerably in the past century spurred on by societal shifts and stunning technological advances. Sir Cyril

Chantler's (1998) oft-quoted summary of the contemporary state of medicine as having shifted from a "simple, ineffective and relatively safe" affair into an enterprise that is "complex, effective, and potentially dangerous" captures the sentiment of how major changes to healthcare delivery, particularly those technologically driven, have impacted practitioners, patients, and society. This seismic shift has disrupted, as Kneebone (2019) explains, long-standing ways of knowing and doing things. Healthcare has had to become more inter-professional and safety-driven not only to be able to manage the complexity of patients with multiple morbidities but also due to the sheer magnitude of diagnostic, therapeutic, and interventional tools available. Such technologic advances provide greater options for care, but they also continually shift the scope and boundaries of work and the nature of roles played by healthcare professionals (O'Brien et al. 2018). Challenges to stable professional cultures have ensued.

Healthcare has also had to become more accountable to the public because of, among other things, the increased complexity of its work and the potential for error (IOM 2000). And, unfortunately, high-profile incidents involving significant harm to patients have occurred at the hands of healthcare providers or systems (Bristol Heart, Staffordshire) due to professional negligence. Additionally, citizens in many societies have choice around where they receive their healthcare and take greater interest in judging the clinical effectiveness of service provision. Beyond increasing accountability and choice, citizens feel increasingly empowered to expect care that takes their needs and expectations into account, altering long established sociocultural dynamics between healthcare professionals and patients (O'Brien et al. 2018).

Healthcare is thus said to be evolving from an enterprise characterized by many as patriarchal, individualistic, provider-centered, and closed to the outside world into something more democratic, team-driven, patient-centered, and transparent. Alongside the related drivers of accountability and patient-safety, Bleakley (2019) argues that this evolution is critical not only for healthcare but also to create an "innovative expansion of medical culture" away from the current form that he argues still "socializes its young into hierarchical structures or eats them whole" (p. 1422). Bleakley's provocative words point us to the essential connection that exists among healthcare practices, healthcare culture, and health-professions education. It likewise draws attention to parallel shifts in higher education where institutions have been pressed to consider similar changes to the dynamics between teachers and learners giving way to more "learner-centered" educational practices.

Influential medical educators surveyed by O'Brien and colleagues (2018) identify a range of prominent drivers in healthcare professions education which include the following: competency-based education, simulation-based education, faculty development, globalization and its implications on workforces, and greater emphasis on curriculum and standards. To this, we would add the ever-growing emphasis placed on the explicit teaching, learning, and assessment of professionalism. The development of each of these educational approaches can be traced back to changing healthcare practices and societal change.

As educators, these trends touch our thinking and actions regularly and raise the following important questions: Does competency-based education promote the development of expert practitioners? Do our learners get more from a placement they do in a low-middle income country than the host? Do our students need to spend a significant portion of their time learning communication skills, or ENT, or the Krebs cycle for that matter? Should simulation replace authentic experiences with patients? Should we focus on educating generalists? Should we resist the standardization of processes? Should practitioners get a formal qualification in healthcare professions education? Should we use active learning, reduce lecturing time, teach outside the written curriculum, use more self and peer assessment, be more inclusive, let students shape the curriculum, and spend limited time engaging in reflection? The list of questions goes on and on.

These concrete questions make sense to many educators, but just below the surface they also present pressing philosophical questions such as the following: What should be learned (by a nurse, a dentist, a midwife, etc.); how it should be learned (for example, by a paramedic or a social worker or a surgeon); what values matter; and what the purpose of education is in relation to practice and its contexts, within and beyond university studies. Crucially, we must ask ourselves, how healthcare and educational practices relate to the overarching concepts of care, risk, quality, and responsibility in healthcare. These are not solely questions for philosophers of education. These questions are at the heart of how practitioners go about working, educating, and responding to the expectations placed on them by their learners, their employers, their professions, and society at large.

Critically, it is individual practitioners who must make sense of and implement initiatives. How we contemplate philosophical questions about the meaning and use of education in relation to our daily practice as teachers, assessors, curriculum developers, and learners is the kind of practical and personal philosophy that Ennis in Lipman (2003) calls the "reasonable, rational thinking that helps us decide what to believe and do" (p. 37).

It is within this landscape that our proposal for a philosophy for healthcare positions itself, broadly embedded within a postpositivist and interpretivist paradigm. The proposal is further influenced by ideas derived from critical theory, as it engages with political questions about who defines healthcare, who defines healthcare professions education, and how their norms can be interpreted in relation to specific sociocultural and political contexts. The central purpose of proposing a philosophy of healthcare professions education is to provide healthcare professions educators with philosophical tools for examining and evolving personal and community practices.

Exemplifying Changing Paradigms in Healthcare Education

As discussed earlier, wider societal trends spur evolution of healthcare and healthcare education. This evolution has come through successive exploration, adoption, and refinement of practices that draw on an increasingly broad range of philosophic paradigms and has been motivated in large part by scholars and research from the healthcare professions' education community. To substantiate this claim, and importantly to consider how practitioners might benefit from developing a philosophy for healthcare, let us consider two evolving patterns in healthcare education, (1) assessment of competence in competency-based education and (2) involvement of patients and learners in health professions' education.

In the first example, greater accountability and complexity in healthcare have given rise to heightened demands for reliable outcomes through demonstration of reliable performance in assessment. What was considered valuable in assessment was what could be shown to be psychometrically sound (i.e., a test or series of tests shows us that this candidate is reliably able to perform a task) and primarily at the level of the individual. In philosophic terms, this represents an ontological, epistemological, and axiological position aligned closely with positivism.

Many healthcare education scholars, chief among them Hodges and Lingard (2012), argue that this position is at odds with the complexity and interdependent nature of healthcare work. In considering individual assessments of competence alone, Govaerts and van der Vleuten (2013) and others have persuasively argued that clinical performance is unstable, heavily dependent on contextual factors and hence should draw further on strategies that acknowledge the performance context and the judgment of various "experts" to provide a holistic picture of learners and their competence. Assessment "quality" in this more socially constructed, interpretivist assessment approach relies on more than just psychometric validity to determine whether a learner should be trusted to provide specific healthcare. It relies on learners and assessors to record and reflect to construct an interpretation that explains performance over time. Reality, and how it is understood, is seen as more complex in this assessment scenario. What is seen as "valued" in the performance and in how its nature is "evidenced" also shifts (Govaerts and van der Vleuten 2013; Cook et al. 2016). Together, a more social-constructivist argument for assessment emerges. This is one which, in principle, we can see materializing in, for example, the UK's most recent Intercollegiate Surgical Curriculum Project assessment program where multi-consultant reports, created at key points in training placements, will now take priority over numeric measures of performance from work-based assessments (ISCP 2021). This is not to say that numbers do not matter but rather that they provide only a partial view of a complex picture of learning and development, a picture that can be complemented by words and discussions about things that are difficult to measure, such as professional values (Ginsburg et al. 2004).

Beyond the broadening of assessment of competence to emphasize qualitative information and expert judgment at the level of the individual, there is also the evolution of learning and assessment approaches to foster the team competence that Lingard (2012) argues is essential to high-quality healthcare, and that by its social nature is difficult to assess in solely psychometric ways. In this space, the "debriefing" community is advancing approaches that draw on a wider range of philosophic positions and related educational practices (Bearman et al. 2019; Schmutz and Eppich 2017). Bearman and colleagues (2019) discuss the culture of debriefing as having emerged from more therapeutic and developmental approaches, for example, in the military where it served to help participants "talk through" difficult missions, concluding that this background has shaped the "assumptions, values and norms" of debriefing facilitators.

In our second example, we consider how healthcare professions education curricula have shifted dramatically in character over the decades to include more patient- and learner-centered perspectives. These far-reaching healthcare and educational approaches have also evolved in practical and philosophical terms over time. The role of patients and learners in shaping their care and education has become increasingly democratic, even though this transition is, as Bleakley (2019), Snow et al. (2019), and others argue, incomplete. Snow et al. (2019) describes a process, based on Arnstein's (1969) Ladder of Citizen Participation, where patient involvement has moved from lower rungs of "consulting" and "placating" (e.g., surveying patients for their views on care/education without necessarily following through on their feedback) to higher levels of "participation" and "citizen control" where hierarchies are broken down and power and responsibility are increasingly shared with or given to patients. This process of moving toward more shared and meaningful participation parallels endeavors in higher education institutions where students are being given more significant roles in developing and evaluating curricula – an approach associated with philosophies that are more social constructivist and critical theory oriented in nature.

In both situations, the evolution of healthcare and healthcare professions education has come through successive exploration and adoption of practices that draw on wider philosophic paradigms, beyond the positivist one that, despite notable progress in some arenas, still tends to dominate the healthcare field toward those that rely on the understanding of context, the participation of stakeholders, and creation of shared, considered judgment. The very notion of professionalism, in keeping with this argument, is shifting its focus from a behavioral one to a virtue-informed one which stresses care, responsiveness, and responsibility toward patients, toward learners, toward one's own profession, and toward society at large.

These paradigmatic shifts require a different kind of healthcare professions education that is more holistic in nature, based on an ability to consider and interrogate "pathologies" not only from a biotechnological viewpoint but also from a sociocultural one, in which both patients and their ailments are situated. This ability we call philosophy for healthcare professions education. We consider this to be both an attitude and a set of tools, inherited from the philosophical tradition, which allows healthcare professionals to look at their patients, learners, and their own field of practice in more complex and helpful ways.

Specific educational philosophies and theories have only been touched upon here. Further reading is warranted to create greater awareness and alignment between personal philosophies and scholarly discourses in education and educational research (Lincoln et al. 2011). Academic Medicine and Advances in Health Sciences Education, for example, have recently published series on philosophies of science and education that provide useful overviews and commentaries (Baker et al. 2021; Varpio and MacLeod 2020; Varpio and Ellaway 2021). Readers may also find chapters from this book, for example, Bezemer's chapter exploring social semiotics or McNaughton's on critical theory, useful in expanding their understanding of educational theories.

Greater familiarity with a wider range of educational philosophies is useful. However, we argue that cultivating an ability to engage with philosophy for education goes beyond this and entails the development of more nuanced and deeper interpretation capabilities of the local and wider contexts on the part of the healthcare professional as well as a disposition to value the insights and contributions of patients and students, along those of established scholars across a variety of disciplinary fields. As Filipe et al. (2017) argue, what is needed is initiatives which can foster an "exploratory space and a generative process that leads to different, and sometimes unexpected, forms of knowledge, values, and social relations." Our proposal to develop a philosophy for healthcare professions education has the potential to create greater exploration of healthcare systems and its underpinning disciplinary fields and value systems, in cooperation with patients and learners, and more agency for the everyday healthcare professions educator. But it is contingent on healthcare professions educators taking on the challenge of developing new knowledge, new habits, and new mindsets. Our suggestion for a philosophy for healthcare professions is a step in this direction.

What Do We Mean by *Philosophy for Healthcare Professions Education*? Why Do We Need It?

Every professional has their tools for thinking, doing, and communicating with their own community of practice. Scientists, for example, use the scientific method and instruments in the laboratory to carry out their experiments; they use critical arguments and evidence to support their scholarship and peer review to ensure and enhance the standards of science. They place high value on these processes and on the nature and quality of knowledge they produce. Doctors, nurses, dentists, physical therapists, pharmacists, and all health professionals have their own material and intellectual tools to carry out their work. Philosophers too possess a toolkit that contains its own instruments and practices which bear similarities and differences to other professions'. Drawing more extensively on the philosopher's intellectual toolkit offers a way forward for refreshing and critically examining current healthcare and healthcare professions education strategies, many of which have been shown to have limitations due to conceptual weaknesses in the approach (Bleakley 2000; Eva et al. 2004; Ginsburg et al. 2004; Greenhalgh et al. 2014) or have had poor (or temporary) uptake by learners and educators or both (Hung et al. 2019; Finlay 2008; Wyer 2019).

It is likely that many people will look at the marriage between philosophy and healthcare and, by extension, health professions education, with surprise and perhaps even suspicion. However, healthcare, as much as other disciplinary and professional fields (such as design, law, the social sciences, etc.), is traversed by philosophical assumptions about its nature, aims, and values. Testimony to this is borne by special academic journals revolving around the link between healthcare and philosophy (such as *Medicine, Healthcare and Philosophy, Philosophy of Medicine* and *The Journal of Medicine and Philosophy,* to mention a few) or dedicated books such as the works by Evans, Louhiala, and Puustinen (2004) and Thompson, Ross, and Upshur (2017).

The link between healthcare, healthcare professions education, and philosophy is generally actualized by moral philosophy, a specific branch of philosophy which deals both with the creation of criteria we use to make decisions about what is good (normative ethics) and how these criteria are applied in relation to concrete situations and problems, to fully appreciate the gamut of ethical issues practice that may surface (applied ethics). Normative and applied ethics can be considered either as separate subfields, or as intertwined enterprises – each of them having their own acolytes, research endeavors, and publications (Donzelli and Spadafora 2021). In turn, philosophy, as a wider field, covers a whole spectrum of intellectual activities which includes interrogating, searching for meaning, critiquing, dissecting, and reassembling, experimenting, and transforming (Fabbrichesi 2017). This is the skill set which we propose to cultivate in healthcare professionals, within and beyond their specialisms, to grapple with the complexity of their work and contribute actively and critically to change, toward more informed and agentic forms of professionalism.

We argue for a philosophy for healthcare professions education. We consider this to be, in the first instance, an exercise in applied ethics through which we reflect on societal trends and professional norms to make them "ours" in relation both to the contexts in which we, as professionals, operate and the conceptual foundations of healthcare. It is both a conceptual and practical exercise, which is meant to reveal the continuous tension underpinning healthcare professions.

We argue that healthcare professionals should keep alive discussions around this tension throughout their academic studies and professional life to interrogate norms and practices through foundational lenses such as cure/care, responsibility, risk, and quality. In doing so, healthcare professionals stand to enrich their understanding and strengthen their ability to take a professional posture also by referring, whenever possible, to the works of experts who have dealt with the matters under consideration. Ethical thinking occurs all the time in healthcare, when a doctor reasons about a specific case, when a nurse interacts with patients, and when a surgeon takes a decision on an action to take. However, this thinking is rarely brought to the surface in a systematic way – it is left dormant and undisclosed because it is claimed of time limitations and other acute pressures, no matter how important it is. Rarely are such matters discussed in staff development, as they are deemed to be time-consuming and not practical; rarely, in our experience, do foundational concepts emerge consciously in healthcare professions education, unless in the form of ad hoc sessions (especially in patient communication and professionalism strands) or as a part of humanities programs. We therefore advocate a more systemic and systematic approach to foundational ethical concepts as the nerve traversing healthcare studies and practice.

As importantly, we consider philosophy for healthcare professions education to be an epistemological reflection on the disciplinary foundations underpinning each field of healthcare practice, to fully appreciate its shifts and actively contribute to these, rather than passively aligning with them. This necessitates both disciplinary and interdisciplinary encounters that can shed light on how a given field is moving, not just from a biotechnical viewpoint, but holistically, in relation to those societal changes in which scientific knowledge and professional practice are embedded. Philosophy for healthcare professions education requires an integration of technical know-how with wider philosophical abilities to question and understand the contexts within which healthcare occurs, which is vital for patient care. As such, it asks for a vigorous engagement with other disciplinary sets, especially those of the humanities and social sciences. This exposes professionals and students to different and integrative ways to look at healthcare, thus widening their knowledge set. As a corollary, it provides them with tools to better embed patient care into wider contexts, thus helping to transform treatment into care (Donzelli and Spadafora 2021; Good 1993). Readers may also be interested in reading related chapters in this book, for example, Harvey, Livesay and Walter, Knight and Papanikitas, and Stephenson and Bliss.

The advantages of adopting the tools of philosophy in healthcare practice and education are therefore multiple. It brings professional practice and thinking back to the foundations of healthcare, providing clarity in the fog of superimposed norms and fast actions, thus enriching understanding, while *actively* assisting with the evolution of the field from an epistemological and axiological viewpoint. In healthcare professions beset by norms and hectic schedules, thinking cogently about one's profession could be a vital motivational exercise as healthcare practice is strongly infused by ethical thinking and questions about the evolution of the field more widely. Adopting a philosophical stance may empower healthcare professionals with the necessary conceptual tools and habits to critique hetero-directed norms, thus making them citizens of their profession rather than just performers.

Additionally, if well embedded within undergraduate and postgraduate curricula, both systemically and systematically, the adoption and cultivation of a philosophy for healthcare would become the axis around which both practitioners and students could reflect on their learning by engaging with foundational concepts as epistemological reflections on the nature and aims of healthcare practice. Taken as a whole, and if well integrated, a philosophy of healthcare professions education could usefully add to technical knowledge; it could become the thread which links together an otherwise crowded and heterogenous curriculum and bring students continuously to the foundational core of their studies and chosen profession.

Experiments are afoot. What follows are two selected examples of healthcare professions education which adopts a philosophy for healthcare professions education, at least partially. Through these examples, we aim to shed light on possible ways forward, toward a healthcare practice and education that are mindful of their conceptual foundations and make these a centerpiece to form well-rounded and ethically formed professionals.

Toward a Philosophy for Healthcare Professions Education Approach: Two Case Studies

Case Study One: Exploring Professional and Educational Values and Identity Through a Philosophical Approach to Practice

In 2016, faculty on the MEd in Surgical Education at Imperial College London developed a curriculum to embrace a more transformative, and values-rich, experience for their students. Most students on the program are surgeons or surgeons in training who start their study having had a long background of more technical rationale, biomedical approaches to practice.

The program team has long taken the view that its students, by "educating" themselves as "educators," are embarking on a process of forming another identity alongside their clinical one and that this will require not only learning new strategies for teaching, assessment and evaluation, new knowledge of applying concepts from educational theories to educational problems, and learning qualitative approaches to creating new knowledge, but also examining and developing their values and epistemological positions over time and alongside the development of new educational approaches (Cuming and Horsburgh 2019).

The program achieves this mainly through three layered and integrated strands: (1) a "bridging" strand that aims to facilitate connections between students' "home" disciplines and those outside it; (2) an educational theory strand for analyzing educational problems, and finally, (3) a strand around reflective practice as and for personal philosophizing. In practice, we initiate these strands in parallel and return to them frequently in a range of formats.

Bridging activities commence early and entail identifying key philosophic positions from the home discipline and comparing these to those from education around specific themes. For example, we ask the students to discuss what they believe to be the main aims, forms of knowledge, skills, and attitudes in surgery and in education and then compare them to our own views of education as professional educators (Di Napoli, personal communication). We engage in similar interdisciplinary discussions as it relates to other topics about the nature of theory, knowledge, research, and quality with a range of professionals, inside and outside health professions education (Kneebone and Schlegel 2021).

The reflective strand challenges students to explore their values and beliefs as educators via a series of structured reflections starting at the commencement of the program and continuing across its different stages. We make use of Gibbs cycle (1988) to prompt the recognition of emotion alongside other more familiar elements of the reflective cycle, and we are deliberate in the structuring of tasks to raise issues around values and beliefs as they relate to becoming a professional and an educator. For example, a reflective task may ask a student to consider an event that shaped them into the professional that they are today. The periodic tasks are guided by discussion with tutors and peers and by criteria we wish to emphasize such as "considers own beliefs, values and assumptions," or "looking from the perspective of other stakeholders and the literature."

Educational theory is explored across the program not only in concentrated ways by dedication of a full module midway through the program, but also in smaller ways, integrated with other activities early on. Importantly in these early days, introducing theories follows more personal, contextualized, and concrete discussions with our students. For example, having started exploring their personal theories and philosophies of learning as emerging alongside professional and academic development, we revisit the area by discussing Jarvis-Selenger and colleagues' (2012) article advocating the introduction of professional identity formation theories in the education and training of healthcare professionals. Selenger's article describes and applies Kegan's stage model and focuses on the concept of "crises" serving as pivotal moments in identity formation. We discuss this theory considering competency-based education and our students' personal experience of making sense of their own professional development.

Together, the introduction of these three pedagogic strands enables us to lay an integrated foundation for the students to explore and challenge their values and beliefs around their profession and education. The activities introduce reflective practice as a flexible and layered activity that can be undertaken alone and with others, through discussions and in writing, considering personal perspectives, while also looking outward to colleagues and the literature to widen the view, including critiques of reflective practice itself (Finlay 2008).

Case Study Two: A Values-Based Philosophic Approach to Professionalism Development

In a second approach to embedding reflection and values-based approaches into faculty development programs, De Cossart and Fish (2019) describe their efforts to engage clinicians in surfacing and reflecting on their values systems through a series of activities carried out in early parts of a program aimed at developing educational supervisors for trainees. They charge their students (senior clinicians) with considering what personal and professional values they bring to doctoring through writing exercises and discussions.

Later in the program, the authors provide their students with a values-based framework to practice their supervisory activities, for example, the case-based discussion (CBD). Carried out by trainees as part of their competency-based assessment program, the CBD provides the trainee and their educational supervisee an opportunity to discuss a case they have recently worked on that has been challenging in some way. It is meant to be formative and yield learning points for the trainee. In the approach taken by De Cossart and Fish (2019), the CBD takes the shape of an intentional and explicit reflective process focused on the "professional values in practice" of the trainee. The case is first considered independently by the trainee, then by the supervisor, and finally through a reflective conversation between trainer and trainee focusing on the ethical dimensions of the clinical case and the trainee's thoughts and actions in response to them. De Cossart and Fish (2019) conceive of this process as "transformational professionalism" as it integrates and makes explicit the personal and professional values that run alongside the technical and rational elements of care.

Toward a Philosophy for Healthcare Professions Education: A Curricular Proposal

The cases above constitute examples of a rigorous attempt being made toward the adoption of a philosophy for education; they contain seminal aspects of it such as comparisons, interdisciplinarity, critical reflections on value systems, construction, and de-construction of the meanings of a specialism, with the aim of nourishing curiosity toward a more holistic and complex understanding of healthcare. Evans et al. (2004) clarifies this perspective as he reflects on medical education:

> If 'health' means that the parts of your body meet the expectations of statistical norms, then a mechanical approach to diagnosis and treatment is perfectly appropriate. However, if 'health' means something more like your ability to experience and engage with the world in a way that you are used to, understand and enjoy, then this has the most profound implications for the preparation, training and post-qualification education of clinical doctors... Our recognition that clinical medicine is bristling with philosophical questions suggests that doctors gain much, and perhaps offer much to their patients subsequently, when they recognize and reflect on these questions in a philosophical spirit... (p. 13)

It is precisely this spirit that we argue healthcare practitioners and educators should adopt a reflective attitude nourished by a broad philosophical practice, which we have named Philosophy for Healthcare Professions Education. This could constitute an important strand in academic and professional education, as the linking element between biotechnical knowledge and professional practice:

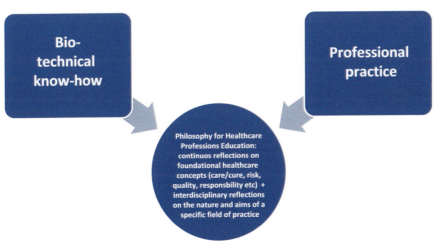

We propose that these three dimensions should be strictly intertwined and become the lynchpin of healthcare professions practice and education. The curricular implications of this proposal are numerous and provide opportunities for clinicians, curriculum developers, and clinical teachers to embed moral and epistemological reflections into everyday practice, through explicit and intentional educative activities such as role modeling and supervisory support for learners around the nature, aims, and ethical dimensions (De Cossart and Fish 2019) of healthcare practice.

What we have tried to do in this chapter is to launch a curricular proposal which may be put into practice as academics and professional developers engage with healthcare practitioners and students and plan their course of study. To us, educational and professional development need to coalesce around foundational concepts in strategic and systematic ways to help present and future healthcare workers inject and refine their own thoughts and meanings into the profession. In other words, we consider philosophy for healthcare practice to be a form of rich reflection on practice, which requires an interdisciplinary and ethical approach, which is broadly in line with philosophical practice, and a different posture toward the pedagogy of professionalism.

We maintain that it is through the infusion and perfusion of these three dimensions that healthcare professionals could better contribute to current debates on healthcare practice in informed ways, rather than being the mere consumers of hetero-directed rules and regulations. Our proposal may therefore be considered a political one, aiming toward a reacquisition of a sense of agency and professional judgment on the part of healthcare professionals. As such, philosophy for healthcare professions education could also contribute to give healthcare professions curricula more coherence and cohesiveness, and revive motivation in students who often, immersed as they are in technical know-how and the learning of norms (without perhaps fully understanding them), become test-fatigued technicians of healthcare, losing sight of what brought them to healthcare in the first place. How to achieve this in practice, in terms of curriculum and professional development, remains a matter of debate, development, and practice.

References

Arnstein SR. A ladder of citizen participation. J Am Inst Plann. 1969;35(4):216–24. https://doi.org/10.1080/01944366908977225.

Baker LR, Phelan S, Woods NN, et al. Re-envisioning paradigms of education: towards awareness, alignment, and pluralism. Adv Health Sci Educ. 2021;26:1045–58. https://doi.org/10.1007/s10459-021-10036-z.

Bearman M, Eppich W, Nestel D. How debriefing can inform feedback: practices that make a difference. In: The impact of feedback in higher education. Cham: Palgrave Macmillan; 2019. p. 165–88.

Bleakley A. Adrift without a life belt: reflective self-assessment in a post-modern age. Teach High Educ. 2000;5(4):405–18.

Bleakley A. Invoking the medical humanities to develop a #MedicineWeCanTrust. Acad Med. 2019;94:1422–4. https://doi.org/10.1097/ACM.0000000000002870.

Chantler S C. Reviews. BMJ. 1998;317:1666. https://doi.org/10.1136/bmj.317.7173.1666b

Cook DA, Ayelet K, Hatala R, Ginsburg S. When assessment data are words: validity evidence for qualitative educational assessments. Acad Med. 2016;91(10):1359–69. https://doi.org/10.1097/ACM.0000000000001175.

Cuming T, Horsburgh J. Constructing surgical identities: becoming a surgeon educator. In: Nestel D, Dalrymple K, Paige J, Aggarwal R, editors. Advancing surgical education. Singapore: Springer; 2019. p. 133–40.

De Cossart L, Fish D. Cultivating a thinking surgeon: new perspectives on clinical teaching, learning and assessment. Shrewsbury: tfm Publishing Limited; 2005.

De Cossart L, Fish D. Supporting the development of professionalism in surgeons in practice: a virtues-based approach to exploring a surgeon's moral agency. In: Nestel D, Dalrymple K, Paige J, Aggarwal R, editors. Advancing surgical education. Singapore: Springer; 2019. p. 303–11.

Donzelli G, Spadafora P. Medicina inedita: uno sguardo nuovo su salute e malattia. Milano: La Nave di Teseo in collaborazione con Fondazione Meyer; 2021.

Englander R, Holmboe E, Batalden P, Caron RM, Durham CF, Foster T, Ogrinc G, Ercan-Fang N, Batalden M. Coproducing health professions education: a prerequisite to coproducing health care services? Acad Med. 2020;95(7):1006–13. https://doi.org/10.1097/ACM.0000000000003137. PMID: 31876565

Eva KW, Cunnington JP, Reiter HI, Keane DR, Norman GR. How can I know what I don't know? Poor self-assessment in a well-defined domain. Adv Health Sci Educ. 2004;9(3):211–24.

Evans M, Louhiala P, Puustinen R, editors. Philosophy for medicine: applications in a clinical context. Abingdon: Radcliffe Publishing; 2004.

Fabbrichesi R. Cosa si fa quando si fa filosofia? Milano: Raffaello Cortina; 2017.

Filipe A, Renedo A, Marston C. The co-production of what? Knowledge, values, and social relations in health care. PLoS Biol. 2017;15(5):e2001403. https://doi.org/10.1371/journal.pbio.2001403.

Finlay L. Reflecting on "reflective practice". In: Paper 52 of Practice-based Professional Learning Centre (PBPL CETL), Open University. 2008. https://oro.open.ac.uk/68945/1/Finlay-%282008%29-Reflecting-on-reflective-practice-PBPL-paper-52.pdf. Accessed 25 June 2021.

Gibbs G. Learning by doing: a guide to teaching and learning methods. London: Further Education Unit; 1988.

Ginsburg S, Regehr G, Lingard L. Basing the evaluation of professionalism on observable behaviors: a cautionary tale. Acad Med. 2004;79(10 Suppl):S1–4. https://doi.org/10.1097/00001888-200410001-00001. PMID: 15383374

Good BJ. Medicine, rationality and experience: an anthropological perspective. New York: Cambridge University Press; 1993.

Govaerts M, van der Vleuten CP. Validity in work-based assessment: expanding our horizons. Med Educ. 2013;47(12):1164–74.

Greenhalgh T, Howick J, Maskrey N. Evidence based medicine: a movement in crisis? BMJ. 2014;348:g3725. https://doi.org/10.1136/bmj.g3725.

Hobbs V. Faking it or hating it: can reflective practice be forced? Reflective Pract. 2007;8(3):405–17.

Hodges BD, Lingard L. The question of competence. New York: Cornell University Press; 2012.

Hung W, Dolmans DHJM, van Merriënboer JJG. A review to identify key perspectives in PBL meta-analyses and reviews: trends, gaps and future research directions. Adv Health Sci Educ. 2019;24:943–57. https://doi.org/10.1007/s10459-019-09945-x.

Institute of Medicine (IOM) Committee on Quality of Health Care in America. In: Kohn LT, Corrigan JM, Donaldson MS, editors. To err is human: building a safer health system. Washington, DC: National Academies Press; 2000. ISBN-10: 0-309-06837-1.

Intercollegiate Surgical Curriculum Project. 2021. https://www.iscp.ac.uk. Accessed 30 Aug 2021.

Jarvis-Selinger S, Pratt DD, Regehr G. Competency is not enough: integrating identity formation into the medical education discourse. Academic medicine. 2012;87(9):1185–90.

Kneebone R. Surgical education: a historical perspective. In: Nestel D, Dalrymple K, Paige J, Aggarwal R, editors. Advancing surgical education. Singapore: Springer; 2019. p. 9–16.

Kneebone R, Schlegel C. Thinking across disciplinary boundaries in a time of crisis. Lancet. 2021;397(10269):89–90.

Lincoln YS, Lynham SA, Guba EG. Paradigmatic controversies, contradictions, and emerging confluences, revisited. In: Denzin NK, Lincoln YS, editors. The Sage handbook of qualitative research. Sage; 2011. p. 97–128.

Lipman M. Thinking in education. New York: Cambridge University Press; 2003.

O'Brien BC, Forrest K, Wijnen-Meijer M, ten Cate O. A global view of structures and trends in medical education. Understanding Medical Education: Evidence, Theory, and Practice. 2018;3:7–22.

Quinn FM. Reflection and reflective practice. In: Davies C, Finlay L, Bullman A, editors. Changing practice in health and social care. London: Sage; 2000. p. 81–90.

Schmutz JB, Eppich WJ. Promoting learning and patient care through shared reflection: a conceptual framework for team reflexivity in health care. Acad Med. 2017;92(11):1555–63.

Shah R, Ahluwalia S, Spicer J. A crisis of identity: what is the essence of general practice? Br J Gen Pract. 2021;71(707):246–7. https://doi.org/10.3399/bjgp21X715745. PMID: 34045243

Snow R, Bearman M, Iedema R. Patients and surgical education: rethinking learning, practice and patient engagement. In: Nestel D, Dalrymple K, Paige J, Aggarwal R, editors. Advancing surgical education. Singapore: Springer; 2019. p. 197–208.

Thompson RP, Upshur RE. Philosophy of medicine: an introduction. New York: Routledge; 2017.

Varpio L, Ellaway RH. Shaping our worldviews: a conversation about and of theory. Adv Health Sci Educ. 2021;26:339–45. https://doi.org/10.1007/s10459-021-10033-2.

Varpio L, MacLeod A. Philosophy of science series: harnessing the multidisciplinary edge effect by exploring paradigms, ontologies, epistemologies, axiologies, and methodologies. Acad Med. 2020;95:686–9.

Wyer PC. Evidence-based medicine and problem based learning a critical re-evaluation. Adv Health Sci Educ. 2019;24:865–78. https://doi.org/10.1007/s10459-019-09921-5.

Part III

Curriculum Considerations in Health Professions Education

Health Profession Curriculum and Public Engagement

31

Maree O'Keefe and Helena Ward

Contents

Introduction	576
Curriculum Development and Implementation	577
Challenges of Finding Appropriate Terminology	577
Models of Public Engagement	578
Public Consultation	579
Public as Expert Advisers on Specific Illness Experiences	580
Public as Partners	580
Sociocultural Theories and Public Engagement	581
Limitations of Public Engagement	582
Public Engagement in the Age of the Internet	583
Conclusion	584
Cross-References	584
References	584

Abstract

Health profession curriculum development and implementation is a dynamic process that requires balancing of many factors. Foremost is the need to ensure students master the requisite competencies to satisfy accreditation agencies and registration bodies regarding quality and safety to practice. In addition, there is a need to ensure that academic standards are maintained so as to satisfy the requirements of relevant qualifications. There is also the need to ensure adequate supervision for students placed in health service work environments. Finally, and very importantly, there is a need to ensure that curriculum content, delivery, and learning outcomes meet the health needs and aspirations of the general community as well as the various health professions.

M. O'Keefe (✉) · H. Ward
Faculty of Health and Medical Sciences, The University of Adelaide, Adelaide, SA, Australia
e-mail: maree.okeefe@adelaide.edu.au; helena.ward@adelaide.edu.au

© Springer Nature Singapore Pte Ltd. 2023
D. Nestel et al. (eds.), *Clinical Education for the Health Professions*,
https://doi.org/10.1007/978-981-15-3344-0_40

In this chapter, we review contemporary understandings of public engagement in health professional curriculum, including the various roles that members of the public can and do play in assisting students to navigate the challenge of moving from theory into practice. Consideration is given to the extent to which different models of public engagement empower members of the public to influence curriculum decision.

In the final section, we contemplate ways in which the emerging digital age may change the landscape with a resulting rethink of public engagement in health profession curriculum. Increasingly the general public will have high levels of digital literacy and come to health care professionals not for knowledge and content, but for advice about managing this data.

Keywords

Health profession · Curriculum · Public engagement · Digital literacy · Patient participation · Patient-centred care · Accreditation · Academic standards · Activity theory · Situated learning · Internet

Introduction

The formation of a health professional is a complex undertaking. There are specific disciplinary knowledge and skills that, for example, doctors, dentists, nurses, and physiotherapists require. In addition, the student needs to be supported in developing their ability to integrate these attributes and apply them in practice in ways that are academically rigorous and at the same time deeply personalized and attuned to the needs of the individual or community receiving care.

In most instances, responsibility for the primary education of the health professional rests with an educational institution such as a university or college. Due to the specific nature of health professions, a close working relationship with health services is required. Clinical work placements are an essential component of health professional education programs. During these placements, students develop their diagnostic, technical, and other clinical skills under appropriate supervision.

Health profession curriculum development and implementation should be a dynamic and constantly evolving process. The health care needs of one community may be quite different to those of another. They are also likely to change over time in ways that may or may not be predictable. A strong connection between education institutions, health services, and the community is essential to ensure current graduating health professionals are well equipped to deliver the health care the community needs and expects.

An understanding of the important role of the community in shaping the health professional curriculum is growing. From early exploration and experimenting with patient participation in developing clinical examination skills (Simpson and House 2002; Towle and Godolphin 2015; Towle et al. 1999; Towle and Weston 2006), through the refinement of understandings of patient-centered care (Barry and Edgman-Levitan 2012; Berntsen et al. 2018; Coylewright et al. 2016; Elwyn et al.

2012, 2014; Ferguson et al. 2013; Martin and Finn 2011; Merlino 2015; Towle et al. 2010), to considerations of the role of the patient in interprofessional collaborative care (Cooper and Spencer-Dawe 2006; Furness et al. 2011; Kvarnström et al. 2012; Pyle et al. 2009; Towle et al. 2014; Towle and Godolphin 2013), there has been a maturing understanding of the importance of a more equitable and balanced relationship between the receiver of care and the giver.

More modern conceptions of public engagement in health profession curricula move away from the somewhat paternalistic and unbalanced power relationships and conceptions of the past (Kilgour 2016; Kvarnström et al. 2012, 2013; Makkar et al. 2018; Nugus et al. 2010, 2018; Regan De Bere and Nunn 2016; Selzer and Charon 1999; Towle et al. 1999) to more equitable and balanced model. Realizing such a model in practice is not without it challenges.

Curriculum Development and Implementation

Although each individual health profession has a unique set of competencies that are required to be achieved by all graduates, there are many common educational considerations across the full range of health professions. A number of factors require consideration and at times, rebalancing of resources and priorities in the development and implementation of curriculum. Firstly, there is a need to ensure that every graduating student has achieved the requisite competence to satisfy the relevant professional accreditation agency and registration body that as a practitioner the graduate will provide safe quality health care. Secondly, for universities and other education providers, there is a need to ensure maintenance of academic standards so as to satisfy the academic requirements of the relevant qualification level. Although the professional requirements of, for example, a graduating nurse will be consistent across all registerable qualifications, universities will have different expectations of graduates of masters degrees as compared with bachelor degrees. Thirdly, for education providers, there is a need to ensure adequate supervision in health service work environments when students are undertaking clinical placement activities. This usually involves a formal arrangement between the education provider and the health service and ideally also includes a positive and collaborative set of relationships between key staff within each institution. Finally, and very importantly, there is a need to ensure that curriculum content, delivery, and learning outcomes meet the health needs and aspirations of the general community as well as the profession.

Challenges of Finding Appropriate Terminology

The issue of terminology regarding public engagement in health care is a complex one. The use of particular terms such as patient, client, consumer, lay person, carer, service user, public, and/or citizen can lead to assumptions about roles, relationships, and hierarchy. It is also important to acknowledge that it is not only the patient or service user who may be involved in public engagement with the heath curriculum.

The roles of care-givers, patient support organizations, and patient advocacy groups are also significant in terms of their impact on patient care and health outcomes (Barr and Elwyn 2016; Haskell and Lord 2017; Regan De Bere and Nunn 2016; Towle and Godolphin 2015).

The phrase "patient engagement" itself has been the subject of scrutiny. Previous descriptions of the patient-health professional relationship included "patient-centered care" and "patient activation," which can be interpreted as viewing the patient in a passive role (Haskell and Lord 2017). Some groups use the term Patient and Public Involvement (PPI) as referring to patients, public, and lay representation. (Regan De Bere and Nunn 2016). The term "public" has been chosen for this chapter where many of all of these terms may apply and is inclusive of all the terms referred to above. Where a particular group is described such as patients or health service clients, then the more specific nomenclature will be used.

Models of Public Engagement

Various models are used to describe the key aspects of public engagement in health profession student education. Some focus on the role of the public in helping students to appreciate patient perspectives and to bridge the gap between theory and practice (Cooper and Spencer-Dawe 2006). Others are built around partnerships where patients work with health professional educators to design and deliver curriculum.

An early paper by Arnstein describes a Ladder of Citizen participation (Arnstein 1969). Making the point the *"there is a critical difference between going through the empty ritual of participation and having the real power needed to affect the outcome of this process"* (p. 216), the author describes a taxonomy of citizen participation. This is captured as a ladder with the lower rungs representing nonparticipation and as the ladder is ascended there are greater degrees of power and control available to the "citizen." The notion of "partnership" while towards the top of the ladder is surpassed by delegated power and ultimately citizen control. While Arnstein's paper is written from the perspective of citizen engagement with public officials and community development, it has some relevance to the contemplation of public engagement in health curriculum.

Echoing some of the earlier thinking by Arnstein and other authors, Towle et al. (2010) proposed a taxonomy to characterize the degree of patient involvement to assist classification of individual initiatives. In attempting to capture a continuum of patient involvement, the "spectrum of involvement" described six levels:

1. Patients create learning materials
2. Volunteer or simulated patients
3. Patients share their experience
4. Patients teach and assess students
5. Patients as equal partners
6. Patients involved in decision making at institutional level

31 Health Profession Curriculum and Public Engagement

Table 1 Examples of public engagement in health profession curriculum

Patient involvement[a]	Examples in health profession education[b]
Create learning materials	Members of the public with chronic illness: Design workshops for students Create patient narratives of their experiences
Act as volunteer or simulated patients	Members of the public act as: Mentors for students Standardized patients
Share experiences	Members of the public are invited to: Participate in surveys Join educational committees
Teach and assess	Members of the public are invited to: Share their experiences of health and illness Provide feedback to students Contribute to clinical assessment grades
Equal partnerships	Members of the public are invited to: Co-create curriculum with academics and clinicians Participate in citizen juries
Involvement in institutional decision making	Institutions establish: Patient/consumer consultative committees Processes for shared curriculum decision making with members of the public Communities of practice for users of health services

[a]Adapted from Towle et al. (2010)
[b]Although presented here as discrete levels, there is a high degree of inter-relation and the educational examples provided will be relevant to more than one mode of patient involvement

together with six attributes each of which might apply to any of the levels: level of active engagement during encounter; duration; patient autonomy, training, and involvement in planning; and institutional commitment to patient involvement. Table 1 provides some examples of public engagement for each of these levels.

At this point it is pertinent to consider the extent to which different models of public engagement deliver any power or control to members of the public in relation to health professional curriculum development. Several different models will be considered below from this perspective.

Public Consultation

Capturing community expectations for the competencies of recently graduated health professions is one method of obtaining insights into the priorities of the public for health curriculum content and/or delivery. It is the case though that public priorities within the community may not match those of educators. Childhood obesity is common and is a significant public health concern. In an attempt to align contemporary medical student child health curriculum with community expectations, parents in the community were invited to share their views on what medical schools should teach (O'Keefe and Coat 2009). The researchers made the implicit assumption that parents also saw childhood obesity in the same light. However, there was great difficulty recruiting sufficient numbers of participants despite exhaustive efforts. Those parents who did participate were more focused on healthy eating and exercise than childhood obesity per se. This recruitment challenge contrasted greatly with the experience of the same research team in a study run shortly afterwards in which parents in the public were invited to share their views on what medical schools should teach students about complementary and alternative medicine (O'Keefe et al. 2009). In the latter instance recruitment proceeded far more smoothly and study participants engaged actively with the topic proposed for investigation.

Public as Expert Advisers on Specific Illness Experiences

Consistent with a patient-centered ethos, individuals with chronic illnesses can be understood to be "experts by experience" in terms of their self-management strategies. When given responsibility for designing and delivering workshops with "power to educate students without the mediation or control of faculty," successful student learning has occurred (Towle and Godolphin 2013, p. 220). In contexts such as this patients are educators, students are learners and co-educators, and doctors support and facilitate the learning process (Bleakley and Bligh 2008).

A further example of success with this approach is provided in an interprofessional Health Mentors program involved users with chronic illnesses (Towle et al. 2014). Members of the public were "experts by experience," acting as mentors for interprofessional student teams. The program handed over *control of the learning to the mentor and their students*" and the faculty role was to support learning (Towle et al. 2014, p. 302). The program was longitudinal, over 16 months, which allowed patients to share their lived experience of chronic illness. Patients appreciated the opportunity to contribute to the students' education, while the students learnt about collaborative patient-centered care. The inclusion of the public voice in developing teaching resources can help overcome the marginalization of users (Kilminster and Fielden 2009).

Public as Partners

One of the central factors in patient-centered care is active involvement in clinical decision making, that is, decisions are guided by the patient's values. This process of shared decision making involves both patient and health professional sharing information and sharing responsibility for the decision that is made (Barry and Edgman-Levitan 2012). Shared decision making can be viewed as engaging the public in the health curriculum, as the focus is on patient agency, rather than the paternalistic model where the health professional decides the best course of action for the patient (Elwyn et al. 2012). One aspect of this agency is recognition of the patient as expert in regard to the lived experience of their health issues (Moreau et al. 2012). A collaborative learning approach to support patient learning approached learning as a social phenomenon with patients involved as equals with health professionals (Myron et al. 2018). As the program developed participants became peers rather than separate groups defined by professions or patient status.

An extension of a co-production model is collaborative deliberation which is based on respecting patient autonomy and agency and supporting patients in considering alternative options when decision making (Elwyn et al. 2014). The model is underpinned by constructive engagement based on respectful and empathic approach to communication as a fundamental part of good deliberation.

Sociocultural Theories and Public Engagement

The use of sociocultural theories such as activity theory allow public engagement to be analyzed as an activity system. Activity theory provides a theoretical framework to analyze learning and change in context, by focusing on factors such as rules, division of labor and the tools or artifacts used (Engeström 1987; Engeström 2001, 2004). One of the powerful aspects of applying activity theory to public engagement with the health curriculum is the ability to explore contradictions, for instance, roles for individuals or groups which are not supported by appropriate tools (Regan De Bere and Nunn 2016). For example, it has been proposed that medical students learn about a patient-centered approach from doctors, than from the patients themselves (Bleakley and Bligh 2008), and this could be extrapolated to other health professions. The application of activity theory in response to this proposal can explore this contradiction and reconceptualize the transformation of professional centered health care to patient-centered health care where the user has an active rather than passive role (Regan De Bere and Nunn 2016).

An interesting corollary is where the public may look to increase their personal agency in selecting health care options by working across different health care providers and modalities including complementary and alternative medicines (O'Keefe and Coat 2010).

Sociocultural theories such as situated learning have been used as a lens to explore how medical students learned "with," not only "about" service users (Rees et al. 2007). In situated learning the focus is on legitimate peripheral participation where participants progress from peripheral to full participation within the community of practice. This process includes issues of power and identity, specifically whether the service user role was passive or active. The study revealed that service users had various roles, including teacher, patient, and learner, and active participation occurred in the educational setting and passive participation in the clinical environment. Both students and service users were trying to move to full participation in the community of medical practice. Viewing patients as educators can cause tension in terms of traditional roles of power and expertise by health professionals. There can be challenges for clinical teachers in relation to giving up control of content and delivery of the curriculum.

One approach to empowering patients is to encourage them to reconstruct their experiences by writing a patient narrative. These narratives can be powerful tools to engage with the patient's lived experience of their illness and clarify what matters to them (Kilgour 2016). These narratives can be incorporated into the health professional curriculum and used as a stimulus for reflection by students on the power differentials between the public and health professions. Patient narratives can be used in health professional education to encourage empathy and move away from conceptualizing the patient as a medical or health problem (Bleakley 2005; Kilgour 2016).

Limitations of Public Engagement

When accessing public expertise, there is a need to clarify whether this is as an expert in their disease, their lived experience as a patient, or their lay (as outside the health professions) viewpoint. There can be a paradox where the service users become integrated into the team to such an extent that they are no longer viewed as patients and are subject to "*a process of role blurring which can shift the practice of involvement away from the rationale for involving them in the first place*" (Martin and Finn 2011, p. 163).

Questions of what constitutes adequate or appropriate representation are also relevant. "Who" is the public, how many patient perspectives should be accessed, and what are the optimal methods of accessing this resource? If only certain sectors of the public are included, there is a risk of generalizing their experiences to all patients if not managed carefully. More powerful voices may be more likely to be heard and influence educational activities (Rowland and Kumagai 2018).

The important issue of finding the "right" patients to consult can be analyzed by looking at what sort of knowledge they can contribute. According to Williamson (2007), doctors have three types of knowledge: (1) personal, (2) specialty, and (3) ethics and values. An individual doctor may integrate all three types of knowledge. However, a patient may only have one type of knowledge. For example, an individual patient may have personal expert knowledge of their own illness, while patient advocates may be able to explain service user perspectives on issues such as confidentiality and informed consent.

A distinction is made by Mooney and Blackwell (2004) between members of the public participating in citizen juries and health consumers, with the former having the possibility of broader vision than health care consumers who may be constrained by specific personal experiences or needs. Such constraints may then flavor the advice provided, in this particular case to the allocation of health care resources. The authors go on to suggest that citizens may be in a stronger position to choose the issues for which they wish their preferences to be counted thereby expressing "preferences for preferences" (p. 255).

Much less attention has been given to questions of accountability within models of public engagement in health profession education. That is does the public have true power in the relationship or can professional "veto" can be exercised in relation to any of the activities listed above.

Public Engagement in the Age of the Internet

Although the Internet is no longer new, the extent to which our everyday activities depend at least in part on digital connectivity is rapidly evolving and increasing. Recognizing the emerging digital age as a powerful influence of public health information has seen a growing literature and the establishment of journals specifically focused on, for example, medical Internet research (J Medical Internet Research, www.jmir.org). There have been long standing calls for the inclusion of the Internet as part of the larger health communication system noting a less regulated and more transactional quality of interaction with digital information (Cline and Haynes 2001). It is noted that new technologies and approaches to communicating information will significantly affect both users and providers of information, shaping what information is available, how it is provided, and who has access (Smith and Dumant 2009). (An excellent example of training and resources for public involvement can be found at https://www.imperial.ac.uk/patient-experience-research-cen tre/ppi/ppi-training/) Improving health literacy across all sectors of the public is a key focus of contemporary health policy (De Rosa and Stribling 2018). These changes are not small and will likely dramatically change the landscape with a resulting rethink of public engagement in health profession curriculum.

Understandably, members of the public look to maximize their health care options and the Internet enables this. If community is looking to increase health care options, health care professionals need to guide and be a trusted advisor. Reassuringly for health professions, this appears to be the current trend in health. Evidence is emerging that although members of the public are increasingly turning to the Internet for information with increasingly sophisticated digital literacy skills, health care professionals are still viewed as important and relevant trusted advisors (Lee et al. 2017; Briones 2015). Future health professionals will need skills in providing advice on choices in relation to safety and efficacy when range of options may come from the Internet. Curriculum developers will need to contemplate ways of preparing future graduates to respond to increasingly diverse requests for guidance and a greater desire by the public to be actively involved in their health care.

Increasingly the general public will have high levels of digital literacy and come to the health care professional not for knowledge and content, but for advice about managing this data. Co-production is seen as active involvement from both patients and health professionals and is based on the interconnectedness of community, healthcare system, professionals, and patients (Haskell and Lord 2017). The aim is to blur "*the lines between clinic and community and encouraging partnerships that take into account the lived reality of all sides*" (Haskell and Lord 2017, p. 103). "E-patients" who use the Internet as a resource for health information sometimes request better care and may become collaborators and advisors for health professionals (Ferguson 2007).

The early sections of this chapter addressed the various ways in which the public may engage in health profession curriculum. It could be argued that each of these modes retained a significant proportion of power and control for the health profession. There is clearly a need to align emerging health issues as identified by education providers with public perceptions and concerns as community may have different answers to problems or place different emphases on the value of solutions. There is a need also to find ways to characterize community expertise and review pathways for public engagement, both existing and emerging.

Conclusion

The digital age and associated empowerment of the public, where the health professional is no longer the gate keeper of information, may represent a true disrupter of current approaches to public engagement in health profession curriculum. The balance of power within the pubic-professional relationship may truly shift to a more neutral zone. What might this mean for the curriculum going forward? It is likely (and not a bad thing) that future health professionals will need: skills in nonjudgemental appreciative enquiry and skillful redirection where unsafe suggestions are raised; high levels of digital literacy; and a strong commitment to community engagement. The pace of change is dramatic and therein lies probably the biggest challenge for health profession curriculum – to evolve quickly. Establishing active partnerships with members of the public would seem the most sensible way forward.

Cross-References

▶ Communities of Practice and Medical Education
▶ Focus on Theory: Emotions and Learning
▶ Future of Health Professions Education Curricula

References

Arnstein SR. A ladder of citizen participation. J Am Plan Assoc. 1969;35(4):216–24.
Barr PJ, Elwyn G. Measurement challenges in shared decision making: putting the 'patient' in patient-reported measures. Health Expect. 2016;19(5):993–1001. https://doi.org/10.1111/hex. 12380.
Barry MJ, Edgman-Levitan S. Shared decision making – the pinnacle of patient-centered care. N Engl J Med. 2012;366:780. https://doi.org/10.1056/NEJMp1109283.
Berntsen G, Høyem A, Lettrem I, Ruland C, Rumpsfeld M, Gammon D. A person-centered integrated care quality framework, based on a qualitative study of patients' evaluation of care in light of chronic care ideals. BMC Health Serv Res. 2018;18(1):479. https://doi.org/10.1186/s12913-018-3246-z.
Bleakley A. Stories as data, data as stories: making sense of narrative inquiry in clinical education∗. Med Educ. 2005;39(5):534–40. https://doi.org/10.1111/j.1365-2929.2005.02126.x.
Bleakley A, Bligh J. Students learning from patients: let's get real in medical education. Adv Health Sci Educ Theory Pract. 2008;13(1):89–107. https://doi.org/10.1007/s10459-006-9028-0.
Briones R. Harnessing the web: how e-health and e-literacy impact young adults' perceptions of online health information. Medicine 2.0. 2015;4:e5.

Cline RJW, Haynes KM. Consumer health information seeking on the Internet: the state of the art. Health Educ Res. 2001;16:671–92.

Cooper H, Spencer-Dawe E. Involving service users in interprofessional education narrowing the gap between theory and practice. J Interprof Care. 2006;20(6):603–17.

Coylewright M, Palmer R, O'Neill ES, Robb JF, Fried TR. Patient-defined goals for the treatment of severe aortic stenosis: a qualitative analysis. Health Expect. 2016;19(5):1036–43. https://doi.org/10.1111/hex.12393.

De Rosa AP, Stribling JC. A case report of health seminars supporting patient education, engagement and health literacy. J Consum Health Internet. 2018;22:238–43. https://doi.org/10.1080/15398285.2018.1513269.

Elwyn G, Frosch D, Thomson R, Joseph-Williams N, Lloyd A, Kinnersley P, . . . Barry M. Shared decision making: a model for clinical practice. J Gen Intern Med. 2012;27(10):1361–7. https://doi.org/10.1007/s11606-012-2077-6.

Elwyn G, Lloyd A, May C, van der Weijden T, Stiggelbout A, Edwards A, . . . Epstein R. Collaborative deliberation: a model for patient care. Patient Educ Couns. 2014;97(2):158–64. https://doi.org/10.1016/j.pec.2014.07.027.

Engeström Y. Learning by expanding: an activity-theoretical approach to developmental research. Helsinki: Orienta-Konsultit; 1987.

Engeström Y. Expansive learning at work: toward an activity theoretical reconceptualization. J Educ Work. 2001;14(1):133–56. https://doi.org/10.1080/13639080020028747.

Engeström Y. New forms of learning in co-configuration work. J Work Learn. 2004;16(1/2):11–21. https://doi.org/10.1108/13665620410521477.

Ferguson T. E-patients: how they can help us heal healthcare. 2007. http://www.e-patients.net

Ferguson L, Ward H, Card S, Sheppard S, McMurtry J. Putting the 'patient' back into patient-centred care: an education perspective. Nurse Educ Pract. 2013;13(4):283–7. https://doi.org/10.1016/j.nepr.2013.03.016.

Furness PJ, Armitage H, Pitt R. An evaluation of practice-based interprofessional education initiatives involving service users. J Interprof Care. 2011;25(1):46–52. https://doi.org/10.3109/13561820.2010.497748.

Haskell H, Lord T. Patients and Families as Coproducers of Safe and Reliable Outcomes. In: Sanchez J., Barach P., Johnson J., Jacobs J. (eds) Surgical Patient Care. 2017 Springer, Cham. https://doi.org/10.1007/978-3-319-44010-1_8.

Kilgour J. Power of the patient voice in medical education. Clin Teach. 2016;13(6):451–3. https://doi.org/10.1111/tct.12487.

Kilminster S, Fielden S. Working with the patient voice: developing teaching resources for interprofessional education. Clin Teach. 2009;6(4):265–8. https://doi.org/10.1111/j.1743-498X.2009.00325.x.

Kvarnström S, Hedberg B, Cedersund E. The dual faces of service user participation: implications for empowerment processes in interprofessional practice. J Soc Work. 2012;13(3):287–307.

Kvarnström S, Hedberg B, Cedersund E. The dual faces of service user participation: implications for empowerment processes in interprofessional practice. J Soc Work. 2013;13(3):287–307. https://doi.org/10.1177/1468017311433234.

Lee K, Hoti K, Hughes JD, Emmerton L. Dr Google is here to stay but health care professionals are still valued: an analysis of health care consumers' Internet navigation support preferences. J Med Internet Res. 2017;19:e210.

Makkar N, Jain K, Siddharth V, Sarkar S. Patient involvement in decision-making: an important parameter for better patient experience – an observational study (STROBE compliant). J Patient Exp. 2018;6(3):231–7. https://doi.org/10.1177/2374373518790043.

Martin GP, Finn R. Patients as team members: opportunities, challenges and paradoxes of including patients in multi-professional healthcare teams. Sociol Health Illn. 2011;33(7):1050–65. https://doi.org/10.1111/j.1467-9566.2011.01356.x.

Merlino J. Making the patient paramount. In: Wartman SA, editor. The transformation of academic health centers. Boston: Academic; 2015. p. 213–9.

Mooney G, Blackwell S. Whose health services is it anyway? Community values in healthcare. Med J Aust. 2004;180:76–8.

Moreau A, Carol L, Dedianne MC, Dupraz C, Perdrix C, Lainé X, Souweine G. What perceptions do patients have of decision making (DM)? Toward an integrative patient-centered care model. A qualitative study using focus-group interviews. Patient Educ Couns. 2012;87(2):206–11. https://doi.org/10.1016/j.pec.2011.08.010.

Myron R, French C, Sullivan P, Sathyamoorthy G, Barlow J, Pomeroy L. Professionals learning together with patients: an exploratory study of a collaborative learning Fellowship Programme for Healthcare Improvement. J Interprof Care. 2018;32(3):257–65. https://doi.org/10.1080/13561820.2017.1392935.

Nugus P, Greenfield D, Travaglia J, Westbrook J, Braithwaite J. How and where clinicians exercise power: interprofessional relations in health care. Soc Sci Med. 2010;71(5):898–909. https://doi.org/10.1016/j.socscimed.2010.05.029.

Nugus P, Ranmuthugala G, Travaglia J, Greenfield D, Lamothe J, Hogden A, ... Braithwaite J. Advancing interprofessional theory: deliberative democracy as a participatory research antidote to power differentials in aged care. J Interprofessional Educ Pract. 2018. https://doi.org/10.1016/j.xjep.2018.09.005.

O'Keefe M, Coat S. Consulting parents on childhood obesity and implications for medical student learning. J Paediatr Child H 2009;45(10):573–576.

O'Keefe M, Coat S. Increasing health-care options: The perspectives of parents who use complementary and alternative medicines. J Paediatr Child H 2010;46(6):296–300.

O'Keefe M, Coat S, Jones A. The medical education priorities of parents who use complementary and alternative medicine. Complementary Health Practice Review 2009;14(2):70–83.

Pyle NR, Arthur N, Hurlock D. Service user positioning in interprofessional practice. J Interprof Care. 2009;23(5):531–3. https://doi.org/10.1080/13561820802565551.

Rees CE, Knight LV, Wilkinson CE. "User involvement is a sine qua non, almost, in medical education": learning with rather than just about health and social care service users. Adv Health Sci Educ. 2007;12(3):359–90. https://doi.org/10.1007/s10459-006-9007-5.

Regan De Bere S, Nunn S. Towards a pedagogy for patient and public involvement in medical education. Med Educ. 2016;50(1):79–92. https://doi.org/10.1111/medu.12880.

Rowland P, Kumagai AK. Dilemmas of representation: patient engagement in health profession education. Acad Med. 2018;93:869–73.

Selzer R, Charon R. Stories for a humanistic medicine. Acad Med. 1999;74(1):42.

Simpson EL, House AO. Involving users in the delivery and evaluation of mental health services: systematic review. BMJ. 2002;325:1265. https://doi.org/10.1136/bmj.325.7375.1265.

Smith S, Dumant M. The state of consumer health information: an overview. Health Inf Libr J. 2009;26:260–78.

Towle A, Godolphin W. Patients as educators: interprofessional learning for patient-centred care. Med Teach. 2013;35(3):219–25. https://doi.org/10.3109/0142159X.2012.737966.

Towle A, Godolphin W. Patients as teachers: promoting their authentic and autonomous voices. Clin Teach. 2015;12(3):149–54. https://doi.org/10.1111/tct.12400.

Towle A, Weston W. Patient's voice in health professional education. Patient Educ Couns. 2006;63(1):1–2. https://doi.org/10.1016/j.pec.2006.08.008.

Towle A, Greenhalgh T, Gambrill J, Godolphin W. Framework for teaching and learning informed shared decision making. BMJ. 1999;319(7212):766.

Towle A, Bainbridge L, Godolphin W, Katz A, Kline C, Lown B, ... Thistlethwaite J. Active patient involvement in the education of health professionals. Med Educ. 2010;44(1):64–74. https://doi.org/10.1111/j.1365-2923.2009.03530.x.

Towle A, Brown H, Hofley C, Kerston RP, Lyons H, Walsh C. The expert patient as teacher: an interprofessional health mentors programme. Clin Teach. 2014;11(4):301–6. https://doi.org/10.1111/tct.12222.

Williamson C. How do we find the right patients to consult? Qual Prim Care. 2007;15(4):195–9.

Teaching and Learning Ethics in Healthcare

32

Selena Knight and Andrew Papanikitas

Contents

Introduction	588
Part 1: Theory	591
What Is the Point of Ethics in Healthcare Curriculum?	591
The Syllabus: What Should Be Taught?	593
Part 2: Practice	595
What Format Should Be Used for Teaching?	595
When Should Ethics Be Taught and Learned?	597
Who Should Teach Ethics?	598
Should Ethics Be Assessed and how?	599
Part 3: Challenges for Ethics Education	600
Concluding Thoughts	601
Key Points	602
Cross-References	603
References	603

Abstract

Ethical issues arise throughout healthcare, and as such ethics teaching has long-standing been an important component of education for healthcare professionals. While much of the way healthcare professionals have "learned" ethics has been informal, increasingly ethics has been formally integrated into the training programs for such healthcare professionals during their training and beyond. Ethics differs significantly from other components of training, for example, being considered more subjective and encompassing complex moral, philosophical, and personal concepts. While lending itself to interesting and stimulating

---

S. Knight (✉)
School of Population Health and Environmental Sciences, King's College London, London, UK
e-mail: selena.e.knight@gmail.com

A. Papanikitas
Nuffield Department of Primary Care Health Sciences, University of Oxford, Oxford, UK
e-mail: andrew.papanikitas@phc.ox.ac.uk

© Springer Nature Singapore Pte Ltd. 2023
D. Nestel et al. (eds.), *Clinical Education for the Health Professions*,
https://doi.org/10.1007/978-981-15-3344-0_43

discussion, ethics can pose challenges for those delivering such education. How such a subject should be taught, when, in what format, and by whom are all important considerations. The purpose and modes of assessment of such a topic are controversial and debated, not least because of a lack of consensus about what the aims of ethics education should be.

This chapter aims to address some of these questions by considering educational theory with a broader discussion of how medical ethics education is and how it ought to be. We consider the theory of ethics education, the practicalities that should be considered in designing and delivering ethics education programs, and finally the challenges faced by ethics educators. We articulate the key issues arising in the phenomenon of ethics education, considering teacher, learner, and higher education institution in a real-world context.

Keywords

Ethics · Interprofessional learning · Assessment · Curriculum

Introduction

In this chapter we reflect on how ethics is, and ought to be, taught and learned in healthcare. There is much about healthcare and medicine that generates ethical issues: a power differential between healthcare professional, patient, and employer; disagreements stemming from culture and diversity; divergent concepts of health; and even the definition of goodness (among others). Healthcare professionals (HCPs) bring their own values to the workplace and are subject to many professional duties – negotiated locally and internationally. There may be circumstances in which these values conflict, giving rise to ethical challenges. The medical profession in particular also carries considerable historical "baggage" – not least the involvement of medical professionals in a number of systematic human rights atrocities in the twentieth century.

Medical ethics is a well-established field. Educational texts of medical ethics are too numerous to cite, whether general or specific to a particular specialty or profession. Similarly, medical ethics (often overlapping with law and professionalism) is found in the formal curricula and codes of practice of medical schools, postgraduate training bodies, and other HCP professional organizations in the West. As examples, the United Kingdom's (UK) General Medical Council (GMC) and Nursing and Midwifery Council (NMC) both are explicit in including ethical principles in their professional codes of practice, as well as requiring that higher education institutions (HEIs) include the subject in teaching (General Medical Council 2013; Nursing and Midwifery Council 2018). This demonstrates the importance attributed by regulators to ensuring HCPs meet not only their professional but also moral and ethical obligations to patients.

Such informal (professional enculturation) and formal (defined by regulator) curricula effectively mandate the inclusion of ethics in healthcare education, in turn requiring that those involved in designing and delivering education to HCPs are appropriately equipped to do so. As with any educationally necessary topic, due consideration must therefore be given to the content of ethics education (syllabus) but also the manner in which it is taught and learned (curriculum). We use curriculum here to refer to a single document or single context, specialty, or profession, and curricula as the plural for reference to multiple distinct contexts such as different medical specialties or healthcare professions. Curricular is used as an adjective to relate to a single curriculum or plural curricula, for example, in discussing curricular practices or issues. In spite of the wealth of literature on ethics as a topic, there is much less on ethics *education* per se. This is reflected in curricular emphases on good ideas and good clinicians, often focusing on professionalism, rather than on how these two concepts should connect. Emmerich comments on a (mistaken) tendency in bioethics to conflate healthcare professionals with applied philosophers and to conflate applied philosophy with the moral and ethical practices embedded within modern medical culture (Emmerich 2013). What should be taught and learned, how should it be taught and learned, and whom should it be taught and learned by? Our perspective (as authors) is mainly (though not exclusively) UK-centric and predominantly medical. While we have considered some other professional and geographical contexts, we hope that readers will engage with the chapter in ways that foster cross-cultural and interprofessional learning.

The provision of ethics education for HCPs varies significantly, both between professions and specialties, and over the course of a career. Recently there has been a concerted effort to include ethics in undergraduate curricula for clinical degrees. We use the term "undergraduate" loosely here to refer to any degree or diploma qualifying a student to enter a healthcare profession. For doctors in the UK as an example, ethics has been a compulsory part of the undergraduate curriculum since 1993, originally mandated by the GMC with subsequent development and revision of a *"Consensus statement by teachers of medical ethics and law"* by the Institute of Medical Ethics (IME) (Consensus statement 1998; Stirrat et al. 2010; Institute of Medical Ethics 2019). Internationally, ethics education has an important place within medical training, with UNESCO adopting the Universal Declaration of Bioethics and Human Rights and subsequent development of a declaration in a Bioethics Core Curriculum adopted by its many member states (United Nations Educational, Scientific and Cultural Organization 2016). This ostensible importance does not mean medical schools have a common approach to its inclusion or status within taught curricula. Even UK medical schools vary widely in how ethics is manifest in their internal curricular documents, taught, and assessed (Brooks and Bell 2017). For other HCPs such as nurses, midwives, physiotherapists, and pharmacists, the provision of ethics education varies even more widely than for doctors. While allied healthcare professional bodies in the Anglo-American West generally incorporate ethics within their guidelines and codes of practice (Nursing and Midwifery Council 2018; Chartered Society of Physiotherapy 2011; Royal Pharmaceutical Society of Great Britain 2018), ethics education does not seem as pervasive as it does for doctors in undergraduate and postgraduate curricula (Hoskins et al. 2018).

Postgraduate medical ethics education seems even less systematic than undergraduate educational settings. In one way this makes perfect sense: qualified HCPs have to balance training and continuous education with full-time jobs and service commitments. It is easier for HCPs and their employers to justify training that relates to everyday tasks and the specific educational needs relating to them – for example, a prescribing course for newly qualified doctors, or an emphasis on areas considered necessary for good governance or by regulatory bodies such as confidentiality and data security (Sokol 2010). Additionally, the learning needs in relation to ethics will vary significantly between HCPs at different stages of their career, and in different specialties with implications for how much, or little, ethics is deemed to be necessary for inclusion (either formally or informally) in postgraduate training. Doctors of different specialties inevitably experience different mixes of ethical issues which can be framed in different ways (Diekema and Shugerman 1997). Some medical specialties have been traditionally identified with an interest in ethics. Examples in the UK include general practice (family medicine) (Misselbrook 2012) and palliative care, where an interest in ethics derives from holistic, psychosocial elements of practice being as important as (if not more important than) biotechnical ones (Reeve 2010). In our own analyses of UK postgraduate medical curricula we find that ethics can be extensive for specialties such as palliative care and general practice. However, in others (such as surgery or pathology in the UK) the provision of ethics education and inclusion in postgraduate training is far less represented in formal curricular documents. Qualified HCPs have a stake in ethical questions with potential professional ramifications when issues are shared or disagreements are discussed. This carries implications in terms of if and how ethics education is most appropriately and effectively delivered at a postgraduate level (Roberts et al. 2005).

A significant portion of ethics "learning" for both doctors and other HCPs has been suggested to arise from day-to-day encounters within the clinical setting and the daily realities of healthcare work. This has been described as the "hidden curriculum" (Hafferty and Franks 1994), which refers to the impact on professionalism which can arise from exposure to informal factors, such as poor role models, or adverse organizational or environmental factors. Hafferty and Franks argued that the hidden curriculum had the potential to subvert what had been taught on formal curricula, and that formal teaching accordingly needed to take account of daily realities of practice. Cribb and Bignold take a more embodied view of the hidden curriculum, using the tension between "objectifying" and "humanizing" orientations of medical culture as a tool to promote reflexivity in research and curricular reform (Cribb and Bignold 1999). A related phenomenon is moral distress, described by Morley et al. as a combination of (Brooks and Bell 2017) the experience of a moral event, (Carresse et al., 2015) the experience of "psychological distress," and (Charon and Fox 1995) a direct causal relation between (Brooks and Bell 2017) and (Carresse et al. 2015) together (Morley et al. 2019). The concept was introduced to nursing by Jameton, who defined it as arising, "when one knows the right thing to do, but institutional constraints make it nearly impossible to pursue the right course of action" (Jameton 1984). Ethics education consequently needs to address the issue of good practice being potentially difficult, unpopular, and sometimes even impossible and (as far as possible) prepare learners for this.

This chapter attempts to merge some educational theory with a discussion of how medical ethics education is and how it ought to be. We first consider the theory behind ethics education, discussing the aims of ethics education and what might be taught. Second, the practicalities of ethics education are discussed, in particular what formats should be used for ethics teaching, when it should be taught, who should teach it, and how it might be formally assessed. Finally, challenges to providing ethics education are outlined with recommendations for overcoming these. It is hoped this chapter will support those delivering ethics education to all HCPs to be able to do so with confidence and in an effective manner.

Part 1: Theory

What Is the Point of Ethics in Healthcare Curriculum?

Ethics is generally viewed as an important component of training for HCPs, with many potential benefits. However, the challenges faced in the provision of ethics education and the lack of a substantial body of empirical evidence regarding its tangible benefits mean there is a lack of consensus about what the specific aims of ethics teaching should be (Carresse et al. 2015). Two main aims have been proposed – first the development of virtuous practitioners and second the teaching of moral reasoning skills (Carresse et al. 2015; Papanikitas and Spicer 2018).

The first proposed aim is that ethics education should strive to create virtuous practitioners, by enabling students to learn how to display and practice virtuous characteristics such as compassion, humility, and honesty (Freeman and Wilson 1994; Pellegrino and Thomasma 1993; Shelton 1999). This approach has been proposed as a way of addressing "moral erosion" (referring to "a gradual erosion of ethical behaviour that occurs in individuals below their level of awareness" (Kleinman 2006)), which healthcare students experience as they progress through their careers and are exposed to increasing professional and ethical challenges (Goldie 2004). The main criticism of a virtue-orientated aim for ethics education is that virtues are part of a person's pre-existing personality or character, which would be selected at the entry point to a training program and cannot easily be "taught" (Carresse et al. 2015). Furthermore, it is unclear how this might be taught, for example, where a student might intrinsically not possess such character traits and thus acquisition of virtues through education might be considered "fake" or disingenuous.

The second proposed aim of teaching medical ethics, which is more commonly focused on curriculum design, is that it should provide HCPs with a set of skills for ethical analysis and decision-making (Eckles et al. 2005). Rather than focusing on character development, the role of ethics education is to equip HCPs with skills, tools, and practical wisdom to be able to identify, prevent, and manage ethical dilemmas faced in practice (Miles et al. 1989; Carresse et al. 2015). This has the appeal of often being considered more achievable, given that it does not rely on the underlying personality and character of the student (which might be pre-determined and harder to mold or alter through educational means) and also that it might be more tangibly taught and assessed.

The above aims, virtue and/or skills, are arguable goods, but their inclusion in educational policy or in the teaching offerings of HEIs requires a more nuanced kind of justification than thinking skills and virtue. This is because education takes place in a material world where resources such as time, space, and money are necessary to allow the education to occur. Education provision may be broadly orientated toward different purposes and, therefore, toward different kinds of purchasers – for example, whoever is putting the resources into paying for teacher-time or making a classroom available. Eisner argued that there are five basic orientations to a curriculum (Eisner 1985). All these orientations have a bearing on ethics education and point to different kinds of markets:

1. An orientation toward the development of *cognitive processes* emphasizes the belief that curriculum and teaching strategy should foster the student's ability to think and reason.
2. *Academic rationalism* argues that the function of education is to foster the intellectual growth of students in those subject matters most worthy of study.
3. *Personal relevance* emphasizes the primacy of personal meaning for the learner and the educator's responsibility to make such meaning possible.
4. *Social adaptation and social reconstruction* collectively are an orientation that derives its aims and content from an analysis of the society that education is designed to serve. Social adaptation aims to prepare learners to meet society's ostensible needs. Social reconstruction aims at learners who will recognize and improve upon the deficiencies in society.
5. *Curriculum as technology* is an orientation that conceives of curriculum planning as a technical undertaking, relating means to ends and standards that have already been formulated.

We suggest that orientation toward cognitive processes, academic rationalism, and personal relevance largely favors a "retail market" – students have potential interests in the self-development, credentialing, or social advantage that education implies. By contrast, social adaptation/reconstruction and curriculum as technology largely favor the institutional/industrial purchaser. This, in effect, represents a divide between "education as personal flourishing" and "education to shape the learner for a function in society." Papanikitas argues that the purpose of ethics education in medicine is the key to the justification for resources invested in it whether this is the cost of venues, teachers, and learning materials, or the investment of time by learners or in voluntary educational activities (Papanikitas 2018).

While many view ethics education as an important and beneficial endeavor, the need for its inclusion in training for HCPs is not universally agreed. Those arguing that teaching philosophical ethics to clinicians is unnecessary essentially follow two lines of argument: the first is that doctors and other HCPs need only follow the ethical consensus negotiated in whichever country they practice, namely following the law, other secondary legislation, and professional codes of practice. In other words, if they know the rules and follow the rules, then that is all that they need to do.

They should not attempt to second-guess societal norms, at least not at the point of care (Savulescu 2006). The second line of argument is that ethics is "common sense" and will take care of itself. A more recent variation of this follows a misinterpretation of Adam Smith in *The wealth of nations*, namely that any self-interested member of the marketplace will behave in a fair and considerate manner in order that they retain the custom of their clients and that rules and ethical principles are therefore unnecessary constraints upon market forces (Papanikitas 2018).

One difficulty encountered by proponents of ethics education is the distinct lack of empirical evidence regarding the tangible benefits of teaching ethics, in terms of benefits experienced both by HCPs (e.g., better physician performance) and by patients (e.g., improved patient outcomes) (Carresse et al. 2015; Siegler 2001; Sokol 2016). One reason for this is that there are significant challenges encountered in evaluating and assessing ethics in the educational context, described in more detail later in this chapter. While a close and important relationship between medical ethics teaching and professionalism is often described, this has not been demonstrated empirically (Carresse et al. 2015). The lack of evidence as to either the benefits of ethics education to patients, or the best elements of education with respect to curriculum, pedagogical approaches, or assessment evaluation, risks a lack of justification for the resources needed. Where there is no rigorous justification for a particular set of educational tools, there is little to prevent educational institutions and learners alike defaulting to the easiest and least costly approach: whether in terms of money, time, or political expediency.

The Syllabus: What Should Be Taught?

Depending on what one deems the aims of ethics education to be, views differ as to what ought to actually be taught as part of an ethics syllabus. There is a lack of consensus and evidence as to whether ethics education should focus on taking a knowledge-based, theoretical-based, or skills-based approach (Hoskins et al. 2018).

A knowledge-based teaching approach prioritizes certain ethical "topics" which are almost universally taught as part of most ethics education programs (e.g., consent, confidentiality, end-of-life decision-making). The teaching of such topics often overlaps with that of other areas such as medical law or professionalism, and so commonly entails simply delivering facts such as current law and prevailing moral custom, rather than exploring a deeper more philosophical approach. This might be necessary in order to provide a foundation of knowledge to which HCPs can refer to, particularly given that at early stages of an HCP's training they are likely to be less autonomous in their clinical practice. This may justify ethics education focusing on a more knowledge-based foundation, as more complex ethical dilemmas might be predominantly addressed by more senior HCPs (Papanikitas and Spicer 2018). However, a legalistic (rule- and guideline-based) approach such as this does not necessarily prepare HCPs for decisions arising when law and policy need not apply, when law and policy are in conflict with other law or policy, and in other situations where there might be other complicating factors.

Consequently, formal ethics education (particularly undergraduate medical school ethics teaching programs) has often additionally adopted a theoretical-based approach, including teaching of moral theories and frameworks. In the Anglo-American setting, ethical approaches touched upon might include deontology, virtues, consequentialism, and contractarianism – in essence the self-same ethical approaches that might underlie anglophone society itself. Over the last 50 years, frameworks have been taught as a way to recognize and reconcile conflicting values and duties. Beauchamp and Childress' Four Principles, for example, frame ethical decisions in terms of beneficence (doing good), non-maleficence (avoiding causing harm), respecting autonomy, and justice (treating equals equally and unequals unequally according to the morally relevant difference) (Hoskins et al. 2018). Another is the ethical grid of Ziegler, Winslade, and Jonsen, which frames ethical decisions in terms of self-explanatory clinical indications, patient preference, quality of life, and contextual features (Jonsen et al. 2010). While frameworks can avoid the need for the teaching of more in-depth philosophical approaches, the focus on them has been criticized because they can be used in a superficial and simplistic manner, and principles or quadrants are prima facie – each is action-guiding unless there is a stronger argument under a different heading. These approaches are best taught as discovery tools, ways of identifying relevant facts, and values leading to the question of what is the right thing to do.

Recently there have been calls for ethics education to help students develop specific and sophisticated moral reasoning skills and behaviors (Hoskins et al. 2018), with significant emphasis on character development (Siegler 2001). This is in part because discrepancies continue to arise between students' knowledge and ability to embody ethical knowledge, skills, and attitudes in practice. For example, while medical students may self-report having good knowledge of ethical topics, in many circumstances they still feel unable to take the morally right course of action (Kong and Knight 2017). Other studies have found that HCPs can report confidence in managing ethical problems and behaving ethically but in fact on evaluation have low overall levels of ethics knowledge (Hoskins et al. 2018). This demonstrates that a combined and multidimensional approach to ethics education is necessary in order to equip future HCPs with knowledge, skills, and behaviors to be able to address dilemmas in practice. In their guide to ethics and law in the undergraduate curriculum, Dowie and Martin use the acronym "GRAPHIC" as a framework for course organization (Dowie and Martin 2011):

- Learning experiences allied to **G**roup working.
- Opportunities for facilitated **R**eflection on learning.
- Coupling of **A**wareness/analysis in ethico-legal reasoning.
- An emphasis on **P**rofessional ethics.
- Attention to the **H**idden curriculum.
- **I**ntegration of ethics and law together, as well as horizontally across specialties. And also, vertically throughout the undergraduate curriculum.
- **C**ontextual learning and assessment that is authentic to clinical situation, and connects with students' own experiences in clinical settings.

Formal curricula are policy documents produced by educational bodies that mandate certain educational syllabus content or modes of learning. These should be distinguished from a number of consensus documents on what medical students and other HCPs should learn about medical ethics and law. Such consensus documents may originate in a conference or organization of teachers, often in consultation with the organizations that produce policy. A key example in the UK is the Institute of Medical Ethics (IME). The IME is a membership organization comprising teachers of and postgraduate researchers in Bioethics, and in recent years produced a "Core Curriculum for Undergraduate Medical Ethics and Law" in 2019, and makes recommendations as to which topics form "the basic elements of an ethics and law education that will prepare students for their first years as a doctor" (Institute of Medical Ethics 2019). However, this document and previous iteration of it going back to 1998 have not necessarily translated into practice, with nearly half of UK medical students still not being taught using discrete defined ethics components with specified ethics learning objectives (Brooks and Bell 2017). Similarly, at a postgraduate level, while each medical specialty in the UK has its own syllabus which almost universally includes ethical topics, the format and the delivery vary significantly, and topics which are included within the syllabus may never formally be taught to trainees in practice. Two core issues are first how accessible is the curriculum to learners, and second how relevant is its content. One study, for example, found that HCPs working in commissioning, while often recalling receiving ethics teaching in their training, describe the topics taught as not being relevant or adequately equipping them for these additional roles (Knight et al. 2020). It may be that those roles were beyond the scope of their training, in which case supplementary education may be helpful.

There are potential benefits to having a defined and institutionally endorsed syllabus for ethics education – consistency of teaching, more consistent and reproducible methods of teaching evaluation, and potential "standardization" which can enable data collection for empirical research into the effectiveness of ethics education. However, the differing emphasis and importance which is placed on ethics education at different career stages and between different specialties and professions makes it unlikely that a universal ethics syllabus for all HCPs, or even for all doctors, would be developed.

Part 2: Practice

What Format Should Be Used for Teaching?

There is no general consensus regarding the format with which ethics education ought to be delivered, and there is a lack of empirical research evaluating different teaching styles and methods (Carresse et al. 2015; Eckles et al. 2005). It is generally recommended that a practical approach should be taken, integrating ethics into practical and clinical aspects of training (Consensus statement 1998; Roberts et al. 2005). This has been proposed as more effective for teaching moral reasoning skills compared with formal didactic teaching methods such as lectures (Sokol 2007) and has also proven more popular with students (Mattick and Bligh 2006). That said, didactic teaching methods such as lectures may still be appropriate for teaching knowledge-based ethics topics, or be necessary where teaching resources are constrained (Mattick and Bligh 2006). We recommend that ethics teaching focuses on everyday issues which are of clinical relevance (Stirrat et al. 2010), with case studies (e.g., discussed in small groups) being particularly effective for teaching (Goldie et al. 2004; Consensus statement 1998; Charon and Fox 1995).

The modality of teaching is likely to have implications in terms of both the resources it requires and also how such teaching may be perceived and engaged with by learners. Lectures may be appropriate for teaching knowledge-based ethics topics but clearly offer less opportunity for the case-based discussion and skills-based learning. Classroom teaching can be beneficial in terms of offering students the opportunity to apply theory to practice and discuss cases with others and thus develop skills in moral reasoning. However, such a format is more effort intensive for the learner and requires more tutors or tutor-time. Simulation, including work with live actors and virtual reality environments, may clothe ethical issues in a real-world context, exposing learning needs and allowing skills to be rehearsed and tested in real time. Other modalities for teaching include self-directed learning (e.g., reading or online learning), or work-place-based learning (e.g., discussing ethical aspects of a supervised consultation). These may be more accessible – fitting around busy clinicians' schedules and clinical commitments. However, to be done well they require some training or expertise on the part of clinical supervisors. E-learning or other "structured discussion tools" may be preferred by education providers (be they HEIs or professional or specialty bodies) as they may require less resources and can be developed "one off" before being reused over and over. However, self-directed learning is not without its downsides – there is a risk that, if mandated, teaching delivered through this format can be viewed as simply an "administrative" exercise because of the lack of face-to-face interaction with an educator, and therefore HCPs may not engage fully with such teaching, or if not mandated it may be skipped altogether, as HCPs prioritize other mandated teaching topics or clinical commitments.

A further consideration is the potential role for interprofessional learning as a context for delivering ethics teaching. Ethical dilemmas do not arise in isolation, faced by solely one individual. A single ethical "case" may affect many different HCPs, each of whom will invariably bring their own experiences, knowledge, and personal moral viewpoints affecting how they approach dilemmas and interact with other team members (Wiles et al. 2016). Consequently, there has been interest in the potential benefits and feasibility of interprofessional ethics education (Engward and Papanikitas 2018). A relative lack of collaboration between different professions in terms of ethics education may reflect potential differences in how different pro-fessions see and learn about ethics (Hanson 2005). Where such collaborations happen, they may be very early in HCPs' undergraduate training and occur at universities which host a variety of healthcare degrees. King's College London in the UK has been a notable example (Whelan et al. 2005). Benefits to teaching ethics in an interprofessional setting may include better communication and collaboration leading to reduced staff burnout and improved patient care (Hanson 2005; Clark et al. 2007). Interprofessional ethics education is advocated as a way of improving team work, with such programs demonstrating improved collaboration between HCPs and resulting in them having a better understanding of the benefits of collaborative working to benefit patients (Machin et al. 2018). It has also been shown to improve HCPs' self-efficacy, confidence in team working, resilience, and personal and professional satisfaction (Clark et al. 2007). Although benefits in terms of translation to patient outcomes are yet to be demonstrated, it would be expected that improving collaboration between different HCPs and encouraging more efficient team-based approaches to patient care will benefit patients.

There are inevitably challenges in delivering ethics education to multiple different professionals – these include recruiting and compensating suitable educators, finding and coordinating time within different curriculums and teaching programs, and varying professional learning and teaching styles. One danger is that interprofessional ethics is seen as an opportunity to reduce costs by delivering a standard lecture to all participating professions that is so focused on core ideas that it fails to engage with any professional group. The benefits and challenges of interprofessional ethics education mirror those of interprofessional education more broadly. Lessons may be taken from what works and what does not to incorporate such an approach into the teaching of ethics.

When Should Ethics Be Taught and Learned?

Formal ethics education has traditionally been focused at an undergraduate or pre-clinical level in medical schools and in other HCP training programs. This is a consequence of the availability of dedicated time in the curriculum which can be allocated to teaching ethics; the availability of specific ethics educators due to affiliation with medical schools, HEIs, or training programs; and the opportunity for those overseeing education to design and deliver a set curriculum and assess students as deemed necessary.

However, there has been criticism of this being the sole approach to ethics education. The literature has described (qualified) doctors feeling ill-equipped to deal with ethical dilemmas faced in practice, despite having received previous ethics teaching at an undergraduate level (McDougal 2009). This indicates a potential need for further ethics support and training post-qualification. This may be even more pronounced for other HCPs, for whom ethics teaching may be less well defined or less structured during their training (e.g., learning on the wards) compared with that experienced by medical students within medical schools, who may have more formal lectures and teaching. Research has also indicated that HCPs undertaking additional roles (e.g., commissioning or involvement with healthcare policy) also describe a lack of ethical knowledge and confidence in their moral reasoning skills, with a desire for further ethics education beyond and outside their clinical training (Knight et al. 2020).

Accordingly, there is an argument for the provision of ethics education for those who have qualified and are now working HCPs, either formally through postgraduate ethics education training programs (e.g., for different medical specialties), or as part of less formal ongoing continuing professional development, to which all HCPs are professionally required to undertake. This may also need to be extended to those HCPs who undertake other roles alongside their clinical one, in which they may face additional ethical issues which might fall outside the remit of traditional ethics education. As already discussed, some postgraduates receive ongoing ethics training (e.g., palliative care specialty doctors, for whom ethics forms a significant component of their postgraduate specialty training curriculum (Joint Royal Colleges of Physicians Training Board 2014)), but for many, once they have completed undergraduate training their ethics education tends to be informally acquired through either self-directed learning or through exposure to the hidden curriculum and role models.

Postgraduate medical ethics education occurs via a variety of media – for example, papers in academic and professional journals, online and face-to-face courses, isolated lectures and their online counterparts, and as part of natural gatherings of HCPs such as added onto or integrated into a medical conference. Conferences should not be overlooked as sites for learning, as participants are often protected from competing work and family commitments (Papanikitas 2016). Moral custom is less "settled" allowing for a fuller exploration of ethical positions. Those delivering ethics education should consider how these alternative media might be utilized in order to support them to provide varied and accessible ethics teaching, particularly in order to overcome some challenges such as lack of time in the curriculum, or the need to encourage self-directed learning.

Who Should Teach Ethics?

"You can teach ethics, you're a GP," one of our colleagues was once told by a university education panel composed almost entirely of hospital XXXX (Papanikitas 2014).

There is perennial debate regarding who is best placed to deliver ethics education, with potential proposed suitable educators including clinicians, philosophers, lawyers, and educationalists. There is increasing consensus that ethics teaching is best provided by a multidisciplinary team comprising a mixture of the above (Eckles et al. 2005). Many of those who teach ethics will have additional roles, which on the one hand means they can offer valuable experience and expertise, but on the other hand can limit their availability to provide teaching. Perhaps as a result of many of those who teach ethics having other roles, many institutions have only been able to have very few, if any, dedicated full-time ethics teachers (Mattick and Bligh 2006).

Training for those who actually teach ethics is often lacking, with no current consensus about what training ought to be provided, nor a generally accepted formal training program for those who deliver teaching (Brooks and Bell 2017). This has the potential to lead to inconsistencies in teaching standards and a lack of a sense of support for those who offer teaching. It has been found that those delivering ethics education often do have formal qualifications in ethics from which ethics knowledge may be drawn (Mattick and Bligh 2006). Additionally, a number of bodies provide useful resources (in UK medicine, e.g., the General Medical Council's ethics learning materials (General Medical Council n.d.), the IME's core content (Institute of Medical Ethics n.d.), and the UK Clinical Ethics Network's educational resources (UK Clinical Ethics Network n.d.)). However, many of these provide resources regarding ethical topics and are knowledge focused, rather than offering training on how best to actually *deliver* effective and engaging ethics teaching to students, trainees, and other learners. For this reason, it may be beneficial to consider how ethics educators may support each other through other means, such as informal or formal networks, in order to be able to share good practice and educational resources.

Should Ethics Be Assessed and how?

Arguably one of the greatest challenges faced by ethics educators is determining if, and if so how, ethics should be assessed. The assessment of "ethics," which by many would be considered a more "subjective" field, differs substantially from the assessment of other scientific or clinical subjects such as anatomy, physiology, or clinical skills, which lend themselves more easily to objective and replicable assessment methods. In general, it is agreed that ethics should be assessed in some form. Doing so may mean students are more likely to take the subject seriously and be motivated for learning, but can also provide feedback on how their skills and knowledge in ethics have developed as a result of their teaching (Molyneux 2018). Assessment may highlight attitudes that are incompatible with good medical practice. Assessment can also be beneficial for allowing evaluation of the curriculum and teaching methods, with subsequent improvements to the design and delivery of ethics education (Eckles et al. 2005). Additionally, there may be the potential for assessment outcomes to be used in empirical research, which may inform future ethics education development and theory and demonstrate tangible benefits of ethics education. However, while there is consensus that ethics assessment is important and generally necessary, there is evidence that students may fail their ethics assessments but still graduate as doctors. This suggests that educational institutions have not yet determined the purpose of ethics assessment and the implication that different results might or should have in practice (Mattick and Bligh 2006).

In terms of actually *how* ethics should be assessed, a number of methods have been employed. The majority of these are summative assessments, attributing a score to the students' learning with examples including short answer questions, essays, multiple choice or extended matching questions, objective structure clinical examinations (OSCEs), portfolios, presentations, written papers, and vivas (Mattick and Bligh 2006). In many cases a combination of these methods is used in order to provide a broad overview of the students' knowledge and skills, with such formats also conforming with those used in other areas of assessment. However, medical schools take a variety of approaches, and a recent UK study found inconsistencies in the way ethics was assessed (Brooks and Bell 2017).

Those engaged in promoting ethics education need to be clear that education for healthcare professionals encompasses knowledge, skills, and attitudes. While personal attitudes may be beyond the reach of educators, their manifestation in professional behaviors is not. Attitudes that are incompatible with practice might be detected at entry onto a vocational course, noticed in class or clinical placements (Whiting 2009).

Part 3: Challenges for Ethics Education

While there are many potential benefits of ethics education, and a wide variety of ways in which ethics might be taught, a large number of challenges remain for those designing and delivering ethics education.

Perhaps the most frequently cited challenge is the lack of resources dedicated to teaching of ethics (Goldie 2000). There is frequently a lack of time and space within the curriculum dedicated to ethics, and particularly post-qualification any time available for ethics education is often overshadowed by clinical commitments, which take priority. Possibly as a result of the difficulties in demonstrating tangible benefits of ethics education and the lack of consensus regarding the purpose and place for ethics assessment, ethics teaching is often deemed to be of lower priority than other areas of health education and may be afforded less time than other areas of training, such as practical or clinical skills. Additionally, certain professions or specialties may place higher or lower priority on the teaching of ethics. There may be a number of reasons for this – the perceived frequency with which dilemmas arise for those of that profession or specialty, the role (or limited role) those professionals may have in making autonomous decisions was faced with a dilemma as part of an interprofessional team, historical or cultural factors affecting the perceived "usefulness" of ethics for those of that specialty, and finally competing learning needs (such as the acquisition of time-intensive practical skills, e.g., in surgical trainees). All these factors mean that ethics educators are frequently stretched with limited time resources, and so delivering ethics teaching of a satisfactory standard can be challenging.

An additional resource frequently lacking for ethics education are trained ethics educators, in particular those who might be able to provide interprofessional ethics teaching (Eckles et al. 2005; Hoskins et al. 2018; Hanson 2005). As already discussed, a multidisciplinary team of educators has been advocated as the preferred skill mix, but such people are often hard to come by and are likely to have other conflicting teaching or clinical responsibilities limiting their availability for ethics teaching. This may be further exacerbated by the lower priority given to ethics teaching compared to teaching of other areas of the curriculum, meaning such teachers are encouraged to teach other topics (e.g., clinical bedside teaching), rather than ethics.

The most significant challenge faced by those designing and delivering ethics education is existential. It relates to the lack of consensus and empirical backing for determining the purpose of it altogether. Teaching ethics, even where it results in "adequate ethical and legal knowledge," may not be sufficient to enable students to act with moral integrity. Medical students have described knowing the correct course of action but being unable to follow it, often due to barriers related to the hidden curriculum, demonstrating a mismatch between education and practice (Kong and Knight 2017). This is also an issue for clinicians who have completed their undergraduate training and even those taking on additional roles (e.g., commissioning, policy-making), who describe facing multiple barriers preventing them from taking what they deem to be the ethical course of action (Knight et al. 2020). Some have argued that if an HCP is professional and clinically competent, then perhaps it does not even matter if they are not "virtuous." Many aspects of ethical practice are not performance related in the same way that other clinical skills might be, and even those that are behavioral might be difficult to measure in any sort of conventional quantitative manner – for example, how would one fairly and accurately assess whether a student demonstrates virtues, humility, or altruism? (Carresse et al. 2015). Assessment of HCP's ethical competence is extremely challenging, with methods of assessment for these higher-level skills having been suggested to lack validity and/or reliability (Molyneux 2018).

Finally, while the multidimensional and multidisciplinary nature of ethics is beneficial, it adds complexity for those designing ethics education. The fact that ethics may encompass so many other areas such as clinical medicine, professionalism, law, humanities, and communication skills means that it does not neatly fit into a specific part of the curriculum. The drive for integration of ethics teaching into clinical and practical aspects of training, and in a longitudinal manner during both undergraduate and postgraduate training, also adds to this complexity. Frequently teaching of ethics is combined with that of law, and while this may be appropriate in some instances, knowledge and understanding of law differ substantially from the skills of ethical reasoning. Similarly, frequently ethics teaching is absorbed within the teaching of professionalism, leading to confusion among students and HCPs as to what in fact even constitutes ethics, or erroneously equating "ethical practice" with simply practice which is medico-legally defensive. The chief danger is that practitioners confuse what they must or must not do with what they ought or ought not to do.

Concluding Thoughts

A number of challenges face ethics educators. Some of these are theoretical – how best to foster the best kind of practitioner and how to share good practice in terms of both clinical practice (content) and medical education (method). Others are structural – a lack of consensus and empirical backing for the purpose of ethics education, and the challenges encountered in delivering ethics teaching due to the multidimensional and multidisciplinary nature of ethics. The material aspects of ethics education cannot be ignored – in any society education consumes resources, even if this is only a finite quantity of time. In the Anglo-American West time is money.

We have assumed that ethics is an integral part of clinical practice (at least for the reason that healthcare can do great, even systematic, harm without morals). This ethics education is essential in order that healthcare professions continue to work with professionalism, with integrity, and in a morally desirable way. Our aim in this chapter has been to articulate the importance of ethics education and providing some direction and ideas to support those who commission and deliver ethics education and assessment. Research and innovation in this area ought to be shared and discussed, and we find (we may also be guilty of this) that authors are quick to decry the lack of work, but this is often because they are simply unaware of it – a point that is made in the section on interprofessional ethics education. For this reason, we would encourage ethics educators to create both formal and informal networks for support and sharing of ideas and methods of teaching. This chapter should be critiqued but also used by academics, educators, and interested practitioners as a treasure map to a rich and developing field.

Key Points

- Ethics education aims to foster virtuous practitioners and provide HCPs with skills in ethical analysis and moral decision-making. There is a lack of empirical evidence as to tangible benefits for patients of teaching ethics. However, it can be justified on the basis of healthcare quality and safety or by using Eisner's five curricular orientations.
- Ethics syllabuses may be knowledge based, theoretical based, or skill based. A skills-based approach might equip learners for confidently approaching dilemmas in practice.
- There are multiple ways to deliver ethics teaching, allowing creativity and versatility for those designing ethics education programs. While there is a lack of consensus as to which format is best, those offering a practical approach focusing on clinically relevant cases and small group discussion have proven more effective and popular with learners. Ethics teaching should be considered in a realistically interprofessional setting.
- There is lack of consensus as to how ethical knowledge skills and attitudes should be assessed and the purpose and implications of such assessments. There is general consensus that formative assessment is helpful, and assessment should be matched to whether knowledge skills or attitudes are being assessed.
- Many of the challenges of ethics education reflect broader challenges in medical education such as how to be interprofessional and how to justify the use of resources in teaching and learning. Ethicists and educationalists can learn from one another.

Cross-References

▶ Arts and Humanities in Health Professional Education
▶ Hidden, Informal, and Formal Curricula in Health Professions Education

References

Brooks L, Bell D. Teaching, learning and assessment of medical ethics at the UK medical schools. J Med Ethics. 2017;43:606–12.
Carresse JA, Malek J, Watson K, et al. The essential role of medical ethics education in achieving professionalism: the Romanell report. Acad Med. 2015;90(6):744–52. https://doi.org/10.1097/ACM.0000000000000715.
Charon R, Fox RC. Critiques and remedies: medical students call for change in ethics teaching. JAMA. 1995;274:767–71.
Chartered Society of Physiotherapy. Code of Members' professional values and behaviour. 2011. https://www.csp.org.uk/publications/code-members-professional-values-and-behaviour. Accessed 7 May 2019.
Clark PG, Cott C, Drinka TJK. Theory and practice in interprofessional ethics: a framework for understanding ethical issues in health care teams. J Interprofessional Care. 2007;21(6):591–603. https://doi.org/10.1080/13561820701653227.
Consensus Statement by teachers of medical ethics and law in UK medical schools. Teaching medical ethics and law within medical schools: a model for the UK core curriculum. J Med Ethics. 1998;24:188–92. https://doi.org/10.1136/jme.24.3.188.
Cribb A, Bignold S. Towards the reflexive medical school: the hidden curriculum and medical education research. Stud High Educ. 1999;24:195–209.
Diekema DS, Shugerman RP. An ethics curriculum for the pediatric residency program: confronting barriers to implementation. Arch Pediatr Adolesc Med. 1997;151:609–14.
Dowie A, Martin A. Ethics and law in the medical curriculum. AMEE guide: curriculum planning. Europe: Association for Medical Education; 2011.
Eckles RE, Meslin EM, Gaffney M, Helft P. Medical ethics education: where are we? Where should we be going? A review. Acad Med. 2005;80(12):1143–52.
Eisner EW. Five basic orientations to the curriculum. In: Eisner EW, editor. The educational imagination: on the design and evaluation of the school programmes. 2nd ed. New York: Macmillan Publishing; 1985. p. 61–85.
Emmerich N. Medical ethics education: an interdisciplinary and social theoretical perspective. 1st ed. London: Springer; 2013. Preface, pvii-ix.
Engward H, Papanikitas A. Interprofessional ethics in everyday healthcare. In: Wintrup J, et al., editors. Ethics from the ground up: emerging debates, changing practices and new voices: London: Red Globe Press; 2018. p. 5–16.
Freeman JW, Wilson AL. Virtue and longitudinal ethics education in medical school. S D J Med. 1994;47:427–30.
General Medical Council. Good medical practice. 2013. https://www.gmc-uk.org/ethical-guidance/ethical-guidance-for-doctors/good-medical-practice. Accessed 29 May 2019.
General Medical Council. Learning materials. n.d.. https://www.gmc-uk.org/ethical-guidance/learning-materials. Accessed 19 May 2019.
Goldie J. Review of ethics curricula in undergraduate medical education. Med Educ. 2000;34:108–19.
Goldie JGS. The detrimental ethical shift towards cynicism: can medical educators help prevent it? Med Educ. 2004;38:232–8.
Goldie J, Schwartz L, McConnachie A, Morrison J. The impact of a modern medical curriculum on students' proposed behaviour on meeting ethical dilemmas. Med Educ. 2004;38:942–9.

Hafferty FW, Franks R. The hidden curriculum, ethics teaching, and the structure of medical education. Acad Med. 1994;69:861–71.

Hanson S. Teaching health care ethics: why we should teach nursing and medical students together. Nurs Ethics. 2005;12(2):167–76.

Hoskins K, Grady C, Ulrich CM. Ethics education in nursing: instruction for future generations of nurses. Online J Issues Nurs. 2018;23(1):Manuscript 3. https://doi.org/10.3912/OJIN.Vol23No01Man03.

Institute of Medical Ethics. Core curriculum for undergraduate medical ethics and law. 2019. http://www.instituteofmedicalethics.org/website/images/IME_revised_ethics_and_law__curriculum_Learning_outcomes_2019.pdf. Accessed 7 May 2019.

Institute of Medical Ethics. Core content. n.d.. http://www.instituteofmedicalethics.org/website/index.php?option=com_content&view=section&id=2&Itemid=3. Accessed 19 May 2019.

Jameton A. Nursing practice: the ethical issues. Englewood Cliffs: Prentice Hall; 1984. p. 6.

Joint Royal Colleges of Physicians Training Board. Specialty training curriculum for palliative medicine 2010 (Amendments 2014). 2014. https://www.jrcptb.org.uk/sites/default/files/2010%20Palliative%20medicine%20%28amendments%202014%29.pdf. Accessed 5 June 2019.

Jonsen A, Siegler M, Winslade W. Clinical ethics: a practical approach to ethical decisions in clinical medicine. 7th ed: McGraw-Hill Education/Medical, London; 2010.

Kleinman CS. Ethical drift: when good people do bad things. JONAS Healthc Law Ethics Regul. 2006;8(3):72–6.

Knight S, Hayhoe B, Frith L, et al. Ethics education and moral decision making in clinical commissioning: an interview study. Br J Gen Pract. 2020;70:690.

Kong WM, Knight S. Bridging the education–action gap: a near-peer case-based undergraduate ethics teaching programme. J Med Ethics. 2017;43:692–6.

Machin LL, Bellis KM, Dixon C, et al. Interprofessional education and practice guide: designing ethics-orientated interprofessional education for health and social care students. J Interprof Care. 2018;26:1–11. https://doi.org/10.1080/13561820.2018.1538113.

Mattick K, Bligh J. Teaching and assessing medical ethics: where are we now? J Med Ethics. 2006;32(3):181–5. https://doi.org/10.1136/jme.2005.014597.

McDougall R. Combating junior doctors' "4am logic": a challenge for medical ethics education. J Med Ethics. 2009;35:203–6.

Miles SH, Lane LW, Bickel J, Walker RM, Cassel CK. Medical ethics education: coming of age. Acad Med. 1989;64:705–14.

Misselbrook D. The BJGP is open for ethics. Br J Gen Pract. 2012;62(596):122.

Molyneux D. Learning from the assessment of ethics in UK general practice. In: Papanikitas A, Spicer J, editors. Handbook of primary care ethics. Boca Raton: CRC Press/Taylor & Francis Group; 2018. p. 269.

Morley G, Ives J, Bradbury-Jones C, Irvine F. What is 'moral distress'? A narrative synthesis of the literature. Nurs Ethics. 2019;26:646–62.

Nursing and Midwifery Council. The code: professional standards of practice and behaviour for nurses, midwives and nursing associates. 2018. https://www.nmc.org.uk/standards/code/. Accessed 21 May 2019.

Papanikitas A. The contributions of general practice as a profession. In: Papanikitas A, editor. From the classroom to the clinic: ethics education and general practice. PhD thesis, Kings College London. 2014. p. 96–101.

Papanikitas A. Education and debate: a manifesto for ethics and values at annual healthcare conferences. Lond J Primary Care. 2016;8(6):96–9.

Papanikitas A. Accounting for ethics: is there a market for morals in healthcare? In: Feiler T, Hordern J, Papanikitas A, editors. Marketisation ethics and healthcare. London: Routledge; 2018.

Papanikitas A, Spicer J. Teaching and learning ethics in primary healthcare. In: Papanikitas A, Spicer J, editors. Handbook of primary care ethics. Boca Raton: CRC Press/Taylor & Francis Group; 2018. p. 229.

Pellegrino ED, Thomasma DC. The virtues in medical practice. New York: Oxford University Press; 1993.

32 Teaching and Learning Ethics in Healthcare

Reeve J. Interpretive medicine: supporting generalism in a changing primary care world. Occas Pap R Coll Gen Pract. 2010;(88):1–20, v.

Roberts LW, Warner TD, Green Hammond KA, et al. Becoming a good doctor: perceived need for ethics training focused on practical and professional development topics. Acad Psychiatry. 2005;29(3):301–9.

Royal Pharmaceutical Society of Great Britain. Medicines, ethics and practice. Edition 42. 2018. https://www.rpharms.com/resources/publications/medicines-ethics-and-practice-mep. Accessed 7 May 2019.

Savulescu J. Conscientious objection in medicine. BMJ. 2006;332:294–7.

Shelton W. Can virtue be taught? Acad Med. 1999;74:671–4.

Siegler M. Lessons from 30 years of teaching clinical ethics. Virtual Mentor. 2001;3(10). https://doi.org/10.1001/virtualmentor.2001.3.10.medu1-0110.

Sokol DK. William Osler and the jubjub of ethics; or how to teach medical ethics in the 21st century. JRSM Open. 2007;100(12):544–6. https://doi.org/10.1177/0141076807100012010.

Sokol D. What to tell junior doctors about ethics. BMJ. 2010;340:c248.

Sokol D. Teaching medical ethics: useful or useless? BMJ. 2016;355:i6415.

Stirrat GM, Johnston C, Gillon R, et al. Medical ethics and law for doctors of tomorrow: the 1998 Consensus Statement updated. J Med Ethics. 2010;36:55–60.

UK Clinical Ethics Network. Educational resources. n.d. Overview. http://www.ukcen.net/education_resources. Accessed 19 May 2019.

United Nations Educational, Scientific and Cultural Organization. Bioethics core curriculum. 2016. http://unesdoc.unesco.org/images/0016/001636/163613e.pdf. Accessed 29 May 2019.

Whelan K, Thomas JE, Cooper S, et al. Interprofessional education in undergraduate healthcare programmes: the reaction of student dietitians. J Human Nutr Dietetics. 2005;18:461–6. https://onlinelibrary.wiley.com/doi/abs/10.1111/j.1365-277X.2005.00650.x

Whiting D. Should doctors ever be professionally required to change their attitudes? Clin Ethics. 2009;4(2):67–73.

Wiles K, Bahal N, Engward H, Papanikitas A. Ethics in the interface between multidisciplinary teams: a narrative in stages for inter-professional education. Lond J Prim Care (Abingdon). 2016;8(6):100–4. Published 2016 Oct 24. https://doi.org/10.1080/17571472.2016.1244892.

Simulation as Clinical Replacement: Contemporary Approaches in Healthcare Professional Education

33

Suzie Kardong-Edgren, Sandra Swoboda, and Nancy Sullivan

Contents

Key Changes in Health Professions Education	608
SBE Was the Right Tool at the Right Time	609
The NCSBN National SBE Study Demonstrated 50% SBE Acceptable Under Certain Conditions	610
Comparing Traditional Clinical and SBE	611
SBE for Patient Safety and Medical Error Awareness	612
SBE Scalability Issues for Large Classes	613
Use of Observer Roles	613
Tag Team Approach	613
Virtual Reality	614
Telesimulation	614
Faculty Workload for SBE	615
SBE Adoption Across the Health Professions	616
Advanced Practice Providers	616
Certified Registered Nurse Anesthetist	616
Physician Assistant Programs (PA)	617
Undergraduate Medical Education	617
Paramedics SBE Utilization	617
Pharmacy Programs	617
Physical Therapy Programs (PT)	618
Increasing Calls for Competent Safe Practitioners	618
Need for Education for the Facilitator Role Across All Disciplines	618
Conclusion	619
Cross-References	620
References	620

S. Kardong-Edgren (✉)
Nursing Operations, Texas Health Resources Harris Methodist Hospital, Ft. Worth, TX, USA
e-mail: skardongedgren@gmail.com

S. Swoboda · N. Sullivan
Johns Hopkins University School of Medicine and Nursing, Baltimore, MD, USA
e-mail: sswoboda@jhmi.edu; nsulliv@jhmi.edu

© Springer Nature Singapore Pte Ltd. 2023
D. Nestel et al. (eds.), *Clinical Education for the Health Professions*,
https://doi.org/10.1007/978-981-15-3344-0_44

Abstract

Anesthesiologists and engineers began developing and adopting SBE in the late 1960s to meet recognized training needs in their discipline. In medicine, as the clinical environment became more restrictive and health professions learners were asked to stop practicing on live patients, simulation-based education (SBE) was adopted as a logical second-best choice for many learning experiences. It did not take long to realize that SBE provided some unique opportunities that traditional clinical could not. The traditional clinical environment could never provide standardization of patient experiences that can be designed and provided in the SBE environment. Additionally, SBE provides opportunities for assessment that would never exist in a hospital or clinic setting. Essentially, SBE can offer the opportunity to practice and evaluate clinical and communication skills in a safe forgiving area, away from real patients.

Keywords

Health professions education · Simulation based education

Key Changes in Health Professions Education

Restrictions proliferated in the USA, on what care health professions students could provide for patients during the 1980s–2000s. The use of passwords to access medications and electronic medical records became ubiquitous, often excluding health professions students from these systems. The decreasing length of patient stay coupled with increasing acuity of patients, and increasing competition for clinical placement sites, all began to severely impact clinical education in what was already a tenuous and questionable system. As patients in the USA began arriving in hospitals in poorer health and with multiple comorbidities in the early 2000s, the 1:10 teacher to student ratio for most US nursing programs came into serious question from a patient safety perspective. Nurse educators asked the logical question, if an experienced nurse could only handle 5 patients, how could a nursing instructor handle 10 novice nursing students who each might take 1–3 patients a piece? In 2004, California became the first state to pass a mandatory 1:6 nurse-patient ratio for general medical surgical nursing wards (https://www.cga.ct.gov/2004/rpt/2004-R-0212.htm). Later this ratio was decreased to 1:5. In medicine, new mandated restrictions on the numbers of hours interns could work in a week impacted their learning opportunities.

Hospital-based education with live patients was seen as the gold standard in the health professions, and had not really been questioned or truly evaluated as there was no clear alternative. In fact, "the current system of education, training, and maintenance of proficiency has itself never been tested rigorously to determine whether it achieves its stated goals: the high-level reviews of the performance of the health care industry suggests it does not" (Gaba 2004). The rare evaluations of clinical education have consistently yielded unsatisfactory results in nursing education (Jayasekara et al. 2018). Recent evaluations have indicated that only 23–28% of new graduate Registered Nurses (RNs) are actually prepared for practice at the level desired by hospitals (Kavanagh and Szweda 2017).

SBE Was the Right Tool at the Right Time

SBE was rapidly adopted between 2000 and 2010 because it was seen as a clear alternative to the breakdown of the traditional clinical placement experience. Increasing enrollments in health professions increased the demand for clinical placements, even as there was a decrease in the availability of traditional clinical placement sites due to the changing landscape of in-hospital care. Patients were being discharged earlier to home and short- and long-term care facilities. Declining birth rates throughout the country limited the availability of clinical placements in pediatric and obstetric units. Cuts in many US state mental health services limited psychiatric unit placements and opportunities. Experiences in nontraditional settings such as clinics, health facilities, home healthcare, and other specialty areas rose, but the availability of these sites remained dynamic.

The work burden placed on traditional clinical placement sites by a continuous flow of students throughout the year also contributed to a rise in staff burnout. With increasing staff turnover, experienced staff were orienting new hospital staff, leaving less space, time, availability, and energy for student learning and mentoring. Increasingly, clinical placements were becoming fee based. Traditionally, site placements were local partnerships between universities and hospitals; however, increasingly this relationship is outsourced to clinical placement organizations. These challenges may delay students' progression throughout the program (Taylor et al. 2017). Well-formulated experiences using SBE were seen as logical solution.

SBE was adopted in nursing programs because faculty could clearly see that it allowed learners to assume full responsibility for a patient care situation without risk to a real patient. Faculty could see and hear what students would do in a given situation without any interference. SBE was ideal as a clinical placement substitute because participants had more time to think; facilitators could repeat changing physiological patient parameters allowing the learner more time to evaluate a clinical situation. "Inexperienced participants may perform tasks that they would not perform in the clinical environment for safety and ethical reasons...SBE is actually better for learning not despite but because of the differences from clinical reality" (Dieckmann 2009). Table 1 compares differences between SBE and traditional clinical placement.

The adoption of SBE for many health professions programs was slowed by the lack of understanding of how best to integrate SBE into an existing curriculum. More barriers included manikin costs and the lack of understanding of the new skills required to teach and successfully facilitate SBE. Many expensive manikins were initially used as high-end task trainers; many others lay abandoned for years in the crates they arrived in.

Table 1 Differences between SBE and clinical education opportunities for all disciplines

SBE	Traditional clinical placement
Deliberately developed	Random access to patients and diagnoses
Learners can truly demonstrate what they know	Learners may require intervention to save a patient
Facilitator requires extra training to move beyond instructor to facilitation	Instructor may be good clinician but not good educator
One on one and scalable to large groups	One on one or scalable to small groups
Diagnoses on demand	Random availability
Practice before meeting a real patient	Application expected without any opportunity for practice ahead of time

Some entrepreneurial health professions educators began experimenting with and developing the nascent pedagogy of SBE. Nursing educators and researchers began experimenting with teaching with SBE, learning new skills such as script writing, moulage, and trouble-shooting electrical and mechanical problems with manikins. These early adopters founded the International Nursing Association for Clinical SBE and Learning (INACSL). This group began to seriously consider the pedagogy of SBE for nursing which led to the development of the INACSL Standards for SBE[SM].

The NCSBN National SBE Study Demonstrated 50% SBE Acceptable Under Certain Conditions

Initially, SBE was used in addition to traditional clinical placements, as there was a lack of understanding about how and when to integrate SBE into a curriculum. As SBE began to proliferate in schools of nursing, many schools asked their local boards of nursing for guidance in the use of SBE for education. No large-scale studies were found in the literature to date to provide guidance so a national study was commissioned by the Boards of Nursing (BON) through the National Council of State Boards of Nursing (NCSBN). After 2 years of planning, 10 schools of nursing from around the USA were chosen to run a cohort study with 3 different conditions running simultaneously in each program, a 10% substitution with SBE (considered the traditional amount of SBE at the time), 25% substitution with SBE for traditional clinical placement, and 50% SBE substituted for traditional clinical placement hours (Hayden et al. 2014). All admitted students in the fall of 2011 at the 10 schools were informed of the study. Those that consented (n = 666) were randomized into a study group and observed for 2 years, until graduation.

Scenarios used in the study were standardized and programmed across all sites. Site coordinators and lab or faculty involved in the study were specifically trained in the same facilitation and debriefing methods. All sites used this one method throughout the study. Using the same standardized tools weekly along with end-of-course evaluations, students were evaluated by their clinical faculty. Findings suggested that up to 50% SBE could successfully be substituted for traditional

Table 2 NCSBN recommendations for using up to 50% SBE

Program preparation	SBE facilitators
Appropriate fiscal, human, and material resources to support SBE	Program based on SBE education theories
Policies and procedures for SBE	Tool designed for evaluation using INACSL standards
Dedicated and trained SBE facilitators	Planned objectives and outcomes communicated to learners prior to SBE
Job descriptions for SBE facilitators	A standardized debriefing method is used
SBE program uses evaluative feedback for quality improvement	A plan for sharing student performance with clinical faculty
INACSL SBE standards used	Planned facilitator evaluation data gathered and retained
Long range plan for SBE use	Program provides a means for faculty education such as webinars, conferences, journal clubs, formal education programs

clinical placement *if* similar conditions were employed within schools of nursing. These conditions are summarized in Table 2 (Alexander et al. 2016).

Many graduates who participated in the NCSBN study were further evaluated through surveys conducted with their nurse mangers at 6 weeks, 3 months, and 6 months after beginning practice as an RN. There were no differences in manager ratings. Study findings provided evidence that SBE was an effective substitute for traditional clinical experiences in pre-licensure nursing education as long as the same standards applied during the study are maintained for SBE experiences.

Comparing Traditional Clinical and SBE

As SBE began to be widely adopted and the pedagogy developed further, questions arose about the time equivalency between SBE and the traditional clinical experience. When discussing replacing clinical with SBE there was only conjecture and opinion about how to compare this equivalence. Breymier (Breymier et al. 2015) found most nursing schools maintained a 1:1 clinical to SBE ratio meaning 1 h of clinical clock time was considered equal to 1 h of SBE when substituting clinical with SBE. Since that time, despite a lack of empirical evidence, some schools adopted a 2:1 ratio (2 h of clinical equals 1 h of SBE) due to the perceived greater intensity of SBE. Educators suggested they did this based on personal observation and a "gut" feeling.

Further questions arose about the quality of experiences available in each venue. Pauly-O'Neill, Prion, and Nyugen (Pauly-O'Neill et al. 2013) compared traditional clinical placements and SBE, with nursing students in their pediatric rotations. They found students engaged in more meaningful work in the SBE setting compared to the traditional clinical setting. Similarly, Sullivan (Sullivan et al. 2019) observed students in their medical surgical rotation. This multisite study compared traditional clinical to SBE using the type and number of educational activities performed in both environments. Learning activities were categorized according to their level on Miller's Pyramid (Miller 1990) to determine the level and quality of the activities. Miller's categories include "knows, knows how, shows how, and does." In the study, "knows" was defined as fact-gathering activities: looking up information in the chart, researching meds, getting report or pre-conference/post-conference activities, and debriefing focused on direct recall. "Knows how" was defined as application of "knows" demonstrated via discussion of the plan of care, pre-conference/post-conference activities, and debriefing focused on interpretation and application. "Shows how" was defined as activities/skills completed with support or supervision. "Does" were activities/skills completed independently. In terms of the level or quality, "knows how" was considered a higher level of cognitive activity than "knows," "does" a higher level of behavior than "shows how." In terms of types and numbers of actual activities, the study found there were more skills, physical assessment, and teaching activities in SBE. In contrast, safety interventions were more common in clinical placements. Sullivan (Sullivan et al. 2019) also found more down time in clinical than in SBE, similar to the findings of Pauly-O'Neill, Prion, and Nyugen (Pauly-O'Neill et al. 2013). When examining activities in terms of Miller's Pyramid, the study found important differences between clinical placements and SBE. The percentage of time in "knows" was higher in clinical placement, while the percentage of "knows how" or application was higher in SBE. This was similar to the work of Ironside et al. (2014) and reflects a focus on tasks rather than clinical reasoning or application of knowledge in traditional clinical education. The percentage of "does" was higher in SBE than in traditional clinical placements. This is not surprising as, in SBE, the student is functioning independently in the role of a nurse.

The Sullivan et al. (2019) study provided evidence supporting a 2:1 clinical placement to SBE ratio; 2 h of traditional clinical is the equivalent of 1 h of SBE. Data indicated students completed more activities independently (does) in approximately one-fifth of the time in SBE as compared to traditional clinical placement. Also, and very importantly, students spent more time and completed more activities in Miller's "knows how" in SBE when compared to traditional clinical placement, indicating a greater focus on clinical reasoning in SBE. This data suggests that SBE is an intense efficient learning environment.

SBE for Patient Safety and Medical Error Awareness

SBE scenarios are being used to enhance the students' experience of safety (high risk, low occurrence) events without causing harm to patients. In the clinical setting, exposure or lack of exposure to safety events is variable. Substitution of clinical placement with simulated scenarios can introduce classic safety issues and provide an opportunity to practice preventing harm to patients by speaking up and also disclosing adverse events. SBE is being used for teamwork and communication practice, ergonomics, and for systems evaluation in the clinical environment. Studies using SBE are examining human factor interactions in the patient care environment (hospital room, ambulance) to enhance design and make recommendations to evaluate the safety and efficiency of space for patient care (Hallihan et al. 2019).

There is currently a national US focus on improvement and prevention of medication and procedural errors. SBE scenarios can provide opportunities for learners to discover the impact of disruptions during medication administration to increase learner awareness of safety and preparation for practice (Hayes et al. 2015). Ford et al. demonstrated that SBE experiences significantly reduce medication administration errors compared to traditional didactic education. The simulated environment provided realistic hands-on training with real-time judgment and psychomotor skills (Ford et al. 2010). Similar results were found when SBE training was utilized for central line insertion. Barsuk et al. (2009) examined the prevalence of procedure complications for central line insertion over a 1-year period. They found that SBE training resulted in fewer complications in the patient care setting.

SBE Scalability Issues for Large Classes

Use of Observer Roles

The question of scalability looms large when trying to provide equivalent SBE experiences for large groups of learners. Multiple learners are often placed in an SBE in various roles such as a main care provider, an assistant, a medication provider, or recorder. This helps to provide engagement and an opportunity for as many participants as possible in the belief that learning primarily happens when participating in the SBE in an active way. In reality, the artificiality of breaking up the role of a single RN into multiple roles often proves to be distracting and unsatisfying for those assigned. Those in the family member roles performed the worst in future SBEs, as they did not feel responsible for learning when in the family member role (Zulkosky et al. 2016). Research indicates that learners in the observer role, observing on a remote television screen or from an observation room, are learning as much and sometimes more than those performing in the SBE (Zulkosky et al. 2016; Johnson 2019; O'Regan et al. 2016; Bong et al. 2017).

Tag Team Approach

The Tag Team SBE (TTS) approach was developed as a way to engage up to 20 learners in a SBE (Levett-Jones et al. 2015). The methodology is adapted from applied theater; learners are reimagined as cast members and the facilitator becomes the play director. Learners and the director can "tag" other learners into or out of an SBE experience, which occurs in two "acts." Act one is the first run through a scenario followed by a brief intermission. The scenario is then repeated, hopefully with improved care and outcomes. Any new actor tagged into the scenario picks up the scene and action where the last actor stepped out. The potential for being called upon at a moment's notice to step into a scene keeps all potential cast members (learners) engaged and following the action. The patient (protagonist) is often a simulated patient. Some students are assigned to the audience role with assignments such as providing feedback to the actors and suggesting changes at the intermission and in the formal debriefing that follows (Levett-Jones et al. 2015; Guinea et al. 2019). A full explanation of this method and all scenarios and cue cards are available online for free at https://www.cqu.edu.au/about-us/structure/schools/nm/SBE/ttpss.

Virtual Reality

The problem of engaging large classes in SBE may ultimately be solved by the large-scale adoption of virtual reality (VR), using headsets which block out all external stimuli and immerse the learner in another world. VR provides both immersion and presence in a game/scenario/experience (Kardong-Edgren et al. 2018). Immersion refers to the psychological reaction induced by a continuous stream of visual and auditory experiences in a virtual environment – the greater the immersion, the greater the presence. Presence refers to the experience of the virtual environment as real. Dang et al. (2018) developed a VR device that allowed students to immerse themselves in a real-time SBE experience by wearing VR headgear that placed the learner in the center of the real-time action. A larger multisite study compared student presence, engagement, and learning in three groups: those actively involved in the SBE, those observing wearing VR goggles, and those observing the scenario using a TV screen for real-time observation. Findings indicated most engagement was in the actual scenario participants followed by the VR group and lastly, by those watching on TV. There was equivalent learning and an increased scenario "presence" in students using an immersive VR headset compared to those observing a SBE on a TV screen. These experiences provide the learner the opportunity to "live in the shoes" of the patient or patient environment which introduces a unique perspective to the clinical setting. Substitution of clinical experiences with VR could enhance a deeper understanding of future patient encounters. These results provide an intriguing opportunity for further exploration and research.

Telesimulation

Telesimulation-based simulation is the process of linking telecommunication and SBE resources to learners at an off-site location to provide education, training, and/or assessment to learners (McCoy et al. 2017a). This methodology along with teledebriefing can combine learners and educators in remote locations and globally for quality experiential learning (Ahmed et al. 2014). Using observation of a live SBE of a critical care case off-site with group debriefing and Google glass in a disaster management triage course have shown educational benefit to medical students and emergency medical services (EMS) providers (McCoy et al. 2017b, 2019). Similarly, telesimulation has been shown to be effective in teaching procedural skills to learners in developing countries (Mikrogianakis et al. 2011). The use of robots in healthcare and the education setting has gained traction. Robotic SBEs increase access to SBE education and can facilitate educational experiences to remote areas and enhance and substitute for clinical experiences (Hayden et al. 2018). This is an innovative solution to decrease the burden of education on working students, cost in time and travel to a clinical site, and can be used to increase the footprint of the educational experience. The efficiency of telesimulation, telehealth, and robotics can be used to bridge the gap of distance, access, and cost. With the growth of all healthcare programs, clinical site availability will continue to be a challenge, thus substitution of simulation, including telesimulation and VR, for clinical experience can expand programs and connect multiple providers caring for complex patients, expand interprofessional education (IPE) programs, and improve communication skills of all providers.

Faculty Workload for SBE

There has been a generalized lack of understanding in many academic institutions that SBE is not a "plug and play" operation and that reading a book or attending one course would not fully prepare a faculty or staff member to be a SBE facilitator. The increasing use of SBE in healthcare education necessitated considerable effort to determine faculty workload (Wilborn et al. 2013). Faculty workloads are never easily defined. They include myriad responsibilities (teaching, clinical practice, research, scholarship, and administrative duties) and vary considerably among institutions (Wilborn et al. 2013; Eisert and Geers 2016; Quilici et al. 2015; Blodgett et al. 2018). Workload formulations exist in the healthcare domain; however, the impact of SBE workload is not well developed and has led to unanticipated cost, time, and burden (Acton et al. 2015). A retrospective review of surgical faculty workload and SBE at a single institution over a 6-year period combined with a survey to program directors of surgical residency education revealed an increase in teaching hours and cost with a need for more instructors (Acton et al. 2015).

In academia, there is no universal definition of faculty workload; thus, recommendations for most workload including SBE workload are in early stages of development and are based on descriptive studies and anecdotal recommendations (Bittner and Bechtel 2017). Factors to consider are the amount of substitution of clinical, faculty to student ratios, SBE to clinical hour ratios, operationalization of the simulated day (length and frequency of the SBE case), preparation, content development, training, and coordinator/director/educator roles. Strategies to address workload can include a dedicated SBE team or faculty workload model to encompass the impact of SBE and these factors (Blodgett et al. 2018; Acton et al. 2015).

SBE Adoption Across the Health Professions

Advanced Practice Providers

Despite a rise in the number of advanced practice programs for advanced nurse practitioners (APNs), enrollment and competition for clinical sites, and qualified preceptors, SBE is currently only used for competency testing, skill-based exercises, and standardized clinical learning. SBE as a substitute for clinical hours is prohibited by regulatory agencies and both the US National Organization of Nurse Practitioner Faculty (NONPF) and the US National Task Force on Quality Nurse Practitioner Education (NTF). APN accreditation and certification organizations require a minimum of 500 practice hours, 600 practice hours for specialty areas (neonatal and women's health) with no substitution of SBE (American Association of Colleges of Nursing 2015).

While there is limited evidence to support the substitution of clinical hours with SBE in APN programs, there is a move to evaluate its feasibility and practicality to meet faculty needs, enrollment numbers, distance learning, clinical placement challenges, and clinical experiences (Anderson et al. 2019; Fulton et al. 2017). A study of NP students' self-report of direct patient care activities during clinical rotations of family nurse practitioners (FNP) and adult geriatric primary care NPs revealed only 34% of students' time in clinical was spent in direct patient care, with variability between the different programs (Fulton et al. 2017). SBE experiences have the ability to provide standardized experiences across programs. A survey of program directors and APN educators including Midwifery, Clinical Nurse Specialists, and Certified Registered Nurse Anesthetists programs in the USA and Canada revealed that 77% of respondents support the substitution of a percentage of clinical hours with SBE (Nye et al. 2019). The US National Board of Certification and Recertification for Nurse Anesthetists (NBCRNA) is currently evaluating a SBE alternative to the computer-based multi-choice exam required for maintenance of certification assessment (MOCA) for certified registered nurse anesthetists (CNRAs) (Karen Plaus, personal communication). A NONPF committee is also currently investigating a research study to investigate the use of SBE.

Certified Registered Nurse Anesthetist

The Council on Accreditation of Nurse Anesthesia Programs (COA) requires a standard number of clinical cases and specialty experiences in the curriculum. While CRNA programs have a rigorous clinical experience requirement, many CRNA doctoral program standards require SBE experiences to be incorporated into the curriculum to prepare students for the delivery of safe and effective patient care (COA n.d.).

Physician Assistant Programs (PA)

A national survey of Physician Assistant Programs (PA) revealed 56–90% of programs utilized SBE experiences depending on their affiliation with academic medical centers (Coerver et al. 2017). Hi-fidelity SBE and task trainers are utilized for skill performance, competencies, and interprofessional experiences; however, regulatory and accreditation agencies of PA programs require supervised clinical practice experiences to meet program objectives (Accreditation Standards for Physician Assistant Education 2018) (ARC-PA).

Undergraduate Medical Education

SBE is routinely incorporated throughout medical education for procedural skills, physical examination, and communication and to provide clinical context for didactic content. Published surveys show SBE use throughout undergraduate medical education across all years of training including subspecialty scenarios (Medical SBE 2011). A variety of technologies including virtual patients, virtual cadavers, and computer-based cases are used to supplement medical educational content (Lipps et al. 2017). Due to work hour restrictions medical students have limited time for hands-on patient care experiences; therefore, procedural skills and patient encounters in SBE can enhance training (Olasky et al. 2019; Buist and Webster 2019). A meta-analysis of first year physicians' ability to assess and manage deteriorating patients found increased knowledge and confidence with the use of SBE. Authors suggested that translating this ability to clinical practice needed more study (Buist and Webster 2019).

Paramedics SBE Utilization

Paramedics were surveyed in a 2015 descriptive study of SBE use in paramedic education (McKenna et al. 2015). Many programs utilized a variety of simulators (i.e., manikins, computer games, and VR); however, 31% of respondents said they had equipment that sat unused in their programs due to lack of training. While most educators were trained by manufacturers of simulators, 19% had no training at all. Only 44% of survey respondents had specific SBE support in their programs and the majority reported SBE was used for skills training rather than for clinical hours.

Pharmacy Programs

SBE is being used more frequently and is growing in pharmacy education. Washington State University and the University of Pittsburgh pharmacy programs were early SBE adopters. The Accrediting Council for Pharmacy Education (ACPE) suggest that a maximum of 60 h of the total required 300 pharmacy clinical hours may be completed in simulated pharmacy care situations. SBE hours cannot substitute for any of the 150 h required for community and institutional health experience (Amy Seybert, personal communication).

Physical Therapy Programs (PT)

SBE experiences are used in PT programs to enhance clinical experiences but are not currently accepted as meeting the standards of a real clinical patient. A systematic review and meta-analysis of empirical studies with simulated (standardized) patients showed a positive impact on the development of PT clinical practice competencies (Pritchard et al. 2016).

Increasing Calls for Competent Safe Practitioners

A move toward an increasing expectation of competency and safety upon graduation from health professions education is being discussed as SBE becomes more sophisticated (Leigh et al. 2016). In nursing, recent aggregate national data from the USA suggests that only 23% of new graduates are prepared to practice safely and independently upon graduation (Kavanagh and Szweda 2017). However, there continues to be a lack of a universally accepted definition of competence, safe practice, and a lack of universally accepted evaluation tools (Leigh et al. 2016; Llewallen and Van Horn 2019). Objective Structured Clinical Examination (OSCE) testing is being used in medicine and paramedicine and gaining favor in nursing as a means to evaluate safety and competency at some level. Along with the call of competency evaluation is the call for graduating a safe novice practitioner. SBE can be used to evaluate new core Entrustable Professional Activities (EPAs) in medical and pharmacy schools. EPAs are designated activities that health profession graduates should be able to independently perform upon graduation to meet performance gaps in residency.

Need for Education for the Facilitator Role Across All Disciplines

In academia and the hospital, there is an increasing recognition that there is a distinct difference between the traditional academic or clinical educator role and the SBE facilitator role. In fact, the SBE facilitator role arguably requires a higher and more skilled level, as often expert clinical knowledge must be combined with skilled facilitation and debriefing knowledge. A review by Topping et al. (Topping et al. 2015) suggested that the ability to (1) plan and design a scenario, (2) create and facilitate a safe learning environment, (3) possess expert clinical knowledge about expected behaviors and outcomes in a scenario, and (4) the demonstration of professionalism were all required for successful SBE education. However, only 60% of those using SBE in prelicensure nursing programs have received formal SBE education (Smiley 2019).

Education programs for SBE educators are available and expanding to meet the need. Several graduate masters level SBE certificates exist. There are more free-standing courses for SBE in educational masters of education programs, and doctoral programs tailoring courses of study to accommodate SBE. An example is the Massachusetts General Hospital Institute of Health Professions (MGHIHP) offering doctoral education in SBE. The University of Washington Center for Health Sciences Education, Research, and Practice website (http://collaborate.uw.edu) offers several brief introductory SBE education training modules. A free seven-module course, Essentials in Clinical Simulation Across the Health Professions, is available from Coursera online. New educational offerings for a fee are available from the INACSL organization (https://www.inacsl.org/education/inacsl-SBE-education-program/). For those feeling well prepared and experienced, the Society for Simulation in Healthcare provides a certification in SBE education, the CHSE, which can be sought after working at least 2 years in SBE educator role.

Conclusion

A recent systematic review evaluated the evidence for SBE as a substitute for clinical practice in prelicensure health professions education (Bogossian et al. 2019). Findings from medicine, nursing, and PT suggested that SBE was beneficial and could be substituted for a "portion" of traditional clinical hours. These authors suggest that SBE is well past its early development and that superiority trials should be conducted to help with expense justification, to overcome current budgetary and manpower barriers. Pragmatically, these authors question why the numbers of clinical hours in the traditional clinical environment required to achieve competency are not yet known; and yet regulatory bodies are currently dictating the number of *SBE* hours that can be substituted for traditional clinical hours.

The largest barriers to the full implementation of SBE integration into healthcare curricula continue to be (1) the continued lag or reluctance of faculty to prepare for or embrace the use of the pedagogy of SBE and (2) the lack of change in budgets, job descriptions, and workload for academics involved in SBE. Entrenched reluctant traditional faculty are a concern. Authors of a recent study concluded there was no evidence to support the number of traditional clinical hours necessary for nursing competency and then suggested that 61–80 clinical hours in pediatrics would be necessary for nursing students to achieve competency in pediatrics (with no evidence) (Bowling et al. 2018). Tradition and emotion are hard to overcome (Harder 2015). However, researchers are beginning to provide nascent evidence for these issues. Eisert and Geers (2016) calculated the actual time and activities involved in both academic and hospital-based SBE. They found only 27% of a SBE practitioner's time was spent actually running and debriefing scenarios. The rest of their time was spent planning scenarios with faculty, coordinating, gathering supplies, cleaning, etc. Blodget et al. (2018) proposed a model for determining workload for faculty involved in SBE. This work is ongoing and will provide a framework and evidence base for administration to make a rational evidence-based calculation of workload.

SBE will continue to evolve and be a major part of future clinical education, in some form, such as manikin based or VR. The human interaction accompanying the use of this method will continue to be critical and require educational preparation beyond what most faculty preparation programs currently provide. Research suggests that better practitioners will result from the widespread adoption of SBE by well-qualified educators and SBE practitioners.

Cross-References

▶ Allied Health Education: Current and Future Trends
▶ Conversational Learning in Health Professions Education: Learning Through Talk
▶ Developing Patient Safety Through Education
▶ Entrustable Professional Activities: Focus on Assessment Methods
▶ Measuring Performance: Current Practices in Surgical Education
▶ Obstetric and Midwifery Education: Context and Trends
▶ Supporting the Development of Professionalism in the Education of Health Professionals

References

Accreditation Standards for Physician Assistant Education 4th edition effective September 1, 2010 approved March 2010, updated March 2018 copyright Accreditation Review Commission on Education for the Physician Assistant, Inc. http://www.arc-pa.org/wp-content/uploads/2018/06/Standards-4th-Ed-March-2018.pdf. Accessed 30 June 2019.

Acton RD, Chipman JG, Lunden M, Schmitz CC. Unanticipated teaching demands rise with SBE training: strategies for managing faculty workload. J Surg Ed. 2015;72(3):522–9. https://doi.org/10.1016/j.jsurg.2014.10.013.

Ahmed R, King Gardner A, Atkinson SS, Gable B. Teledebriefing: connecting learners to faculty members. Clin Teach. 2014;11(4):270–3. https://doi.org/10.1111/tct.12135.

Alexander M, Durham CF, Goldman N, Hooper JI, Jeffries PR, Kardong-Edgren S, Kesten KS. et al. NCSBN SBE guidelines for prelicensure nursing education programs. (2016). https://www.ncsbn.org/16_SBE_Guidelines.pdf. Accessed 11 July 2019.

American Association of Colleges of Nursing. White paper: current state of APRN clinical education. Available at http://www.aacn.nche.edu/APRN-White-Paper.pdf. Published 2011. Published 2015. Accessed 28 June 2019.

Anderson M, Campbell SH, Nye C, Diaz D, Boyd T. SBE in advanced practice education: let's dialogue! Clin Sim Nurs. 2019;26:81–5. https://doi.org/10.1016/j.ecns.2018.10.011.

Barsuk JH, McGaghie WC, Cohen ER, O'Leary KJ, Wayne DB. SBE-based mastery learning reduces complications during central venous catheter insertion in a medical intensive care unit. Crit Care Med. 2009;37(10):2697–701.

Bittner N, Bechtel C. Identifying and describing nurse faculty workload issues: a looming faculty shortage. Nurs Ed Perspec. 2017;38(4):171–6. https://doi.org/10.1097/01.NEP.00000000000 00178.

Blodgett NP, Blodgett T, Kardong-Edgren SE. A proposed model for SBE faculty workload determination. Clin Sim Nurs. 2018;18:20–7. https://doi.org/10.1016/j.ecns.2018.01.003.

Bogossian FE, Cant RP, Ballard EL, Cooper SL, Levett-Jones TL, McKenna LG, Ng LC, Seaton PC. Locating 'gold standard' evidence for SBE as a substitute for clinical practice in pre-licensure health professional education: A systematic review. J Clin Nurs. 2019; Accepted manuscript. https://doi.org/10.1111/jocn.14965.

Bong CL, Lee S, Ng ASB, Allen JC, EHL L, Vidyarthi A. The effect of active (hot seat) versus observer roles during SBE-based training on stress levels and non-technical performance: a randomized trial. Adv Sim. 2017;2:7. https://doi.org/10.1186/s41077-017-0040-7.

Bowling AM, Cooper R, Kellish A, Kublin L, Smith T. No evidence to support number of clinical hours necessary for nursing competency. J of Ped Nurs. 2018;39:27–36. https://doi.org/10.1016/j.pedn.2017.12.012.

Breymier TL, Rutherford-Hemmings T, Horsely TL, Atz T, Smith LG, Badowski D. Substitution of clinical experience with SBE in prelicensure nursing programs: A national survey in the United States. Clin Sim Nur. 2015;11(11):472–8. https://doi.org/10.1016/j.ecns.2015.09.004.

Buist N, Webster CS. SBE training to improve the ability of first-year doctors to assess and manage deteriorating patients: a systematic review and meta-analysis. Med Sci Ed. 2019;29:1–13. https://doi.org/10.1007/s40670-019-00755-9.

COA. Response Regarding the Use of SBE. https://www.coacrna.org/about/Pages/COA-Position-Statements.aspx. Accessed 4 July 2019.

Coerver D, Multak N, Marquardt A, Larson EH. The use of SBE in physician assistant programs: a national survey. J Phys Ass Educ. 2017;28(4):175–81. https://doi.org/10.1097/JPA.000000000 0000173.

Dang B, Palicte JS, Valdez A, O'Leary-Kelley C. Assessing SBE, virtual reality, and television modalities in clinical training. Clin Sim Nus. 2018;19:30–7. https://doi.org/10.1016/j.ecns.2018.03.001.

Dieckmann P. Using SBE for education, training and research. Miami: Pabst Science Publishers; 2009.

Eisert S, Geers J. Pilot-study exploring time for SBE in academic and hospital-based organization. Clin Sim Nurs. 2016;12(9):361–7. https://doi.org/10.1016/j.ecns.2016.04.005.

Ford DG, Seybert AL, Smithburger PL, Kobulinsky LR, Samosky JT, Kane-Gill SL. Impact of SBE-based learning on medication error rates in critically ill patients. Intensive Care Med. 2010;36(9):1526–31. https://doi.org/10.1007/s00134-010-1860-2.

Fulton CR, Clark C, Dickinson S. Clinical hours in nurse practitioner programs equals clinical competence: fact or misnomer? Nurs Ed. 2017;42(4):195–8. https://doi.org/10.1097/NNE.0 000000000000346.

Gaba D. The future vision of SBE in health care. BMJ Qual Saf. 2004;13:i2–i10.

Guinea S, Andersen P, Reid-Searl K, Levett-Jones T, Dwyer T, Heaton L, Flenady T. SBE-based learning for patient safety: the development of the tag team patient safety SBE methodology for nursing education. Collegian. 2019;26(3):392–8. https://doi.org/10.1016/j.colegn.2018.09.008.

Hallihan G, Caird JK, Blanchard I, Wiley K, Martel J, Wilkins M, Thorkelson B, Plato M, Lazarenko G. The evaluation of an ambulance rear compartment using patient SBE: issues of safety and efficiency during the delivery of patient care. Appl Ergon. 2019;81:102872. https://doi.org/10.1016/j.apergo.2019.06.003.

Harder N. Replace is not a four letter word. Clin Sim Nurs. 2015;11:435–6. https://doi.org/10.1016/j.ecns.2015.07.001.

Hayden J, Smiley RA, Alexander M, Kardong-Edgren S, Jeffries PR. The NCSBN National SBE Study: a longitudinal, randomized, controlled study replacing clinical hours with SBE in prelicensure nursing education. J Nurs Reg. 2014;5(2):S3–S64.

Hayden EM, Khatri A, Kelly HR, Yager PH, Salazar GM. Mannequin-based teleSBE: increasing access to SBE-based education. Acad Emer Med. 2018;25(2):144–7. https://doi.org/10.1111/acem.13299.

Hayes C, Power T, Davidson PM, Daly J, Jackson D. Nurse interrupted: development of a realistic medication administration SBE for undergraduate nurses. Nurs Ed Tod. 2015;35(9):981–6. https://doi.org/10.1016/j.nedt.2015.07.002.

Ironside PM, McNeilis AM, Ebright P. Clinical education in nursing: rethinking learning in practice settings. Nurs Out. 2014;62:185–91. https://doi.org/10.1016/j.outlook.2013.12.004.

Jayasekara R, Smith C, Hall C, Rankin E, Smith M, Visvanathan V. The effectiveness of clinical education models for undergraduate nursing programs: A systematic review. Nur Ed Prac. 2018;29:116–26. https://doi.org/10.1016/j.nepr.2017.12.006.

Johnson BK. SBE observers learn the same as participants: the evidence. Clin Sim Nurs. 2019;33:26–34. https://doi.org/10.1016/j.ecns.2019.04.006.

Kardong-Edgren S, Breitkreutz K, Werb M, Foreman S, Ellertson A. Evaluating the usability of a second-generation VR game for refreshing sterile urinary catheterization skills. Nur Ed. 2018; Published ahead of print. https://doi.org/10.1097/NNE.0000000000000570.

Kavanagh JM, Szweda C. A crisis in competency: the strategic and ethical imperative to assessing new graduate nurses' clinical reasoning. Nurs Ed Per. 2017;38(2):57–62. https://doi.org/10.1097/01.NEP.0000000000000112.

Leigh G, Stueben F, Harrington D, Hetherman S. Making the case for SBE-based assessments to overcome the challenges in evaluating clinical competency. Int J Nurs Ed Scholarsh. 2016;1:27–34. https://doi.org/10.1515/ijnes-2015-0048.

Levett-Jones T, Andersen P, Reid-Searl K, Guinea S, McAllister M, Lapkin S, Palmer L, et al. Tag team SBE: an innovative approach for promoting active engagement of participants and observers during group SBE. Nur Ed Prac. 2015;15:345–52. https://doi.org/10.1016/j.nepr.2015.03.014.

Lipps JA, Bhandary SP, Meyers LD. The expanding use of SBE for undergraduate preclinical medical education. Int J Acad Med. 2017;3(1):59. https://doi.org/10.4103/IJAM.IJAM_40_17.

Llewallen LP, Van Horn ER. The state of the science on clinical evaluation in nursing education. Nurs Ed Per. 2019;40(1):4–10. https://doi.org/10.1097/01.NEP.0000000000000376.

McCoy CE, Sayegh J, Alrabah R, Yarris LM. TeleSBE: An innovative tool for health professions education. AEM Ed Train. 2017a;1(2):132–6. https://doi.org/10.1002/aet2.10015.

McCoy CE, Sayegh J, Rahman A, Landgorf M, Anderson C, Lotfipour S. Prospective randomized crossover study of teleSBE versus standard SBE for teaching medical students the management of critically ill patients. AEM Ed Train. 2017b;1(4):287–92. https://doi.org/10.1002/aet2.10047.

McCoy CE, Alrabah R, Weichmann W, Langdorf MI, Ricks C, Chakravarthy B, Anderson C, Lotfipour S. Feasibility of teleSBE and google glass for mass casualty triage education and training. West J Emer Med. 2019;20(3):512–9. https://doi.org/10.5811/westjem.2019.3.40805.

McKenna KD, Carhart E, Bercher D, Spain A, Todaro J, Freel J. SBE use in paramedic education research (SUPER): a descriptive study. Prehosp Emerg Care. 2015;19(3):432–40. https://doi.org/10.3109/10903127.2014.995845.

Medical SBE in Medical Education: Results of an AAMC Survey September 2011 Association of American Medical Colleges https://www.aamc.org/download/259760/data/medicalSBEinmedicaleducationanaamcsurvey.pdf. Accessed 4 July 2019.

Mikrogianakis A, Kam A, Silver S, Bakanisi B, Henao O, Okrainec A, Azzie G. TeleSBE: an innovative and effective tool for teaching novel intraosseous insertion techniques in developing countries. Acad Emer Med. 2011;18(4):420–7. https://doi.org/10.1111/j.1553-2712.2011.01038.x.

Miller GE. The assessment of clinical skills/competence/performance. Acad Med. 1990;65(9):S63–7.

Nye C, Campbell SH, Hebert SH, Short C, Thomas M. SBE in advanced practice nursing programs: A north-American survey. Clin Sim Nurs. 2019;1(26):3–10. https://doi.org/10.1016/j.ecns.2018.09.005.

O'Regan S, Molloy E, Watterson L, Nestel D. Observer roles that optimize learning in healthcare SBE education: a systematic review. Adv Sim. 2016;1:4. https://doi.org/10.1186/s41077-015-0004-8.

Olasky J, Kim M, Muratore S, Zhang E, Fitzgibbons SC, Campbell A, Acton R. ACS/ASE medical student SBE-based skills curriculum study: implementation phase. J Surg Ed. 2019;76 (4):962–9. https://doi.org/10.1016/j.jsurg.2019.01.014.

Pauly-O'Neill S, Prion S, Nguyen H. Comparison of quality and safety education for nurses (QSEN)-related student experiences during pediatric clinical and SBE rotations. J Nur Ed. 2013;52(9):534–8. https://doi.org/10.3928/01484834-20130819-02.

Pritchard SA, Blackstock FC, Nestel D, Keating JL. Simulated patients in physical therapy education: systematic review and meta-analysis. Phys Ther. 2016;96(9):1342–53. https://doi.org/10.2522/ptj.20150500.

Quilici AP, Bicudo AM, Gianotto-Oliveira R, Timerman S, Gutierrez F, Abrão KC. Faculty perceptions of SBE programs in healthcare education. Int J Med Ed. 2015;6:166–71. https://doi.org/10.5116/ijme.5641.0dc7.

Smiley RA. Survey of SBE use in prelicensure nursing programs: changes and advancement, 2010–2017. J Nurs Reg. 2019;9(4):48–61. https://doi.org/10.1016/S2155-8256(19)30016-X.

Sullivan N, Swoboda SM, Breymier T, Lucas L, Sarasnick J, Rutherford-Hemming T, Budhathoki C, et al. Emerging evidence toward a 2:1 clinical to SBE ratio: a study comparing the traditional clinical and SBE settings. Clin Sim Nurs. 2019;30:34–41. https://doi.org/10.1016/j.ecns.2019.03.003.

Taylor C, Angel L, Nyanga L, Dickson C. The process and challenges of obtaining and sustaining clinical placements for nursing and allied health students. J Clin Nurs. 2017;26 (19–20):3099–110. https://doi.org/10.1111/jocn.13658.

Topping A, Buus Boje R, Rekola L, Hartvigsen T, Prescott S, Bland A, Hope A, et al. Towards identifying nurse educator competencies required for SBE-based learning: a systemized rapid review and synthesis. Nur Ed Tod. 2015;35:1108–13. https://doi.org/10.1016/j.nedt.2015.06.003.

Wilborn TW, Timpe EM, Wu-Pong S, Manolakis ML, Karboski JA, Clark DR, Altiere RJ. Factors influencing faculty perceptions of teaching workload. Cur Iss Pharm Teac Lear. 2013;5(1):9–13. https://doi.org/10.1016/j.cptl.2012.09.011.

Zulkosky KD, White KA, Price AL, Pretz JE. Effect of SBE role on clinical decision-making accuracy. Clin Sim Nurs. 2016;12(3):98–106. https://doi.org/10.1016/j.ecns.2016.01.007.

Teaching Simple and Complex Psychomotor Skills

34

Delwyn Nicholls

Contents

Introduction	626
Psychomotor Skills in Health Education	627
Defining a Psychomotor Skill	627
The Rationale for Classifying a Psychomotor Skill	628
Determining Whether a Psychomotor Skill Is Simple or Complex	628
The Motor Learning Theory and Pedagogical Approaches Used to Teach Psychomotor Skills	630
The Stages of Skill Acquisition Motor Learning Theories Which Inform Current Skill Teaching Approaches	630
The Two-Step Model to Teach Psychomotor Skills	632
Contemporary Models to Guide the Teaching and Learning of Psychomotor Skills	632
Three-Stage Approach to Teaching a Psychomotor Step	634
Conclusion	641
Cross-References	641
References	641

Abstract

Executing a psychomotor skill requires the use of the health professional's upper limbs and the processing, by the brain, of the sensory information related to the skill execution. Psychomotor skills can be classified as either simple or complex.

Delwyn Nicholls: deceased.

Electronic supplementary material: The online version of this chapter (https://doi.org/10.1007/978-981-15-3344-0_45) contains supplementary material, which is available to authorized users.

D. Nicholls (✉)
College of Nursing and Health Sciences, Flinders University, Adelaide, SA, Australia

Sydney Ultrasound for Women, Sydney, NSW, Australia
e-mail: delinicholls@hotmail.com

© Springer Nature Singapore Pte Ltd. 2023
D. Nestel et al. (eds.), *Clinical Education for the Health Professions*,
https://doi.org/10.1007/978-981-15-3344-0_45

There have been very few published resources which have enabled educators to reliably and reproducibly classify a psychomotor skill. The lack of information is problematic for educators teaching psychomotor skills. This is because, the research outcomes and efficacy of using a pedagogical approach are being reported for psychomotor skills of varying complexity. The following chapter provides one approach to classify a psychomotor skill. It is an important and antecedent step to perform, by the educator, before advancing to teaching the psychomotor skill. This is because, when the skill is complex there is a growing body of literature which suggests that an alternative pedagogical approach should be used to the traditional or two-step skill teaching model. The two-step model involves the educator performing a skill demonstration and a simultaneous verbal overlay of the skill steps. Followed by the learner practicing the skill. The following chapter outlines the theory related to teaching a psychomotor skill and then explores additional pedagogical approaches to use when the skill has been classified as being complex.

Keywords

Psychomotor skills · Skill classification · Teaching model · Education · Complex skill · Simple skill

Introduction

Teaching psychomotor skills for many health professionals is a complex and challenging task. It is a challenge logistically, because the psychomotor skills curriculum continues to expand, while allocated teaching time and clinical skills teaching opportunities on-the-job are contracting. Consequently, many educators, seek out opportunistic moments to teach psychomotor skills. There is an additional challenge for many experienced educators. This is because, most educators usually commence their clinical teaching role without having completed formal educational training. Additionally, many professions and their professional associations do not have the training and financial resources to provide the initial training to teach health professionals the knowledge and skills that are needed for their clinical teaching role.

Michels, Evans, and Blok point out that performing a clinical skill involves the health professional being able to: synthesize and recall the knowledge and the underlying theory to perform the skill, apply clinical reasoning skills, justify decision-making approaches, communicate with the patient, execute the required psychomotor skill for the clinical scenario, and use acceptable professional practice attitudes and norms for the clinical practice scenario (Michels et al. 2012). Therefore, one dimension of the clinical teaching role involves educators teaching the psychomotor skills that are required for professional practice. The teaching of the psychomotor skill should be separated from the other knowledge domains to limit the effects of cognitive overload (van Merriënboer and Sweller 2010). Yet, many health professional educators clump these domains together and they often try to teach all the information, at the same time, in one session. There is now convincing motor learning theory and practice evidence to clearly debunk this teaching approach. However, many educators continue to do so as they have not been taught an alternative method.

A psychomotor skill is also referred to in the literature as a technical, procedural, or clinical skill (Kovacs 1997; Grantcharov and Reznick 2008). Therefore, this chapter will use the term psychomotor skill to refer to these synonyms for a psychomotor skill. The psychomotor skills that are used by each profession are unique. Educators across the health professions may conclude that the process to teach a psychomotor skill changes when they teach surgical, physiotherapy, podiatry, or ultrasound psychomotor skills; however, the major steps used to teach the discipline specific skills does not change. A structured and methodical approach is required to teach all psychomotor skills. The approach varies slightly when more complex skills are to be taught and learned. Nevertheless, there is a basic approach that should be used, and the steps to teach a psychomotor skill are premised on the motor learning theories and principles related to understanding how psychomotor skills are acquired, performed, and learned.

This chapter explores the pedagogical approaches that are required to intentionally teach a complex psychomotor skill. The phrase "clinical educator" will be used throughout the chapter to refer to anyone involved in supporting the development of clinical skills. There is a strong emphasis placed on first explaining the motor learning theory required to teach a psychomotor skill, and to practically apply this theory. A three-stage approach will be presented to guide the teaching and learning of a psychomotor skill. Each of the stages needed to teach a psychomotor skill will be reviewed and described. However, before beginning to teach a psychomotor skill, the educator must first determine whether the skill to be taught is simple or complex. This is because many of the skills that are taught in clinical practice are complex; therefore, several of the teaching steps used to teach these skills need to be further modified. There is very little practical guidance in the literature that explains and outlines how to teach complex skills, and why these modified instructional approaches are required. It is important for educators to be cognizant of these teaching practices and then apply these approaches in their clinical practice.

Psychomotor Skills in Health Education

Defining a Psychomotor Skill

A psychomotor skill involves the voluntary, goal directed, mental activities and limb movements which enable the execution of a movement pattern that is safe and efficient for each clinical situation (Nicholls et al. 2014).

The Rationale for Classifying a Psychomotor Skill

Health professionals use a mixture of open and closed psychomotor skills and these can be further classified as simple or complex (Sattelmayer et al. 2016). There is a dearth of literature which provides a classification system to identify those simple and complex skills which are performed by health professionals. Indeed, many health professional authors use both terms without definition and justification. This practice suggests that educators may have an implied or tacit understanding of the characteristics and attributes of simple and complex skills. This assumption is problematic, as what one educator considers an example of a simple skill frequently differs to their peers. For example, most educators would agree that taking a patient's blood pressure is an example of a simple skill. However, other educators and researchers assert that performing laryngeal mask airway insertion on a manikin, a far more complex task, is also an example of a simple skill (Orde et al. 2010).

The arbitrary practice of classifying simple and complex skills, by educators, is problematic but also understandable. This is because, there is very little health and medical education literature which outlines the need for a classification. Further, there is no resource which identifies the attributes related to performing a simple and complex skill. There is an emerging body of literature which suggests that the pedagogical approaches required to teach simple and complex skills differ (Wulf and Shea 2002; van Merriënboer et al. 2006; Brydges et al. 2007; Sigrist et al. 2013a). Therefore, health professional educators, from all disciplines, require an evidenced-based approach to classify the skills they intend to teach. The following section provides a method to categorize simple and complex skills.

Determining Whether a Psychomotor Skill Is Simple or Complex

It is important to be able to correctly classify and categorize simple skills to enable effective teaching of these skills. Yet, there is very little health professional literature which describes and outlines the characteristics associated with learning and performing a simple or complex skill. Therefore, the metrics and attributes identified in the motor learning domain literature have been reviewed. This knowledge has been integrated with health professional literature to provide criterion that enable a skill to be identified and classified.

The features and attributes that enable a psychomotor skill to be categorized as a simple skill, include:

- Their execution involves one degree of freedom or one combination of joint movements to perform the skill (Wulf and Shea 2002). For many health educators, this definition is difficult to understand and apply to those skills that are performed in a health professional's clinical practice.
- They require small amounts of practice to reach a predefined standard of performance (Wulf and Shea 2002; van Merriënboer et al. 2006).

34 Teaching Simple and Complex Psychomotor Skills

- They are usually comprised of one sub-part which contain no more than nine skill steps (van Merriënboer and Sweller 2010).
- They can be taught and learned in one teaching session.
- That teaching and learning of a simple skill places modest cognitive demands on the learner's attention, memory, and central processing unit (Sweller 1993; van Merriënboer and Sweller 2010).
- They are usually performed with minimal practice variation.
- That demonstration of the skill enables the observer to see and perceive *all* the movements required to perform the skill.

Complex psychomotor skills present a far great challenge to categorize. Complex skills have been classified by researchers from the motor learning domain, using a catalogue of metrics for several decades (Wulf and Shea 2002; Spittle 2013; Schmidt et al. 2019). The metrics used to classify a complex skill include reaction time, response errors/variability, movement time, and degrees of freedom (usually more than three) (Wulf and Shea 2002). However, these metrics lack application and relevance to categorize complex skills performed by health professionals. This is because, the equipment may limit the range of movements, or the number of degrees of motion freedom during the skill execution; for example, when performing a laparoscopic examination (Spruit et al. 2014). Additionally, metrics such as response errors or reaction and movement time will also vary for each clinical encounter due to fetal movement, patient anatomical variability, or patient voluntary and involuntary movements.

Most of the psychomotor skills performed by health professionals are randomly and arbitrarily classified by health educators and researchers. The current classification approach is subjective; consequently, it lacks consistency and reliability. The process to identify and classify a complex psychomotor skill begins by deconstructing the knowledge, skills (psychomotor and communication), and professional practice attitudes that are needed to perform the task. The processing of each of these cognitive and knowledge domains places large demands on the learner's attention and the finite capacity of the working memory (van Merriënboer and Sweller 2010; Leppink and Heuvel 2015). The limitations of the working memory need to be at the forefront of the considerations when a health educator uses a pedagogical approach to teach a complex psychomotor skill.

A complex psychomotor skill is multidimensional and multipart, and it is these domains or dimensions of performance that enable a complex skill to be identified and classified. For example, Raman and Donnon (2008), from the discipline of gastroenterology, point out that performing a complex skill such as colonoscopy, involves the cognitive, technical, and process domains. While, Nicholls et al. (2014) argue that most complex skills involve visuospatial and visuomotor skills, in order to be able to process and interpret real-time sensory feedback that is generated as a skill is being performed. Finally, van Merriënboer, Kester, and Paas (2006) state that performing a complex skill involves the execution of many linked sub-parts which are prone to practice variation.

Therefore, the attributes that enable a complex skill to be identified include:

- They require a large volume of precursor knowledge to be able to: conceptualize; perform; modify; or stop the skill (Raman and Donnon 2008): the theoretical knowledge linked to being able to perform a complex task is often dense, copious in quantity, and difficult to learn.
- They involve the learner developing the technical skills to use, maneuver, clean, and care for the equipment to perform the task (Raman and Donnon 2008).
- They involve developed visuospatial and/or visuomotor ability to interpret, analyze, and discriminate the visual and other sensory information generated throughout the execution of the skill (Nicholls et al. 2014; Spruit et al. 2014).
- Their execution involves co-occurring verbal communication with a conscious patient. For example, being able to explain the procedure to the patient (Silverman and Wood 2004), obtain consent, and describe the indications and contra-indications before performing the examination (Raman and Donnon 2008; Bearman et al. 2011).
- Their execution involves many sub-parts and they are usually prone to practice variation (van Merriënboer et al. 2006).
- They present a pedagogical challenge to teach using traditional skill teaching approaches (Wulf and Shea 2002; Magill 2011); this is because, the fine motor movements that are essential for the execution of the skill are small in magnitude; consequently, they may not be disclosed and visually perceived through one or even several skill demonstrations. Therefore, additional pedagogical approaches are needed by the educator to communicate these movements to the learner.

Collectively, these task attributes enable a complex skill to be identified and classified. This is one method that clinical educators can use to categorize a complex skill. The step to providing a transparent approach to classify a complex skill is an important step for health professional educators seeking to compare research outcomes of specific pedagogical approaches. This is because, the learning effect from using a pedagogical approach can now be compared for simple or complex skills. The research outcomes can now be equitably evaluated for a known skill classification.

The Motor Learning Theory and Pedagogical Approaches Used to Teach Psychomotor Skills

The Stages of Skill Acquisition Motor Learning Theories Which Inform Current Skill Teaching Approaches

In the twentieth century, motor learning theorists proposed that a learner's psychomotor skill acquisition occurred in phases or stages, and they proposed a range of models which outlined the varying number of stages over which the skill acquisition and learning occurred (for a review see Simpson 1966; Fitts and Posner 1967; Gentile 1972; Harrow 1972). The model by Fitts and Posner (1967) has endured in the literature. These authors propose that psychomotor skill acquisition occurs in three stages. The first or cognitive stage of the model by Fitts and Posner (1967) involves the learner understanding the task and the motor movements required to execute the skill. The educator commences by demonstrating and describing the skill steps to perform the task. At this stage, the learner performs the skill imperfectly and erratically. This is because, the combination of motor movements needed to perform the skill, referred to as the motor program, have not yet been encrypted into the motor cortex or further refined with intentional practice. Without this program, the learner has no way of comparing the real-time outcome of their movements with those that are needed to execute the skill. In the very early stages of acquiring a psychomotor skill, the learner is rarely aware of their skill performance errors; further, performance errors cannot be self-corrected. Therefore, the educator needs to provide immediate error correcting feedback to the learner to ensure that skill errors are fixed in real-time, and the skill is practiced correctly. There is another outcome from providing error-correcting feedback, and that is to ensure the schema for the skill, and the motor program are not encrypted with error. The second stage, or the integration (also referred to as the associative stage) stage, relies on the learner deliberately practicing the skill, and receiving end-task feedback. The learner remains in this stage of skill acquisition much longer than the other stages. Indeed, the learner may remain in this stage for weeks or months when the skill is complex (Spittle 2013).The learner is now able to perform the skill steps correctly using efficient movement patterns. With continued practice, the learner develops the ability to detect and correct errors. The third, final, or autonomous stage is only achieved with ongoing practice. Intentional practice of the skill progresses the learner's performance and it becomes smoothly executed and with the correct skill sequencing and timing. The movement patterns and motor program to perform the skill have become encrypted and learned. The learner can now focus on improving the speed and accuracy of the skill. The learner should be able to demonstrate that they can repeatedly recall and practice the skill without error. After this, the skill must be practiced in different clinical scenarios to gain the practice experience to be able to modify the skill execution with varied presentations. Simultaneously, the learner's attention is no longer focused on the procedural knowledge related to skill production; therefore, other dimensions of the task such as decision-making or communication with the patient can now be attended to. This is because, there is limited literature to suggest that gaining proficiency in the verbal communication skills to communicate with a patient, as the skill is performed, is more challenging for the student to learn than the psychomotor skill (Silverman and Wood 2004; Nicholls et al. 2018). Therefore, skills which require synchronous communication skills need to be partitioned into the psychomotor and communication skills-required to execute the task. After this step, the psychomotor skill is first taught, followed by the co-occurring communication skills and vocabulary linked to performing the skill (for a detailed review see Nicholls et al. 2018).

Fitts and Posner (1967), and many other authors, have proposed models for acquiring psychomotor skills that are based on established motor learning theories. However, a limitation of these models is that they provide very little detail about the instructional steps to be used by health professionals. Subsequently, several authors involved in the teaching of psychomotor skills have published models which are premised on these theories of motor skill acquisition (Walker and Peyton 1998; George and Doto 2001; Nicholls et al. 2016). The primary tenet of the published teaching models is that learning a psychomotor skill is maximized when a series of instructional steps are used to teach the manual movements required to execute the skill, and that the skill is only learned through intentional and purposeful practice. Additionally, ongoing skill development is reliant on the educator providing end-task or terminal feedback to foster the learner to reflect on their performance. Despite these models being published, there is anecdotal evidence to suggest that clinical educators to continue to use the two-step or traditional skill teaching model to teach psychomotor skills.

The Two-Step Model to Teach Psychomotor Skills

Most clinical educators use a teaching approach that mirrors how they were taught, and for many educators they were taught the psychomotor skills required for clinical practice using the two-step or master-apprentice skill teaching model. The master-apprentice skill teaching approach involves the learner observing an expert demonstration of the skill while the educator provides an accompanying description of the skill steps. Next, the learner practices the skill with a variable amount of supervised practice. This model has been used to teach simple and complex skills that are used by health professionals. However, the use and application of the two-step model to teach the multidimensional and continuous, or complex, skills such as those used to perform interventional, surgical, endoscopy, colonoscopy, physiotherapy, and ultrasound scanning skills is now being challenged (Nicholls et al. 2016). This is because, when a skill is both new and complex there is a growing body of research which suggests that alternative pedagogical approaches should be used to teach and learn complex skills. As, working memory has a limited and finite capacity (van Merriënboer and Sweller 2010), and this limitation remains even when the learner is intelligent and educated. Consequently, when the theory and the steps to perform the whole skill are taught, to a novice, in one session the capacity of working memory may be exceeded (van Merriënboer and Sweller 2010). Also, providing just one skill demonstration may be insufficient to visually communicate the combination, magnitude, and sequencing of the motor movements needed to perform the skill.

Contemporary Models to Guide the Teaching and Learning of Psychomotor Skills

Clinical educators have had the choice of many skill-teaching models to use as a guide to teach profession-specific psychomotor skills. In addition to the 2-step model, there are the 4-step (for a review see Walker and Peyton 1998), 5-step (for a review see George and Doto 2001), and the 11-step model (for a review see Nicholls et al. 2016) used to teach psychomotor skills. In particular the model proposed by Nicholls et al. (2016) is intended for the teaching of complex psychomotor skills. The steps to teach and learn a psychomotor skill are outlined in Table 1. Importantly, the steps to teach a psychomotor skill can also be divided into three stages. Using this three-stage approach helps the educator to break down the

Table 1 A comparison of the instructional steps used to teach psychomotor skills when using the 2-step, 4-step, 5-step, and 11-step models. For consistency the synonyms used to represent each step, by the authors, are included

Stages to teach and learn a psychomotor skill	Model/instructional steps	Two-step or traditional approach	Four-step – authored by Walker and Peyton (1998)	Five-step – authored by George and Doto (2001)	11-step – authored by Nicholls et al. (2016)
Stage one	Educator performs task analysis				x
Prior to teaching the skill	Establish learner's prior knowledge and skill level				x
	Pre skill conceptualization of what the skill execution involves, looks, sounds, and feel like. Contra-indications of when not to perform the task are taught			x	x
Stage two	Silent demonstration-learner observes		x	x	x
	Demonstration-verbalization of skill steps by the educator	x	x	x	x
The steps required to teach a psychomotor skill	Immediate error correction of learner's verbalized or executed skill steps			x	x
	Limit guidance and coaching				x
	Verbalization of skill steps by the learner – then educator performs the steps		x	x	x
	Learner verbalizes the skill steps prior to executing the step		x	x	x
Stage three	Learner intentionally practices the skill	x	x	x	x
Skill practice and feedback	Educator provides post skill execution feedback				x

teaching and learning of a psychomotor skill. Each stage involves the educator and/or learner performing several steps. Using this approach provides structure to the teaching of the psychomotor skill and this is important for educators who are beginning their clinical teaching role.

Three-Stage Approach to Teaching a Psychomotor Step

Stage One – The Steps Required Before Commencing Teaching a Psychomotor Skill

The first stage of teaching a psychomotor skill involves tasks that the educator performs before they teach the psychomotor skill. This is an important and distinct step that is antecedent to teaching the learner the steps to perform the skill, which occurs in the next or second stage. Step one commences with the educator identifying the psychomotor skill that they intend to teach. The next step involves deconstructing the skill into the domains of knowledge, psychomotor skills, communication skills, and the professional practice attitudes that are needed to perform the skill. Ordering the content that is to be taught, first knowledge, then psychomotor, followed by communication skills, and finally professional practice attitudes, helps educators to organize and layer the teaching of the information and skills to support the teaching of the clinical skill. The theory related to the execution of the skill must be taught in advance of the educator teaching the psychomotor skill. Likewise, the glossary of words that accompany the execution of the task, when the patient is awake, must also be taught before the learner is taught the skill to communicate with the patient (Nicholls et al. 2018). Clinical educators should try to use a variety of educational approaches to ensure that adult learners remain engaged and motivated while learning the theory and skills to perform a psychomotor skill. Therefore, it is best to use differing media, resources, and activities to ensure the curriculum of prerequisite knowledge before teaching the psychomotor skill.

The next step in this stage involves performing task deconstruction and task analysis. Task analysis involves breaking the skill into the skill steps and knowledge that are required to perform the task (Sullivan et al. 2008). Whereas task deconstruction involves breaking the task down into the sub-tasks, and then deconstructing each sub-part into seven to nine steps (van Merriënboer et al. 2006; Sullivan et al. 2008; van Merriënboer and Sweller 2010). Experts who teach psychomotor skills have become automated. Sullivan et al. identified that experts teaching procedural skills; for example, colonoscopy, failed to recall and teach 50% of the steps (Sullivan et al. 2008). Additionally, only 57% of the critical cognitive decisions that accompany the skill execution were verbalized (Sullivan et al. 2008). In contrast, once cognitive task analysis was performed this improved the recollection and teaching of the skill steps to approximately 70% (Clark et al. 2012). The omission by the educator to teach all the skill steps is problematic for novices, as they have insufficient knowledge of the task to be able to splice into the skill sequence the required skill steps. Therefore, providing the learner with a censored and correct video

34 Teaching Simple and Complex Psychomotor Skills

resource, which includes *all* the skill steps, may be one approach to overcome this teaching and learning limitation. Other benefits derived from using cognitive task analysis include: the educator identifying those skills that are less and more complicated and then scaffolding their teaching from simple to complex, so segments of a task can be taught in smaller and opportunistic teaching moments. All available teaching time is used, no matter how small. To do so, progressively whittles away at the remaining skills and knowledge to be taught. Additionally, teaching complex theory or psychomotor skills in chunks that are "bite-sized," and using approaches which do not overcomplicate the content, further diminishes the possibility of cognitive overload occurring, which has been shown to protract skill learning (van Merriënboer and Sweller 2010).

It is important to establish the learner's prior skill learning as this avoids teaching previously learned skills and information. Task analysis elicits and identifies the knowledge and skills required to perform the clinical skill. Then, these domains can be compared to the student's evidence of prior learning. The advantage of performing this step is that teaching time, which is a limited resource, can be then devoted to novel content, which has not yet been taught.

The final step in this stage, pre-skill conceptualization, is devoted to ensuring that the learner is aware of both their clinical environment and how to use, care, and clean equipment. In many teaching settings, it is assumed that the learner can turn on and use the equipment. However, when the information has not been previously taught to the learner, this information is not known. So, it is an important and distinct step to teach all facets of the knowledge related to the use and operation of the equipment, before beginning to teach the skill.

Stage Two – The Steps Required to Teach a Psychomotor Skill

The second stage to teaching a psychomotor skill involves four steps and is based on the need for the learner to see and then hear each step required to perform the skill. Before teaching the skill, it is important to explain to the learner the instructional steps that will be used to teach the psychomotor skill and what they are required to do at each step. It is also essential to explain, that as the skill is being taught, only the information related to teaching the skill steps will be described. Other enquiries will be discussed after the practical teaching session has finished.

The practical steps to teach a psychomotor skill start by silently demonstrating the psychomotor skill with the correct sequencing and timing. The human brain is adept at recognizing and then remembering the motor patterns that are required to execute a psychomotor skill; however, to do so the skill must first be observed. So, the purpose of this step is to demonstrate what the skill execution looks like as well as communicating the magnitude and the combination of motor movements needed to perform the skill correctly – also referred to as a model or standard of performance (Nicholls et al. 2016).

The second step involves repeating the skill demonstration and only describing each of the steps as they are executed. It is important not to provide the learner with any other superfluous or extraneous information as the steps are being described.

The additional information can interfere or even hinder the learning process (Schmidt et al. 2019).

The third step requires the learner to recall and describe the steps to perform the skill, with the correct sequence and timing, prior to the educator performing each step. The purpose of verbalizing each skill step before it is performed is to get the learner to think "out-loud," and to check that they have correctly comprehended the motor movements needed to execute the task. At this time, incorrectly described skill steps are immediately corrected by the educator and the step is then restated correctly. At this third step, there is a further opportunity for the learner to observe the motor movements that are needed to perform the skill.

The final step involves the learner describing each skill step before they execute the accompanying step. Immediate error correction is again provided by the educator when the skill step is incorrectly described or executed. Consequently, the skill step should be correctly restated and/or reperformed. Error correction feedback is essential when a learner is first acquiring the cognitive and psychomotor skills to perform a task. The feedback maybe in the form of verbal instruction (Ong et al. 2016) or physically correcting skill execution errors. This is because learners are not yet aware of their practice errors, nor can they correct them (Magill 2011; Schmidt et al. 2019).

Performing a skill demonstration has two intended learning goals, and for each goal there are assumptions made by the educator and learner. The first goal is that the skill demonstration provides a standard of performance or what the skill should look like. The accompanying assumption is that all the motor movements that are required to perform the skill are known by the educator in advance of teaching the skill. However, when a skill is complex and prone to practice variation (due to patient build, anatomical variation, or unexpected clinical practice findings) the skill practice will necessarily be modified to suit the clinical scenario. The second goal from performing the skill demonstration is that it will visually convey the combination of motor movements needed to execute the steps. The assumption of this goal is that *all* the motor movements that are needed to perform the skill will be visible at the time of the skill demonstration. The large movements are readily visible. However, many of the fine motor movements which are controlled by the small muscles of the hands and fingers are so slight that they are not perceived through vision alone. Consequently, these movements remain unseen and latent to the learner at the time of skill demonstration. So, when a complex skill involves very small motor movements, the educator is frequently required to use additional pedagogical approaches, other than skill demonstration, to teach the skill. There is very little health professional literature which describes these limitations and provides the research outcomes from using alternative teaching approaches to support the teaching and learning of a complex psychomotor skill.

Simulation is increasingly being used to support the acquisition of a range of skills using high and low fidelity phantoms. A benefit of using this approach is that the educator can ensure that the teaching session is learner rather than patient centered. Skill sequences can be repeatedly rehearsed and practiced by the learner. Initial skill acquisition errors can be made without fear of harming the patient.

Additionally, error-correcting feedback can be provided without causing patient anxiety. It is important though that skill practice is scaffolded to include authentic practice opportunities to ensure the learner is exposed to the inevitable realities of the clinical environment.

When Skill Demonstration Does Not Allow a Learner to Get the Idea of the Movement

Psychomotor skills that involve small and imperceptible motor movements require alternative pedagogical approaches to be used; for example, tactile modelling, physical guidance, or verbal guidance. These pedagogical approaches provide sensory information to the learner, about the motor movements needed to execute the task. Once the learner understands the motor movements required to perform the skill, they can then attempt to replicate these actions.

The use of tactile modelling and physical guidance involves the educator and learner having physical contact with each other. Tactile modelling involves the learner placing their hand over the educator's while the skill is performed in authentic or simulative practice (O'Connell et al. 2006). Whereas, physical guidance involves the educator placing their hand over the learners, so the learner's movements are guided to assist the skill execution (Dresang et al. 2004; O'Connell et al. 2006). Physical guidance provides a type of sensory feedback to the learner; therefore, to avoid overloading the learner with several types of sensory feedback concurrently, it is usually performed silently (Sutkin et al. 2015).

Ong, Dodds, and Nestel (2016), from a surgical background, propose that physical guidance is a potent and adjunctive pedagogical approach to teach psychomotor skills. This is because, physical guidance can provide the learner with kinesthetic understanding of the type, timing, and magnitude of the motor movements required to execute the skill. The sensory information is referred to as in-task feedback. While, verbal direction can also be used to guide and orientate the motor movements to the learner, when they are known by the educator. These instructional approaches (refer to Fig. 1) can be used in isolation or in combination, when teaching a complex psychomotor skill, *during the very early stages* of teaching and learning a psychomotor skill; after which, these supportive behaviors should be faded (White et al. 2016). The tapering of the in-task sensory feedback is necessary to ensure the learner has the opportunity to integrate the other accompanying sensory feedback that is linked to the task practice and not to become reliant on one mode of feedback (Blandin et al. 2008).

When the skill is simple, there is a large body of research which suggests that concurrent or in-task augmented feedback, in the form of guidance and coaching, should be limited (Salmoni et al. 1984; Walsh et al. 2009); especially when the skill is simple (Sigrist et al. 2013a). This is because, the learner's performance of a simple skill is enhanced, during skill practice, when they are provided with verbal guidance and coaching, and physical guidance from the educator. The in-task feedback becomes relied upon to perform the task and it is detrimental to the *long-term* learning of the skill, this phenomena is referred to as the guidance hypothesis (Salmoni et al. 1984; Marchal-Crespo et al. 2010).

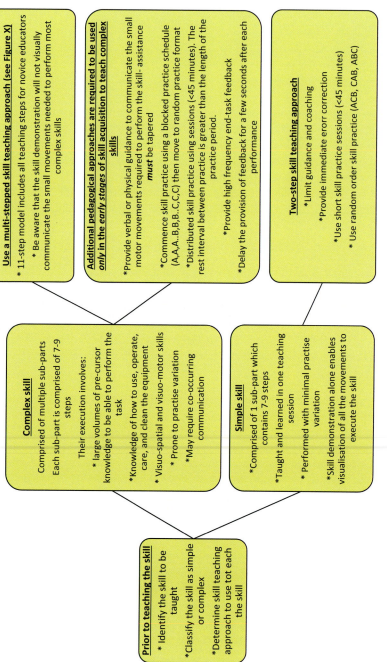

Fig. 1 A stepped approach to guide the classification of psychomotor skills and the suggested pedagogical approaches to use to teach simple and complex psychomotor skills

It is important that educators explain to their learners that they may use modelling or physical guidance to support their teaching approach and the role for using the approach, prior to doing so. It is essential that educators gain consent from the learner to physically touch their learner, as psychomotor skills are acquired and practiced. It is also essential for the educator to wear a glove when physical contact is made with the learner to model appropriate practices in their use of touch.

Stage Three – Skill Practice and Feedback

Psychomotor skills are acquired over time through intentional and deliberate skill practice (Ericsson et al. 1993). To be able to perform a psychomotor skill, the learner must first create a schema or motor map for the skill. The schema is stored in memory as a motor program (Schmidt et al. 2019). The creation of a motor program involves three progressive stages: encoding, consolidation, and retrieval (Kantak and Winstein 2012).

Skill *encoding* occurs during the acquisition phase of learning and it requires that the skill is diligently practiced using multiple, shorter practice sessions of less than 45 min duration (White et al. 2016) that are distributed over time (Poole 1991; DeBourgh 2011; Kantak and Winstein 2012). The goal of the learner, at this stage, is to *consolidate* their knowledge of the task and to get the idea of the motor movements that are needed to execute the skill. Therefore, using blocked practice, or repeatedly practicing the same task (A,A,A, B,B,B, C,C,C), may be beneficial to the learner when they are initially gaining an understanding of the motor movements to execute complex tasks (see Fig. 1). During the skill encoding phase, the learner does not have the capacity to identify or correct errors. This is because, the schema for the skill is still incomplete (van Merriënboer and Sweller 2010; Sattelmayer et al. 2016). Therefore, all skill performance errors must be immediately corrected to ensure the skill is correctly practiced and learned which results in an error free motor map being encrypted in the motor cortex. For all skills, memory consolidation and long-term learning of the skill occurs following intentional, repeated, random (ABC, BAC, ACB), and variable practice (Kantak and Winstein 2012; Sattelmayer et al. 2016). The skill movements and actions that are required to execute the task begin to become known. During this stage, there are small gains in proficiency for long periods of skill practice. *Retrieval* of the motor movements is only made possible by ongoing and intentional skill practice; after which, the skill becomes encrypted and learned. A learned skill is retained in long-term memory and it is then capable of being recalled and importantly modified for the practice conditions (Kantak and Winstein 2012). Further, as the skill becomes proficiently practiced and learned, this frees up space in working memory to attend to other aspects of task practice (Spruit et al. 2014); for example, communicating with the patient and/or other health professionals who may be involved in the skill.

The Role of Feedback in Skill Acquisition

Motor skill acquisition is reliant upon task practice and feedback (Archer et al. 2015). Feedback refers to the information that learners receive from within (referred to as intrinsic feedback) or from an external source (referred to as extrinsic augmented feedback) (Spittle 2013). Intrinsic sensory feedback is derived from the learners' own sensory realm and can be in the form of visual, auditory, tactile, or proprioceptive information. Extrinsic feedback is information provided to the learner about their performance and it may come from the educator or from another source (Poole 1991; Winstein 1991; Walsh et al. 2009). Information can be provided to the learner as the task is progressing, referred to as concurrent feedback; or alternatively, at the conclusion of the skill performance, referred to as end-task or terminal feedback (Walsh et al. 2009).

Terminal or end-task feedback refers to information about the learner's task performance and it should be withheld until the conclusion of the skill practice (Salmoni et al. 1984). This is because the learner can focus on practicing the skill and become acquainted with the sensory, motor, and tactile skill elements that are linked to task execution (Salmoni et al. 1984; Schmidt and Lee 1999; Lean et al. 2016). Lean et al. (2016) explored the learning outcomes from using different, continuous in-task and end-task feedback formats to teach medical students spinal anesthesia on a manikin. They found that those students who received end-task feedback demonstrated superior long-term procedural learning and skill retention compared to those who received in-task feedback. A learned skill is capable of being recalled from long-term memory and then performed beyond the practice period.

The frequency that in-task concurrent and end-task feedback is provided to the learner varies according to whether the skill is simple or complex. When the skill is simple, the provision of very frequent terminal feedback has been found to have a detrimental impact upon the long-term learning of the skill (Sigrist et al. 2013a). When a complex psychomotor skill is being learned, a relatively high feedback frequency has been shown to be beneficial for learning skills which are complex, or a skill sub-part is complex (Sigrist et al. 2013b). This is because the feedback helps to consolidate and refine the motor program for the skill. A 100% relative feedback frequency refers to the provision of terminal feedback after every practice trial. The benefits of using high frequency feedback, when the skill is complex, are realized by the learner during the initial stages of skill acquisition when largest motor learning gains are made across the skill acquisition curve (O'Connor et al. 2008). Bosse et al. (2015) concluded that end-task feedback after every practice trial (100% feedback frequency), when learning to perform nasogastric tube insertion on a manikin, resulted in the learners' having superior skill performance and smoother motor actions compared to learners receiving a 20% feedback frequency. There is an ill-defined point during the stage of skill acquisition where the terminal feedback should be faded (Sigrist et al. 2013a; Sattelmayer et al. 2016).

Fading feedback refers to decreasing the provision of feedback over time (Sigrist et al. 2013a). Using this approach provides the learner with the opportunity to develop their own intrinsic feedback about their performance (DeYoung 2003) and minimizes dependence on others. During this period, when the learner's skill is being consolidated, it is suggested that the educator should also delay the provision of terminal motor learning feedback for a few seconds. This hiatus in communication gives the learner time to assess their movement outcomes and errors, and it also develops the skill to self-assess their practice performance (Walsh et al. 2009; Sigrist et al. 2013a). Additionally, no feedback trials are required for the learner to develop their learning autonomy, to consolidate their learning, and to recall the skill at future practice performances (Sigrist et al. 2013b).

Perceived Challenges for Educators

An enduring perception by educators is that using an alternative pedagogical approach to the traditional two-step method takes too much additional teaching time (Orde et al. 2010). This assumption is unmerited, and it is a potential barrier to educators using a four-step approach to teach complex psychomotor skills. This is because, limited research by Orde et al. (2010) and Krautter et al. (2011) suggests that similar teaching times were needed to teach laryngeal mask insertion and gastric tube insertion on manikin, using the two-step and four-step teaching approaches.

Conclusion

Psychomotor skills can and should be classified as simple or complex before they are taught. Clinical educators require knowledge of the pedagogical approaches to teach psychomotor skills, particularly those skills which are complex. Nuanced teaching approaches are needed by educators to maximize the learning of complex psychomotor skills. The two-step skill teaching model has limited application when teaching complex skills. Therefore, additional pedagogical approaches have been presented to support the teaching of complex skills. However, when the skill is complex, it is important to point out that further research is now required to determine how some of these suggested pedagogical approaches affect a leaner's skill performance and long-term skill retention.

Cross-References

▶ Cognitive Neuroscience Foundations of Surgical and Procedural Expertise: Focus on Theory
▶ Simulation as Clinical Replacement: Contemporary Approaches in Healthcare Professional Education
▶ Simulation for Procedural Skills Teaching and Learning

References

Archer E, van Hoving DJ, de Villiers A. In search of an effective teaching approach for skill acquisition and retention: teaching manual defibrillation to junior medical students. Afr J Emerg Med. 2015;5(2):54–9.

Bearman M, Anthony A, Nestel D. A pilot training program in surgical communication, leadership and teamwork. ANZ J Surg. 2011;81(4):213–5.

Blandin Y, Toussaint L, Shea CH. Specificity of practice: interaction between concurrent sensory information and terminal feedback. J Exp Psychol Learn Mem Cogn. 2008;34(4):994–1000.

Bosse HM, Mohr J, Buss B, Krautter M, Weyrich P, Herzog W, et al. The benefit of repetitive skills training and frequency of expert feedback in the early acquisition of procedural skills. BMC Med Educ. 2015;15:22.

Brydges R, Carnahan H, Backstein D, Dubrowski A. Application of motor learning principles to complex surgical tasks: searching for the optimal practice schedule. J Mot Behav. 2007;39(1):40–8.

Clark RE, Pugh CM, Yates KA, Inaba K, Green DJ, Sullivan ME. The use of cognitive task analysis to improve instructional descriptions of procedures. J Surg Res. 2012;173(1):e37–42.

DeBourgh GA. Psychomotor skills acquisition of novice learners. A case for contextual learning. Nurse Educ. 2011;36(4):144–9.

DeYoung S. Teaching strategies for nurse educators. Upper Saddle River: Prentice Hall; 2003. p. 280.

Dresang L, Rodney W, Dees J. Teaching prenatal ultrasound to family medicine residents. Fam Med. 2004;36(2):98–107.

Ericsson KA, Krampe RT, Tesch-Romer C. The role of deliberate practice in the acquisition of expert performance. Psychol Rev. 1993;100:364–406.

Fitts PM, Posner MI. Human performance. Belmont: Brooks/Cole; 1967.

Gentile AM. A working model of skill acquisition with application to teaching. Quest. 1972;17:3–23.

George JH, Doto FX. A simple five-step method for teaching technical skills. Fam Med. 2001;33:577–8.

Grantcharov T, Reznick R. Teaching rounds: teaching procedural skills. Br Med J. 2008;336:1129–31.

Harrow AJ. A taxonomy of the psychomotor domain. New York: David McKay; 1972.

Kantak SS, Winstein CJ. Learning–performance distinction and memory processes for motor skills: a focused review and perspective. Behav Brain Res. 2012;228(1):219–31.

Kovacs G. Procedural skills in medicine: linking theory to practice. J Emerg Med. 1997;15(3):387–91.

Krautter M, Weyrich P, Schultz J-H, Buss SJ, Maatouk I, Jünger J, et al. Effects of Peyton's four-step approach on objective performance measures in technical skills training: a controlled trial. Teach Learn Med. 2011;23(3):244–50.

Lean LL, Hong RYS, Ti LK. End-task versus in-task feedback to increase procedural learning retention during spinal anaesthesia training of novices. Adv Health Sci Educ. 2016;22:713–21.

Leppink J, Heuvel A. The evolution of cognitive load theory and its application to medical education. Perspect Med Educ. 2015;4(3):119–27.

Magill RA. Motor learning and control: concepts and applications. 9th ed. New York: McGraw-Hill; 2011. p. 466.

Marchal-Crespo L, McHughen S, Cramer SC, Reinkensmeyer DJ. The effect of haptic guidance, aging, and initial skill level on motor learning of a steering task. Exp Brain Res. 2010;201(2):209–20.

Michels ME, Evans DE, Blok G. What is a clinical skill? Searching for order in chaos through a modified Delphi process. Med Teach. 2012;34:e573–81.

Nicholls D, Sweet L, Hyett J. Psychomotor skills in medical ultrasound imaging: an analysis of the core skill set. J Ultrasound Med. 2014;33:1349–52.

Nicholls D, Sweet L, Muller A, Hyett J. Teaching psychomotor skills in the twenty-first century: revisiting and reviewing instructional approaches through the lens of contemporary literature. Med Teach. 2016;38(10):1056–63.

Nicholls D, Sweet L, Muller A, Hyett J. A model to teach concomitant patient communication during psychomotor skill development. Nurse Educ Today. 2018;60:121–6.

O'Connell M, Lieberman LJ, Petersen S. The use of tactile modeling and physical guidance as instructional strategies in physical activity for children who are blind. J Vis Impair Blind. 2006;100(8):471–7.

O'Connor A, Schwaitzberg SD, Cao CGL. How much feedback is necessary for learning to suture? Surg Endosc. 2008;22(7):1614–9.

Ong C, Dodds A, Nestel D. Beliefs and values about intra-operative teaching and learning: a case study of surgical teachers and trainees. Adv Health Sci Educ. 2016;21(3):587–607.

34 Teaching Simple and Complex Psychomotor Skills

Orde S, Celenza A, Pinder M. A randomised trial comparing a 4-stage to 2-stage teaching technique for laryngeal mask insertion. Resuscitation. 2010;81(12):1687–91.

Poole J. Application of motor learning principles in occupational therapy. Am J Occup Ther. 1991;45(6):531–7.

Raman M, Donnon T. Procedural skills education – colonoscopy as a model. Can J Gastroenterol. 2008;22(9):767–70.

Salmoni AW, Schmidt RA, Walter CB. Knowledge of results and motor learning: a review and critical reappraisal. Psychol Bull. 1984;95(3):355–86.

Sattelmayer M, Elsig S, Hilfiker R, Baer G. A systematic review and meta-analysis of selected motor learning principles in physiotherapy and medical education. BMC Med Educ. 2016;16:15.

Schmidt RA, Lee TD. Motor control and learning: a behavioural emphasis. Champaign: Human Kinetics Publishers; 1999.

Schmidt R, Lee T, Winstein C, Wulf G, Zelaznik H. Motor control and learning: a behavioural emphasis. 6th ed. Champaign: Human Kinetics; 2019. p. 532.

Sigrist R, Rauter G, Riener R, Wolf P. Augmented visual, auditory, haptic, and multimodal feedback in motor learning: a review. Psychon Bull Rev. 2013a;20(1):21–53.

Sigrist R, Rauter G, Riener R, Wolf P. Terminal feedback outperforms concurrent visual, auditory, and haptic feedback in learning a complex rowing-type task. J Mot Behav. 2013b;45(6):455–72.

Silverman J, Wood DF. New approaches to learning clinical skills. Med Educ. 2004;38(10):1021–3.

Simpson E. The classification of educational objectives, psychomotor domain. Urbana: University of Illinois; 1966. p. 45.

Spittle M. Motor learning and skill acquisition: applications for physical education and sport. South Yarra: Palgrave Macmillan; 2013. p. 514.

Spruit E, Band G, Hamming J, Ridderinkhof KR. Optimal training design for procedural motor skills: a review and application to laparoscopic surgery. Psychol Res. 2014;78(6):878–91.

Sullivan ME, Ortega A, Wasserberg N, Kaufman H, Nyquist J, Clark R. Assessing the teaching of procedural skills: can cognitive task analysis add to our traditional teaching methods? Am J Surg. 2008;195(1):20–3.

Sutkin G, Littleton EB, Kanter SL. How surgical mentors teach: a classification of in vivo teaching behaviors. Part 2: physical teaching guidance. J Surg Educ. 2015;72(2):251–7.

Sweller J. Some cognitive processes and their consequences for the organisation and presentation of information. Aust J Psychol. 1993;45:1–8.

van Merriënboer JJG, Sweller J. Cognitive load theory in health professional education: design principles and strategies. Med Educ. 2010;44(1):85–93.

van Merriënboer JJG, Kester L, Paas F. Teaching complex rather than simple tasks: balancing intrinsic and germane load to enhance transfer of learning. Appl Cogn Psychol. 2006;20 (3):343–52.

Walker M, Peyton R. Teaching in theatre. In: Peyton R, editor. Teaching and learning in medical practice. Rickmansworth: Manticore Europe Limited; 1998. p. 171–80.

Walsh CM, Ling SC, Wang CS, Carnahan H. Concurrent versus terminal feedback: it may be better to wait. Acad Med. 2009;84(10 Suppl):S54–7.

White C, Rodger M, Tang T. Current understanding of learning psychomotor skills and the impact on teaching laparoscopic surgical skills. Obstet Gynaecol. 2016;18:53–63.

Winstein CJ. Knowledge of results and motor learning – implications for physical therapy. Phys Ther. 1991;71(2):140–9.

Wulf G, Shea CH. Principles derived from the study of simple skills do not generalize to complex skill learning. Psychon Bull Rev. 2002;9(2):185–211.

Developing Professional Identity in Health Professional Students

35

Kathleen Leedham-Green, Alec Knight, and Rick Iedema

Contents

Introduction and Overview	646
Conceptions of Professional Identity	648
Professional Identity as "Ideal": A Collective Contract with Society	648
Professional Identity as "Self and Other": Tribes and Siloes	648
Professional Identity as an Expression of Status: Hierarchies and Power	649
Professional Identity as a Coping Strategy: Depersonalization and Detachment	649
Professional Identity as How we are Perceived by Others: Culture and Identity	650
Professional Identity as Contextual and Situated: A Sociocultural Perspective	650
Professional Identity and Role Fluidity: Chimera and Chameleon	651
Professional Identity as a Transcendent Attribute: Fact or Fiction?	652
Professional Identity Formation	652
Identity Formation as Socialization	653
Identity Formation as Transformation	653
Curricular Positioning	654
Framing Professional Identity within Curriculum Design	654
A Model to Aid Curriculum Planning	656
Focused Strategies for Educators	656
Access to Role Experiences	656
Multi-Professional Simulation	657
Safe Reflective Spaces and Protected Time	658
Responding to the Hidden Curriculum	658
Communities of Practice and Activity Theory	659
Mentoring and Role Modelling	659

K. Leedham-Green (✉)
Medical Education Research Unit, Imperial College London, London, UK
e-mail: K.leedham-green@imperial.ac.uk

A. Knight
School of Population Health and Environmental Sciences, King's College London, London, UK
e-mail: alec.knight@kcl.ac.uk

R. Iedema
Centre for Team-Based Practice & Learning in Health Care, King's College London, London, UK
e-mail: rick.iedema@kcl.ac.uk

© Springer Nature Singapore Pte Ltd. 2023
D. Nestel et al. (eds.), *Clinical Education for the Health Professions*,
https://doi.org/10.1007/978-981-15-3344-0_46

Assessment Practices	660
Student Engagement	661
Conclusion	661
Cross-References	662
References	662

Abstract

Professional identity formation is a relatively new area of interest within health professional education, gaining academic attention after the Carnegie Foundation Report on Medical Education of 2010 called for its introduction into medical curricula in the United States. This chapter presents a critical discussion, introducing various schools of thought, and provides theoretically informed suggestions for practice. The authors explore both conventional identity formation and more complex modern reconfigurations of healthcare professional identity. The chapter starts with an overview of different stances on what professional identity means, drawing on a variety of literatures including sociological and organizational scholarship. Next, a range of theories of identity formation are presented, including socialization and transformation. A matrix model is introduced to inform curricular planning, which can be used flexibly within different institutions or contexts. The authors discuss and critique a number of focused strategies for educators including role modeling, mentoring, reflective practice, responding to the hidden curriculum, authentic role experiences and simulation-based education, communities of practice and activity theory, student engagement, and assessment practices. The chapter concludes with possible future directions in healthcare professional identity education. Kathleen Leedham-Green is a research fellow in the Medical Education Research Unit at Imperial College London with interests in the social and behavioral aspects of clinical practice as well as healthcare innovation and quality. Alec Knight is a postdoctoral researcher and educator at King's College London with interests in health services research, applied psychology, medical education, public health, health policy, and implementation science. Rick Iedema is professor and director of the Centre for Team-Based Practice and Learning in Health Care at King's College London.

Keywords

Professional identity formation · Curriculum design

Introduction and Overview

Kathleen Leedham-Green is a research fellow in the Medical Education Research Unit at Imperial College London with interests in social and behavioral aspects of clinical practice as well as healthcare innovation and quality. Alec Knight is a postdoctoral researcher and educator at King's College London with interests in health services research, applied psychology, medical education, public health, health policy, and implementation science. Rick Iedema is professor and director of the Centre for Team-Based Practice and Learning in Health Care at King's College London.

Professional identity formation is a relatively new research area within health professional education. The overwhelming majority of articles on the topic have appeared since the Carnegie Foundation Report on Medical Education of 2010 (Irby et al. 2010). This report was commissioned for the 100th anniversary of the Flexner Report of 1910 and called for the reform of medical education in the United States and Canada, which it argued had changed little in a century. It explicitly called for professional identity formation to be included in medical curricula. Irby et al. defined identity formation as "the development of professional values, actions and aspirations," clarifying the aspirational aspects as "excellence, humanism, accountability and altruism."

The report's curricular recommendations on identity formation were

- Providing formal ethics instruction, storytelling, and symbols (honor codes, pledges, and white coat ceremonies).
- Addressing the underlying messages expressed in the hidden curriculum and striving to align the espoused and enacted values of the clinical environment.
- Offering feedback on, reflective opportunities for, and assessment of professionalism in the context of longitudinal mentoring and advising.
- Promoting relationships with faculty members who simultaneously support learners and hold them to high standards.
- Creating collaborative learning environments committed to excellence and continuous improvement.

In the intervening 20 years since the report's publication, almost 200 articles, reviews, and commentaries have appeared within the health professions literature, taking a variety of stances on what is to be achieved and developing perspectives on how it may be realized.

Our aim in writing this chapter was not to provide a recipe for how to define, teach, or assess professional identity; rather, it was to present a critical discussion, introducing various schools of thought, and to provide theoretically informed suggestions for practice. The chapter explores both conventional identity formation and more complex modern reconfigurations of healthcare professional identity. First, we present an overview of different stances on what professional identity means, drawing on a variety of literatures including sociological and organizational scholarship. Second, we explore theories of identity formation including socialization and transformation. Third, we introduce a model to inform curricular planning, which can be used flexibly within different institutions or contexts. Fourth, we discuss and critique a number of focused strategies for educators including role modelling, mentoring, reflective practice, responding to the hidden curriculum, authentic role experiences and simulation-based education, communities of practice and activity theory, student engagement, and assessment practices. Finally, we present our conclusions and possible future directions in healthcare professional identity education.

Conceptions of Professional Identity

To understand how professional identities are formed, it is necessary to first consider what professional identity is. Rather than take a simplistic stance on this, we have drawn a range of perspectives, which we present under separate subheadings.

Professional Identity as "Ideal": A Collective Contract with Society

Clinical professions, like legal, religious, and other expert professions, are characterized by a lengthy period of study and a set of standards and skills defined by a governing body that novices must adhere to. The caring professions are also often typified as vocations ("something that you are") rather than occupations ("something that you do"). This intersection between one's identity and the defined or presumed attributes, beliefs, values, motives, and experiences of one's profession can be said to be one's individual professional identity (Schein 1978).

Idealized views of how identities are intertwined with behavior (how what one does is related to who one is) have much sway in the public imagination. These idealized views have important implications for educators and for interprofessional practice generally. The expectations of society on a professional group are often explicitly referred to in the codes of practice of its governing body. For example, the United Kingdom's Royal College of Physicians expects its members to adhere to "a set of values, behaviours, and relationships that underpins the trust the public has in doctors" (Royal College of Physicians 2005). Similarly, the Nursing and Midwifery Council promotes its standards as being those "that patients and members of the public tell us they expect from health professionals" (Nursing and Midwifery Council 2018). These ideals carry weight not just for the profession and for its standing in society but also for healthcare students and trainees, as they orient themselves to what it means to be a healthcare professional. Indeed, they are critical to enabling students and trainees to develop their professional identity: "the 'self' who participates in everyday social interaction can do so only through its recognition of certain cultural norms, values and ideals" (Abbinnett 2003). These norms, values, and ideals publicly legitimize an individual's identity and position in social and organizational terms. They act not only as an explanatory background to our actions and decisions but also as a definitive frame of reference for actions and decisions that do not accord with relevant standards or prevailing expectations.

Professional Identity as "Self and Other": Tribes and Siloes

A second perspective on professional identity is one that embodies the prevailing views held within their profession, as well as the group's views of other healthcare professionals. Such views may express ideal values and norms but may also reveal a more functional understanding of what it means to be a healthcare professional. For example, Lingard et al. conducted a study asking surgeons and surgical nurses to watch excerpts of tense conversations around the operating table and to discuss what they understood to be the underlying values and motivations behind what was said. Interestingly, participants identified along professional lines, giving their "side" more complex, noble intentions and the other side shallower stereotypical motivations: the surgeon just wants to make money, while the nurse just wants to finish their shift (Lingard et al. 2002). This finding highlights that identification is a social process. It also suggests that a normative definition of the self may be accompanied by a delegitimation of those who identify with different practices, values, and norms. This phenomenon has been referred to as "professional inclusivity," where members are expected to socialize with people within the same profession. Its obverse is "social exclusivity," which is the tendency not to socialize with people from other professions (Iedema and Jorm 2018). Professional inclusivity and exclusivity are terms that capture and highlight the problems linked to identification, such as interprofessional siloes and cross-professional status contests. Such dynamics risk impacting negatively on the high levels of communication and collaboration that are critical to safety in clinical care environments.

Professional Identity as an Expression of Status: Hierarchies and Power

A third perspective on identity can be found among sociologists of medicine and of healthcare. Freidson argued that medical professional identity was as closely tied to status in the labor market as it is to expert skill and ethical values (Freidson 1970). He saw identity as a complex phenomenon encompassing interests that are economic (income), social (power control), and expert professional (skills and knowledge). Zola also regarded professionalization in healthcare as overlapping with "medicalization." In other words, the processes of enacting medicine and healthcare conspire to convert people's daily existence into a manifestation of either health or illness (Zola 1972). Zola further described the accrual of status to a profession according to its tendency to medicalize pathology. Illich argued that modern medicine, with its customs and rituals, was in effect expropriating health as a commodity handed out by doctors, and by turning patients into consumers, doctors were actually destroying society's capacity for health (Illich 1976). Such sociological critiques have contemporary relevance when considering the ongoing privileging of high-end medicine and expensive kinds of clinical care over primary care and community services (Wass and Gregory 2017).

Professional Identity as a Coping Strategy: Depersonalization and Detachment

Psychoanalyst Menzies Lyth offers a related perspective (Menzies 1960). She approached professional identity from the perspective of the work that healthcare professionals were called on to do and the stresses and conflicts that such work entailed. She construed clinicians' identity as a complex psychological dynamic that enabled them to excuse and cope with the more overwhelming aspects of everyday care work: "I deal with death, distress and intimate parts of people because I am a nurse." Menzies Lyth found clinicians' detachment from the pain of patients was coupled with a denial of their own emotional stress. This, she found, affected not only the clinician-patient relationship but also the clinician-clinician relationship. She described how the separation between personal and professional identities caused heightened anxiety, particularly for junior clinicians who might have unrealistic expectations placed on them. Identifying as a professional may be accompanied by a feeling that one should possess all the competencies of that professional group. Menzies Lyth was able to use the detachment created by professional identity to construct an explanatory analysis for a variety of dysfunctional behaviors and coping mechanisms, including the paradox of simultaneously overestimating and undervaluing other clinicians' abilities.

Professional Identity as How we are Perceived by Others: Culture and Identity

Another strand in professional identity theory relates to culture and identity and ranks self-other relationships as foundational to identity formation and to identity itself. Here, identity formation and identity are not just developmentally conditional on growth of the subject himself/herself, but on how the subject is perceived and judged (supportive or otherwise) by others. Identity formation is thus "a process 'located' in the core of the individual and yet also in the core of his [sic] communal culture" (Erikson 1968, p. 62). Abbinnett notes that how we view ourselves is influenced by our reaction to how we are treated by others (Abbinnett 2003). He discusses the stress caused by attempting to contain or deny the impacts of seeing how others view oneself. Popular culture and media can impact on how individuals are treated on account of their profession. For example, stereotypical portrayals within popular media of gender within nursing (Weaver et al. 2014), or professionalism amongst social workers (Gibelman 2004), are likely to have negative impacts on those identifying within those professions.

Professional Identity as Contextual and Situated: A Sociocultural Perspective

Conceptions of professional identity, and what it is to be a healthcare professional, have evolved over time and between different cultures and groups. Learners might also identify differently during different stages of training. For example, an individual may ascribe to different social norms about how one should dress as a medical student, as postgraduate trainee, and as a consultant. This leads us to reflect on how conceptions of what it is to be a good healthcare professional are not objective, but a product of the sociocultural conditions in which they are produced. Another example involves the professional identity of pharmacists, which has been affected by the rise of the pharmaceutical industry. Graduating pharmacists may differentially identify as apothecaries, hospital scientists, clinicians responsible for patient outcomes, or merchants (Kellar 2019).

Mehta argues that the advent of dissection into Western medical education was facilitated by Cartesian dualism, the separation of mind and body (Mehta 2011). Foucault also described the medical profession's attitude to the corpse and thus death as medicine's "absolute point of view over life" and fundamental to understanding the profession's identity within society (Foucault and Sheridan 2003, p. 155). Through this lens, the role of the healthcare professional is reduced to what they can do for bodies, or parts of bodies, rather than what they can do for the person: the treatment of disease rather than the creation of health and the "care/cure dichotomy" (Treiber and Jones 2015). Since the 1960s, there has been a concerted effort to recreate a more humanistic professional identity within healthcare: reintegrating the mind with the body and the person with the patient, and simultaneously acknowledging the subjectivity and identity of healthcare professionals (Armstrong 2002).

Current challenges to identity within healthcare professions include the shift from the clinician as an autonomous and sometimes idiosyncratic professional toward a culture of micro-management, monitoring, and incentivization (Iedema 2006). There are calls to reconcile this battleground in the interests of care quality (Berwick 2016). We should expect these evolutions in identity to continue as the healthcare context itself evolves.

Professional Identity and Role Fluidity: Chimera and Chameleon

Professional identity is shifting from clearly delineated role-based structures toward a flexible, multi-stranded, and potentially noncoherent behavioral repertoire: a beast composed of many animals (chimera) or a beast that changes its appearance according to context (chameleon). Professional boundaries are being reframed as clinicians are increasingly expected to attend to holistic patient needs, rather than deliver profession-led services. Rising care complexity has meant that clinicians must reconcile themselves with competing demands (multiple patients, comorbidities, specialty priorities), challenging contexts (resource constraints, management targets, understaffing), and pervasive uncertainties (organizational, scientific, and pragmatic). There is an ever-increasing range of stakeholders involved in patients' care (interpreters, patient liaison officers, quality and safety managers, etc.). This has produced an emphasis on the skills required for relationships and communication across different clinical-technical and sociocultural domains. Multiple members of the healthcare team are now operating with overlapping roles relating to clinical decision-making, prescribing, health promotion, and the extent to which they address a patient's psychological or social needs (Nancarrow and Borthwick 2005).

Professional Identity as a Transcendent Attribute: Fact or Fiction?

The final conception of professional identity presently discussed is the tacit assumption that professional identity transcends other forms of identity such as race, religion, class, gender, and sexuality. In other words, one's professional attributes are more important than one's personal attributes in both clinician-patient and clinician-clinician interactions. Cohen described this primacy of professional identity as "subordinating all other relevant roles to the professional identity. The higher the status of the profession, the more this process of subordinating all other relevant roles will be allowed" (Cohen 1981, p. 177). However, as there are changes in the demographic mix of people entering different professional groups, and yet inertia in professional identity formulations, this suggests that there may be persistent and pervasive influences of variables such class, gender, race, or ethnicity on professional identity.

Intersectionality is the notion that we have multiple social identities that are not independent and contribute to how we are perceived, valued, and treated by others (Crenshaw 1991). This supposition has been supported empirically in a study exploring factors influencing professional identity in first year health and social care students. Adams and colleagues concluded that "gender stereotypes, together with masculine/feminine traits and designations, have implications with regard to intergroup relations, and hence to the way in which professional identity is acted out" (Adams et al. 2006, p. 63). The authors cite related research suggesting that gender is an important determinant of the frequency and nature of interprofessional interactions (Kendrick 1995) and that gender is activated in the course of social perception (Brewer 1988). Volpe and colleagues found that only 10 of 92 articles included in their review of professional identity formation examined the intersection of personal demographics with professional identity (Volpe et al. 2019). This raises the issue of whether our ideas about professional identity formation are socioculturally biased, which disadvantages trainees from nontraditional backgrounds and thus preserves the status quo. Volpe and colleagues' review also reveals how underrepresented minorities report having to repress their personal attributes (gender, race, ethnicity, class, sexuality) in order to succeed and how a lack of role models and social exclusion cause some to self-select out of certain professions. Their review reveals how professional identity as a transcendent attribute, where professionals are valued according to what they do, rather than who they are, is an ideal rather than a reality, and in an era of identity politics and populism, it is perhaps at risk.

Professional Identity Formation

Having presented a range of critical perspectives on professional identity, this section moves on to discuss theories on how professional identities are formed.

Identity Formation as Socialization

Goldie describes various perspectives on identity formation including socialization, whereby students learn to adhere to, internalize, or reject prevailing sociocultural norms (Goldie 2012). In this way, novices rework their identity until it fits into their social surroundings through a process of experimentation and feedback. They ultimately learn to express themselves in a way that is socially acceptable, observing the consequences of their own behaviors. They can also see how they are treated by others because of their professional role and see the social consequences of others' behaviors, including through vicarious experience, storytelling, and cautionary tales. What was initially a behavioral performance eventually becomes habitual as their professional identity becomes an integral part of who they are. This socialization model accounts for how professional identity can be transmitted forward onto novices. It relies heavily on the existence of positive role models and positive role experiences, as part of the experimentation process is likely to include emulation of aspects of seniors' conduct. The impacts of negative role modelling and suboptimal role experiences can, to a certain extent, be mitigated through the provision of safe reflective spaces, supporting the novice in rejecting rather than adopting those behaviors (Leedham-Green et al. 2019).

Identity Formation as Transformation

Jarvis-Selinger and colleagues suggest that mature shifts in identity are a much deeper form of learning than internalizing social norms (Jarvis-Selinger et al. 2012). Within health professional education, there are transformations that can happen to learners. These might be the by-product of finally grasping a concept where the learner suddenly understands an idea or integrative theory that explains an aspect of their practice, or a transformative experience such as cadaveric dissection or attending their first crash call. Such transformative learning experiences are so called because they fundamentally change the learner and cannot be unlearned (Mezirow 1990). Ultimately, the learner may find himself or herself identifying within a narrow group of peers not necessarily based on professional boundaries, but also boundaries based on experiences, expertise, discourse, and interests, as an educator, innovator, or researcher.

Perceptual shifts are described by Meyer and Land in their theory of threshold concepts (Meyer and Land 2005). True perceptual shifts do not occur very often, and can be profoundly unsettling, opening up new affective and cognitive domains. Perkins introduced the concept of "troublesome knowledge" as a precursor to transformation (Perkins 1999). It is called troublesome because it does not fit into the learner's current conceptual understanding. For example, a healthcare student may fixate on their role as healer and find the patient with chronic symptoms or a dying patient outside their perceptual understanding of their role and therefore troublesome. Nursing students might see the provision of traditionally physician-led therapies as outside their professional role, requiring a perceptual shift in what it means to be a nurse before truly engaging in this learning (Hurley 2013). To progress from one identity to another involves transitioning through an in-between space or the liminal state (Turner 1987). This is a transitional place in which students see the need to let go of an earlier identity, but still have not quite grasped and integrated the new identity. The role of the educator is then to guide students safely across boundaries into a new space. These shifts in identity are likely to be greatest at transitional moments, such as from school to higher education (Nyström 2009), as well as from higher education to the clinical workplace, from trainee to professional, or from professional to retiree. A true shift in perspective often involves new ways of talking, so that the "cadaver" becomes the "donor's body." You can be socialized into using this language, but ultimately, it entails a shift in perception.

Atherton describes how learners might resist identity transformation, as this type of learning involves loss: there is destabilization as the old self is lost, disorientation while in a liminal state, and the hard work of reorientation as a new self is constructed (Atherton 1999). Land et al. argue that the liminal state is an uncomfortable and vulnerable one and that students are unlikely to progress independently across these thresholds without expert support, as the knowledge they need to progress might be outside their previous understanding of their world. They argue for educators to promote a "positive psychology" of hope, self-efficacy, and coherence to support learners through the emotional cost of transformation (Land et al. 2016).

Curricular Positioning

Whether one sees professional identity formation as a process of socialization or transformation or as a combination of both, there are considerations for curricular planning and positioning which we now present.

Framing Professional Identity within Curriculum Design

The multiplicity of perspectives on professional identity raises important questions on how to frame professional identity formation within curricular design. There are likely to be multiple perspectives on what professional identity is and how it is formed, and educators will need to be both critical and creative about how institutions set about professionalizing healthcare students.

Education on professional identity that simply reiterates the formally articulated codes of conduct of a profession is likely to yield curricula that induct students into idealized forms of professional identity. As such, the teaching will not give emphasis to the more pragmatic and even dysfunctional aspects of their profession. Therefore, teaching may risk alienating students if they are unable to reconcile the espoused ideal with what they see practiced, if they are unable to criticize what they perceive to be adverse influences, or if they are unable to reconcile their personal identity within the prevailing sociocultural norms of their profession. Trying to mold students toward an institutionally predefined concept of professional identity may also be problematic for numerous other reasons, for example, alienating students if educators appear to be prejudging their sense of self and their motivations or to be imposing reductive judgments about who students will become, what they should do, and why.

Teaching that emphasizes professional identity as an expression of sociological status, the medicalization of everyday life, or as a way of coping with unpleasant tasks may also be limited. Such an approach may not give due attention to the high standards, altruistic aims, and demanding practices defining the profession. It risks glossing over professionals' vocational calling and their commitment to self-sacrifice and others' well-being. Emphasizing the complexity and instability of contemporary healthcare practice may highlight the increasing number of competencies and selves required for being a good clinician. However, as the boundaries of professional roles stretch and blur, this may risk the very formation of a professional identity.

Looking at students' perspectives on being professionalized, Birden and Usherwood found that medical students arrived with pre-formed conceptions of professionalism and professional identity and resented being taught to become professional (Birden and Usherwood 2013). Their qualitative study across three medical schools identified the following themes: First, students seemed confident in their developing professional identities and held a pragmatic conceptual framework (definition) of professionalism based on their experience and reflection. Second, students had a low regard for the professionalism teaching they had experienced and for the ways in which professionalism had been assessed in their learning programs. Third, students had learned to "game the system," giving assessors the results on reflective writing assignments that they believed their assessors wanted to hear and that would gain them a pass. Fourth, students saw the situations they experienced in clinical placements as being far more complex than the ones they were presented with in teaching sessions, which they considered superficial or trivial. Fifth, students considered experiential learning – observing good professional practice – to be the best way (some viewed as the only way) to learn professionalism. And finally, students consolidated what they learned, and formed their individual mental model of professionalism, through discussion and reflection with their peers in medical school. These findings suggest that learning happens through authentic role experiences and reflective discussion rather than in the classroom. This has implications for differential attainment based on inclusivity and reaffirms that attempts to teach and assess professionalism and professional identity directly are complex and may even be counterproductive.

To avoid caricaturizing and devaluing professional identity formation, curriculum designers might instead consider fostering criticality and an appreciation of complexity in their students. Approaches might include fostering the articulation of multiple perspectives through humanities-based approaches to clinical education (Zahra and Dunton 2017), fostering student engagement in curriculum design and delivery (Mann 2001), acknowledging and addressing challenges to inclusivity

(Aysola et al. 2018), and using students' lived experiences of the clinical workplace as foci for reflective deliberations and debrief (Leedham-Green et al. 2019).

A Model to Aid Curriculum Planning

Identity as an educational goal is problematic for a variety of reasons, some of which are discussed above. Although problematic, it does not mean that professional identity formation is not important. Students may take time to internalize and enact the espoused values and behaviors of their chosen profession and may need support to develop an aspirational professional identity that feels congruent for them. Identity formation therefore requires educators to think about the topic in a different way to traditional competency-based education.

Depending on one's stance on professional identity formation, the role of the educator may not be to teach people what or how to be; rather it may be to support the development and enactment of a personally congruent positive identity. This requires curriculum planners to attend to the behavioral and contextual drivers of identity formation.

As with any complex intervention, there is unlikely to be a single solution, and curricular activities are more likely to be successful if they target multiple drivers across multiple domains (Pai et al. 2018). Behavioral change theory, rooted in health psychology, tells us to attend to participants' capabilities, opportunities, and motivations (Michie and Johnston 2012). A complementary model, Bronfenbrenner's ecological model (Bronfenbrenner 1994), describes how interventions can be targeted at different interconnected levels: personal, interpersonal, team, organizational, and societal.

By combining the two models, it is possible to create a grid comprised of discrete cells, within which educators can list a range of actions designed to support professional identity formation across multiple domains (Fig. 1). The grid's contents, completed here for illustrative purposes, will need to be considered locally, taking into consideration local resources, team dynamics, and organizational priorities. The grid's purpose is to stimulate curricular planning that considers a broad range of potential interventions.

Focused Strategies for Educators

This section outlines in greater detail some of the strategies listed in Fig. 1 to promote professional identity formation in health professional education.

Access to Role Experiences

Access to role experiences and role models is an essential component of professional identity formation (Cruess et al. 2008). The contours of professional identity can

35 Developing Professional Identity in Health Professional Students

	Personal	Interpersonal	Team	Organisational	Societal
Capability	Knowledge of team roles and expectations Recruitment based on orientation to role	Collaborative skills and proficiencies Interpersonal respect and inclusivity	Address inter-professional power imbalances Interprofessional respect and inclusivity	Address the hidden curriculum Unconscious bias training Protected time for clinical teaching	Acknowledge and respond to societal influences, for example marketization of healthcare
Opportunity	Access to authentic role experiences	Mentoring Personalised support through transitions	Legitimate junior team roles Safe reflective spaces Multi-professional simulation	Students as co-creators of curricular content Longitudinal placements and apprenticeship learning	Opportunities for learner engagement within wider society, for example volunteering
Motivation	Encouragement, rewards, sanctions Imagining self within role Building confidence and self-efficacy	Visible role models Coaching approaches to supervision and remediation	Team feedback Team building	Assessment culture that supports complexity and uncertainty Personal choice in professional developmental activities	Recognise and reward wider societal engagement

Fig. 1 An example of a curricular planning grid across behavioral and contextual domains

never be exhaustively delineated through formal or even informal instruction. Exactly what the role model articulates about the profession may not be the principle influence, as much as the student's observations of their seniors in role. Becoming a healthcare professional thus requires participation in the profession's *in situ* practices in order to appreciate and act on their complexities and to understand the evolving character of the contemporary clinician's identity. Role experiences are contingent on novices being granted access to that practice by those who determine and maintain its boundaries and entry points. This might be a practical boundary, such as passing an exam, or a social entry point, such as inclusion into a reflective discussion after a difficult operation. Addressing the privileging of inclusion to certain demographics can be informed by the literature on retention and success in higher education (Thomas et al. 2017).

Multi-Professional Simulation

Given the complexities of clinical care, it is not surprising that the deployment of experiential learning opportunities including simulation-based education is gathering pace. There are however gaps between simulation and actual clinical-professional practice and between formal debrief and informal workplace learning. Simulation-based education inevitably loses some of the full complexity of clinical settings, and participants' simulated conducts are unlikely to project the full range of conducts and responses elicited in real time amidst emergent care circumstances. Nonetheless, it has the potential to open up opportunities for transferrable learning about professional identity including perpetual shifts relating to hierarchy, leadership, and distributed expertise. Simulation-based education as an opportunity for identity formation may not be effective if it is limited to the reproduction of ideal-type conducts and identities. It loses validity if it becomes a self-referential condition that no longer bridges to the real world (Bligh and Bleakley 2006). For simulation to be meaningful, fidelity becomes less about the physical replication of reality and more about the functional representation of real-world cues and stimuli (Hamstra et al. 2014).

Safe Reflective Spaces and Protected Time

The quality of debrief following simulation-based education is seldom replicated in the rushed but potentially valuable conversations that happen in real time in the clinical workplace. Students entering the workplace for the first time will have fresh eyes on the idiosyncrasies and peculiarities of workplace practice. Learners may have questions about real-time practices encountered on placements that carry great significance for them, including questioning the moral-ethical dimensions of care. Students may not feel safe questioning their seniors in the workplace and therefore would benefit from the creation of safe reflective spaces. For example, a student might ask how a patient can be expected to assume responsibility for negotiating their subsequent referrals and shared decision-making after having been informed they have metastatic cancer and is clearly consumed by emotion. These kinds of questions make it possible for the learner to negotiate and navigate the emotional and moral dimensions of care in addition to the clinical-technical dimensions of care. These impact on their ability to invest themselves fully in the priorities and prerogatives of the clinical workplace and ultimately to align their personal identity with that of their profession. Protected time to support students in processing troublesome knowledge is needed. Creation of safe reflective spaces that are shared by both faculty and students is a challenge. The evidence emerging on student involvement in Schwartz Rounds is promising (Zervos and Gishen 2019), as is research on strategies for facilitating authentic reflective practice (Wald 2015).

Responding to the Hidden Curriculum

The hidden curriculum is a term used to describe the learning that happens outside planned educational activities (Hafferty and O'Donnell 2015), for example, learning through observing interprofessional behaviors in the workplace or absorbing tacit rules and conventions. Hidden curricula are inevitable and can have both positive and negative impacts on student learning and therefore warrant careful examination. In order to study the hidden curriculum in relation to professional identity formation, educators need to develop strategies to explore the clinical learning environment through the eyes of their students (Leedham-Green et al. 2019). The hidden curriculum can never be eliminated, but Haidet and Teal suggest that interventions should instead be directed upstream toward the forces fostering the hidden curriculum and downstream toward mitigating its impacts (Haidet and Teal 2015). Examples relating to professional identity formation might include support for better role modelling through protected time for clinical teaching or through the provision of safe, reflective spaces to process difficult workplace experiences.

Communities of Practice and Activity Theory

Creuss et al. suggest that attending to the determinants of identity formation at a team level can be informed by the literature on communities of practice (Cruess et al. 2019). Wenger describes how learning is socially constructed, shifting the analytic focus from the individual as learner to learning as participation in a social world. Wenger critiques the theoretical inadequacy of blaming the marginalized for being marginal. He describes how identity is formed through access to competence and experience, and "mutual engagement around a joint enterprise," and gradual movement from the periphery to the center of a community of practice (Wenger 1998, p. 214). This is challenging in an undergraduate context unless there are stable teams that students can be invited to join, longitudinal placements for students within those teams, and opportunities for students to engage in legitimate team roles.

Research on longitudinal integrated clerkships is therefore likely to be helpful, whereby students undertake their core clinical learning within a single team rather than rotate through specialties, with responsibility for patients rather than for tasks (Hirsh et al. 2012). Bates et al. found explicit links between competency and identity in a longitudinal integrated clerkship (Bates et al. 2013). Longitudinal relationships between preceptors and students also allow team members to make informed entrustment decisions (Hirsh et al. 2014). This means that participation can be pitched at a level that stretches the student without compromising their ability to complete a task safely with support at hand at the zone of proximal development (Vygotsky et al. 1978). Where there is no "team" and activities are organized around fluid combinations or "knots" of professionals that form and reform depending on the task, this becomes doubly complicated. Bleakley suggests that student identity formation in this context needs to be informed by activity theory (Engeström 1999) where students learn through engagement in multi-professional activities (Bleakley 2011), for example, an operation rather than engagement in a surgical "firm." This requires clarity of handover regarding entrustment decisions as teams dissolve and reform.

Mentoring and Role Modelling

On an interpersonal level, interventions to support professional identity formation include mentoring and role modelling. If these are left to grow organically, there is a risk that they favor hegemony over diversity. Edmunds et al., in their systematic review of gender in clinical academia, found informal networks tend to favor those with highest social capital, while learners with low social capital tend not to ask powerful incumbent mentors to support them (Edmunds et al. 2016). Furthermore, a lack of diverse role models can result in disidentification, compensatory behaviors, and stereotype threat. The literature on retention and success within higher education has recommendations for how mentoring and role modelling can be facilitated to promote inclusivity and more equitable educational attainment (Thomas et al. 2017). Unconscious bias training is another potentially fruitful area for action (Sukhera and Watling 2018).

Assessment Practices

Identity itself is a social construct, and attempts to measure it as an attribute through validated scales will only be as valid as the constructs the scale is based on. This is further complicated by the fact that as soon as any scale becomes a target, either for faculty or for students, it is unlikely to remain a valid test of the underlying quality it was designed to measure.

Any test based on observation is fundamentally a test of behavior rather than identity. Behaviors therefore are an indirect measure of professional identity and require interpretation. If a student fails to enact professional ideals in a given situation, there may be many explanations, such as a failure of understanding or skills, or an indication of a wider cultural, educational, or contextual problem, and not necessarily a failure of identity formation.

Rather than trying to measure professional identity formation, we suggest assessment practices focus on providing opportunities and motivation for engagement in complex learning and engagement in the workplace, for example, an assessment that requires learners to reflect on team dynamics and implications for patient safety in the operating theater.

The creation of larger healthcare schools has led, particularly in medicine, to an assessment culture dominated by machine-marked written examinations and structured tests of isolated clinical skills. The prevailing assessment paradigm within medical education has become one of performative measurement to predefined standards, which favors rote learning over the development of cognitive maturity or criticality. There is a risk that these students retreat from learning in the workplace if examinations favor memorization of clinical guidelines and textbook performances of individual rather than team skills.

This entrenched assessment paradigm disadvantages teaching and learning in the humanities and the behavioral and social sciences (Litva and Peters 2008). In an overcrowded curriculum, many students will necessarily prioritize activities that allow them to progress over more optional complex learning activities (Cilliers et al. 2012). There is a call to reduce the burden of assessment while simultaneously increasing the complexity of assessment modalities to support assessment in authentic contexts where standardization is impossible (Van Der Vleuten et al. 2017). There is a need to acknowledge that in many contexts, reductionism in the pursuit of objectivity risks losing validity.

There is an emerging literature on integrative assessments (Crisp 2012) and programmatic assessment (Schuwirth and Vleuten 2019), as well as the maturing literature on how portfolios can be redesigned to support authentic, complex learning (Driessen 2017). Educators may find these more appropriate assessment modalities to promote the behaviors and workplace-based activities that drive positive professional identity formation.

Student Engagement

Engaging students as partners in educational design is a growing movement (Peters et al. 2019). There are likely to be multiple benefits in students co-designing their own professionalization curricula, potentially in collaboration with patients or other interprofessional students. Students are likely to view their curriculum through a forward-looking rather than retrospective lens, as well as attending to the perceived value and authenticity of assessments. Co-design can work on an individual as well as curricular level. Goldie describes a postmodernist stance on professional identity formation, where the educator's role is to support graduates in constructing their own professional identity, developing attributes that feel authentic to them (Goldie 2012). This stance might involve co-designing opportunities for learning that strengthen their sense of personal identity within their work context, for example, through research activities or projects that feel congruent to their intrinsic values and motivations.

Conclusion

Educating healthcare professionals in ways that enable them to retain and enact aspirational professional identities within the demands of contemporary healthcare remains a complex issue. This chapter has examined professional identity as ideal, as well as the more pragmatic identities as enacted within the challenges of a modern healthcare context. We have touched on critical aspects relating to hierarchies and inclusion and the future of professional identity as role boundaries blur in response to rising care complexity and holistic rather than siloed approaches to patient care. In addition to providing a range of perspectives on healthcare identity and the dynamics of its formation, this chapter has set out a range of parameters and enabling strategies to support identity formation within health professional curricula while acknowledging the challenges that these phenomena pose for novices, including the hidden curriculum. We have called for educators to enact the epistemologies of the behavioral and social sciences as well as the humanities in designing their professionalization curricula, rather than the prevailing paradigm that is more suited to the biomedical sciences, particularly in relation to educational goals and assessment. Finally, we have provided a flexible framework for educators that targets multiple behavioral and contextual domains, so that strategies to enable the formation and enactment of a personally congruent professional identity can be considered within a variety of healthcare professional contexts. There will always be developments and challenges for how novices professionalize and for how educators educate. Looking forward into a challenging and uncertain future for health and healthcare, supporting students in developing a positive identity and outlook, through expertise, criticality, and cognitive maturity is an important strategy with the potential for enduring positive impacts.

Cross-References

▶ Communities of Practice and Medical Education
▶ Contemporary Sociological Issues for Health Professions Curricula
▶ Focus on Selection Methods: Evidence and Practice
▶ Focus on Theory: Emotions and Learning
▶ Hidden, Informal, and Formal Curricula in Health Professions Education
▶ Programmatic Assessment in Health Professions Education
▶ Simulation as Clinical Replacement: Contemporary Approaches in Healthcare Professional Education

References

Abbinnett R. Culture and identity: critical theories. London: Sage; 2003.
Adams K, Hean S, Sturgis P, Clark JM. Investigating the factors influencing professional identity of first-year health and social care students. Learn Health Soc Care. 2006;5:55–68.
Armstrong D. A new history of identity. London: Palgrave Macmillan; 2002.
Atherton J. Resistance to learning: a discussion based on participants in in-service professional training programmes. J Vocat Educ Train. 1999;51:77–90.
Aysola J, Barg FK, Martinez AB, Kearney M, Agesa K, Carmona C, Higginbotham E. Perceptions of factors associated with inclusive work and learning environments in health care organizations a qualitative narrative analysis. JAMA Netw Open. 2018;1:e181003.
Bates J, Konkin J, Suddards C, Dobson S, Pratt D. Student perceptions of assessment and feedback in longitudinal integrated clerkships. Med Educ. 2013;47:362–74.
Berwick DM. Era 3 for medicine and health care. JAMA. 2016;315:1329–30.
Birden HH, Usherwood T. They liked it if you said you cried: How medical students perceive the teaching of professionalism. Med J Aust. 2013;199(6):406–9. [published Online First: 2013/09/17]
Bleakley A. Learning and identity construction in the professional world of the surgeon. In: Fry H, Kneebone R, editors. Surgical education: theorising an emerging domain. Dordrecht: Springer; 2011.
Bligh J, Bleakley A. Distributing menus to hungry learners: can learning by simulation become simulation of learning? Med Teach. 2006;28:606–13.
Brewer MB. A dual process model of impression formation. Hillsdale: Lawrence Erlbaum Associates, Inc.; 1988.
Bronfenbrenner U. Ecological models of human development. Read Dev Child. 1994;2:37–43.
Cilliers FJ, Schuwirth LW, Herman N, Adendorff HJ, Van Der Vleuten CP. A model of the pre-assessment learning effects of summative assessment in medical education. Adv Health Sci Educ Theory Pract. 2012;17:39–53.

Cohen HA. The Nurse's quest for a professional identity. Menlo Park: Addison-Wesley Publishing Company, Medical/Nursing Division; 1981.

Crenshaw K. Mapping the margins: intersectionality, identity politics, and violence against women of color. Stanford Law Rev. 1991;43:1241–99.

Crisp GT. Integrative assessment: reframing assessment practice for current and future learning. Assess Eval High Educ. 2012;37:33–43.

Cruess SR, Cruess RL, Steinert Y. Role modelling – making the most of a powerful teaching strategy. BMJ. 2008;336:718–21.

Cruess SR, Cruess RL, Steinert Y. Supporting the development of a professional identity: general principles. Med Teach. 2019;41:641–9.

Driessen E. Do portfolios have a future? Adv Health Sci Educ. 2017;22:221–8.

Edmunds LD, Ovseiko PV, Shepperd S, Greenhalgh T, Frith P, Roberts NW, Pololi LH, Buchan AM. Why do women choose or reject careers in academic medicine? A narrative review of empirical evidence. Lancet. 2016;388:2948–58.

Engeström Y. Activity theory and individual and social transformation. In: Perspectives on activity theory. New York: Cambridge University Press; 1999. p. 19.

Erikson EH. Identity: youth and crisis. Oxford, UK: Norton & Co.; 1968.

Foucault M, Sheridan A. The birth of the clinic: an archaeology of medical perception. London: Routledge; 2003.

Freidson E. Profession of medicine: a study of the sociology of applied knowledge. Mead: Dodd; 1970.

Gibelman M. Television and the public image of social workers: portrayal or betrayal? Soc Work. 2004;49:331–4.

Goldie J. The formation of professional identity in medical students: considerations for educators. Med Teach. 2012;34:E641–8.

Hafferty FW, O'donnell JF. The hidden curriculum in health professional education. Dartmouth College Press; 2015.

Haidet P, Teal CR. Organizing chaos: a conceptual framework for assessing hidden curricula in medical education. The hidden curriculum in health professional education. Dartmouth College Press; 2015.

Hamstra SJ, Brydges R, Hatala R, Zendejas B, Cook DA. Reconsidering Fidelity in simulation-based training. Acad Med. 2014;89:387–92.

Hirsh D, Walters L, Poncelet AN. Better learning, better doctors, better delivery system: possibilities from a case study of longitudinal integrated clerkships. Med Teach. 2012;34:548–54.

Hirsh DA, Holmboe ES, Ten Cate O. Time to trust: longitudinal integrated clerkships and entrustable professional activities. Acad Med. 2014;89:201–4.

Hurley J. Perceptual shifts of priority: a qualitative study bringing emotional intelligence to the foreground for nurses in talk-based therapy roles. J Psychiatr Ment Health Nurs. 2013;20: 97–104.

Iedema R. (Post-) bureaucratizing medicine: health reform and the reconfiguration of contemporary clinical work. In: Gotti M, Salanger-Meyer F, editors. Advances in medical discourse analysis: oral and written contexts. Bern: Peter Lang; 2006. p. 111–31.

Iedema R, Jorm C. Nurturing anaesthetic expertise: on narrative, affect and professional inclusivity. Commun Med. 2018;15:53–64.

Illich I. Limits to medicine medical Nemesis: the exploration of health. London: Boyars; 1976.

Irby DM, Cooke M, O'brien BC. Calls for reform of medical education by the Carnegie Foundation for the Advancement of Teaching: 1910 and 2010. Acad Med. 2010;85:220–7.

Jarvis-Selinger S, Pratt DD, Regehr G. Competency is not enough: integrating identity formation into the medical education discourse. Acad Med. 2012;87:1185–90.

Kellar J. Who are we? – the evolving professional role and identity of pharmacists in the 21st century. In: Babar Z-U-D, editor. Encyclopedia of pharmacy practice and clinical pharmacy. Oxford: Elsevier; 2019.

Kendrick K. Nurses and doctors: a problem of partnership. In: Soothill K, Mackay L, Webb C, editors. Interprofessional relations in health care. London: E. Arnold; 1995.

Land R, Meyer JH, Flanagan MT. Threshold concepts in practice. Springer; 2016.

Leedham-Green KE, Knight A, Iedema R. Intra- and interprofessional practices through fresh eyes: a qualitative analysis of medical students' early workplace experiences. BMC Med Educ. 2019;19:287.

Lingard L, Reznick R, Devito I, Espin S. Forming professional identities on the health care team: discursive constructions of the 'other' in the operating room. Med Educ. 2002;36:728–34.

Litva A, Peters S. Exploring barriers to teaching behavioural and social sciences in medical education. Med Educ. 2008;42:309–14.

Mann SJ. Alternative perspectives on the student experience: alienation and engagement. Stud High Educ. 2001;26:7–19.

Mehta N. Mind-body dualism: a critique from a health perspective. Mens Sana Monogr. 2011;9:202.

Menzies IEP. A case-study in the functioning of social systems as a Defence against anxiety: a report on a study of the nursing service of a general hospital. Hum Relat. 1960;13:95–121.

Meyer JHF, Land R. Threshold concepts and troublesome knowledge (2): epistemological considerations and a conceptual framework for teaching and learning. High Educ. 2005;49:373–88.

Mezirow J. How critical reflection triggers transformative learning. In: Fostering critical reflection in adulthood, vol. 1. San Francisco: Jossey-Bass; 1990. p. 20.

Michie S, Johnston M. Theories and techniques of behaviour change: developing a cumulative science of behaviour change. Health Psychol Rev. 2012;6:1–6.

Nancarrow SA, Borthwick AM. Dynamic professional boundaries in the healthcare workforce. Sociol Health Illn. 2005;27:897–919.

Nursing & Midwifery Council. The code: professional standards of practice and behaviour for nurses, midwives and nursing associates. London: Nursing & Midwifery Council; 2018.

Nyström S. The dynamics of professional identity formation: graduates' transitions from higher education to working life. Vocat Learn. 2009;2:1–18.

Pai M, Schumacher SG, Abimbola S. Surrogate endpoints in global health research: still searching for killer apps and silver bullets? BMJ Glob Health. 2018;3:e000755.

Perkins D. The many faces of constructivism. Educ Leadersh. 1999;57:6–11.

Peters H, Zdravkovic M, João Costa M, Celenza A, Ghias K, Klamen D, Mossop L, Rieder M, Devi Nadarajah V, Wangsaturaka D. Twelve tips for enhancing student engagement. Med Teach. 2019;41:632–7.

Royal College Of Physicians. Doctors in society: medical professionalism in a changing world. London. Royal College of Physicians of London; 2005.

Schein EH. Career dynamics: matching individual and organizational needs. Reading: Addison Wesley Publishing Company; 1978.

Schuwirth LWT, Vleuten CPMVD. Current assessment in medical education: programmatic assessment. J Appl Test Technol. 2019;20:2.

Sukhera J, Watling C. A framework for integrating implicit Bias recognition into health professions education. Acad Med. 2018;93:35–40.

Thomas L, Hill M, O'mahony J, Yorke M. Supporting student success: strategies for institutional change. What Works; 2017.

Treiber LA, Jones JH. The care/cure dichotomy: nursing's struggle with dualism. Health Soc Rev 2015;24(2):152–62. https://doi.org/10.1080/14461242.2014.999404

Turner V. Betwixt and between: the liminal period in rites of passage. In: Betwixt and between: patterns of masculine and feminine initiation. La Salle: Open Court; 1987. p. 3–19.

Van Der Vleuten C, Sluijsmans D, Joosten-Ten Brinke D. Competence assessment as learner support in education. In: Competence-based vocational and professional education. Cham: Springer; 2017.

Volpe RL, Hopkins M, Haidet P, et al. Is research on professional identity formation biased? Early insights from a scoping review and metasynthesis. Med Edu. 2019;53(2):119–32. https://doi.org/10.1111/medu.13781

Vygotsky LS, Cole M, John-Steiner V, Scribner S, Souberman E. Mind in society: development of higher psychological processes. Cambridge, MA: Harvard University Press; 1978.

Wald HS. Professional identity (trans)formation in medical education: reflection, relationship, resilience. Acad Med. 2015;90:701–6.

Wass V, Gregory S. Not 'just' a GP: a call for action. Br J Gen Pract. 2017;67:148–9.

Weaver R, Ferguson C, Wilbourn M, Salamonson Y. Men in nursing on television: exposing and reinforcing stereotypes. J Adv Nurs. 2014;70:833–42.

Wenger E. Communities of practice: learning, meaning, and identity. Cambridge: Cambridge University Press; 1998.

Zahra FS, Dunton K. Learning to look from different perspectives – what can dental undergraduates learn from an arts and humanities-based teaching approach? Br Dent J. 2017;222:147–50.

Zervos M, Gishen F. Reflecting on a career not yet lived: student Schwartz rounds. Clin Teach. 2019;16:409–11.

Zola IK. Medicine as an Insitution of Social Control. Sociol Rev. 1972;20:487–504.

Hidden, Informal, and Formal Curricula in Health Professions Education

36

Lisa McKenna

Contents

Introduction 668
Defining the Hidden Curriculum 668
The Hidden Curriculum in Health Professions Education 670
Professionalism and Role Modelling 670
Hidden Curriculum and Behavioral Skills 672
The Hidden Curriculum in Peer Interactions 673
How the Hidden Curriculum Operates in Clinical Settings 673
The Role of the Patient in the Hidden Curriculum 674
Risks and Challenges in the Hidden Curriculum 674
Harnessing Positive Aspects of the Hidden Curriculum 675
Practical Approaches for Managing the Hidden Curriculum in Clinical Practice 676
Conclusion 677
Cross-References 677
References 677

Abstract

The existence of the hidden curriculum has been documented in educational literature for a number of decades. This concept largely refers to unintended learning occurring alongside that which is intended and formally delivered. Since the 1990s, a body of literature has evolved examining the hidden curriculum in the education of health professionals, particularly in the disciplines of nursing and medicine. Much of this has examined how the hidden curriculum operates in professional socialization and values development in practice-based settings. This chapter examines this body of literature and explores the concept of the hidden

---

L. McKenna (✉)
School of Nursing and Midwifery, La Trobe University, Melbourne, VIC, Australia
e-mail: l.mckenna@latrobe.edu.au

© Springer Nature Singapore Pte Ltd. 2023
D. Nestel et al. (eds.), *Clinical Education for the Health Professions*,
https://doi.org/10.1007/978-981-15-3344-0_47

curriculum, along with its potential benefits and challenges. In addition, the chapter explores how the hidden curriculum has been described across different learning contexts. Finally, it provides insights on how educators can harness the hidden curriculum to enhance student learning outcomes.

Keywords

Collateral learning · Hidden curriculum · Health professions education · Unintended curriculum · Vicarious learning

Introduction

The existence of a hidden curriculum has been described in education literature for decades. Over more recent decades, the hidden curriculum has also found its way into health professional literature, predominantly in the disciplines of nursing and medicine. For practice-based disciplines, the hidden curriculum is experienced primarily as the student negotiates between learning in the academic setting and what they witness within the unpredictable practice setting, that is, from concept-driven understandings to everyday variations in the real-world context. Traditionally, literature around the hidden curriculum in the health professional literature has focused on professionalism and role attributes, and often imparted from professional to student. Recent developments in thinking around the topic suggest that multiple hidden curricula exist in other types of learning, including between learners themselves. Undoubtedly though, overall focus on the hidden curriculum has been directed towards learning related to clinical practice.

This chapter explores the nature of the hidden curriculum in health professions education. By its nature in those disciplines, the focus is largely placed upon clinical or practice-based learning, whether in simulated learning environments or actual practice settings. The chapter begins by exploring the emergence of the concept of the hidden curriculum and related concepts, then examines how hidden curricula operate within health professions education. It concludes by exploring how the positive aspects of hidden curricula can be harnessed to enhance clinical learning outcomes and effective professional socialization.

Defining the Hidden Curriculum

Extensive consideration is given by course developers, clinicians, academics and accreditation bodies to the development of curricula for health professional students. This consideration involves the development of theoretical and practice learning experiences to prepare graduates who are competent to practice in their disciplines, and for professional registration in many disciplines. Learning is designed around structured learning experiences with measurable outcomes. However, this intended, explicitly defined curriculum only accounts for a part of what students will learn during their courses. In the background, other learning is informed by the hidden curriculum, and sometimes through multiple hidden curricula, operating. The hidden curriculum represents unintended learning outcomes acquired outside of the prescribed curriculum. For that reason, the hidden curriculum has been identified by some authors as the unintended curriculum. Chen (2015) suggests the hidden curriculum is composed of two elements, namely, "the absence of intentionality and the lack of awareness." (p. 8). By this, Chen was meaning that some of what students learn may not necessarily be what educators intend, and educators may be unaware of the full scope of what they are teaching students, namely, through their behaviors and actions. Hafferty (1998) distinguished between the concept of the hidden curriculum and informal curriculum. He viewed the hidden curriculum as being structural aspects that support learning, such as assumed professional norms, rituals, and customs, impacting on socialization, and viewed the informal curriculum as those processes in which students are immersed "at the level of interpersonal interactions" (p. 404). More recently, numerous authors have developed on Hafferty's ideas (Hafferty and O'Donnell 2015). According to Mulder et al. (2019), this means that the hidden curriculum operating in a particular clinical context "refers to the transfer of the culture of that workplace" (p. 36), while Karnieli-Miller et al. (2010) see the informal curriculum as the interpersonal processes in which the student interacts, namely, with health professionals, patients, and their families. Hence, overall, it appears that there are some definitional differences surrounding the concept of the hidden or informal curriculum, yet authors concur that the nature of learning is unintended or prescribed. Despite this, the hidden curriculum does enable unique and important insights into the "interactional nature of education" (Semper and Blasco 2018).

The idea that learning takes place beyond the intended curriculum is not new. As early as 1938, Dewey coined the concept of collateral learning, stating that this type of "learning in the way of formation of enduring attitudes, of likes and dislikes, may be and often is much more important than the spelling lesson or lesson in geography or history that is learned." (p. 20). In the context of health professional education then, it needs to be carefully considered by educators. Adding further complexity to this, learning via the hidden curriculum can occur with some intention, or by vicarious learning. The concept of vicarious learning has been well described in health professional education. Roberts (2010) describes the process of vicarious learning as how students utilize the experience of others for their own learning. For example, Stegmann et al. (2012) compared learning by doing and vicarious learning in simulated (standardized) doctor-patient interactions. They found that learning vicariously resulted in better student learning outcomes than learning by doing, reinforcing that learning by watching others can be an effective way to learn. Furthermore, a systematic review conducted by O'Regan et al. (2016) found that vicarious learning outcomes in healthcare simulation were enhanced through the use of observer tools and clarity about the observer role.

The Hidden Curriculum in Health Professions Education

The hidden curriculum can manifest itself in different ways, through practice, language and rituals. Hence, it can exist and underpin learning in a variety of ways in the education of health professions and in both educational and practice settings. Educators are becoming increasingly aware of its existence and influence on learning with extensive research emerging in health professional education, particularly from the disciplines of nursing and medicine. While in the health professions, the hidden curriculum is largely reported in practice-based learning, it can also be found in formal teaching and learning contexts, such as through unintended messages, including off-the-cuff statements, made during lectures or other academic teaching encounters (Chuang et al. 2010). It might also be delivered via presentation of cases with particular racial, gender, or cultural stereotypes, or stories and anecdotes (Hafferty and Franks 1994), or perspectives. In one Canadian study, Phillips and Clarke (2012) identified the hidden curriculum in the medical classroom. Students in their study reported conflict between the values being shared by the presenter and those of the institution via comments about marginalized people from lower socio-economic groups, or where the presenter's values differed from those of students.

Professionalism and Role Modelling

It is often through the hidden curriculum that health professional students learn about the expected behaviors of their profession and become socialized within that profession. As such, studies have suggested that students value the informal, hidden curriculum in developing their professional roles. According to Phillips (2013), "the values students absorb are those modelled by their teachers and colleagues, whether these comply with institutional mission statements, goals and codes of conduct or not" (p. 124). In Australia, Ozolins et al. (2008) interviewed medical students from first to fourth year using focus groups about their perceptions of the hidden curriculum. Students reported that it was through this learning that they actually learnt about how to behave as doctors. In the United States, Bandini et al. (2017) examined faculty and student perceptions of challenges encountered by students in caring for critically ill patients, and specifically influences of the hidden curriculum. Within this area, the hierarchy of medicine, role modelling of behaviors, research versus clinical work, and the hidden curriculum's importance emerged as key aspects. Students described how they learnt about power and hierarchy in the hospital and their role within that. They identified "good" behaviors where clinicians acted as good role models as well as "bad" behaviors such as belittling or objectifying patients. Students also identified learning what excellent patient care was and how to be compassionate, person-centered, how to listen to patients, and teamwork. Hence, the values and behaviors that were modelled before them directly influenced their own development. Similarly, in their study on medical students' learning experiences around professionalism, Karnieli-Miller et al. (2011) found that the hidden curriculum strongly influenced learning around respect, communication, responsibility, and caring.

The impact of negative role modelling through the hidden curriculum was specifically identified in one Brazilian study. In that study, Silveira et al. (2018) explored the impact of the hidden curriculum on medical students' professional identity development. They found that medical students were expected to "speed up" their work to ensure they were able to see as many patients as they could, rather than focus on their own learning. They experienced negative role modelling whereby patients were seen to be dehumanized, and practice that contradicted what they had been taught in the university which impacted on the students' overall wellbeing. Furthermore, medicine was demonstrated by doctors as being primarily commercial in nature, rather than a discipline with a sense of purpose and meaning. Such negative aspects of the hidden curriculum have the potential to lead to poor practices being reinforced or even questioning of career choice. Students may believe that they need to become resilient and adopt those values they are seeing operationalized in practice, having a very real impact on their learning and professional development (Phillips and Clarke 2012). Providing educators with training around educator professionalism has been identified as a possibility for enhancing focus on students and their learning needs (Glicken and Merenstein 2007).

Cultural influences play a large role in how and what students learn in clinical placements. Cultural differences between the academic- and practice-based settings may lead to further divide between formal and hidden curricula. Mossop et al. (2013) described a cultural web of factors influencing learning in clinical settings, consisting of core assumptions, routines, rituals, systems of control, and organizational and power structures that students need to learn at a local level. In another aspect of culture, formal contemporary health professional curricula place significant emphasis on cultural competence education. However, this may not necessarily be seen by students, or experienced by students from other ethnicities, in practice and in the delivery of culturally appropriate care (Paul et al. 2014). These authors argue that for cultural inequities to be addressed, the formal, informal, and hidden curricula need to become congruent.

The impact of role modelling in the hidden curriculum may not only be experienced by students. In a study of new graduate nurses in New Zealand, Hunter and Cook (2018) examined professional socialization and factors influencing professional development. Here, the hidden curriculum played a major part as graduate nurses reported learning how to act by watching other clinical nurses, in particular in the area of professionalism. They reported watching how other nurses interacted with patients, demonstrated calmness and effective time management. By watching many different nurses, they were able to discern the professional behaviors and attributes that they wanted to emulate. It was identified that where they witnessed repeated poor behaviors that these may influence the graduate nurse's own practice in a negative way.

The hidden curriculum often plays out in aspects of professional roles and attitudes. Phillips and Clarke (2012) undertook a qualitative study to examine teachers' behaviors in three Canadian medical schools. The researchers spoke with medical students about learning environments in relation to issues of equality, openness, values, discrimination, and perceptions of different types of doctors. They found that, despite organizational values, students had experienced being exposed to teachers' negative biases and personal beliefs, including around diverse groups in the community, denigration of female and family doctors and focus on patient diagnosis rather than patient-centeredness that was part of the formal curriculum. As a result, students were confronted with views that conflicted with their own personal values, were confused or challenged or resisted the ideas being presented. The study suggests that while students learn from the intended curriculum, they may regularly have to negotiate hidden curricula that they encounter.

Hidden Curriculum and Behavioral Skills

Over recent years, there has been a focus in health professions education on development of behavioral (also known as nontechnical) skills for ensuring patient safety and quality of care (Murphy et al. 2019). Behavioral skills refer to "the cognitive, social and personal resource skills that complement technical skills, and contribute to safe and efficient task performance." Such skills include situation awareness, decision-making, communication, and teamwork (Flin et al. 2013) and can be found embedded in the professional competency standards for a range of health disciplines (Peddle et al. 2018). Such skills are commonly identified within discussions around the hidden curriculum. In a US study, fourth year medical students reported that observing physicians and residents in interactions with patients did not always reinforce what they had learnt pre-clinically in medical school. As a result, at times they felt confused about what effective interviewing skills were (Rosenbaum and Axelson 2013). The nature of professional demeanor and communication styles with patients were key observations influencing medical students' learning in community-based clinical placements in a study by Thiedke et al. (2004). Similarly, nursing and midwifery students were found to be strongly influenced in their communication skills from what they experienced between teachers, nurses and doctors in providing patient education (Azadi et al. 2017).

Teamwork, too, emerges in discussions around the hidden curriculum. In a study exploring ward rounds in a pediatric clinical teaching unit, Doja et al. (2018) described observing rules around the medical team. They reported the nature of the team dynamics as occurring in a hierarchy with students knowing when they could speak up and ask questions. Nursing participants in the study by Hunter and Cook (2018) reported needing to work through the complexities of teamwork to enable them to work as effective team members but having to negotiate different personalities, hierarchical structures, other behaviors, and power relations. On the other hand, radiology resident programs in a study by Van Deven et al. (2013) in Canada found that a hidden curriculum of isolation operated whereby there was little teamwork and collaboration.

The Hidden Curriculum in Peer Interactions

The hidden curriculum is most often described as being delivered by academic or clinical staff. Little has been written around peer-to-peer transmission of hidden curricula (Halfer et al. 2011) which is also possible. In nursing and paramedic education, McKenna and Williams (2017) found that a hidden curriculum operated in near-peer teaching. In clinical learning laboratories, final year students were engaged in teaching clinical skills to first year students. In addition to the intended skills learning, it was found that junior students used the opportunity to explore aspects with their peers that they could not legitimately do with their academic teachers, utilizing the experience to explore aspects about the course more broadly, what to expect in clinical placement experiences and how to negotiate difficult or confronting practice situations into the future.

How the Hidden Curriculum Operates in Clinical Settings

The hidden curriculum can play out in numerous ways in clinical contexts. One of these is through the observational learning of health professionals engaging in their clinical work. Using ethnography, Webster et al. (2015) undertook a study to explore optimal interprofessional education between physicians in the emergency department and those in general internal medicine and how these impacted on residents and trainees. The researchers uncovered a hidden curriculum operating in how care delivery was viewed. They deemed that the concept of efficiency had greater importance than education in delivering "good patient care," and that ongoing references to patients with high needs were being termed as "failure to cope" reflecting that they impacted on efficiencies in delivery of care. Such views had the potential to impact on the way care was observed by residents and trainees and the researchers highlighted that "failure to cope" was not a recognized medical diagnosis so not taught in the classroom.

Another way that the hidden curriculum plays out in clinical education is through differing expectations of learners in the clinical setting between those educators delivering the academic curriculum and those working in practice. This is particularly evident in nursing. In the United Kingdom, Allan et al. (2011) described how, despite having specific learning outcomes to achieve in their supernumerary clinical placements, nursing students were expected to provide clinical care as nurses, not students, with the emphasis being on labor that they provided and not on their education. The authors argue that the nature of their status being supernumerary was not seen to be legitimate within the clinical setting, where one need to be seen to be working. The hidden curriculum enforced that the students were workers in that context, and not learners. Similarly, in a study conducted in Pakistan, nursing students were commonly used as adjunct staff despite being insufficiently educated to do so. This limited students' learning and opportunities to observe other activities from which they could learn (Jafree et al. 2015).

Using an ethnographic approach, Doja et al. (2018) conducted observations of interactions between medical students, residents, and attending staff during clinical rounds in a tertiary pediatric unit to explore how aspects of the hidden curriculum were enacted. They reported observing clear hierarchy within the team, whereby there were particular "rules" about who spoke and how each responded, and that physical positioning of the team reinforced a person's place in the hierarchy. They reported that students had clearly learned when it was appropriate to speak and how to demonstrate engagement.

The Role of the Patient in the Hidden Curriculum

While much has been written about the hidden curriculum, particularly relating to clinical learning, the patient or client is largely missing from the discussions. There is a clear gap in regard to what hidden curricula the patient brings to the learning process and a need for further research to understand this aspect. Despite this, there is reference to the patient in some of the hidden curriculum literature as a subject. In an ethnographic study exploring ten medical teams in two large US tertiary teaching hospitals, Higashi et al. (2013) identified that the hidden curriculum existed in determining patients' worthiness to receive treatment. Medical students in the study spoke about how they learned from senior physicians that certain patients, such as those considered to be "nice," wealthy, or suffering from conditions not resulting from their habits, were more deserving of care than others, such as frequently admitted patients, drug addicts, the elderly, and homeless people. Despite some students, trying to reject such values, the hospital and medical hierarchies meant that this was largely impossible to achieve. Similarly, medical students in Canada were exposed to the concept of a "good" patient as one who prioritized their health and self-care to manage their condition (Stergiopoulos et al. 2018).

Risks and Challenges in the Hidden Curriculum

The hidden curriculum that students encounter along their educational journeys has the potential to pose both personal risk and challenge. Different messaging may lead to confusion or conflict, internal or external, through tensions in beliefs, values, or what is being taught. Using qualitative methodology, Balboni et al. (2015) sought to examine the role of religion and spirituality for medical students and how these were negotiated as they encountered aspects of the hidden curriculum. Overall, they identified three domains where religion and spirituality were important in the socialization process and negotiating the hidden curriculum. Firstly, they found that experiences could challenge students' personal identities and impact their self-confidence, but religion and spirituality had the potential to offer some protection in managing emotional stress in caring for patients, enhanced ability to be compassionate and navigate challenging relationships, as well as achieving work-life balance. It also enhanced coping when dealing with patients who were suffering. In another study, medical students reported grappling with holding onto their personal and professional values in experiences where these were placed into conflict (Gaufberg et al. 2010). Given the potential person conflict that may arise from the hidden curriculum, there is a need to equip health professional students with strategies to enable them to manage their emotional responses to what they see in practice, and potential burnout and compassion fatigue (Bandini et al. 2017).

Harnessing Positive Aspects of the Hidden Curriculum

The existing literature presents examples of both positive and negative outcomes of the hidden curriculum. Certainly, both aspects present powerful learning opportunities if recognized and managed appropriately by educators and clinicians. In their study with medical students, Bandini et al. (2017) recognized that the hidden curriculum was an important component in students' professional role development, offering opportunities for reflections on self and others. These authors identified that students were not passive in receiving the hidden curriculum, rather internalized what they were learning. Chuang et al. (2010, p. 316.e4) suggest some strategies for harnessing and shaping learning within the hidden curriculum in the context of clinical learning:

1. Establish a climate that is cooperative, respectful, and supportive that includes learners, and where possible, patients.
2. Recognize and use sentinel events.
3. Role model desired attributes and behaviors, providing commentary on these.
4. Promote active learner engagement that facilitates human elements of care.
5. Act practically and with relevance, through humanistic approaches, communication skills, and strategies that enhance outcomes.
6. Apply a variety of strategies to promote learning and reflect different learning approaches.

The hidden curriculum has the potential to be a powerful learning strategy. It can be a highly challenging and emotional part of students' overall learning as they develop their professional values and socialize into their chosen profession. For this reason, effective support from educators is important as they make sense of what they hear and see, particularly in the professional practice setting in order to make sense of their experiences and how to effectively utilize them. According to Aultman (2005):

> Uncovering the hidden curriculum and understanding its effects on medical students and their relationships with others is a challenge requiring a collective commitment between educator and student through which a better understanding of diverse values and beliefs, within and external to the curriculum, can be achieved. (p. 264)

Furthermore, the identification of positive role models to support student learning is beneficial. To enable this, there needs to be a process of educating academics and clinicians to identify hidden curricula to enable them to work with students in critically evaluating their experiences to promote the positive and reject the negative components of hidden curricula encountered in every learning experience. In addition, clinicians need to encouraged to reflect on their practice, values, and beliefs and how these may impact on learners around them.

Practical Approaches for Managing the Hidden Curriculum in Clinical Practice

While aspects of the hidden curriculum may be challenging to manage, there are some practical approaches that may enable learners to grasp the positive aspects of the hidden curriculum and mitigate potential negative effects. Holmes et al. (2015) propose a four-step approach for assisting students to reflect on aspects of the hidden curriculum as they move into the practice setting:

1. Priming: Preparing the student for the hidden curriculum and addressing pressures to conform
2. Noticing: Assisting students to have situation awareness about pressures to conform
3. Processing: Reflecting on the situation, their actions, thoughts, and how they might approach similar situations in future
4. Choosing: Assisting students to make "intentional and informed decisions" about the behaviors they adopt (pp. 1365–1366)

Practically there are a number of strategies that clinical educators and clinicians can implement to support learning within the practice setting, including:

- Closely monitor what learners are exposed to in the clinical setting and identify where hidden curricula may exist and cause potential issues for students.
- Acknowledge students' perspectives and where tensions might arise.
- Promote critical reflection on students' experiences and highlight the learning that can be drawn from them.
- Guide learners towards positive, professional role models.
- Allow students to have time for open debriefing of practice experiences.
- Ensure a culture of safety and openness where negative experiences can be carefully understood and relayed back to individuals concerned.
- Utilize elements of the hidden curriculum as formal learning experiences through group discussions.
- Encourage opportunities to learn from peers about their clinical experiences as a safe way to acknowledge fears, apprehension, and issues and learn to deal with difficult situations.

Conclusion

The operation of the hidden curriculum has been described in health professional literature for a number of decades. Evidence of its existence can be found in both academic and practice learning settings. While it is largely unintended, learning from the hidden curriculum can be profound and powerful. Most research discusses its impact on aspects of professional socialization. While it can present challenges, and in some instances have negative outcomes, learning from the hidden curriculum can be harnessed into effective learning outcomes. While much is known, there still remains a distinct need for more evidence into how it operates and how it can be effectively utilized and managed, particularly in health disciplines other than nursing and medicine. Furthermore, there is a need for more research around the patient contribution to learning from the hidden curriculum.

Cross-References

▶ Conversational Learning in Health Professions Education: Learning Through Talk
▶ Developing Care and Compassion in Health Professional Students and Clinicians
▶ Developing Professional Identity in Health Professional Students
▶ Focus on Selection Methods: Evidence and Practice
▶ Focus on Theory: Emotions and Learning
▶ Learning and Teaching at the Bedside: Expert Commentary from a Nursing Perspective
▶ Medical Education: Trends and Context
▶ Obstetric and Midwifery Education: Context and Trends
▶ Supporting the Development of Patient-Centred Communication Skills
▶ Supporting the Development of Professionalism in the Education of Health Professionals

References

Allan HT, Smith P, O'Driscoll M. Experiences of supernumerary status and the hidden curriculum in nursing: a new twist in the theory-practice gap? J Clin Nurs. 2011;20:847–55. https://doi.org/10.1111/j.1365-2702.2010.03570.x.

Aultman JM. Uncovering the hidden medical curriculum through a pedagogy of discomfort. Adv Health Sci Educ. 2005;10:263–73.

Azadi Z, Ravanipour M, Yazdankhahfard M, Motamed N, Pouladi S. Perspectives of nursing and midwifery students regarding the role of the hidden curriculum in patient education: a qualitative study. J Educ Health Promot. 2017;6:108. https://doi.org/10.4103/jehp_jehp_37_17.

Balboni MJ, Bandini J, Mitchell C, Epstein-Peterson ZD, Amobi A, Cahill J, Enzinger AC, Peteet J, Balboni T. Religion, spirituality and the hidden curriculum: medical student and faculty reflections. J Pain Symptom Manag. 2015;50:507–15.

Bandini J, Mitchell C, Epstein-Peterson ZD, Amobi A, Cahill J, Peteet J, Balboni T, Balboni MJ. Student and faculty reflections of the hidden curriculum: how does the hidden curriculum shape students' medical training and professionalization? Am J Hosp Palliat Med. 2017;34:57–63.

Chen C. Do as we say or do as we do? Examining the hidden curriculum in nursing education. Can J Nurs Res. 2015;47:7–17.

Chuang AW, Nuthalapaty FS, Casey PM, Kaczmarczyk JM, Cullimore AJ, Dalrymple JL, Dugoff L, Espey EI, Hammoud MM, Hueppchen NA, Katz NT, Peskin EG. To the point: reviews in medical education – taking control of the hidden curriculum. Am J Obstet Gynecol. 2010;203:316:e1–6.

Dewey J. Experience and education. Indianapolis: Kappa Delta Pi; 1938.

Doja A, Bould MD, Clarkin C, Zucker M, Writer H. Observations of the hidden curriculum on a paediatric tertiary care clinical teaching unit. Paediatr Child Health. 2018;23:435–40. https://doi.org/10.1093/pch/pxx206.

Flin R, O'Connor P, Crichton M. Safety at the sharp end: a guide to non-technical skills. Cornwall: Ashgate; 2013.

Gaufberg EH, Batalden M, Sands R, Bel SK. The hidden curriculum: what can we learn from third-year medical student narrative reflections? Acad Med. 2010;85:1709–16.

Glicken AD, Merenstein GB. Addressing the hidden curriculum: understanding educator professionalism. Med Teach. 2007;29:54–7. https://doi.org/10.1080/01421590601182602.

Hafferty FW. Beyond curriculum reform: confronting medicine's hidden curriculum. Acad Med. 1998;73:403–7.

Hafferty FW, Franks R. The hidden curriculum, ethics teaching, and the structure of medical education. Acad Med. 1994;69:861–71.

Hafferty FW, O'Donnell JF, editors. The hidden curriculum in health professional education. New Hampshire: Dartmouth College Press; 2015.

Halfer JP, Ownby AR, Thompson BM, Fasser CE, Grigsby K, Haidet P, Kahn MJ, Hafferty FW. Decoding the learning environment of medical education: a hidden curriculum perspective for faculty development. Acad Med. 2011;86:440–4.

Higashi RT, Tillack A, Steinman MA, Johnston CB, Harper GM. The 'worthy' patient: rethinking the 'hidden curriculum' in medical education. Anthropol Med. 2013;20:13–23.

Holmes CL, Harris IB, Schwartz AJ, Regehr G. Harnessing the hidden curriculum: a four-step approach to developing and reinforcing reflective competencies in medical clinical clerkship. Adv Health Sci Educ. 2015;20:1355–70. https://doi.org/10.1007/s10459-014-9558-9.

Hunter K, Cook C. Role-modelling and the hidden curriculum: new graduate nurses' professional socialisation. J Clin Nurs. 2018;27:3157–70.

Jafree SR, Zakar R, Fischer F, Zakar MZ. Ethical violations in the clinical setting: the hidden curriculum learning experience of Pakistani nurses. BMC Med Ethics. 2015;16:16. https://doi.org/10.1186/s12910-015-0011-2.

Karnieli-Miller O, Vu TR, Holtman MC, Clyman SG, Inui TS. Medical students' professionalism narratives: a window on the informal and hidden curriculum. Acad Med. 2010;85:124–33.

Karnieli-Miller O, Vu TR, Frankel RM, Holtman MC, Clyman SG, Hui SL, Inui TS. Which experiences in the hidden curriculum teach students about professionalism? Acad Med. 2011;86:369–77.

McKenna L, Williams B. The hidden curriculum in near-peer learning: an exploratory qualitative study. Nurs Educ Today. 2017;50:77–81. https://doi.org/10.1016/j.nedt.2016.12.010.

Mossop L, Dennick R, Hammond R, Robbé I. Analysing the hidden curriculum: use of a cultural web. Med Educ. 2013;47:134–43. https://doi.org/10.1111/medu.12072.

Mulder H, ter Braak E, Chen C, ten Cate O. Addressing the hidden curriculum in the clinical workplace: a practical tool for trainees and faculty. Med Teach. 2019;41:36–43. https://doi.org/10.1080/0142159X.2018.1436760.

Murphy P, Nestel D, Gormley GJ. Words matter: towards a new lexicon for 'nontechnical skills' training. Adv Simul. 2019;4:8.

O'Regan S, Molloy E, Watterson L, Nestel D. Observer roles that optimise learning in healthcare simulation education: a systematic review. Adv Simul. 2016;1:4.

Ozolins I, Hall H, Peterson R. The student voice: recognising the hidden and informal curriculum in medicine. Med Teach. 2008;30:606–11. https://doi.org/10.1080/01421590801949933.

36 Hidden, Informal, and Formal Curricula in Health Professions Education

Paul D, Ewen SC, Jones R. Cultural competence in medical education: aligning the formal, informal and hidden curricula. Adv Health Sci Educ. 2014;19:751–8.

Peddle M, Bearman M, Radomski N, McKenna L, Nestel D. What non-technical skills competencies are addressed by Australian standards documents for health professionals who work in secondary and tertiary clinical settings? A qualitative comparative analysis. BMJ Open. 2018;8: e020799. https://doi.org/10.1136/bmjopen-2017-020799.

Phillips SP. Blinded by belonging: revealing the hidden curriculum. Med Educ. 2013;47:122–5.

Phillips SP, Clarke M. More than an education: the hidden curriculum, professional attitudes and career choice. Med Educ. 2012;46:887–93. https://doi.org/10.1111/j.1365-2923.2012.04316x.

Roberts D. Vicarious learning: a review of the literature. Nurse Educ Pract. 2010;1:13–6.

Rosenbaum ME, Axelson R. Curricular disconnects in learning communication skills: what and how students learn about communication during clinical clerkships. Patient Educ Couns. 2013;91:85–90. https://doi.org/10.1016/j.pec.2012.10.011.

Semper JVO, Blasco M. Revealing the hidden curriculum in higher education. Stud Philos Educ. 2018;37:481–98. https://doi.org/10.1007/s11217-018-9608-5.

Silveira GL, Campos LKS, Schweller M, Turato ER, Helmich E, de Carvalho-Filho MA. "Speed up!" The influences of the hidden curriculum on the professional identity development of medical students. Health Prof Educ. 2018. https://doi.org/10.1016/j.hpe.2018.07.003.

Stegmann K, Pilz F, Siebeck M, Fischer F. Vicarious learning during simulations: is it more effective than hands-on learning? Med Educ. 2012;46:1001–8.

Stergiopoulos E, Fernando O, Martimianakis MA. "Being on both sides": Canadian medical students' experiences with disability, the hidden curriculum, and professional identity construction. Acad Med. 2018;93:1550–9. https://doi.org/10.1097/ACM.0000000000002300.

Thiedke C, Blue AV, Chessman AW, Keller AH, Mallin R. Student observations and ratings of preceptor's interactions with patients: the hidden curriculum. Teach Learn Med. 2004;16:312–6.

Van Deven T, Hibbert K, Faden L, Chhem RK. The hidden curriculum in radiology residency programs: a path to isolation or integration? Eur J Radiol. 2013;82:883–7. https://doi.org/10.1016/j.ejrad.2012.12.001.

Webster F, Rice K, Dainty KN, Zwarenstein M, Durant S, Kuper A. Failure to cope: the hidden curriculum of emergency department wait times and the implications for clinical training. Acad Med. 2015;90:56–62. https://doi.org/10.1097/ACM.0000000000000499.

Arts and Humanities in Health Professional Education

37

Pam Harvey, Neville Chiavaroli, and Giskin Day

Contents

Introduction	682
A Health Humanities Perspective	682
A Clinical Encounter	682
A Humanities Lens	683
Why Health Humanities?	685
Learning and Teaching Strategies	688
The Tolerance of Ambiguity in Healthcare	691
Unstructured Learning Moments	692
A Clinical Encounter Revisited	693
Conclusion	694
Cross-References	695
References	695

Abstract

This chapter provides a perspective on clinical education through the lens of the humanities. It discusses enhancing clinical expertise by focusing learning on affective aspects of a learner's discipline, assisting their development as effective health professionals.

P. Harvey (✉)
La Trobe Rural Health School, La Trobe University, Bendigo, VIC, Australia
e-mail: p.harvey@latrobe.edu.au

N. Chiavaroli
Department of Medical Education, University of Melbourne, Melbourne, VIC, Australia
e-mail: n.chiavaroli@unimelb.edu.au

G. Day
Imperial College London, London, UK
e-mail: giskin.day@imperial.ac.uk

© Springer Nature Singapore Pte Ltd. 2023
D. Nestel et al. (eds.), *Clinical Education for the Health Professions*,
https://doi.org/10.1007/978-981-15-3344-0_49

Keywords

Health humanities · Humanities lens · Phronesis · Epistemological education

Introduction

The health humanities are an evolving area of scholarship and educational practice at the intersection of humanities and healthcare. It takes an interdisciplinary approach towards understanding the complexities of health and illness, the humanistic factors that influence the lived experience of those involved, and the contexts in which these occur. Education through the health humanities provides a way of making meaning using disciplines traditionally aligned with the arts and humanities, challenging notions that the necessary clinical skills of health professionals need only be learned through scientific knowledge and teaching clinical skills.

The health humanities are not new to health professional education. What began as "medical humanities," and became more inclusive of other health disciplines (Jones et al. 2017), is now part of the curriculum of many health professional schools, either integrated into core curricula or offered as an elective. The health humanities promised to assist learners to better manage the challenges and uncertainties of health practice through educational experiences that reflect the kinds of reasoning which underlie good clinical practice (Boudreau 2015).

A Health Humanities Perspective

A Clinical Encounter

Fourth year undergraduate medical student, Dana, is on the medical ward under the supervision of a registrar. Dana prepared to present Mrs. Thelma Bright to her clinical supervisor with the following information:

> Mrs Thelma Bright is a 78-year-old woman admitted yesterday after a fall at home. She was discovered by a neighbor after failing to bring in her recycling bin. It is estimated that Mrs Bright was not found for 24 h after her fall. Ambulance officers responded to the neighbor's telephone call and presented to the rural town 45 min later. Mrs Bright was assessed as responsive, with a Glasgow Coma Scale reading of 11. There was obvious deformity in her right wrist. She was transferred to a regional hospital and diagnosed with a right fracture of the radius and ulna, dehydration, and cachexia. Her wrist was immobilized and she responded to treatment in the emergency department, with her GSC revised to 13. Comorbidities include Type II diabetes, diverticulitis, and early stage dementia.

In Mrs. Bright's notes, Dana discovered an advance care plan in her records that stated she wanted medical treatment only if it would sustain her current quality of life. Her substitute decision-maker was listed as a son who was unable to be present until the next day. There were no other contacts listed in her record. A previous occupational therapy visit to her home reported that there were multiple safety concerns in Mrs. Bright's house but, at the time, a cognitively competent Mrs. Bright had refused any modifications.

As Dana stood at the nurse's station reading these notes, Mrs. Bright began to call out for pain relief. Dana notified a nurse who said pain relief was not due for another 2 h. An emergency call was made to another bed, and staff became busier. Mrs. Bright was still yelling when Dana's supervisor returned but Dana felt unable to mention her concerns until the registrar had attended to other patients. "She's had all the pain management possible for the moment," the registrar said. "She'll just have to cope."

Dana left the ward to attend tutorials and didn't return until the next day. Overnight, Mrs. Bright had a cardiac arrest and the team interpreted her written wishes as "no CPR." Mrs. Bright died shortly before Dana arrived. As Dana stood with the nurses at the central station, Mrs. Bright's son arrived looking flustered. Although he was taken to a private interview room, Dana could still hear him reacting angrily to news of his mother's death. The registrar shrugged when Dana looked at him. "It's difficult," he said, rubbing his face with his hand. "I might react the same way if it was my mother in there."

Dana remained at the desk as the son came out and went into his mother's room, emerging 2 min later and leaving the ward. She could see the corner of Mrs. Bright's bed and a nurse beginning to take care of the body. This was not how she imagined the care of a patient would go and she didn't know how to feel.

A Humanities Lens

The above fictional case is an amalgamation of student experiences, but the presentation of Mrs. Bright fits a typical standard medical paradigm. The patient is presented as a biomedical "problem" – a case of loss of consciousness, for which there are several possible differential diagnoses and underlying causes. The broken wrist complicates this presentation, as do other comorbidities. While the hospital team is presented as focussing on Mrs. Bright's immediate medical needs (restoration of full consciousness and stabilization of her fracture), Dana is portrayed as noticing important aspects, empathizing, and struggling to process several ethical, professional, and psychosocial aspects of Mrs. Bright's care. While this vignette was created specifically for the purposes of this chapter, this tension is by no means uncommon for medical and healthcare students (Ginsburg and Lingard 2011; Monrouxe et al. 2014).

Such tensions offer important opportunities for a humanities-related perspective on medical and health professional training. Dana's discovery of the advance care plan (a written document expressing a person's wishes for their end of life care) raises important considerations – ethical, functional (that is, determining quality of life), social, and legal issues which require understanding beyond biomedicine and clinical procedures. Mrs. Bright's previous refusal to allow modifications to her home might also raise further medicolegal and psychosocial issues (for example, regarding her cognitive functioning) which could influence how the advance care plan is interpreted and acted upon.

Dana's communication and articulation of her concerns to the hospital staff (including her own supervisor) introduces important system-level issues, complicated by Dana's status as a medical student. While the decision to hold off further pain management may well be defensible from a medical perspective, Dana's instinctive empathy is to be commended. Clearly, broader ethical and professional issues remain over how well the health system manages high-quality, compassionate care during busy periods, both in this case and more generally. Finally, from a pedagogical and professional development perspective, Dana's presence during the unfolding of the situation clearly presents a significant learning moment for her, and the scholarly literature is increasingly clear that these are moments that can be critical for students' professional identity formation (Monrouxe et al. 2014; Monrouxe and Rees 2012; Kay et al. 2018; Lundin et al. 2018). The supervisor's frank admission in relation to the son is commendable and could provide an important example of humanistic concern and empathy for Dana.

There is no doubt that many clinical supervisors are instinctively attuned to these sorts of challenges and teaching moments, and can and do assist health professional students through them. These moments are not always reflected in the taught or formal curriculum, which we now know can have major implications for how such affective and professional matters are perceived by students and supervisors alike (Hafferty and Franks 1994; Martimianakis et al. 2015). A number of teachers and practitioners of the health humanities have presented detailed and passionate rationales as to how humanities content, methods, and/or perspectives can facilitate student learning in medical and health professional education (Blease 2016; Tsevat et al. 2015; Bleakley 2015; Doukas et al. 2013; Kumagai 2017; Chiavaroli et al. 2018). Many go further to argue that the humanities can help students to learn to prepare for clinical placements and to learn to know and think like clinicians, drawing on the humanities' content and methods which emphasize and explore the ambiguous, the experiential, the particular, and the qualitative aspects of phenomena as a complement to the more positivistic and generalizable knowledge and ways of thinking of the bioscientific and clinical foundations of medicine. Such claims can be described as "epistemological," and we will explore these further in the next section.

Specifically, a humanities-informed perspective could have helped an educator focus on both the broader professional aspects and clinical complexities of the situation, including:

- Dana's thoughts and uncertainty about the status and impact of the advance care plan
- Dana's concerns about Mrs. Bright's pain (and lack of response of the staff)
- Dana's inability to bring the full extent of her concerns to the registrar's attention
- Her status on the ward as a medical or health professional student
- Dana's struggle to understand the clinical management priorities of the staff

- The difficulty of communicating bad news to family and the challenge of dealing with their response
- The emotional impact of the whole event on Dana, as a medical student and as a fellow human being.

While some of the above clearly involve specific clinical and medical features of Mrs. Bright's condition and situation, the majority concern *affective* aspects of a student's learning and development as a professional, such as Dana's final reflection on how events unfolded for Mrs. Bright. Therefore, they are likely not very amenable to didactic or clinically oriented responses by clinical supervisors; as deeply personal, emotional, and "embodied" experiences (Shapiro and Stolz 2019), approaches which value and explore empathy and understanding of patients' perspective would seem to be more useful here. The humanities can help clinicians tap into this level of response.

Let us leave Dana for now and turn to consider the status of health humanities in health and medical education.

Why Health Humanities?

The inclusion of the study of humanities in health professional curricula has had an uneven trajectory. Its successes have depended on the curriculum policies of individual medical schools, and often the enthusiasm of individuals willing to make a case for curriculum change. Fox has traced the origins of the medical humanities in the United States to a 1960s campaign for courses in "human values in medicine" (Fox 1985). In the United Kingdom, the General Medical Council's 1993 guidelines for outcomes for medical education (General Medical Council 1993) gave an impetus to the field when stating that arts and humanities be included in special-study options that were to make up a third of the undergraduate curriculum. Since the 1990s, courses have been offered in Australia and New Zealand, as well as many countries across Europe. An account of the development of medical humanities in Hong Kong, Taiwan, and China is given by Wu and Chen (2018), and initiatives in India are described by Shankar (2016). Initiatives in Africa are described in a special issue of the journal *Medical Humanities* (Various 2018). In spite of these initiatives, Dana would have been unlikely to have had exposure to humanities-type teaching at medical school. She may have been offered the opportunity to do a module in medical history or medicine and literature, but these are likely to have been optional on top of an already busy curriculum, or offered in competition with more apparently medically "useful" courses.

Journals, books, and medical humanities associations report a plethora of case studies on teaching humanities for students in medicine, nursing, dentistry, pharmacy, and allied professions. As Ousager and Johannessen have pointed out in their literature review of humanities in undergraduate education, many reports are descriptive of teaching models and justifications, rather than demonstrations of impact (Ousager and Johannessen 2010). The case for making space for the arts and humanities in already crowded curricular tends to be based on arguments that biomedical education is reductionist and in danger of depersonalizing medicine. The humanities are often construed as a corrective to a curriculum that trains doctors to be diagnostically skilled but uninspired, focused on treating diseases rather than healing individuals.

Another trend gaining traction is for the term "medical humanities" to be replaced, or supplemented, with "health humanities" (Jones et al. 2017). The word "medical" is argued to be insufficiently inclusive of allied health professionals, informal caregivers, patients, and those focused on health and wellbeing rather than just medical care (Crawford et al. 2015a; Jones et al. 2014a). Indeed, the humanities have been active in health professional teaching well before the name change (Parlow and Rothman 1975; Neidle 1982; Thow and Murray 1991; Bumgarner et al. 2007). The International Health Humanities Network (2019), funded mainly by the Arts & Humanities Research Council, is the nexus for this contemporary interdisciplinary work.

While few would argue that biomedical sciences are devoid of imagination and creativity, the case is often made that pedagogy in the sciences emphasizes the internalizing of bodies of knowledge by students rather than grappling with concepts such as uncertainty, lived experience, and the contextual contingencies of medicine (Day 2016). It is not surprising, then, that humanities and the arts, in which the emphasis is often on process – interpretation, acknowledgement of subjectivity, critical reflection – are seen as adjunct to the sciences.

While undoubtedly successful in gaining a foothold for the humanities in medical curricula, this complementary approach has been criticized for failing to "disrupt an intellectual economy in which all animating liveliness is accrued by the humanities, and all hard-nosed scientific expertise by the biomedical sciences" (Viney et al. 2015). Research into the intellectual underpinnings of the culture, social, and historical dimensions of medicine received a major boost in 2008 in the UK when the Wellcome Trust (Wellcome 2019) announced expanded funding streams for the medical humanities. Under the umbrella of the "critical medical humanities," spearheaded by the Institute for Medical Humanities at Durham University (2019), UK, proponents call for disciplinary "entanglement," rather than the hitherto dominant ideology of "integration" of humanities and medical science.

As alluded to earlier, an important rationale for the humanities in health professional education can be considered "epistemological," in the sense of helping students (and practitioners) to learn and better understand how to think like a clinician. Such a view goes beyond the traditional rationales for the medical/health humanities that offered essentially intrinsic or instrumental rationales for the field. Rather, it focuses on the required knowledge, reasoning, and thinking practice that makes for good clinical practice (Boudreau 2015; Kumagai 2017; Macnaughton 2000; Chiavaroli 2017; Solomon 2008). This involves much more than science-based knowledge or logico-deductive reasoning, as Montgomery argues in her influential book "How Doctors Think" (2006). Clinical reasoning, she writes, is "flexible, interpretive, ineradicably practical." For Kumagai (2017), such reasoning involves "encouraging engagement with complexity and ambiguity; seeing past the surface to historical and societal influences and causes; and encouraging an awareness of the multiple, unique voices and perspectives of patients." Such an approach applied to clinical education, we suggest, would be more educationally meaningful and personally supportive than one aimed at simply helping students understand the clinical details of patient presentations or learn their place in the health system as a medical student.

These epistemological considerations draw on a relatively long tradition in educational philosophy and the humanities of distinguishing between the *idiographic* and the *nomothetic*; or more simply, between the particular and the general. Biomedical knowledge privileges, indeed relies on, the latter, so that a medical treatment or clinical technique that works in one context is likely to generalize sufficiently to help other patients in a different context but with a similar condition. A good thing, too: health practice would be unsustainable if every case had to be approached from first principles every time. And yet, in some ways, every patient must be approached anew, at least from a holistic and patient-centered paradigm. This is where the humanities are a vital part of a health professional education. The humanities privilege the particular, the "individual and contextual factors that make a particular situation or experience qualitatively different from another" (Chiavaroli 2017; Bruner 1985). Different patients may share the same disease, but as the revered Canadian medical educator William Osler (1849–1919) sagely noted long ago, "it is much more important to know what sort of a patient has a disease than what sort of a disease a patient has."

Aristotle has bequeathed an Ancient Greek concept for such situationally sensitive clinical perspective – *phronesis*, or "practical wisdom." Many scholars and practitioners alike regard this as the essence of clinical practice: being able to recognize and incorporate the contextual, situational, and particular aspects of a presentation, while drawing on the clinically relevant, generalizable aspects which will enable evidence-based management (Chiavaroli and Trumble 2018; Neighbour 2016; Davis 1997; Kinsella and Pitman 2012). As important as clinical guidelines and algorithms have been in standardizing practice around the world, with indisputable improvements in certain patient outcomes, health practice which seeks to draw on an ethical, empathic, and situationally sensitive perspective of the patient remains the hallmark of professionalism (Kinsella and Pitman 2012). Phronesis, then, is the process of determining the appropriate action to take when "knowledge depends on circumstance" (Montgomery 2006). Health professionals should recognize in this phrase the very language frequently used in competency statements that purport to represent a profession's particular knowledge and competencies, or indeed, its epistemology. Consider how frequently the professions resort to phrases such as "appropriate," "relevant," and "suitable" as indicators of, and placeholders for, clinical and professional judgment; necessarily so, since like algorithms, such statements can never capture the actual and myriad factors that go into making the right decision at the right time. It is the humanities, with its disciplines and methods focused on analyzing, interpreting, and understanding human personal and social experience, which can help train our minds to look for, and be sensitive to, data at this level. It is exactly the alternative perspective that scientific knowledge and reasoning needs to provide health practice with a balanced and complementary foundation of knowledge, reason, and thinking.

So, let's return for a moment to Dana. We left her with particular dilemmas – uncertainty about aspects of Mrs. Bright's care, an inability to situate herself more powerfully on the ward as a team member, and the professional and personal challenges of highly emotive situations.

Applying a broader, humanities-oriented perspective to Dana's preparation for practice as a health professional student, her education so far may not have equipped her to cope with and learn from the reality of patient care and its accompanying affective impact. She has the clinical knowledge to accurately report Mrs. Bright's presenting issues to the clinical supervisor, and to formulate Mrs. Bright's management requirements. Tension was generated when Dana struggled to process the complex psychosocial and ethical aspects of the situation. Would the "entanglement" (Viney et al. 2015) of the health humanities into her curriculum have given her strategies for enhanced clinical practice? We think so: but what would this education look like?

Learning and Teaching Strategies

If Dana's educators decided to modify the health professional curriculum by entangling the health humanities, they may have included material such as literature, visual arts, or music. Applying another discipline's teaching paradigm into health professional education is not a new concept (Lake et al. 2015; Jones et al. 2019) and is used with the expectation that the application of a different lens to education will enrich student learning and professional development.

There are a multitude of practical examples from the literature of teaching incorporating the arts and humanities, used in different ways and for different purposes. The following provide some ideas and strategies which health professionals may use in their teaching. Evaluating these strategies will depend on the contexts in which they are delivered.

Close Noticing

The concept of "close noticing" arises from the need for health professionals to practice critical observation and *notice* their patients' presentation for diagnostic acumen (Bleakley 2015). It focuses on health professionals' use of their *senses* and their ability to be *sensitive* (that is, ethically and humanely aware of a situation). Bleakley (2015) regards close noticing as the core of work done by artists and art critiques, making the techniques these professions use as highly suitable for the training of clinicians.

There have been visual arts-based educational programs reported in the health profession educational literature (Braverman 2011; Boisaubin and Winkler 2000). Many focus on improving the observational skills – the visual literacy – of health professional students and also the ability to interpret and describe their observations. Others emphasize the development of empathy (Sampson et al. 2018; Yang and Yang 2013) and communication skills.

Borromeo et al., report on a visual arts-based training program for dentistry students studying the management of special-needs patients (Borromeo et al. 2014). The program aimed to improve students' ability to notice relevant information, that is, to see behind clinically focused areas such as the mouth to the individual as a whole. Students participated in several 2-h sessions involving analytical observation of artworks in an art gallery space and group discussions. At the end of these sessions, students reported that they had learned new skills in visual observation that they could apply to special-needs patients.

Naghshineh et al. used an arts-observation teaching technique called Visual Thinking Strategies (VTS) with a group of medical students to develop critical thinking and communication skills, and improve visual literacy (Naghshineh et al. 2008). Students were assigned either to be trained in this method or attend regular medical education sessions then tested against observational criteria. Students trained in VTS had improved observational skills. VTS has also been used for specific visual literacy needs such as improving clinical observation in dermatology (Gurwin et al. 2018).

What this training has in common is applying arts-based critical thinking to improve the critical reasoning of health professional students. Each involves "close noticing" for meaning-making. The use of our senses, not only limited to sight, in clinical judgment is a professional aesthetic that Bleakley suggests would complement more strictly analytical decision-making methods (Bleakley 2015).

Close Reading

The term "close reading" arises from literary scholarship and advocates close attention to more than the words in a text but also its tone, context, and representation (Shapiro et al. 2015). For example, medical educator Rita Charon suggests that training in close reading assists the interpretation of all textual matter, from fiction to clinical artefacts such as X-rays (Charon 2006). Developing this skill is part of *narrative competence*, or the ability to interpret the stories of the person and their illness within a situational context.

The use of literature in health professional courses has a history in the USA that dates back to the 1970s. The types of genres vary. Stories from patients (illness narratives or pathographies) and those from health professionals are common, particularly when the aim is to elicit responses about people's experiences of illness and healthcare. In the scholarly literature, there are recurring novels, short stories, and poems that lend themselves to these experiences. *The Doctor Stories* by William Carlos Williams is frequently used as an example of the social barriers between the patient and their carers, and the experience of dying (McLennan 1996; Charlton and Verghese 2010; Williams 1984/1932); as is *Wit* a play by Margaret Edson which has also successfully been adapted for film (Gottlieb 2018; Shapiro 2016).

By closely examining texts for their form and content, other elements are revealed. The act of reading itself is an active pursuit, as the reader interprets the text and creates meaning from it. In a sense, the reader uses cognitive and imaginative processes to position the text for understanding. The stories of Sherlock Holmes by Arthur Conan Doyle (a medical practitioner himself) have been used to study clinical reasoning (Montgomery 2000); Aldous Huxley's *Brave New World* to study bioethics (Yates 2013); and poems such as Raymond Carver's *What the Doctor Said* (Carver 2008) can be used to examine patient–clinician relationships. The choice of text will depend upon the learning objectives of the session.

A growing genre of literature is the "medical work memoir." These are often didactic about lessons learned from experience making them attractive reads for students eager to benefit from the first-hand accounts of professionals. Henry Marsh's accounts of dealing with fallibility in brain surgery, *Do No Harm* (Marsh 2014) and *Admissions* (Marsh 2018), are popular choices. The story of Paul Kalanithi's transition from doctor to patient in *When Breath Becomes Air* (Kalanithi 2016) wrestles with issues of medical hierarchy and when "too much information" becomes psychologically unhelpful. *The Language of Kindness* by nurse Christie Watson (2018) gives an insight into the highs and lows of caring for patients at their most vulnerable. Adam Kay's "secret diaries" of his medical training, *This is Going to Hurt* (Kay 2018), is both extremely funny and very poignant. The study of medical memoirs, and extracts from them, provides an opportunity to discuss the ethical implications of writing about patients, e.g., when does a memoir have to be so heavily fictionalized to protect patient identities that it no longer becomes "true"? At what point does writing about patients and colleagues become exploitative? Do candid admissions of medical mistakes damage public trust in medicine, or does honesty about medicine as a fallible enterprise serve as valuable reality check?

Close noticing and close reading are teachable skills if teachers themselves have strategies to do so. Having art and literature teachers involved in health professional education already occurs, particularly in universities that encourage interdisciplinary and interfaculty collaboration. It is also possible for clinician-teachers to upskill in arts and humanities methods. Having broader capabilities as teachers may give health professional students more scope to manage the discomfort and ambiguity of healthcare.

The experience of exploring difficult issues associated with healthcare through close noticing and close reading in an educational setting opens opportunities for conversations with students about ethically fraught situations: conversations they may recall and draw on when faced with complex situations on the wards. Had Dana studied a text such as *The Death of Ivan Ilych,* a novella by Tolstoy, it may have resonated with her in the face of Mrs. Bright's predicament. She may have recalled the loneliness felt by Ilych when his family appeared indifferent to his suffering. The story may have given Dana the confidence to approach Mrs. Bright and offer solace by merely being a comforting presence. If the reading had been supplemented with, say, the writings of Atul Gawande – especially his book *Being Mortal* (Gawande 2015) – Dana might have felt less overwhelmed by the situation and more comfortable with end-of-life issues. Crucially, she would have had the opportunity to talk through concepts around quality of life in the care of the elderly so that she could feel better emotionally prepared to interact with Mrs. Bright in a compassionate, humanistic way.

Learning and Practicing Empathy

If we add to the practices of close noticing and close reading, the idea of close listening, we approach the concept of empathy in health care, commonly defined as a multidimensional construct with cognitive, affective, behavioral, and moral components (Jeffrey 2016). There was a time (especially in medical education and practice) when its value or appropriateness was debated, challenged by the alternate principle of "clinical detachment" (Garden 2007). These days, wariness tends to be negated by increasing evidence of the powerful therapeutic effects of clinical empathy (Hojat 2016), and thankfully rare but disturbing evidence of the opposite effect when health system factors lead to emotionally uninvolved care (Weir et al. 2015; Halligan 2013). In terms of both education and practice, empathy is today regarded as a fundamental component of high-quality and effective health care (Hojat 2016); yet, alarmingly, some evidence points to its decline through the course of training across health professions (Sherman and Cramer 2005; Neumann et al. 2011; Nunes et al. 2011; Ward et al. 2012).

Importantly, then, one of the most consistent and particular claims of the medical/health humanities has been its capacity to promote and teach empathy to medical and health professional students (Garden 2007; Jones et al. 2014b), and evidence is accumulating to support such claims, through the use of the various genres and methods representative of the humanities (Darbyshire 1994; Graham et al. 2016; Muszkat et al. 2013; Shapiro et al. 2004; Wilby 2011; Zazulak et al. 2017; Bal and Veltkamp 2013). Essentially, the humanities seek to understand human experience; in the context of health professional education, one of the most clinically useful and relevant applications of this is to help practitioners (and students) better attend to the patient's needs. This is more than just good communication skills, although undoubtedly important in themselves; genuine empathy helps the "epistemological" focus of the clinical interaction (Chiavaroli 2017; Hooker 2015), encouraging and assisting the clinician to be mindful of, and seek to better understand, the patient's experience and perspective of their illness, and their particular social circumstances. We see this clearly in Dana's intuitive responses to Mrs. Bright's situation and discomfort – her request for more pain medication, her focus on the son's reactions, her sense of emotional ambiguity at the end – all responses which, in the light of the above findings of empathy decline, take on a particular importance, and vulnerability. The imperative for clinical supervisors to nurture such instinctive responses, and help transform them into useful clinical learning experiences, cannot be overestimated.

The Tolerance of Ambiguity in Healthcare

Of related interest to health professional educators is how learners become comfortable accepting that ambiguity and uncertainty form much of the context in which healthcare occurs (Simpkin and Schwartzstein 2016). Researchers have investigated whether this tolerance is an inherent characteristic of an individual, leading to them specializing in particular disciplines (Geller et al. 1990), or an attribute that can be enhanced with teaching. Tolerance of ambiguity is also associated with the development of empathy: and an increased empathetic response to challenging or ambiguous circumstances is a significant factor in healthcare communication (Bentwich and Gilbey 2017).

In Dana's situation, ambiguity surrounded Mrs. Bright's circumstances. The black-and-white application of healthcare principles, such as providing appropriate and effective pain management, did not seem to provide a solution. Instead, there was uncertainty as to why Mrs. Bright had not responded; and the marginalization of Dana's position as a member of the healthcare team. Her clinical supervisor, reacting to his own workload and supervisory pressures, had a less-than-empathetic response to Dana's concern, adding to her confusion.

Tolerance of the grey-scale reality of healthcare is seen as an important skill, and one that can be taught through the health humanities. Visual skills training, for instance, has been used to not only improve visual literacy and observation skills but also as an effective way for students to accept "multiple meanings" of a situation (Bentwich and Gilbey 2017), thus increasing their tolerance of ambiguity. Similarly, the development of narrative competence through close reading encourages health professionals to "recognise, absorb, interpret, and be moved by the stories of illness" (Charon 2006), approaching the uncertainty within the experience of illness with empathy and openness.

All of these different aspects of learning about clinical and/or health practice can be subsumed under the banner of professional formation. The humanities are focused on and furnished with the particular methods and perspectives that help explore and understand human experience. This provides innumerable opportunities to think through and discuss collaboratively the kinds of issues and considerations which health professionals need to understand and manage on a daily basis. In this sense, the humanities provide a "social laboratory" (or perhaps better, a *collaboratory*) for students to initially learn professionalism, safely and supportively, if set up and managed appropriately, before (or alongside) applying and translating such learning into the clinical setting. This sense of safety also applies to supervisors, and ultimately patients. A number of published resources provide examples and outlines of materials and methods which can be used or adapted to support a humanities-based professionalism curriculum, so we refer the reader to some of this literature (Jones et al. 2014b; Bates et al. 2013; Cole et al. 2015; Crawford et al. 2015b; Monrouxe and Rees 2017; Peterkin and Brett-MacLean 2016; Peterkin and Skorzewska 2018), and return to Dana to consider how the situation may have played out differently, from a humanities-informed and professional learning perspective.

Unstructured Learning Moments

What of Dana's workplace learning, the opportunities that the supervisor on the ward failed to seize in the face of Mrs. Bright's death? Is the clinical placement, where theory and practice meld together to inform effective practice, a suitable location for the sensibilities of the health humanities?

In Dana's situation, the clinical supervisor had many opportunities to support and reinforce key professional learning. Dana was left with many uncertainties, some of which were exacerbated by her supervisor's responses. With humanities-based learning and a broader approach to supervision, could the learning experience have turned out differently for Dana?

We are not suggesting that the health humanities are a panacea for the complexities of health professional education. Imagine, though, if humanities-based perspectives such as close noticing and close reading had been an explicit part of the curriculum and clinical supervisor's training. Dana's dilemmas may have been recognized and addressed more clearly and explicitly. She queried Mrs. Bright's pain management, not because she thought she had the decision-making power to give more pain relief, but because she was responding humanely to a person's cry for help. It may have been the case that Mrs. Bright could not have had more medication, but that was probably not what Dana was thinking. She was *bearing witness* to a person's expressed pain then not being recognized as the witness. If the supervisor had noticed this, he may have given more thought to what his student was saying: *how do we provide comfort to Mrs Bright?* A response may have included clinical aspects of managing pain, but may have also addressed the role of a health professional in providing other care to Mrs. Bright.

A Clinical Encounter Revisited

Fourth-year undergraduate medical student, Dana, is on the medical ward under the supervision of a registrar. Dana prepares to present Mrs. Thelma Bright to her clinical supervisor with a summary of information required for him to consider Mrs. Bright's management. Once she has done that, Dana writes in her "parallel chart" as encouraged by her supervisor, that is, her personal reflection of her encounter with Mrs. Bright for later discussion:

> Mrs Thelma Bright looks very frail and tiny in her bed. She's the same age as my grandmother so I was expecting someone as independent and strong as Granny. I can imagine how scary and painful it must have been for Mrs Bright to lie on the floor alone for so long. Her face is still pinched and she hardly opens her eyes so I wonder whether she knows where she is. Perhaps she still thinks she's on the floor of her home.

In Mrs. Bright's patient record, Dana discovers an advance care plan that stated Mrs. Bright's wishes that she only wanted medical treatment if it would sustain her current quality of life. Considering that Mrs. Bright had recently been living independently at home, Dana concludes that a good quality of life would mean the ability to return to as much independence as possible but wonders whether any health professional has talked this through with Mrs. Bright. Real end-of-life care situations are new to Dana but she remembers being introduced to the topic through reading both clinical accounts and other literature in tutorial discussions. A critical reading of *Being Mortal* brought about discussions of contemporary medical practice and death and dying, informing Dana of the need to consider healthcare management, ethical concerns, and a patient's wishes in the context of best care. That Mrs. Bright's son was unable to be present until the next day understandably complicated matters.

As Dana is standing at the nurse's station reading these notes, Mrs. Bright begins to call out for pain relief. Dana notifies a nurse who informs her that pain relief is not due for another 2 h. Although Dana understands the pharmacological concerns, she thinks that Mrs. Bright might find some consolation in someone sitting with her and perhaps acknowledging her suffering. When Dana's supervisor returns, he commends her compassion, recognizes her concerns and says, "Mrs Bright's had all the pain management possible for the moment but perhaps we could organize someone to spend some time with her. I will ask one of the nurses or arrange the chaplain to visit."

Dana leaves the ward to attend tutorials and doesn't return until the next day. Overnight, Mrs. Bright has a cardiac arrest and dies shortly before Dana arrives. As Dana stands with the nurses at the central station, Mrs. Bright's son arrives looking flustered. Although he is taken to a private interview room to talk to the consultant, Dana could still hear him reacting angrily to news of his mother's death. She understands a bit more deeply how challenging delivering bad news is but understands and accepts the son's emotions while her supervisor explains the care Mrs. Bright had received. Narrative competence was crucial in such a volatile situation as was close noticing, married with a high degree of empathy.

Dana remains at the desk as the son came out and went into his mother's room, emerging 2 min later and leaving the ward. She could see the corner of Mrs. Bright's bed and a nurse beginning to take care of the body. Dana had never seen a real dead body but she had been involved in studying representations of death and dying through art. It struck her that health professionals had the opportunity to approach Mrs. Bright's final moments with respect and dignity, and the solemnity the occasion deserved. Dana knew that she would still find the scene confronting but that her contribution to this aftercare was important.

When Dana meets her supervisor later that day, she has a number of questions for him, both clinical and professional. Alongside some of the biomedical management explanations of Mrs. Bright's care, she is keen to understand how health professionals manage the ethical and emotional care of their patients and themselves, and how she could apply this to herself as she works towards becoming a qualified health professional.

Conclusion

Dana's initial experience on the ward introduced some unintended consequences. The workplace, embroiled in busy-ness and process, was not something she had encountered before and her teaching to date had not provided her with tools or strategies to manage. The valuable learning opportunities that could have taken place were instead swamped by the struggle to balance teaching with a full clinical workload, a situation experienced by many clinician-teachers.

While the health humanities are not a panacea to the reality of workplace-based health professional education, they help better prepare a learner for the complexity of healthcare. While much teaching focuses on diagnosis and management, contemporary learners need more in their toolbox to work effectively with patients, carers, and the rest of the healthcare team. Likewise, teachers and supervisors need a range of strategies to assist learners in developing into competent health professionals. Entangling the health humanities into undergraduate, postgraduate, and professional education, while being challenging, may well enhance clinical practice for the twenty-first century.

Cross-References

▶ Interprofessional Education (IPE): Trends and Context
▶ Transformative Learning in Clinical Education: Using Theory to Inform Practice

References

Bal PM, Veltkamp M. How does fiction Reading influence empathy? An experimental investigation on the role of emotional transportation. PLoS One. 2013;8(1):e55341.

Bates V, Bleakley A, Goodman S. Medicine, health and the arts: approaches to the medical humanities. London: Routledge Chapman and Hall; 2013.

Bentwich ME, Gilbey P. More than visual literacy: art and the enhancement of tolerance for ambiguity and empathy. BMC Med Educ. 2017;17(1):200.

Bleakley A. Medical humanities and medical education. London: Routledge; 2015.

Blease C. In defence of utility: the medical humanities and medical education. Med Humanit. 2016;42(2):103–8.

Boisaubin EV, Winkler MG. Seeing patients and life contexts: the visual arts in medical education. Am J Med Sci. 2000;319(5):292–6.

Borromeo M, Gaunt H, Chiavaroli N. The visual arts in health education at the Melbourne dental school. In: McLean CL, editor. Creative arts in humane medicine. Edmonton: Brush Education Inc; 2014. p. 40–55.

Boudreau JD. Fuks A. the humanities in medical education: ways of knowing, doing and being. J Med Humanit. 2015;36(4):321–36.

Braverman IM. To see or not to see: how visual training can improve observational skills. Clin Dermatol. 2011;29(3):343–6.

Bruner J. Narrative and paradigmatic modes of thought. In: Eisner E, editor. Learning and teaching the ways of knowing. 84th yearbook of the National Society for the study of education. Chicago: University of Chicago Press; 1985.

Bumgarner GW, Spies AR, Asbill CS, Prince V. Using the humanities to strengthen the concept of professionalism among first-professional year pharmacy students. Am J Pharm Educ. 2007;71(2):Article 28.

Carver R. What the doctor said. Acad Med. 2008;83(4):420.

Charlton B, Verghese A. Caring for Ivan Ilyich. J Gen Intern Med. 2010;25(1):93–5.

Charon R. Narrative medicine: honoring the stories of illness. New York: Oxford University Press; 2006.

Chiavaroli N. Knowing how we know: an epistemological rationale for the medical humanities. Med Educ. 2017;51:13–21.

Chiavaroli N, Trumble S. When I say...phronesis. Med Educ. 2018;52:1005–7.

Chiavaroli N, Huang CD, Monrouxe LV. Chapter 16 Learning medicine with, from and through the humanities: Tim Swanwick KF, O'Brien B., Understanding medical education: evidence, theory and practice. 3rd ed West Sussex: Wiley Blackwell; 2018

Cole T, Carlin N, Carson RA. Medical humanities: an introduction. Cambridge: Cambridge Press; 2015.

Crawford P, Brown B, Baker C, Tischler V, Abrams B. Health Humanities. London: Palgrave Macmilla UK; 2015a. p. 1–19.

Crawford P, Brown B, Baker C, Tischler V, Adams B. Health humanities. London: Palgrave Macmillan; 2015b.

Darbyshire P. Understanding caring through arts and humanities: a medical/nursing humanities approach to promoting alternative experiences of thinking and learning. J Adv Nurs. 1994;19 (5):856–63.

Davis FD. Phronesis, clinical reasoning, and Pellegrino's philosophy of medicine. Theor Med. 1997;18(1–2):173–95.

Day G. Establishing a pulse: arts for reflection, resilience, and resonance in STEM education. Int J Soc Polit Community Agendas Arts. 2016;11(4):1–9.

Doukas D, McCullough LB, Wear S, Lehmann L, Nixon LL, Carrese J, et al. The challenge of promoting professionalism through medical ethics and humanities education. Acad Med. 2013;88(11):1624–9.

Durham University. Institute for Medical Humanities. 2019. Available from: https://www.dur. ac.uk/imh/

Fox DM. Who we are: the political origins of the medical humanities. Theor Med. 1985;6:327–42.

Garden RE. The problem of empathy: medicine and the humanities. New Lit Hist. 2007;38(3): 551–67.

Gawande A. Being mortal. London: Wellcome Collection; 2015.

Geller G, Faden RR, Levine D. Tolerance for ambiguity among medical students: implications for their selection, training and practice. Soc Sci Med. 1990;31(5):619–24.

General Medical Council. Tomorrow's Doctors: recommendations on undergraduate medical education. London: General Medical Council; 1993.

Ginsburg S, Lingard L. 'Is that normal?' Pre-clerkship students' approaches to professional dilemmas. Med Educ. 2011;45:362–71.

Gottlieb CM. Pedagogy and the art of death: reparative readings of death and dying in Margaret Edson's *Wit*. J Med Humanit. 2018;39(3):325–36.

Graham J, Benson LM, Swanson J, Potyk D, Daratha K, Roberts K. Medical humanities coursework is associated with greater measured empathy in medical students. Am J Med. 2016;129(12):1334–7.

Gurwin J, Revere K, Niepold S, Bassett B, Mitchell R, Davidson S, et al. A randomized controlled study of art observation training to improve medical student ophthalmology skills. Ophthalmology. 2018;125(1):8–14.

Hafferty FW, Franks R. The hidden curriculum, ethics teaching, and the structure of medical education. Acad Med. 1994;69(11):861–71.

Halligan A. The Francis report: what you permit, you promote. J R Soc Med. 2013;106(4):116–7.

Hojat M. Empathy in health professions education and patient care. Cham: Springer International Publishing; 2016.

Hooker C. Understanding empathy: why phenomenology and hermeneutics can help medical education and practice. MED HEALTH CARE PHIL. 2015;18:541–52.

International Health Humanities Network. 2019 [cited 2019 30 August]. Available from: http://www.healthhumanities.org

Jeffrey D. Clarifying empathy: the first step to more humane clinical care. Br J Gen Pract. 2016;66(643):e143–e5.

Jones T, Wear D, Friedman LD. The why, the what and the how of the medical/health humanities. Health humanities reader. New Brunswick: Rutgers University Press; 2014a.

Jones T, Wear D, Friedman LD. Health humanities reader. New Brunswick/London: Rutgers University Press; 2014b.

Jones T, Blackie M, Garden R, Wear D. The almost right word: the move from *Medical* to *Health* humanities. Acad Med. 2017;92(7):932–5.

Jones EK, Kumagai AK, Kittendorf AL. Through another lens: the humanities and social sciences in the making of physicians. Med Educ. 2019;53(4):328–30.

Kalanithi P. When breath becomes air: what makes life worth living in the face of death. London: Vintage; 2016.

Kay A. This is going to hurt: secret diaries of a junior doctor. London: Picador; 2018.

Kay D, Berry A, Coles NA. What experiences in medical school trigger professional identity development? Teach Learn Med. 2018;31(1):17–25.

Kinsella EA, Pitman A. Phronesis as professional knowledge: practical wisdom in the professions. Rotterdam: Sense Publishers; 2012.

Kumagai AK. Beyond "Dr. feel-good": a role for the humanities in medical education. Acad Med. 2017;92(12):1659–60.

Lake J, Jackson L, Hardman C. A fresh perspective on medical education: the lens of the arts. Med Educ. 2015;49(8):759–72.

Lundin RM, Bashir K, Bullock A, Kostov CE, Mattick KL, Rees CE, et al. "I'd been like freaking out the whole night": exploring emotion regulation based on junior doctors' narratives. Adv Health Sci Educ. 2018;23(1):7–28.

Macnaughton J. The humanities in medical education: context, outcomes and structures. Med Humanit. 2000;26:23–30.

Marsh H. Do no harm: stories of life, death and brain surgery. London: Weidenfeld & Nicolson; 2014.

Marsh H. Admissions: a life in brain surgery. London: Weidenfeld & Nicolson; 2018.

Martimianakis MA, Michalec B, Lam J, Carrie C, Taylor J, Hafferty FW. Humanism, the hidden curriculum, and educational reform: a scoping review and thematic analysis. Acad Med. 2015;90(11 Suppl):S5–S13.

McLennan MF. Literature and medicine: some major works. Lancet. 1996;348:1014–6.

Monrouxe LV, Rees CE. "It's just a clash of cultures": emotional talk within medical students' narratives of professionalism dilemmas. Adv Health Sci Educ. 2012;17(5):671–701.

Monrouxe LV, Rees CE. Healthcare professionalism: improving practice through reflections on workplace dilemmas. Oxford: Wiley; 2017.

Monrouxe LV, Rees CE, Endacott R, Ternan E. Even now it makes me angry': health care students' professionalism dilemma narratives. Med Educ. 2014;48:502–17.

Montgomery K. Sherlock Holmes and clinical reasoning. In: Hunsaker Hawkins A, Chandler McEntyre M, editors. Teaching literature and medicine. New York: The Modern Language Association; 2000. p. 299–305.

Montgomery K. How doctors think: clinical judgment and the practice of medicine. New York: Oxford University Press; 2006.

Muszkat M, Yehuda AB, Moses S, Naparstek Y. Teaching empathy through poetry: a clinically based model. Med Educ. 2013;44(5):503.

Naghshineh S, Hafler JP, Miller AR, Bianco MA, Lipsitz SR, Dubroff RP, et al. Formal art observation training improves medical students' visual diagnostic skills. J Gen Intern Med. 2008;23(7):991–7.

Neidle EA. Bringing humanities into dental education: a modest experiment. Mobius. 1982;2 (3):89–104.

Neighbour R. The inner physician: why and how to practice 'Big picture Medicine'. RCGP: London; 2016.

Neumann M, Edelhauser F, Taushel D, Fischer MR, Wirtz M, Woopen C, et al. Empathy decline and its reasons: a systematic review of students with medical students and residents. Acad Med. 2011;86(6):996–1009.

Nunes P, Williams S, Sa B, Stevenson K. A study of empathy decline in students from five health disciplines during their first year of training. Int J Med Educ. 2011;2:12–7.

Ousager J, Johannessen H. Humanities in undergraduate medical education: a literature review. Acad Med. 2010;85(6):988–98.

Parlow J, Rothman A. Attitudes towards social issues in medicine of five health science faculties. Soc Sci Med. 1975;8(6):351–8.

Peterkin A, Brett-MacLean P. Keeping reflection fresh: a practical guide for clinical educators. Kent: Kent State University Press; 2016.

Peterkin AD, Skorzewska A. Health humanities in post-graduate medical education. Oxford: Oxford University Press; 2018.

Sampson S, Shapiro J, Billimek J, Shallit J, Youm J. Medical student interpretation of visual art: who's got empathy? MedEdPublish [Internet]. 2018;7(3):68 p.

Shankar PR. Medical humanities in medical schools in India. Arch Med Health Sci. 2016;4(2):166.

Shapiro J. Commentary on *Wit*. Acad Med. 2016;91(11):1523.

Shapiro L, Stolz SA. Embodied cognition and its significance for education. Theory Res Educ. 2019;17(1):19–39.

Shapiro J, Morrison E, Boker J. Teaching empathy to first year medical students: evaluation of an elective literature and medicine course. Educ Health. 2004;17(1):73–84.

Shapiro J, Nixon LL, Wear SE, Doukas DJ. Medical professionalism: what the study of literature can contribute to the conversation. Philos Ethics Humanit Med. 2015;10:1–8.

Sherman JJ, Cramer A. Measurement of changes in empathy during dental school. J Dent Educ. 2005;69:338–45.

Simpkin AL, Schwartzstein RM. Tolerating uncertainty – the next medical revolution? N Engl J Med. 2016;375(18):1713–5.

Solomon M. Epistemological reflections on the art of medicine and narrative medicine. Perspect Biol Med. 2008;51(3):406–17.

Thow M, Murray R. Medical humanities in physiotherapy: education and practice. Physiotherapy. 1991;77(11):733–6.

Tsevat RK, Sinha AA, DasGupta S. Bringing home the health humanities: narrative humilty, structual competancy, and engaged pedagogy. Acad Med. 2015;90(11):1462–5.

Various. Special issue: medical and health humanities in Africa – inclusion access and social justice. Med Humanit. 2018;44(4)

Viney W, Callard F, Woods A. Critial medical humanities: embracing entanglement, taking risks. Med Humanit. 2015;41:2–7.

Ward J, Cody J, Schaal M, Hojat M. The empathy enigma: an empical study of decline in empathy among undergraduate nursing students. J Prof Nurs. 2012;2012:28–34.

Watson C. The language of kindness: a nurse's story. London: Chatto & Windus; 2018.

Weir JM, Aicken MD, Cupples ME, Steele K. From Hippocrates to the Francis report – reflections on empathy. Ulster Med J. 2015;84(1):8–12.

Wellcome. Research in the humanities and social sciences. 2019. Available from: https://wellcome.ac.uk/what-we-do/our-work/research-humanities-and-social-sciences

Wilby M. Teaching others to care: a case for using the humanities. Int J Human Caring. 2011;15(4):29–32.

Williams WC. The doctor stories. New York: New Directions Books; 1984/1932.

Wu H, Chen J. Conundrum between internationalisation and interdisciplinarity: reflection on the development of medical humanities in Hong Kong, Taiwan and China. MedEdPublish [Internet]. 2018;7(46). Available from: https://www.mededpublish.org/manuscripts/1920

Yang K-T, Yang J-H. A study of the effect of a visual arts-based program on the scores of Jefferson scale for physician empathy. BMC Med Educ. 2013;13:142.

Yates SM. Bioethics and medical issues in literature. San Francisco: University of California Medical Humanities Press; 2013.

Zazulak J, Sanaee M, Frolic A, Knibb N, Tesluk E, Hughes E, et al. The art of medicine: arts-based training in observation and mindfulness for fostering the empathic response in medical residents. Med Humanit. 2017;43(3):192–8.

Debriefing Practices in Simulation-Based Education

38

Peter Dieckmann, Rana Sharara-Chami, and Hege Langli Ersdal

Contents

Introduction	700
Vignettes	701
Analytical Categories	702
People	703
Content	705
Interaction Patterns	707
Physical Context	709
Organizational Context	709
Application of the Analytical Categories to Different Practices	709
Summary	711
Conclusion	712
Cross-References	712
References	712

P. Dieckmann (✉)
Copenhagen Academy for Medical Education and Simulation (CAMES), Center for Human Resources and Education, Herlev and Getofte Hospital, Herlev, Denmark

Department of Quality and Health Technology, Faculty of Health Sciences, University of Stavanger, Stavanger, Norway

Department of Clinical Medicine, University of Copenhagen, Copenhagen, Denmark
e-mail: mail@peter-dieckmann.de

R. Sharara-Chami
Department of Pediatrics and Adolescent Medicine, American University of Beirut, Beirut, Lebanon
e-mail: rsharara@aub.edu.lb

H. L. Ersdal
Department of Quality and Health Technology, Faculty of Health Sciences, University of Stavanger, Stavanger, Norway

Department of Anaesthesiology and Intensive Care, Stavanger University Hospital, Stavanger, Norway
e-mail: hege.ersdal@safer.net

© Springer Nature Singapore Pte Ltd. 2023
D. Nestel et al. (eds.), *Clinical Education for the Health Professions*,
https://doi.org/10.1007/978-981-15-3344-0_51

Abstract

In this chapter, we describe overarching categories that can be used to describe and analyze debriefing practices across a variety of settings: the people involved, the content discussed, the interaction patterns between participants, the physical characteristics, and the organizational context. We develop these categories from fictitious case examples and provide theoretical foundations for the categories, namely, through the lens of Activity Theory. Activity Theory emphasizes the motive-guided and goal-oriented human being, acting in a social and physical context to reach these goals. Understanding the interplay of motives, goals, and context of human action is important to optimize debriefing practice. Finally, we apply the categories derived to another fictitious case example to explore their analytical value.

Keywords

Debriefing · Simulation · Work-as-done · Social Practice

Introduction

For a long time, debriefing has been considered the "heart and soul" of simulation-based training (Rall et al. 2000), often inspired by debriefings run in the aviation industry (McDonnell et al. 1997; Fanning and Gaba 2007; Dismukes et al. 2006). Countless workshops and numerous publications emphasize the importance that practitioners and scientists place on debriefings. Within the context of this chapter, we use the word "debriefing" to describe the reflective phase after a simulation-based learning event (Dieckmann 2009). Typically, but not always (Kun et al. 2019; Kang and Yu 2018; Oikawa et al. 2016; Boet et al. 2011), this is a group-based discussion of the preceding simulation scenario more or less focusing on pre-defined learning goals and investigating different points of view in terms of description and assessment of the events during the preceding simulation (Fanning and Gaba 2007; Dieckmann et al. 2008; Rudolph et al. 2006; Eppich and Cheng 2015a; Steinwachs 1992).

From a practical point of view, debriefing is integrated into a context that needs to be considered when describing debriefing practices. How the debriefing unfolds is influenced by the events in the scenario, which in turn is influenced by how participants perceived the scenario briefing, or by the kind of atmosphere created in the course opening, to name a few cross connections within the different phases of the simulation setting (Dieckmann 2009). These connections would need to be considered to describe, understand, and optimize debriefing practices. This chapter will only focus on the debriefing as following scenario-based simulations.

From a theoretical standpoint, debriefing provides the reflection component of the experiential learning paradigm. It allows participants to shift perspective from acting to reflecting upon action, to discuss different interpretations of scenario events, as well as to investigate short-, mid-, and, to some extent, long-term consequences of actions taken. The dynamics in a debriefing are different from those in the scenario (there is usually less stress during the debriefing than during the scenario itself). In many instances, the group composition changes, as people who were observers during the scenario become actively included in the debriefing and are encouraged to contribute (Zottmann et al. 2018). Potentially, the location can change from the simulation room to the debriefing room. Many interaction techniques are employed to allow for a wealth of learning opportunities at the individual, team, and organizational levels. Interesting insights can be derived not only from exchanging novel ideas and establishing new mental connections, but also from taking a fresh look on what has been considered "practice" for some time (Iedema et al. 2013; Dieckmann et al. 2017).

Debriefing practices vary in many respects. We here describe and take a critical look at some techniques without necessarily including all the ones available. The selection is based on our experience and our knowledge of the literature. By offering a few examples of different simulation experiences, we represent only snapshots of the huge variety of techniques used in practice. Our approach provides an illustration of the analytical categories that we shall use in the remaining of chapter.

Vignettes

The vignette described here is fictitious in the sense that it did not happen as described, but is composed of elements that regularly happen during simulation practice. We have constructed it in a way that allows us to demonstrate the analytical categories in the following discussion.

Denmark

Five participants, all doctors in their first year, take part in a course aimed to optimize interprofessional collaboration during critical care. Four of the participants were active in the last scenario. One took the role of the "senior physician," being called into the room about halfway through the scenario. One took the role of the less experienced physician being called into the scenario in the beginning by the two role-played nurses. The patient had an asthma attack that was quickly recognized, and the "nurses" called for help early. The attack was quite resistant to treatment, and therefore, the less experienced physician called in the more experienced colleague quickly. Together, intensely involving one of the nurses in the discussion, the team optimized the treatment and could eventually help the patient. One debriefer is leading the debriefing. She is a resident training in anesthesiology and has finished her third year in the specialist education. She feels rather comfortable with the scenario, as she ran it many times before, and it usually provides good points for discussion. About 5 min after the debriefing started, the simulation operator, who is a medical student, also enters the debriefing room and starts the video recording of the scenario. He then sits close to the computer, listening to the discussion and waiting to manage the replay of the video recording.

The goal for the debriefing is defined as getting a systematic approach to treating asthma and to collaborate with the team members in a way that supports speaking up, in case a team member has safety relevant information. The debriefing is set to last about 45 min and lunch is the next point on the course agenda. The debriefing is conducted in a small room without windows within the simulation center. The debriefer likes to let participants develop their own thoughts and leaves them plenty of space for open discussion. Today, she happens to struggle with time management in this set up as she finds it difficult to interrupt participants, even if they start discussing issues not directly related to the scenario at hand. So, some discussions she feared stayed a bit superficial. On the other hand, she is pleased to see how nicely participants picked up on some of the terms discussed earlier – for example, "situation awareness." At times, she would like to discuss also the team issues further, but does not really feel prepared to do so. She is proud of how well the participants exchanged their views with each other. At times, she could lean back a bit and just let the discussion flow, and often, there are so many great ideas flying back and forth – at times almost too many – making her head spin. She is happy that she was assigned to the facilitator course by the institution that hosts the simulation course. This way, she gets a feel to how deep she should go with the discussion. Situation awareness and decision-making, beyond the medical issues, are what she likes to discuss best – as do her participants. The elements in those skills seem rather clear to her. Teamwork often feels a bit less clear, although she knows from experience that it is important. But now it is already time for lunch, so she rushes to formulate some "take-home messages" and is happy that everyone said a bit, even though with some of the issues, she would have loved to dig a bit deeper, but can't, as lunch break will not happen if she is late with her course. There are so many participants today that there would be a long waiting time because of the limited space in the canteen.

Analytical Categories

If you work with simulation-based debriefings, you might see some similarities and some differences to your own practice from the vignette: you might recognize some elements and some interaction patterns – others might be unknown, even strange in your eyes. There are myriad variations in simulation practices. In previous works, we considered simulation as a social practice – the rule-based interaction of human beings with each other and the environment (Dieckmann 2009; Dieckmann et al. 2007, 2017, 2018). Describing a social practice entails describing its elements and how they interact with each other. We will try to identify some elements and their interactions that we see relevant for debriefing practice. Again, we do not aim for completeness but rather for illustration.

Gaba (2007) described eleven dimensions that can be used to describe simulation as a social practice, including, for example, the purpose of the simulation, the experience level of the participants, or technology applied. This chapter focuses in

38 Debriefing Practices in Simulation-Based Education

Table 1 Analytical categories to describe debriefing with examples

People	Directly involved: debriefers, debriefees, operators
	Indirectly involved: course director, center director, patients, relatives
Content	Diagnosis, treatment, nursing aspects, situation awareness, decision-making, effectiveness, cost considerations, wishes for changes
Interaction patterns	Types, sequences, duration
The physical characteristics	Rooms, furniture, light, equipment
Organizational context	Organizational embedding, curricular integration, time available, resources

more detail on the debriefing and therefore adds more dimensions – that partly overlap with Gaba's dimensions.

Table 1 provides an overview of the analytical categories we use to describe debriefing as a social practice.

People

First, there are *people* involved, the debriefer, the "active participants" – some of them in their "actual role" (as young physicians) and some of them in "played" roles (the "experienced" physician and the "nurses") – the observer, and the simulation operator. There are even more people involved in an indirect fashion, without being physically present in the debriefing room. The scenario is part of a course that was designed by a "course director," who hired the debriefer and explained to her how to run it. The course director reports to the leader of the simulation institute, often discussing resources needed for the course. The leader, on the other hand, tries to place the institute on the map of the larger organization it is part of, fighting for resources on this level. There are also the patients who will be cared for later by the course participants and the relatives of these patients. This collection might be sufficient to demonstrate that the people involved are a relevant category to be considered in the work around debriefing practice; and those directly or indirectly involved and who could influence the debriefing practice have to be distinguished from those who do not.

Many different models were used when trying to describe, understand, and predict the actions of those involved. Some models propose more stable "traits" (Barrick and Mount 1991), even personalities (Rothmann and Coetzer 2003; Myers and Myers 1995), when describing people and their actions. Other models propose that it is the interaction of the people and their environment that explains human actions. We mostly work with models of the latter category, especially building on the work of Lewin (1943), Lahlou (2017), Leontyev (1978) and Engeström (Engeström et al. 1999, 2007).

Kolbe and colleagues drew on systemic family theory and applied basic assumptions and techniques to debriefings in healthcare (Kolbe et al. 2013). The point here is to recognize that interactions within the simulation setting are fundamentally influenced by basic assumptions which those involved hold about other human beings, themselves, how people act, change, learn, etc. Reflecting on one's own assumptions in this regard is important in the process of development as a professional facilitator. These basic assumptions could also be considered as the "frames" people hold, a term many debriefers are familiar with from a well- recognized paper by Rudolph and colleagues (Rudolph et al. 2006). We support the idea that it is not only participants' assumptions that should be investigated, but also those of the simulation facilitators (Rudolph et al. 2013).

Activity Theory was discussed in the context of simulation practice (Eppich and Cheng 2015b) and is a promising approach to structured debriefings. Activity Theory underlines what motives simulation participants followed during the scenario and what concrete goals they tried to achieve. It helps describe how those involved interacted with each other, with the environment, and how they used tools, distributed work, etc. (Eppich and Cheng 2015b).

A very helpful element in Activity Theory is the distinction of three analytical levels: (1) motive-based activities, (2) goal-oriented actions, and (3) context-sensitive operations. When considering the motives and related activities people fulfill in simulations and debriefings, a fundamental difference between simulation-based learning and clinical practice becomes evident. In clinical practice, most healthcare professionals work with the motive of helping patients and their relatives under the given circumstances of the system. In healthcare simulation, their motive (ideally) is to learn how to help patients better. This difference is fundamental, and neglecting it lies at the heart of many discussions between facilitators and participants around "unrealistic scenarios" and other forms of interaction discrepancies. Participants are promised a certain learning setting through flyers, emails, and courses and hence form motives accordingly. Once in the debriefing, however, they are (sometimes) assessed within a frame that belongs to the working activity, not the learning activity. Issues of efficiency, correctness, etc. are at times discussed not to actually help participants learn but to prove that facilitators are the better clinicians. This becomes even more pronounced when participants take a role that is not theirs in clinical practice. If a young physician is debriefed as a "nurse" in the debriefing (because she/he took this role during the scenario), it might be less effective since his/her basic motive was not nursing work but learning with role play for his/her own role as physician. Consider the speak-up dynamic in the vignette: Imagine that one of the participants was instructed to speak-up (or not) in a certain situation and he/she may or may not have followed this instruction. These instructed actions may or may not be representative for what the participant would actually have done in clinical practice. This difference needs to be acknowledged and communicated in order to avoid conflicts and confusion due to a mix in activities.

Most human beings in most situations pursue several goals at the same time. Our debriefer, for example, tries to stir the discussion away from teamwork. She realizes the importance of teamwork in patient care but at the same time feels insecure about facilitating a relevant discussion. She protects her self-image and avoids conflict by not addressing a content she does not feel comfortable with. So, to understand debriefing practices, it would be important to consider more than one layer of motives and goals: what people want to achieve professionally versus what drives them on a personal level. This distinction became clear also in an interview study, where an inexperienced debriefer described a successful debriefing as one in which participants would not ask questions that the debriefer could not answer (Dieckmann et al. 2009).

The many layers of motives and goals potentially involved in simulation practice bring up the importance of the societal relevance of simulation. Simulation activities are financed, built, and maintained in order to fulfill a societal purpose that aims at increasing safety and quality of care for patients and their relatives and to improve the effectiveness of care processes, among others. This notion is important especially in those cases, where there is conflict between the people involved. Sometimes facilitators get into conflict with a participant, where it becomes about "who is right." Taking the societal charge for simulation into account, this interaction would loosen up the relevance which it holds from the personal frames of those involved (Dieckmann and Krage 2013). From the societal level, it does not seem relevant to investigate who was right in this case. For simulation practice, the reflection about the different frames of reference is an important first step before consciously selecting the frame of reference when designing, conducting, and evaluating simulation settings.

Also, the assumptions about how human beings learn play a role in debriefing and how simulation courses are run. In two previous studies, we could, for example, show that some types of simulation-based courses can best be described by referring to their behavioristic assumptions about learning, while others can best be described by constructivist assumptions (Dieckmann et al. 2018; Rasmussen et al. 2013). In behavioristic-oriented courses, there is a tendency to clearly define "right" and "wrong," and a focus is placed on repeated activity with short corrective and supporting feedback. Constructivist-oriented courses, on the other hand, seem to focus more on describing advantages and disadvantages of different ways of acting and often tend to place more emphasis on reflective discussions over concrete actions (Dieckmann et al. 2018; Rasmussen et al. 2013).

The operator in our vignette is an illustration that we do not always consider all members of a social practice – in this case, the operator is a person with a big potential for change in healthcare. The operator might actually be the person who sees the scenario most often run by a whole range of different teams of healthcare professionals. He or she will, by just being there and observing the scenario, learn a lot and may see the impact of different ways of working together on patient safety and quality of care many times. Actually, pre-graduate students might benefit tremendously from the various roles they can take during simulation-based education (Viggers et al. 2020).

Content

The next analytic category we discuss is *content*. We will leave the question of who decides which content is to be discussed in a debriefing to the *interaction* section.

The "content" question fundamentally addresses what is seen worthy of discussion during the limited (and precious) time available to debriefers and participants. In other words, it is defining which competence(s) participants should acquire. Healthcare competence is a construct under constant change (Hodges 2006). In our perception, in recent years, the scope of discussion shifted. In the early days of simulation, the so-called technical/medical issues were in vogue (Owen 2016). Then the focus expanded to include the so-called "nontechnical skills" (Flin et al. 2008) and issues of "crisis resource management" (Gaba et al. 2015), and now the distinction is being questioned and the discussion seems to be shifting to become a blend of many different aspects of competence into one model (Murphy et al. 2019; Glavin 2011a, b; Flin et al. 2010; Glavin and Maran 2003). This discussion, however, is beyond the scope of this chapter.

We would like to set the focus on a micro level and point out a potential problem – the problem of conceptual clarity of the discussions during debriefings. A previous study showed that the depth of reflection during debriefings may not be as anticipated (Kihlgren et al. 2015). Discussions in debriefings investigated were somewhat superficial. This finding led us to analyze debriefing interactions in more detail. In a so far unpublished study, we wrote down verbatim "take-home messages" from debriefings. These sentences were agreed upon as relevant and correct by the facilitator and participants during the debriefing. However, when we showed these sentences to clinicians and debriefers, they rejected the sentences in their actual form unanimously as they considered them too imprecise or (at least partly) wrong. Obviously, it is not fair to take such a sentence out of the context of a debriefing, yet the strong rejection was so clear that we raise the concern that, at times, the debriefing discussions are not sharp enough – especially, where it comes to the human factor-related issues (like decision-making, situation awareness, teamwork, etc.). The discussions of these complex topics do not always reflect the state-of-the-art research in human factors, psychology, and other related fields. For example, many a times during debriefing, it is (more or less explicitly) assumed that "more is more": the more summaries you do, the better; the more you involve your team members, the better. In practice, the relationship seems more complex: there is an optimum number of summaries (over-summarizing might limit the amount of real "work") and involvement of the team members (involving them too much might get in the way of care). The application of nontechnical skills most often seems to follow an "inverted U-shape" – more is better until the optimum amount is reached beyond which "more" becomes detrimental to performance. In our experience, this is left implicit too often. Such implicit aspects, we assume, would not be accepted in cardiology or neurology discussions around patients (or within any other healthcare discipline for that matter). We would like to point out that we need the debriefing practice to become sharper around all related competences, not "only" around diagnosis and treatment. This might mean that there's a need to revise faculty development programs to also include human factors and related issues and to find effective ways of collaborating across professions and disciplines. An important point to highlight: becoming conceptually sharper does

38 Debriefing Practices in Simulation-Based Education

not (or should not) mean to become less kind and to compromise psychological safety in the learning environment.

Interaction Patterns

The discussion does not always go as planned during a debriefing and *interaction patterns* during debriefings are one way of describing debriefings in practice. Often, but not always, the learning goals for the scenario provide guidance for what should be discussed. In some instances, pre-planned goals do not guide the discussion or do so only very loosely. In a study, we found that debriefings originally aimed at "crisis resource management" as learning goals, in fact, focused substantially on technical–medical issues (although it was not always easy to distinguish both aspects) (Dieckmann et al. 2009). Such deviations may be positive for the learning of participants but may also be negative and may stem from underlying dynamics; some are justified professionally, whereas some flow from personal preferences. For debriefing practice, it seems important to understand which dynamic actually manifested itself in any given debriefing.

One possible scenario is that the facilitator tried to focus on the learning goal without success. This often happens if participants have different learning interests or needs from what the scenario offers (the needs analysis for the scenario might not have been optimal). The debriefer might initiate discussion of a certain topic, but the participants might insist to discuss another.

Another possible scenario where such underlying dynamics unfold is when the debriefer simply disagrees with the learning goals originally set by the course (and the course director). Healthcare professionals, especially those who freely decide about intervention and management of care in their clinical work, often seem to have independent viewpoints on educational issues as well and may or may not be willing to comply with the actual planned scenarios. An example of this dynamic is when faculty members twist the debriefing towards their own interests and areas of expertise, irrespective of the contents previously planned. Obviously, this could be challenging for other involved faculty members, the courses themselves and scenarios as certain learning goals need to be achieved before moving on to different aspects or levels of the educational experience. The only way to recognize such deviations seems to be direct observations or video recordings of debriefings that are used for assessment and feedback. The implication for faculty development programs is to agree on concepts and on ways of handling concept–related disagreements and conflicts. That's where the leadership and management of course directors become especially crucial in identifying ways to make sure that agreements are in place and that they are put into practice.

The interaction patterns in our categorization also include the diverse debriefing structures and recipes (Rudolph et al. 2006, 2007, 2008; Brett-Fleegler et al. 2012; Cheng et al. 2015, 2016; Maestre and Rudolph 2015; Auerbach et al. 2018; Odreman and Clyens 2019). In our view, a rather old paper by Steinwachs still covers the essence of most of these structures, when proposing three different phases in debriefings (Steinwachs 1992). In the description phase, participants discuss what happened during the scenario, what they considered important for them, and how they felt. They do so in a collective, overview-oriented level, basically creating a table of content of interesting aspects from the preceding scenario. In the following analysis phase, certain aspects of the scenario are discussed in more detail. This discussion (of certain aspects in detail) differentiates the different debriefing structures and their underlying theoretical assumptions about human actions and human learning as described in the *people* category. In the third phase, participants reflect on what they can take out of the scenario.

Debriefing practices within these phases vary considerably, and they might have different names in the different phases: the facilitator might tell the participants what they did well or not so well or he/she might ask them to describe their own view around these issues; the leader during the simulation scenario might be in the center of the discussion or he/she might choose to listen to what the team members have to say; the content focus might shift throughout, giving more weight to certain discussions over others; the team might seek consensus around certain aspects or nurture diversity of views. Several papers try to describe debriefing practice in more detail, for example, who speaks with whom about what in a debriefing (Dieckmann et al. 2009), how debriefing interactions unfold in different cultures (Ulmer et al. 2018), how people interact in debriefings with each other and with the material they have available (Nystrom et al. 2016), how facilitators' questions are related to the discussions and reflections during debriefings (Kihlgren et al. 2015; Husebo et al. 2013), if and how video is used during debriefings (Johansson et al. 2017), and what kind of thought and emotions facilitators might experience during debriefing (Rudolph et al. 2013).

On the other hand, a significant body of work in the literature tries to set evaluation criteria and assessment methods of debriefings (Brett-Fleegler et al. 2012; Bortolato-Major et al. 2019; Johnston et al. 2018; Kim and De Gagne 2018; Thompson et al. 2018; Bae et al. 2019; Zhang et al. 2019).

From our perspective, it seems important to adapt the interaction style implemented in the debriefing to the context in which it took place. Each educational healthcare system has some traditional norms, values, and beliefs and is undergoing unique development processes. In any research, the issues of external validity would need to be considered to avoid promoting certain approaches that worked in one context to another context without making necessary adaptations. For us, it was a mind-opening input by a participant in a workshop about culture in debriefings who said: "Are you aware that the whole idea of debriefing – the verbal reflection about action – is a western idea?" (Dong 2013); up until that point in time, we had not really realized this so clearly. We believe that as simulation educators, we need to make sure not to let go of well-working traditions only because we learned of debriefing strategies that work well but that might be foreign to local traditions. In our own faculty development programs, we try to work with participants to identify adaptation needs and ways to achieve them.

Physical Context

The *physical context* has an impact on debriefings similar to any learning setting. A recent book discusses simulation and debriefing practices from a socio-material perspective (Dahlgren et al. 2019). How people sit (in classroom style or in a circle around a table – whether there is a table or not, etc.), how much space there is for debriefing, and whether material can be displayed and other physical characteristics of the room impact interactions in line with socio-material assumptions (Nystrom et al. 2016; Dahlgren et al. 2019). The impact of the physical context on debriefing is significant in those instances where there is a noticeable distance between the simulation room and other rooms – including the debriefing room – requiring "transport times," which tend to be forgotten during course planning and could easily contribute to time pressure during the course.

Organizational Context

This is the last category and we use it to discuss debriefing practice *organizational context*. The vignette illustrated different organizational layers that are relevant to the facilitator, to the course director, to the simulation center director, all the way to the political level of the country where the center operates. The different stakeholders might have different agendas and matching those often requires various balances and compromises. One prominent effect of these concerns is the balance between learning goals and content and the available time to deliver them. When "selling" courses, simulation enthusiasts are easily biased into promising a large amount of learning goals and covered content. When putting this into practice, a practical consideration is time pressure, resulting, often, in shallow discussions, as there is simply not enough time to cover the promised topics to any sufficient extent.

Application of the Analytical Categories to Different Practices

We have described some analytical categories that can be used to reflect on simulation practice. In the last part of this chapter, we apply them to debriefings in different contexts. The descriptions are, again, fictitious and are created to emphasize differences in practice, but are composed of elements that happened or that we considered as functional based on our experience in working in this context for some time. We use the categories to describe practice difference in different countries and different settings. The next step is to interpret the differences and how they came about. The differences might, for example, stem less from the practice taking place in different countries, than from comparing center-based simulations to in situ simulations. Although we provide substantial information about the scenario and the course setting in our vignettes, we focus on the debriefing here. We specifically apply the categories only to the information contained in the vignettes. To collect more information, other types of information sources might be necessary – here, we only want to demonstrate the categories' potential to systematize the description of debriefing practice(s).

Lebanon

It's Wednesday at noon, time for an in situ simulation session on the general pediatrics ward. The case chosen for today is a child with status asthmaticus. The team is a multidisciplinary team composed of two junior residents, one senior resident and two nurses. They have the option to call the pediatric intensive care unit physicians if needed (a second-year resident, a third-year resident, and a fellow) and the pediatric intensive care unit nurses, and they have the option to call their attending physician. The simulation is taking place in the procedure room on the wards, and the debriefer is an experienced pediatric intensivist who regularly runs in situ simulations and has run this same scenario multiple times before. The scenario this time ran well in terms of medical management, but roles were not strictly assigned, one of the medications was not ordered correctly but was nonetheless administered by the nurse. Also, the attending was not called at any point, and when they elected to call the intensive care team, roles became even less clear and medications were ordered "in the air."

After the simulation ended, the team moved to a conference room on the wards in order to start the debriefing. There was no option to play the video recorded during the simulation but still photographs were taken to illustrate the physical dynamics and interactions during the simulation among the different members of the team.

The goal for the debriefing is defined as getting a systematic approach to treating asthma and to collaborate with the team members in a way that supports speaking up, in case a team member has safety relevant information. The debriefer used a debriefing technique that would help her uncover frames of thoughts and behaviors behind the observed actions during the simulation. Despite wanting to focus on communication and speaking up, participants spent a long time in the emotional release phase and in discussing the clinical case per se. The debriefer found herself leading a lot of the interactions in order to discuss nontechnical skills, and there wasn't much exchange between participants but rather between individual participants and the debriefer. Take-home messages included some technical guidance and less focus on nontechnical skills. The debriefer made a point to come back to these issues next time around with that same team.

The analytical categories allow to describe debriefings as they unfold in practice and can stimulate reflections about the different elements of debriefing practices and how they interact with each other. In Table 2 we used them to compare Denmark to Lebanon.

38 Debriefing Practices in Simulation-Based Education

Table 2 Comparison of debriefing practices in Denmark and Lebanon along the categories developed

Category	Denmark	Lebanon
People	Debriefer with relatively little more clinical and simulation experience than participants but feeling comfortable with the scenario Participants take different roles in terms of profession and/or experience level Observer during the scenario becomes active during the debriefing Operator, who learns a lot about the scenarios and in the debriefing discussions	Debriefer Participants, who had their own "roles" during the scenario and who know the department better than the debriefer. All were active during the scenario
Content	Systematic approach to treat a child with status asthmaticus Collaboration between team members that supports speaking up in in case of safety relevant cases Debriefer supports the discussion of those parts of the learning goals, she is especially familiar with Take-home messages stay superficial	Systematic approach to treat a child with status asthmaticus Collaboration between team members that supports speaking up in case of safety relevant cases Take-home messages focus on the treatment aspects
Interaction Patterns	Debriefing set to last about 45 min Struggle with time management, so discussions become superficial Debriefer happy about recognition of learning in the participants Participants discuss with each other – possibly too much for the debriefers taste	Techniques to uncover the frames of participants which lie behind the actions of participants Participants discuss other issues than debriefer would like to focus Attempt of the debriefer to control the content of the debriefing, resulting in one on one interaction between the debriefer and various participants Debriefer intends to come back to the cognitive and social skills in following debriefings
The physical characteristics	Small room, no windows in the simulation center	Conference room on the ward Still photographs from the scenario
Organizational context	Debriefing part of regular and established courses	The debriefing takes place in the context of an established in situ simulation program in the hospital

Summary

We described fictitious but plausible examples of debriefing practice. We analyzed one vignette for analytical categories to describe debriefing practices and defined those categories as people, content, interaction patterns, the physical characteristics, and the organizational context. In the second vignette, we showed how these categories can be used to reflect upon and describe debriefing practices and to compare different contexts along the lines of the dimensions contained.

Conclusion

The categories for describing debriefing practice that we developped in this chapter and applied in different context can be used to sharpen the analytical approach to describing debriefing practices.

Cross-References

▶ Debriefing Practices in Simulation-Based Education
▶ Embedding a Simulation-Based Education Program in a Teaching Hospital
▶ Focus on Theory: Emotions and Learning
▶ Social Semiotics: Theorizing Meaning Making

References

Auerbach M, Cheng A, Rudolph JW. Rapport management: opening the door for effective debriefing. Simul Healthc. 2018;13(1):1–2.

Bae J, Lee J, Jang Y, Lee Y. Development of simulation education debriefing protocol with faculty guide for enhancement clinical reasoning. BMC Med Educ. 2019;19(1):197.

Barrick MR, Mount MK. The big five personality dimensions and job performance: a meta-analysis. Pers Psychol. 1991;44(1):1–26.

Boet S, Bould MD, Bruppacher HR, Desjardins F, Chandra DB, Naik VN. Looking in the mirror: self-debriefing versus instructor debriefing for simulated crises. Crit Care Med. 2011;39 (6):1377–81.

Bortolato-Major C, Mantovani MF, Felix JVC, Boostel R, Silva A, Caravaca-Morera JA. Debriefing evaluation in nursing clinical simulation: a cross-sectional study. Rev Bras Enferm. 2019;72(3):788–94.

Brett-Fleegler M, Rudolph J, Eppich W, Monuteaux M, Fleegler E, Cheng A, et al. Debriefing assessment for simulation in healthcare: development and psychometric properties. Simul Healthc. 2012;7(5):288–94.

Cheng A, Palaganas J, Eppich W, Rudolph J, Robinson T, Grant V. Co-debriefing for simulation-based education: a primer for facilitators. Simul Healthc. 2015;10(2):69–75.

Cheng A, Morse KJ, Rudolph J, Arab AA, Runnacles J, Eppich W. Learner-centered debriefing for health care simulation education: lessons for faculty development. Simul Healthc. 2016;11 (1):32–40.

Dahlgren MA, Rystedt H, Felländer-Tsai L, Nyström S, editors. Interprofessional simulation in health care. Materiality, embodiment, interaction. Cham: Springer Nature Switzerland; 2019.

Dieckmann P. Simulation settings for learning in acute medical care. In: Dieckmann P, editor. Using simulation for education, training and research. Lengerich: Pabst; 2009. p. 40–138.

Dieckmann P, Krage R. Simulation and psychology: creating, recognizing and using learning opportunities. Curr Opin Anaesthesiol. 2013;26(6):714–20.

Dieckmann P, Gaba D, Rall M. Deepening the theoretical foundations of patient simulation as social practice. Simul Healthc. 2007;2(3):183–93.

Dieckmann P, Reddersen S, Zieger J, Rall M. A structure for video-assisted debriefing in simulator-based training of crisis resource management. In: Kyle R, Murray BW (eds). Clinical Simulation: Operations, Engineering, and Management. Burlington: Academic Press; 2008. p. 667–676.

Dieckmann P, Molin Friis S, Lippert A, Ostergaard D. The art and science of debriefing in simulation: ideal and practice. Med Teach. 2009;31(7):e287–94.

Dieckmann P, Patterson M, Lahlou S, Mesman J, Nystrom P, Krage R. Variation and adaptation: learning from success in patient safety-oriented simulation training. Adv Simul (Lond). 2017;2:21.

Dieckmann P, Birkvad Rasmussen M, Issenberg SB, Soreide E, Ostergaard D, Ringsted C. Long-term experiences of being a simulation-educator: a multinational interview study. Med Teach. 2018;40(7):713–20.

Dismukes RK, Gaba DM, Howard SK. So many roads: facilitated debriefing in healthcare. Simul Healthc. 2006;1(1):23–5.

Dong C. Personal communication in the context of a debriefing workshop. 2013.

Engeström Y, Miettinen R, Punamaki-Gitai R-L. Perspectives on activity theory. Cambridge: Cambridge University Press; 1999. xiii, 462 p. p.

Engeström Y, Kerosuo H, ProQuest (Firm). Activity theory and workplace learning. Bradford: Emerald Group Publishing; 2007. Available from: http://ebookcentral.proquest.com/lib/abdn/detail.action?docID=320648

Eppich W, Cheng A. Promoting Excellence and Reflective Learning in Simulation (PEARLS): development and rationale for a blended approach to health care simulation debriefing. Simul Healthc. 2015a;10(2):106–15.

Eppich W, Cheng A. How cultural-historical activity theory can inform interprofessional team debriefings. Clin Simul Nurs. 2015b;11(8):383–9.

Fanning RM, Gaba DM. The role of debriefing in simulation-based learning. Simul Healthc. 2007;2(2):115–25.

Flin RH, O'Connor P, Crichton M. Safety at the sharp end: a guide to non-technical skills. Aldershot/Burlington: Ashgate; 2008. x, 317 p

Flin R, Patey R, Glavin R, Maran N. Anaesthetists' non-technical skills. Br J Anaesth. 2010;105(1):38–44.

Gaba DM. The future vision of simulation in healthcare. Simul Healthc. 2007;2(2):126–35.

Gaba DM, Fish KJ, Howard SK, Burden AR, Gaba DM. Crisis management in anesthesiology. 2nd ed. Philadelphia: Elsevier/Saunders; 2015. xxii, 409 pages

Glavin RJ. Human performance limitations (communication, stress, prospective memory and fatigue). Best Pract Res Clin Anaesthesiol. 2011a;25(2):193–206.

Glavin RJ. Skills, training, and education. Simul Healthc. 2011b;6(1):4–7.

Glavin RJ, Maran NJ. Integrating human factors into the medical curriculum. Med Educ. 2003;37(Suppl 1):59–64.

Hodges B. Medical education and the maintenance of incompetence. Med Teach. 2006;28(8):690–6.

Husebo SE, Dieckmann P, Rystedt H, Soreide E, Friberg F. The relationship between facilitators' questions and the level of reflection in postsimulation debriefing. Simul Healthc. 2013;8(3):135–42.

Iedema R, Mesman J, Carroll K. Visualising health care practice improvement: innovation from within. London: Radcliffe Publishing; 2013. 211 s. p.

Johansson E, Lindwall O, Rystedt H. Experiences, appearances, and interprofessional training: the instructional use of video in post-simulation debriefings. Int J Comput-Support Collab Learn. 2017;12(1):91–112.

Johnston S, Coyer FM, Nash R. Kirkpatrick's evaluation of simulation and debriefing in health care education: a systematic review. J Nurs Educ. 2018;57(7):393–8.

Kang K, Yu M. Comparison of student self-debriefing versus instructor debriefing in nursing simulation: a quasi-experimental study. Nurse Educ Today. 2018;65:67–73.

Kihlgren P, Spanager L, Dieckmann P. Investigating novice doctors' reflections in debriefings after simulation scenarios. Med Teach. 2015;37(5):437–43.

Kim SS, De Gagne JC. Instructor-led vs. peer-led debriefing in preoperative care simulation using standardized patients. Nurse Educ Today. 2018;71:34–9.

Kolbe M, Weiss M, Grote G, Knauth A, Dambach M, Spahn DR, et al. TeamGAINS: a tool for structured debriefings for simulation-based team trainings. BMJ Qual Saf. 2013;22(7):541–53.

Kun Y, Hubert J, Bin L, Huan WX. Self-debriefing model based on an integrated video-capture system: an efficient solution to skill degradation. J Surg Educ. 2019;76(2):362–9.

Lahlou S. Installation theory. The societal construction and regulation of behaviour. Cambridge: Cambridge University Press; 2017.

Leont'ev AN. Activity, consciousness, and personality. Englewood Cliffs: Prentice-Hall; 1978.

Lewin K. Defining the 'field at a given time.'. Psychol Rev. 1943;50(3):292–310.

Maestre JM, Rudolph JW. Theories and styles of debriefing: the good judgment method as a tool for formative assessment in healthcare. Rev Esp Cardiol (Engl Ed). 2015;68(4):282–5.

McDonnell LK, Jobe KK, Dismukes RK. Facilitating LOS debriefings: a training manual. Moffett Field, CA, USA: Ames Research Center; 1997.

Murphy P, Nestel D, Gormley GJ. Words matter: towards a new lexicon for 'nontechnical skills' training. Adv Simul (Lond). 2019;4:8.

Myers IB, Myers PB. Gifts differing: understanding personality type. Mountain View: Davies-Black Pub; 1995. xxiii, 228 p. p.

Nystrom S, Dahlberg J, Edelbring S, Hult H, Dahlgren MA. Debriefing practices in interprofessional simulation with students: a sociomaterial perspective. BMC Med Educ. 2016;16:148.

Odreman HA, Clyens D. Concept mapping during simulation debriefing to encourage active learning, critical thinking, and connections to clinical concepts. Nurs Educ Perspect. 2019. https://doi.org/10.1097/01.NEP.0000000000000445. [Epub ahead of print]

Oikawa S, Berg B, Turban J, Vincent D, Mandai Y, Birkmire-Peters D. Self-debriefing vs instructor debriefing in a pre-internship simulation curriculum: night on call. Hawaii J Med Public Health. 2016;75(5):127–32.

Owen H. Simulation in healthcare education. New York: Springer Science+Business Media; 2016. pages cm p.

Rall M, Manser T, Howard SK. Key elements of debriefing for simulator training. Eur J Anaesthesiol. 2000;17(8):516–7.

Rasmussen MB, Dieckmann P, Barry Issenberg S, Ostergaard D, Soreide E, Ringsted CV. Long-term intended and unintended experiences after Advanced Life Support training. Resuscitation. 2013;84(3):373–7.

Rothmann S, Coetzer EP. The big five personality dimensions and job performance. SA J Ind Psychol. 2003;29:1. 2003

Rudolph JW, Simon R, Dufresne RL, Raemer DB. There's no such thing as "nonjudgmental" debriefing: a theory and method for debriefing with good judgment. Simul Healthc. 2006;1 (1):49–55.

Rudolph JW, Simon R, Rivard P, Dufresne RL, Raemer DB. Debriefing with good judgment: combining rigorous feedback with genuine inquiry. Anesthesiol Clin. 2007;25(2):361–76.

Rudolph JW, Simon R, Raemer DB, Eppich WJ. Debriefing as formative assessment: closing performance gaps in medical education. Acad Emerg Med. 2008;15(11):1010–6.

Rudolph JW, Foldy EG, Robinson T, Kendall S, Taylor SS, Simon R. Helping without harming: the instructor's feedback dilemma in debriefing–a case study. Simul Healthc. 2013;8(5):304–16.

Steinwachs B. How to facilitate a debriefing. Simul Gaming. 1992;23(2):186–95.

Thompson R, Sullivan S, Campbell K, Osman I, Statz B, Jung HS. Does a written tool to guide structured debriefing improve discourse? Implications for interprofessional team simulation. J Surg Educ. 2018;75(6):e240–e5.

Ulmer FF, Sharara-Chami R, Lakissian Z, Stocker M, Scott E, Dieckmann P. Cultural prototypes and differences in simulation debriefing. Simul Healthc. 2018;13(4):239–46.

Viggers S, Østergaard D, Dieckmann P. How to include medical students in your healthcare simulation centre workforce. Advances in Simulation. 2020;5(1):1.

Zhang H, Morelius E, Goh SHL, Wang W. Effectiveness of video-assisted debriefing in simulation-based health professions education: a systematic review of quantitative evidence. Nurse Educ. 2019;44(3):E1–6.

Zottmann JM, Dieckmann P, Taraszow T, Rall M, Fischer F. Just watching is not enough: fostering simulation-based learning with collaboration scripts. GMS J Med Educ. 2018;35(3):Doc35.

Written Feedback in Health Sciences Education: "What You Write May Be Perceived as Banal"

39

Brian Jolly

Contents

Introduction	718
What Is Written Feedback?	720
Why Is Written Feedback Important?	720
Modes of Written Feedback	720
Comments on Work (Activities, Status, or Output)	720
Reflective Modes (Self and Other)	722
Report Cards	722
Social and Other Media	723
Where Have We Got To	723
Where To from Here	724
Generating Guidelines on Written Feedback	724
Systematic and Conceptual Reviews	725
Studies in the Medical Context	731
Charting the Best Course in Written Feedback	735
General Issues	735
Structuring Written Feedback	736
Conclusion	738
Cross-References	738
References	739

Abstract

This chapter reviews salient literature on the use of written feedback and distils some advice from the research to guide teachers in the health sciences as to what might work best for them. There are contradictions in this field, both in the research findings and in theoretical perspectives. There are two ways to use this

---

B. Jolly (✉)
Faculty of Health and Medicine, University of Newcastle, Newcastle, NSW, Australia

School of Rural Medicine, University of New England, Armidale, NSW, Australia
e-mail: brian.jolly@newcastle.edu.au

© Springer Nature Singapore Pte Ltd. 2023
D. Nestel et al. (eds.), *Clinical Education for the Health Professions*,
https://doi.org/10.1007/978-981-15-3344-0_52

chapter. Some readers may be interested in the points raised in the studies reviewed as well as in practical advice, because these studies cover a wide range of contexts, and some advice may not work in all settings. Other readers may go straight to the distillation, and if they hit a concept that requires explanation may go back to find it in the discussion.

Keywords

Feedback dialogue · Structured feedback · Balanced feedback · Self-regulation · Task-based feedback · Understanding feedback

Introduction

The quote about banality in the title of this chapter is taken from an example of actual written feedback from a teacher to a student in a study by Sellbjer (2018). It shows how easy it is to make a pig's ear of feedback, when a silk purse opportunity is afforded. The feedback is essentially content-free and emotionally draining. The research in that paper looked at the feedback given to students who had failed one or more examinations in a teacher training program. The comment "banal," and its probable impact illustrate several concepts that have come to the fore in the last decade since a major theoretical reconceptualization of feedback theory (see Boud and Molloy 2013). These include, to name a few, the importance of positive as well as negative messages, the emotive-cognitive nexus involved in feedback, the inappropriate use of "final" vocabulary (Boud 1995; Rorty 1989), the concepts of feedforward and dialogic feedback, and the focus on self-regulation in academic tasks, on the part of both teacher and student.

Written feedback is used in very different ways in health professions education, depending on discipline, context, academic and workplace culture, and its role in curriculum. Traditionally, written feedback has been a one-way process from teacher to student, and in many disciplines bears the brunt of any student–teacher interaction that is possible, given large student numbers (Nicol 2010). Clinical education has frequently been protected from having large numbers of students because of the typical quota system of titrating student intake against both clinical need and the existence of a finite number of employment or training positions and subsequent opportunities for specialty training. Nevertheless, some degree of increase, sometimes dramatic, in numbers of students is occurring across all health disciplines. For example, Australia has doubled the number of students in medical schools over a 10-year period while the increase (if any) in staffing has not been of that order, so the potential for intensive personalized feedback (of any sort) is under considerable threat.

Furthermore, most clinical education takes place in a socially intense environment where, despite the need for extensive documentation of processes and outcomes, verbal interaction in person, by "phone or digital" means, is the norm. Nevertheless, with the advent of workplace-based assessment (Weller et al. 2017; Burch 2019), at both undergraduate and specialty training levels, affordances for the use of written feedback, sent and received digitally using conventional and/or social media, are increasing. Also writing emails, or "texting," has replaced many other forms of communication. So, there is a high likelihood that feedback will be delivered in written form, but not in hard copy. It is against this milieu of rapid but disruptive progress, with increasing complexity, amidst mounting pressure to do more with less, that this section has been written.

Before interpreting the best way to approach written feedback, there is a need to acknowledge that research in this area is relatively young and frequently appears contradictory. The reasons for this are varied and may involve the complex interdependencies within academic institutions and the disciplinary contexts that influence students' perspectives (O'Donovan et al. 2019). These include the mode of feedback used (written, oral, etc.), how it fits into the curriculum and its assessment strategies, the relationships between students, their peers and the faculty, and how assessment-wise the students are. Nevertheless, almost indisputably, the literature is clear that the most influential factor, when it comes to improving the performance of students at academic tasks, is the feedback they receive. Hattie (Hattie 2009; Hattie and Gan 2011) reports, in an extensive review synthesizing over 800 meta-analyses, that feedback is the most powerful single influence that makes a difference to student achievement. However, there is evidence that not all "feedback" results in improved performance (see Price et al. 2010; Rust et al. 2005 for a complete discussion). The tendency has been for the ineffectiveness of feedback to be attributed to characteristics associated with student perceptions or staff's ineptitude, for example, when feedback is vague, misunderstood, too late, or not read. Moreover "when the emphasis of the marking is on the mark or grade, it may be perceived to relate to the student's personal ability or worth, rather than just to the individual piece of work, and in such situations poor marks can damage the student's self-efficacy" (Rust et al. 2005, p. 234).

Yet even careful research in ostensibly similar locations or disciplines gives rise to different results. For example, there is no clear indication on whether students prefer, or perform better, using written vs digital technology-delivered feedback (Hilton and Rague 2015; Morris and Chikwa 2016; Ryan et al. 2016; Deeley 2018). So, there are major contextual factors at play, and the research paradigms are eclectic; hence there are few, if any, replications of studies. The traditional modes of education in a discipline may also have a function in this diversity. For example, nursing education has relatively short periods of clinical placement compared to medicine, which uses immersion in working environments to a much greater extent, and opportunities for effective feedback may differ both in mode and in quantity. Furthermore, there is limited research on written feedback in the health disciplines, but much more beyond those, and this chapter tries to encompass that breadth.

What Is Written Feedback?

Written feedback is information about student performance conveyed by prose, through email, sms text, letters, reports, notes on documents, hard or soft, and other means of production. It also includes information given using predesigned rubrics, forms, or score sheets that might contain a tick in a box against a particular criterion or characteristic to indicate whether the work being assessed has that attribute. It incorporates exemplar outputs, such as model answers, given to students after assignments are submitted, to indicate what the constituents of an appropriate completed assignment might be. When such things are distributed beforehand to students, this "feedback" is sometimes called "feedforward" (Ion et al. 2017).

Why Is Written Feedback Important?

Written feedback is important because it has distinctive characteristics. It is usually, or can easily be made, private. Some research recommends that, even when receiving praise, students prefer this to be done quietly and privately (Sharp 1985). In written feedback, it is possible to make clear that the information is addressed to an individual or specific group (such as a student project group or a course design team). Consequently, although written feedback can be confidential, unlike real-time verbal feedback which disappears as soon as it is spoken, it is traceable. So, knowing who gave it, when, to whom, under what circumstances, and its reported content, can be substantiated. Written feedback is helpful when a response from the recipient is not expected or needed immediately. It is also useful when the provider of the feedback hopes for a considered response and will follow this up, such as when reviewing a journal article for publication. Most importantly, written feedback is useful when further work is expected, that would itself take written forms, or when the complexity of the task might require a number of issues to be dealt with. Another advantage is that written feedback can be accessed on multiple occasions when needed. For example, feedback to educational institutions from regulatory, accrediting, or quality assurance bodies is almost always given in writing even if a prior comprehensive verbal report has been delivered.

Modes of Written Feedback

Comments on Work (Activities, Status, or Output)

In many disciplines, especially where student assignments are a common part of the curriculum, comments on students work, using track changes in e-documents, or writing on hard copies, is the typical mode of feedback. In medical courses, especially in clinical settings, such assignments are infrequent largely because, it is assumed, clinicians are time-poor in relation to the effort that such feedback entails. Studies of written feedback on workplace-based clinical exercises such as the Mini-

CEX (Norcini et al. 1995), while not uniform in outcome, suggest that the quality of feedback is not optimal. Bing-You et al. (2018) performed an extended scoping review of articles describing feedback on a number of modes, including the Mini-CEX and report cards (see below), as well as formal written feedback. They found a number of features that, in their view, contributed to inadequate feedback. Leniency bias, with feedback providers being reticent to give "any or even minimally (p. 658)" negative feedback to the learners, occurred in 37% of articles reviewed, most commonly in routine written feedback. However, the Mini-CEX mode was the most likely to contain negative feedback. Low-quality feedback (limited in amount or too general or did not conform to guidelines) occurred in 24% of studies reviewed and half of those did not include action plans (a feedforward mechanism) or mention of any previously identified action plans. Sixteen percent (16%) of articles indicated challenges with the faculty members' capacity to provide feedback. Faculty, even those who were experienced teachers did not use forms appropriately, or did not provide adequate feedback after training. When a handwritten method was the means for communicating feedback, there was frequent illegibility of the information.

The gender of feedback givers also impacted on the quantity and detail of feedback, with females tending to give and take on more feedback (see also discussion below). The authors recommended that "it is unrealistic to expect to uniformly and consistently raise the level of feedback competency for all faculty. A unique (narrowed down) group of medical educators working closely with learners may be required for feedback to be successful" (p. 660). Page et al. (2019) found even worse performance by UK faculty in a study of 500 written feedbacks randomly sampled from a set of 2500 direct observations of procedures by radiologists in training: 97% of these contained written feedback but the number of instances of high-quality feedback was only 5%. The authors also identified that, from a utility perspective, 7–13% of feedback elements were recorded at the very end of placements, or retrospectively, presenting no opportunity for trainees to improve their performance during their placements. In contrast, a Malaysian study of 33 students undertaking a series of Mini-CEXs with 14 family medicine practitioners found good quality feedback (Awang Besar et al. 2018). Although the forms collected evidence in written form, this was communicated to students verbally and the conversations recorded for the study. The feedback given was thus more dialogic (97% of 33 interviews), contained positive elements (91%) as well as faculty-generated plans for improvement (91%). However, student-generated plans were only observed in 36%, and only 24% of students were asked if they wanted to ask questions.

An Australian study in a dispersed clinical placement program, across a large rural footprint (Harvey et al. 2013), used textual analysis to examine the structure and content of written feedback statements in 1000 Mini-CEX records (about 30 Mini-CEX each contained in a personal logbook) from 33 undergraduate medical students during their 36-week placement. Only 40% of records had written comments, with an average length of 12 statements per logbook, equivalent to about or just under one statement every two Mini-CEXs. Moreover, about 20% of these comments had no evaluative or judgmental value, consisting of one or two word statements, for example, "review of chest pain" or "imparting information" (Harvey et al. 2013, Table 1, p. 1011). Fewer than might be expected at this stage of training (52 of 404 statements) had statements with specific goals for improving student clinical performance, and there was little inclusion of forward-focused, action-orientated learning goals. Very similar results were obtained in a study by Nesbitt et al. (2014), who analyzed 250 records of supervised learning events (Mini-CEX equivalents). Of these 63% were categorized by the authors as "weak." Just under half of those were left blank, and one-third were nonspecific using words such as "keep practicing." There were some mitigating factors in this research. Students may have also received verbal feedback that was not captured by the study, and assessors may not have had time to fill in the forms. There is a view that supervised learning events may just be regarded as a check box activity. Nevertheless, there were examples of "strong" feedback such as exhorting a student to use "a systematic approach to CVS examination to make sure relevant aspects are not forgotten: e.g. measuring BP, collapsing pulse and radio-radial delay"(p. 242).

Reflective Modes (Self and Other)

Portfolios, and/or logbooks, are generally regarded as means to provide feedback in a more holistic manner than comments about individual tasks (e.g., one Mini-CEX) can achieve. However, in the study discussed above (Harvey et al. 2013), logbook feedback entries were sparse. Portfolios have been variously described as "shopping trolleys full of outputs" (Endacott et al. 2004) up to self-reflective journals chronicling educational pathways or development (Heeneman and de Grave 2017). In this latter mode, the use of reflection is identified as an essential part of the process, and one that provides the most potential for learning (Chertoff et al. 2016). Most assessment methods in health care education now include an element of reflection, but the portfolio is probably the most intense and concentrated pathway to reflection. In some e-portfolios, reflection is divided into a private folder, and a shared one which can be marked or reflected on by a second party (peer, tutor, assessor etc.). Research on feedback in the context of portfolio assessment is scarce and was initially spasmodic (Lawson et al. 2004; Gough and Hamshire 2012) and is only just being developed systematically (Babovič et al. 2019). However, some research on the engagement of students with feedback highlighted that an "assessment portfolio" was both a potentially useful device (ranked 4th of 10 options) and a feasible option (ranked 3rd of 10) (Winstone et al. 2017; see also Winstone and Nash 2019).

Report Cards

Report cards are hard copy or e-mediated modes of summarizing a professional's performance on the job as they go through a placement or undertake work tasks. They typically involve a series of short statements or a checklist "posted" into an actual or virtual box which is then accessed by a supervisor or the student/trainee to review the feedback. They are most commonly used in high complexity, interprofessional clinical environments for charting individuals' or teams' performance over time (see Cheung et al. 2016). Unlike in-training evaluation reports (ITERs), which are aggregate end-of-clinical placement or junior doctor rotations' assessments, daily encounter cards (DECs) are completed immediately following a clinical encounter, therefore standing a better chance of minimizing recall bias and facilitating assessments based on observation of actual performance. The authors demonstrated that a valid, reliable, and predictive evaluation of multiple DECs was possible using a simple additional summarizing tool, the Completed Clinical Evaluation Report rating, and that feedback to the trainees could be achieved using this overarching instrument.

Social and Other Media

It is noteworthy that social media platforms (e.g., *WhatsApp*) and personal media (smartphones) have received much interest as potential modes of both healthcare professions education and feedback. A number of projects and reviews have appeared, usually started by local enthusiasts, who use the need to engage with "millennials" as a rationale for using platforms and devices to transport written or graphic material directly to the user, (see Coleman and O'Connor 2019). This field is developing rapidly, but as yet its use and exposure as a primary source of feedback information and dialogue has not been extensive.

Barrett et al. (2018) implemented an open access "minute" feedback system for a surgery clerkship in a university-affiliated tertiary care institution. Using commercially available survey software, students were enabled to request feedback from faculty and doctors in training, with whom they were interacting on a daily basis. The student could choose a skill (physical examination, patient history, oral presentation, technical skill, or general performance) on which they required feedback via an emailed response. They were also able to add free text elaboration to their request. When a request was sent, the clinician received an email with a link to a survey in which they both rated and gave two to three sentences of free text feedback on the selected skill. The time required for completion of feedback was around one minute. Over 520 days, 5195 requests were sent with 3123 responses. The average request submission per student was 18.7, more from females, and the response rate was around 60%, more by males. Both students and faculty/clinicians entered "feedback fatigue" over the course of the clerkship, as requests and responses dropped by 13% over time. Nevertheless, the authors were confident that positive clerkship ratings over time suggested that this system provided more feedback than previous approaches at their hospital, and it continues to be used.

Where Have We Got To

To reflect the title of the chapter, feedback as currently provided, and as evidenced by research literature, seems to be somewhat of a sow's ear rather than the educational silk purse it is claimed to be. To paraphrase the Scottish proverb, although many studies contain examples of best-practice feedback-giving, its nature frequently makes it useless for its intended purpose. Most of the available research has focused on the provider's end of the interaction and not on the students' receptivity or the dialogue between student and feedback giver. There also seem to be some environmental factors impacting feedback generation that stem from the individual healthcare discipline, the clinical context, the volume of clinical placement available to students, and the historical organization of curriculum for each discipline. For example, while in healthcare feedback is regarded as weak and too infrequent, some academic and vocational disciplines such as humanities, art, graphic design, media studies, and architecture courses hold the two-way "conversation" as a valued methodology. It is not surprising, therefore, that these courses get high ratings from students on the value of "feedback" as part of the Good Teaching Scale of the course experience questionnaire (Graduate Careers Australia 2012). This lack of opportunity for students to respond may account for many of the studies in which "feedback" has been shown to be absent or ineffective (Carless et al. 2011).

The remainder of this chapter explores how to conceptualize and use written feedback to best effect.

Where To from Here

The "one-way" mode of feedback in higher education shares the same disadvantages as one-way road traffic management. Traffic is easily jammed or held up by extraneous events; in the case of feedback, this would include its failure to be provided, its delay or lack of clarity, and its aberrant focus. And, because there is no flexibility to alter the route, the learner is basically hemmed in to follow a certain itinerary until, if ever, the next feedback opportunity is reached. By contrast, using strategies that seem to be valued by teacher and students alike can build on the notion that feedback is a cyclical process, not merely the provision of information and judgement, and that learners need to internalize the expectation of seeking and using information from peers and teachers, and deliberately pursue further feedback on their work after initial feedback has been integrated into it. For a more extensive discussion of these issues, readers are referred to previous work (Jolly and Boud 2013). In the most interactive or efficacious models of student-directed learning, such as problem-, case-, or team-based learning (see Parappilly et al. 2019), feedback perhaps should be conceptualized as ideally a learner-managed process, or at least a learner-engaged activity (Tai et al. 2018; Telio et al. 2015; Molloy et al. 2020). These approaches suggest that there are windows of opportunity during which comments from others are useful, can be acted on, and the feedback loop closed.

Generating Guidelines on Written Feedback

Research on written feedback has increased dramatically in the last 7 years: Searching the unqualified word "feedback" alone in the title of educational research articles listed in Scopus yielded 3,500 hits in 2013 and 5,000 hits in 2020. By contrast, the number of articles with "written feedback" in the title was 55 in 2013 and 132 in 2020. This strongly implies that how feedback is given is not often made explicit, nor researched, in articles on this topic. Nevertheless, some research findings are emerging, and in this section recent systematic and conceptual reviews are summarized, models of giving feedback that can assist how the written message is crafted and shared are presented, and specific applications in context are discussed.

Systematic and Conceptual Reviews

Teacher and Student Factors

As discussed in the preceding section, researchers have focused frequently on trying to identify the attributes and skills of teachers who are successful at giving feedback. Critics have pointed out that this approach is limited because it stems merely from an attempt to make delivery of the "one-way traffic" mode of feedback from teacher to student more effective (Boud and Molloy 2013; Ajjawi and Boud 2017). However, as far as written feedback is concerned, the fact that it can be poorly crafted, misunderstood, and/or ignored warrants attention to make these inhibitors of "delivery" less problematic. After all, a two-way conversation cannot be had if participants cannot make themselves understood. For reasons of space, in the following discussion, details of literature search strategies and inclusion/exclusion criteria will not be given.

Archer's (2010) review forms a bedrock for recent developments in thinking on feedback. As far as teacher/student factors are concerned, his discussion of "the self" in feedback is astute. Recognizing that there was very little evidence in medical education for the effectiveness of self-assessment, he identifies that our behavior and performance are informed significantly by our unconscious minds. This impacts through an insentient drive towards self-preservation, and that explains why feedback that threatens self-esteem or contains mostly unconditional praise may be less effective. The medical world has, in the past, been awash with esteem-threatening feedback (Seabrook 2004; Lempp and Seale 2004), but this has been mainly in the face-to-face domain. Nevertheless, because of this instinct for self-preservation, recipients of negative feedback frequently attribute it, or the behavior that is the target of the feedback, to external factors and reject personal responsibility; this is known as fundamental attribution error.

To avoid this, Archer suggests that, because self-assessment is akin to the unachievable holy grail of self-knowledge, it is inappropriate to continue to pursue this activity so enthusiastically. Instead, it is better for learners to consult others who epitomize reliable and valid external sources. He acknowledges that many learners will need to be supported both in their motivation to seek, and in gaining affordance of, external feedback as they move from ipsative assessment to routine autonomous feedback-seeking activity. As Archer says, "By learning about our abilities, not ourselves, through external feedback we are then able to better self-monitor" (2010, p. 104). This accords with Hattie's (2009; Hattie and Timperley 2007) notion that in feedback processes, comments on the "self" are best used as a last resort, and only to engage students in reflection about self-regulation.

Archer's review also deals with the need for goal setting. The learner's acceptance of feedback depends on its specificity, salience, and source, which must be credible. Acceptability is increased if the relevance of the feedback is underpinned by goal setting. These goals should be personally meaningful and constructed to be achievable. They may be learning- or performance-orientated. Learning goals are founded in a personal desire to develop and apply more advanced knowledge and skills, undertaken in the belief that cognitive functioning is flexible. Performance orientation reflects a desire to demonstrate competence to others and to be positively evaluated by them.

Agius and Wilkinson (2014) systematically reviewed and evaluated literature investigating the views of students and staff in nursing education on written feedback. They aimed to explore students' expectations of and staff's views on written academic feedback and isolate some strategies to improve feedback in nursing education.

Twenty-one studies were reviewed, with well over half coming from the UK and Australia. The importance students attribute to receiving positive comments alongside critical ones was emphasized by students, and an imbalance was generally perceived as unhelpful. However, critical comments were useful if presented in an understanding and encouraging nature and motivated students to stick to their studies when their performance on assessment was less than expected. Notably, lecturers' perspectives about balancing positive and negative comments were not addressed in any of the reviewed studies. The concept of balanced feedback is described by a group of well-respected researchers as "a myth" (Molloy et al. 2020). They note the "obsession" with feedback delivery skills, and the flawed conclusion that "saying the right words at the right time is all that is necessary to help our learners improve" (p. 35). Their proffered alternative to this approach is the concept of debriefing, from work using simulation in learning. They also advocate using an explicitly values-based approach, where "a commitment to respecting learners and understanding their perspective" is made a ground rule for interaction. They further recommend that the feedback or debriefing session should encourage reciprocal vulnerability between teacher and student, and that this can work as a mechanism for development of both participants. The concept of "ground rules" has been common in small group teaching, such as PBL, but less so in written feedback. However, for students, the importance of balance is that it gives them the opportunity to understand the difference between an acceptable and an inadequate level of performance, and one that could be better, in order to discriminate between descriptive comments and critical ones. And there are other reasons for balance. A number of studies identify that the impact on affect engendered by poorly constructed or hastily compiled written feedback can serve as an impediment to its worth (e.g. Sargeant et al. 2011; Chong 2018). Students who are upset or enraged by feedback typically tend not to respond by trying harder. Chong, in a review of this area (2018, p. 190), points out that students' negative responses to feedback provided by teachers become more evident when the tone of the feedback is "definite, cynical and full of criticism." Even mildly offended students may be reluctant to engage in constructive activity around improving their work or engaging in dialogue about it.

In a review by Agius and Wilkinson (2014), students were appreciative of focus and precision in teachers' comments. Only one teacher-focused study captured information about their views on generalized feedback. In that study, institutional pressure to give timely feedback resulted in the use of "cut-and-pasted," brief, and unspecific feedback, producing a standardized format. One big disadvantage of written feedback, especially that delivered by e-media, is that it is often done quickly, and may use drop-down menus of comments that may seem flexible to the teacher, but will be exactly the same, word for word, for many students. Why would recipients of such feedback perceive it as if there had been individual attention given to their work? Students can recognize when they have been fobbed off with a cut-and-pasted feedback "slogan." And communication between students comparing the slogans they get makes this more irksome for them. It certainly does not reflect "respect and understanding" or "reciprocal vulnerability" on the part of the teachers.

Lecturers' writing was identified as difficult to decipher in 6 of 21 studies reviewed, and academic jargon was indicated as the main reason for misunderstanding feedback. In one study, because oral feedback was perceived to be easier to understand than written feedback, the nursing students preferred it.

Marginal comments were preferred to feedback on cover sheets. Providing detailed feedback was weakened by time limitations and large classes, and when students did not collect marked essays, teachers perceived that their efforts were being undervalued by students who were only interested in marks. They also perceived that giving marks hampers students' engagement with feedback.

Eleven studies indicated that students' value, and expect, feedback that incorporates advice for improvement: the feedforward feature of feedback. When this guidance was worded in the form of imperatives rather than suggestions, students showed resistance to taking it on. However, two studies indicated that previously given guidance for improvement was not prevalent (followed up) in subsequent written comments. While most students expected comments on written work, most lecturers covered in the research did not give any.

Three studies reviewed identified that teachers recognized that feedback should be timely, acknowledging that prompt return of feedback would be of benefit to students. However, in one of these studies, teachers ascribed less relevance to timeliness with summative feedback because they perceived it to be too late for students to act upon the feedback. All assessment should generate feedback.

Teachers generally recognized that learners had difficulty understanding academic discourse. Twelve studies suggested that students valued extensive, detailed feedback. Students thought that effort by the assessor in feedback should equal that of the student in producing the work, and they took comments with examples and explanations as evidence of more profound engagement from lecturers, as opposed to just having grammatical corrections. Agius and Wilkinson (2014, p. 558) concluded that "Guidance on criteria and academic discourse, therefore, needs to be provided to students. In line with student-centred learning, adopting strategies that increase student engagement with the standards and criteria of assessment performance, such as the use of exemplars and self- and peer-assessment, help students become familiar with the language and with how to utilise the criteria."

The systematic review by Bing-You et al. (2018) has previously been mentioned in connection with the discussion of comments made on work submitted. Their findings on gender impacts illustrate the inconsistency of research in this area. Although finding that gender had an impact reported by seven articles, in one study with medical students on clinical placement using feedback cards, fewer recommendations for improvement were noted with gender concordant pairs, but in another, gender concordant female pairs resulted in more detailed goals. Other studies in the review were more coherent around gender differences. In a study of multisource feedback (MSF) to residents on interprofessional behaviors, the female raters scored residents in multiple specialties lower than the male ones. In another MSF article, male obstetrics and gynecology residents received more negative feedback from (predominantly female) nurses than did their female equivalents. Another study on case presentations showed that male first-year medical students were more likely than female students to provide critical feedback to peers. A study reporting on written summative feedback showed that third-year female medical students were more likely than males to seek out this information.

Canning (2018) performed a quick review of feedback literature to inform practice as part of the University of Southampton Sharing Practice in Enhancing and Assuring Quality (SPEAQ) project. (http://blog.soton.ac.uk/gmoof). His conclusions include the observation that feedback which is relevant in terms of the assessment may not be relevant in the context of the needs of the individual students being assessed. He also identified that students should have access to all comments made about a particular assignment or task, not just their own. This is because there will be issues and/or particular standards of work which the individual student may not be aware of, so was not included in their submission. But alerting them to these possibilities would be beneficial. Moreover, students, as well as teachers, could provide feedback on drafts of each other's work, and they may learn more by discussing this in small groups before doing so. Group essays may also be a good way to use written feedback as a direct input into developing better work.

Other Factors

Evans (2013) undertook a comprehensive review of assessment-related feedback, based on 460 papers sourced from systematic and snowballing approaches. Of these papers, 360 were empirical studies and 80 were theoretical treatises. As background, she indicates, for example, that there have been recommendations from higher education institutions to provide more oral as opposed to written feedback, and that more illumination is needed by students to enable them to gain independence in learning, and that the division between formative and summative assessment is too great. This suggests that perspectives on feedback are still buttressed by too limited conceptions of the purposes of feedback. In other words, building dependence on teacher-mediated feedback too rigidly into assessment systems will inhibit the movement of students to more autonomous activity. Evans' review identified a number of significant issues that impact on strategies for written feedback, albeit against a background of deficiencies in research that included inadequate description in some studies of the feedback intervention, and frequent dependence on self-judgments for effectiveness outcomes. Drawing on the theoretical sector of literature, she identifies principles of feedback practice that include the following which have direct relevance to written feedback:

- Ensuring all resources are available to students via virtual learning environments, and via other sources, from the start of a program to enable students to take responsibility for organizing their own learning
- Clarifying with students the different forms and sources of feedback available including e-learning opportunities
- Clarifying the role of the student in the feedback process as an active participant with sufficient knowledge and IT skills to engage in feedback
- Providing opportunities for students to work with assessment criteria and to work with examples of good work
- Giving clear and focused feedback on how students can improve their work including signposting the most important areas to address (see also next section)
- Ensuring support is in place to help students develop self-assessment skills including training, for example, in peer written feedback (See Evans 2013, p. 79)

Several studies have indicated that students vary in their capacity to respond to feedback and that this is related to the degree that they trust the source, whether that is peer- or faculty-mediated (e.g., Tsui and Ng 2000). Students also sometimes take away interpretations from feedback that may not be the messages intended by the giver. Hyland (2013) points out from an interview study of 24 Hong Kong-based students, studying in English, that they often had the impression that before they had written anything, their teachers had told them that their English did not matter, what mattered was the application of knowledge. Hyland goes on to suggest that if assessors ignore things like grammatical expression in feedback this "runs the risk of devaluing the importance of rhetorical appropriacy in disciplinary argument. It says, in effect, that 'content' can be created independently of the language which conveys it: that meaning and form are separate things" (Hyland 2013, p. 182). Hyland feels that writing is too often regarded as an autonomous skill rather than a disciplinary practice that is dependent on using the right terminology and grammatical construction. So, while students recognize the importance of good writing as a way to engage with readers, they fail to extend that skill within disciplinary conventions.

In a complex and extensive project, Nelson and Schunn (2009) studied the effect of various elements of written feedback on its implementation. They studied five features of feedback: summarization, specificity, explanations, scope, and affective language. The first four of these are in the cognitive domain, while the fifth touches on the socioemotional domain, described by Chong, above. Summarization relates to whether the feedback contains a summary of what the feedback receiver is trying to achieve, for example, "your article is striving to redress the balance between formative and summative assessment." Specificity addresses the extent of the details included in the feedback. Of course, specificity stretches across a continuum and contains at least three foci within it. In the study, these were identified as problem identification, providing solutions, and indicating the location of the problem and/or solution. In addition, a further component is explanation. In explanation, the feedback giver may include a direction, and either does or does not elaborate on why the directive is needed. The example given by the authors (p. 379) is "a reviewer may suggest, 'Delete the second paragraph on the third page.'" This may or may not be accompanied by an explanation, for example, "because it interrupts the flow of the paper." If the elaboration is not there, the writer might not follow the advice because they do not know why it is beneficial to the work.

The "scope" in Nelson and Schunn's model relates to the extent to which feedback is about the whole work or small foci within it (global vs local). Local scope would be advice to rewrite a sentence. Global scope would be a judgment about the forcefulness or quality of the whole essay/assignment/report. The final element studied was "affective language." Affective language in feedback might include isolated praise or criticism, and inflammatory or mitigating language (both praise and correction together). The phrase "What you write may be perceived as banal" would be inflammatory. The statement "But I don't think so" would be mitigation. The authors examined the correlations between the above feedback features, and feedback implementation rates. A large dataset of online peer-reviews of a six-to-eight page argument-driven essay, from a single (nonmedical) course in the USA was analyzed to link style of giving feedback and the resulting paper revisions. Each essay was reviewed by six peers. A total of 140 reviews were analyzed. The authors found that only one factor had a statistically significant relationship. A writer was 10% more likely to make changes when a solution was offered than when it was not offered. There was not even a trend of a positive effect for the other variables. However, the authors also looked at students understanding of and agreement with the feedback. Understanding of the problem did have a significant relationship. A writer was 23% more likely to implement the feedback if they understood the problem. Moreover, when summarization provided solutions and localization (indicating where solutions could be found), this significantly increased problem understanding. A writer was 16% more likely to understand the problem if a summary was included, 14% more likely if a solution was provided, and 24% more likely if a location to the problem and/or solution was provided. Paradoxically, the existence of explanation of the problem was significantly related to problem understanding but in an inverse direction: students were 17% more likely to **misunderstand** the problem if an explanation to the problem was provided. Summarizing with solution identification and location (this was wrong, you should have done that, and here's where you can find out how) was offset by elaborate or even **any additional** explanation. This may explain why much feedback is regarded as uninterpretable by students (Marbouti et al. 2019).

Other researchers classified mediators (personal attributes or world views) that appeared to impact on written feedback from five experienced teachers (Dunworth and Sanchez 2018). These mediating attributes were identified from a qualitative analysis both of feedback statements and of initial open and subsequent stimulated-recall interviews based on the statements. Three overlapping mediators were identified: experiential, social and environmental perspectives. "Experiential mediators," include those which appeared to be drawn from beliefs, understandings, and perspectives based on the experience of the educators when they had been students, and also from their "practice" as teachers and writers of academic texts. The second element, "social mediators" related to how participants described their adaptation of feedback and discourse practices to align with those of their colleagues or peers. This was formed from the cultural milieu of the educational program in which they were collectively engaged and teaching. The third category, "environmental mediators," referred to factors predating the individual participants' involvement in their program, or factors which were external and outside their immediate control and imposed upon them, such as institutional assessment policy, the need to address assessment criteria, the limits on time, the class size, the depth of written feedback needed, and the existence of benchmarked templates for and modes of feedback. The authors of this study stress the need to consider that staff feedback practices cannot be viewed in a "stand-alone" way as part of a faculty member's teaching repertoire. The way that academics give feedback is grounded in a complex system of constraints, opportunities, and stimuli within a wide cultural context. This included their past individual experience and practice, which had helped mold academics' views on how they should behave, but also existing structures and artefacts, and the varied other individuals, who contribute to creating the institutional norms by which feedback practice is itself conceptualized. This study demonstrates that, in this setting, staff were sensitive to how they constructed their feedback, for example, the phrases and affective language, in ways that they believed were appropriate to the context of the feedback situation. This raises an important issue. While feedback is a vital centerpiece of student experience, it can only take that role if the curriculum gives it the opportunity and the space to do so. Thus, discrete one-off assessment "events," with no opportunity for students to respond or lack of teacher follow-up of those students' responses to feedback, will not permit feedback the freedom to become effective.

Studies in the Medical Context

Dekker et al. (2013) in a medical context looked at which characteristics of feedback could be distinguished in written feedback provided by 23 medical educators making comments on students' reflective writing and which of those were perceived as stimulating, maintaining, and improving students' reflective processes. They showed that the characteristics of comment could be described in three dimensions: its format (statement versus question), its focus (on the level, or sophistication, of students' reflection,) and its (affective) tone (positive versus negative). Furthermore, comments phrased as a question and in a positive tone were judged as stimulating reflection more than comments framed as a statement or a negative imputation, respectively. Moreover, the effect sizes were 0.86 (large) for format of the feedback comment, 0.42 (moderate) for the tone of the feedback.

Duijn et al. (2017) performed a multicenter focus group study of students' perceptions of meaningful feedback on entrustable professional activities. Although it is not clear whether the authors were studying responses to written or oral feedback, analysis of the discussions identified that students wanted personal rather than group feedback, and from a reliable source – "a person who knows what is expected in such an activity" (p. 260), and that written feedback alone was not enough. Students expected supervisors to provide an oral explanation of written feedback, and if feedback was given on mistakes, this should include a discussion of the context in which they were made. In addition, feedback should include an indication of the student's ability to act unsupervised, and given before a mistake was to be made. Clearly such "just in time" communication can be made in writing.

Bok et al. (2016) in a qualitative interpretive study based on interviews with 14 experienced clinical teachers found that the balance between Mini CEX-based written and oral feedback was frequently shifted towards the latter. This was because the teachers were supposed to document the narrative feedback; due to workload, they frequently asked students to document the feedback and then submit it in their portfolio electronically for approval. This meant that sometimes the Mini-CEX became more of a self-evaluation in contrast to a scaffold containing clues for improvement. The study also suggested that the Mini-CEX, being a short sample of clinical activity, may have constrained some elements of feedback on generic skills and clinical competence development in shorter attachments. The faculty felt that they could only focus on the task rather than the improvement of the student across the board.

Hewson and Little (1998) analyzed narratives of incidents of feedback experienced by 83 academics from the US, Canada, and the UK, who were learning how to be better medical interviewers, and how to teach these skills to others. At the end of the 1-week course, each member provided a short narrative of two examples, one of which they judged as personally helpful, and the other as personally unhelpful. They also rated their own narratives using a semantic differential scale based on literature-supported recommended vs non-recommended techniques/attributes, for example, "being judgmental vs being non-judgmental" (p. 112). The manner in which feedback was provided strongly affected participants' perceptions, for example, helpful incidents were associated with techniques such as "giving feedback lovingly, supportively, and caringly," "being gentle and not hitting someone over the head with his or her mistakes," and "being concerned to understand the other person's position" (p. 113). Feedback that included specific suggestions for improvement was seen as very important. One participant was "amazed to see how much genuine caring can be manifested by strangers, and how helpful it can be" (p. 113). Poor feedback was characterized, for example, by not eliciting a person's ideas, feelings, or goals; or by another participant projecting his or her own safety issues onto others. The authors then refined their findings by comparing them to or infusing them with concepts from constructivist learning and teaching theory. Despite them analyzing written feedback, their model favors direct face to face discussion in giving feedback. However, it might be adaptable to a written or partially written framework. A six-stage model was developed.

1. Create an appropriate climate and orientate students to the focus of the event
2. Elicit the students' self-assessments
3. Diagnose the "gaps" and give feedback
4. Get the students to create a feedback plan
5. Set a goal for the application of the plan
6. Review the session to check students' understanding of the feedback

Research has shown that the quality of written feedback can be assessed reliably, and that faculty can improve their feedback if its quality is fed back to them over time (Bartlett et al. 2017). General practitioners (GPs) undertaking workplace-based assessments (WBA) with students gave written feedback on their skills. An instrument was created to rate the quality of the written comments. The instrument was discussed with GP tutors during faculty development activities (meetings and routine teaching review visits) so that they were familiar with the content and how quality was being assessed. At the end of each of three academic years, each practice teaching student was scored on six separate feedback deliverables and mean scores calculated. These scores were then presented as a "league table" showing the mean score for each practice, using identification numbers. Practices were aware of their own identifier. Mean quality scores were fed back to 85 practices for the first time at the end of the academic year, after which the mean score for all practices rose by 1.4 points from 3.7 to 5.1 (6-point scale). During the next year, three practices had specific faculty support focusing on their activities in the WBA which had been triggered by their poor scores on the instrument. For these practices, the mean score rose from 0.6 to 5.6. A year later, the mean score had stabilized to 4.7. In another study (MacNeil et al. 2019), the authors showed that it is possible to foster meaningful feedback if faculty establish a trusting relationship with the resident, base their feedback on direct observation, and support resident learning. However, in this study almost all the feedback modes were conversational, and moreover, residents perceived the Mini-CEX to be constrained by the checklist style feedback that resulted from the interaction and, as such, most often described it as not being an opportunity for meaningful feedback. This highlights the inadvisability of relying to any great extent on written feedback in the clinical setting.

Previously discussed studies (Nelson and Schunn 2009; Hewson and Little 1998) identified the need to ensure students understood feedback, and that explanation from teachers was sometimes counterproductive in that process. One mode of achieving better understanding is to get students to engage in peer-to peer discussion of feedback they have received. Schillings et al. (2019) explored whether peer-to-peer dialogue between students, about faculty's' written feedback, enhanced their understanding of it. In a pretest- posttest design with mixed methods involving health science students, the teachers attended a 1-hour session on how to provide students with written feedback, this involved the concepts of feed-up, feedback, and feed-forward. Students' conversations were conducted according to the four-step model of Sargeant et al. (2011). In step one of this model, the teacher provided written feedback as described above. Students were then asked to read the feedback provided by the teacher on their own assignment and on the assignments of their peers in the group. Students received no training in advance. At the start of the conversation session, students were asked to follow the three subsequent steps of Sargeant et al.'s (2011) model, which were:

1. The facilitator explored students' initial reactions regarding the written feedback by asking about their first impression of this written feedback.
2. Students discussed the content of their teachers' written feedback with each other.
3. Then, students offered each other additional guidance on how to proceed or move forward.

The overall perceived instructiveness of the teachers' written feedback was statistically significantly higher after the peer-to-peer dialogue session as compared to the perceived instructiveness before the dialogue. However, the original quality of the teachers' written feedback was also perceived to be an important factor in the overall instructiveness of the peer dialogue.

Evaluations of feedback given by senior medical staff to junior staff or students has attracted some research attention. Jackson et al. (2015) investigated feedback given to 228 internal medicine residents, with a total of 6,603 evaluations by 334 attendings. Of these, 1,387 (21%) had no written feedback. From the remainder, the authors looked at a randomly selected sample of 500 monthly written comments on residents' performance. These were qualitatively coded and rated as high-, moderate-, or low-quality feedback by two reliable (kappa = 0.94) independent coders. Among 500 randomly selected written comments, there were 2,056 unique expressions, and of these 49% were coded as nonspecific statements or were comments about resident personality. Both aspects of feedback not highly regarded as useful (Hattie and Timperley 2007). Only 16% concerned patient care, 14% were focused on interpersonal communication, 7% on medical knowledge, 6% professionalism, and 4% each on practice-based learning and systems-based practice. Most comments (65%) were rated as moderate quality and only 22% were rated as high quality, with the remainder as low quality. Attendings who provided high-quality feedback rated residents statistically and meaningfully significantly lower in all six of the competencies covered by the feedback and had a greater range of scores than other attendings.

A study of the quality of feedback provided in the logbooks of preclinical undergraduate students learning in a clinical skills laboratory was undertaken (Abraham and Singaram 2019). The authors found that student's perceptions of logbook feedback in their setting was vague and inconsistent (Abraham and Singaram 2016); therefore, the authors attempted to make the logbook feedback more effective. A "feedforward" three-step strategy on what was done well, what was not done well, and what could be improved was incorporated into the logbook. This allowed clinicians and peers to provide students with learning goals/action plans targeting the performance assessment process and not just the assessment product. The authors identified that adding this strategy to the logbooks increased the overall quality of feedback. This was seen in both peers' and tutors' feedback, because the task was described, and the gap between mastery and current performance identified. This was then translated into action plans. Peers were more diligent than tutors in providing all three steps in written form.

Faculty development may be needed to achieve improvements in feedback. Salerno et al. (2003) evaluated the impact of three 1.5 hour faculty development workshops, partially based on the one-minute preceptor model (Gatewood and De Gagne 2019), on written feedback from encounter cards during an ambulatory internal medicine clerkship, using a pre-post mixed methods design. They found more frequent and more specific feedback after the intervention, but no difference in either "attitudinal" feedback, which was rare in any case, or corrective feedback. The percentage of feedback spent "just providing the grade" decreased, while specific formative feedback, linked to specific student behaviors, increased, and this was in line with previous work (Holmboe et al. 2001). In common with the above finding, Gul et al. (2016) working with teachers from nursing, applied linguistics, medicine, and education departments in higher education providers situated in Karachi identified, through self-reported data, that formal training in giving feedback was perceived as critical to the quality of that feedback. However, they also found that the available time, the relationship between teachers and students, and the policies and culture of the institutions had an impact. In addition, there were disciplinary differences: notably, teachers from nursing provided written feedback most frequently, then education and linguistics, and medical teachers the least.

Charting the Best Course in Written Feedback

In this section, I will attempt a distillation that would allow clinical teachers to improve their written feedback. As noted above, evidence is not clear-cut, and models vary, contexts change and students are diverse (Rae and Cochrane 2008). Also, some health professions have an obdurate history of toxicity in their educational cultures that clearly may inhibit any single teacher's capacity to deliver feedback in an appropriate way (Arluke 1980; Lempp and Seale 2004; Fnais et al. 2014; Halim and Riding 2018).

General Issues

First and foremost, any feedback event (written or otherwise) needs to be set in a learning culture that fosters opportunities for dialogue about and iterative approaches to assessment. So written feedback should be seen as part of a feedback strategy within the curriculum and as a process – a cycle – not simply the provision of information and judgment. Furthermore, democratizing opportunities for feedback is important. This means sourcing it from all stakeholders: the students themselves, peers, supervisors, and teachers and most importantly patients. Opportunities for written feedback may be more difficult with some stakeholders. In addition, through learning activities that highlight feedback, students and trainees need to build the capacity to effectively seek and utilize information from others, usually by having their tasks and reconstructions of those tasks become the object of further feedback.

This requires learning and assessment tasks in the curriculum to be broken down so that feedback can be given more effectively. For example, in our MD program (5 years) at the University of Newcastle, students perform a research project (over years 3 and 4) in a group of four to five members. They have to undertake a focused literature review after a systematic search strategy, with faculty feedback on these steps. Then, they write an outline and then a draft research proposal, which are faculty and peer-reviewed, and a final proposal in which they make clear how they have dealt with the feedback received, which is then reviewed by an independent staff member, who also has access, if needed, to all the research project proposals of the whole cohort. Students receive some guidance on how to give constructive feedback. This all sounds onerous, but it is not that time-consuming spread over large time span, and faculty were impressed by how good the peer feedback was.

Also, ideally any feedback process needs to be managed by the learner or, if that is challenging in the clinical setting, become at least a learner-engaged activity so that when windows of opportunity arise during clinical attachments they can be seized by students. In this way, comments and messages from others who are not necessarily "the teacher" of the moment are received, can be acted on, and the feedback loop closed. Try not to repeat bad exemplars of feedback that you may have received as a student (see points 2 and 7 below).

Structuring Written Feedback

From discussion in the main part of this chapter, an image of ideal written feedback **can be discerned.**

1. Choose as many foci for the feedback as seem warranted by the task undertaken. These can (and possibly should) include:
   (a) Comments on the task itself (its best and worst features)
   (b) Analysis of the process of getting to that point (how and why the task has been done well or inadequately)
   (c) Identification of the role of self-regulation by the student in completing the task (decisions the student made about their planned activity to get the task done/not done)

   Also plan to give the students opportunities to ask themselves questions rather than simply direct them to further practice. Examples of (a) might be "you introduced yourself effectively to the patient by doing x, y and z. You washed your hands before starting. I think you missed out important aspects of the family history; can you identify what those were?"

   Examples of (b) might include "Since I last saw you, you must have done several abdominal exams, your flow and speed has increased, and if you do a few more you will be adequately competent and also efficient. I also noticed your palpation technique has improved and that takes practice, so well done there."

Examples of (c) would be "I've seen you on the ward a lot more than last week, so I think that's made a difference, and you've stayed once or twice to ensure you see things. It all adds up to an improved patient encounter."

2. Choose a format for giving the feedback

The above advice could have been given verbally. But, if a Mini-CEX was the focus of this task, then the likelihood would be that it would be entered in an electronic form of some kind. This would help with its legibility and permanence. If the student was leaving the attachment soon after the feedback was given, then writing it down somewhere (via email or SMS text) might offer advantages to the student. A lot of devices now have voice to text translator software that can provide written or editable copies of a spoken text.

If marking a written piece uses both summaries and comments in the margins to address specific elements and be precise so "I think this is the wrong reference" becomes "This concept is much better addressed in Talley and O'Connor, maybe have a look at that" or "Improve your CVS examination" becomes "Try to practice a systematic approach to CVS examination to make sure relevant aspects are not forgotten: for example, measuring BP, collapsing pulse, and radio-radial delay."

If using a learning management system (e.g., Blackboard), try to avoid using only the drop-down or cut-and-paste feedback phrases.

In brief, in the feedback, use summarization (with solution identification and location), be specific, provide explanation in plain language, indicate the scope of your comments (whole task or subcomponent), and use encouraging affective language.

3. Make sure the message is clear, without using jargon (either educational or medical). Sometimes, assessors can be so much more experienced than the learners that they forget to simplify the terminology.

4. If a grade has been given, make sure the written feedback is commensurate with it. If possible, embed the grade given within the written feedback so that the student has to read through most of it before finding the grade (or separate the grade from the feedback in time).

5. Try to use feed-forward directives, such as "next time you do this task, try to incorporate a more complete family history because, with these autoimmune disorders, that can be quite important." This entails direction, but in a non-dogmatic manner.

6. Do not use "final vocabulary" and absolute vague words such as excellent, poor, good, banal, well structured. When you have written the feedback, go back over it and look for such words. Erase them and replace with a description of why the task was good/bad/indifferent/banal. So "Your introduction was good" would become "You introduced yourself effectively to the patient by telling them your name, and checking on theirs, smiling, offering a seat, asking them their preferred mode of address, and starting with a very open question." This takes

only 25 seconds longer to write, even less with predictive text or voice recognition.

7. Frequent exchange between student and teacher, or feedback dialogue, whether written or verbal, will need support and many learners will need to be encouraged both around their motivation to seek, and in gaining affordance for external feedback. This will need reassuring learning environments, underpinned by ground rules about civility, manner of exchanges, teamwork, acceptance of feedback, and goal setting. It will also need attention to the delivery of balanced feedback to illustrate the difference between under and adequate or excellent performance. Teachers will need support also to engage in reciprocal vulnerability.

8. Use every assessment as a source of feedback, irrespective of the quantum or stakes of the assessment event. So, allocate time in the curriculum and assessment tasks for this to happen. Where possible, use model answers in this process (Huxham 2007), and provide examples of excellence by getting students to share their work and the feedback they received and how they responded.

9. If possible, choose a model for giving feedback that best fits the type of assessment. Elaborate models are fine (Boud and Molloy 2013), but there may be urgencies or extraneous factors that prevent their ubiquitous usage. Models can be easily found in the existing literature (Jolly and Boud 2013; Sargeant et al. 2011; Hattie and Timperley 2007; Pendleton et al. 2003)

10. Give feedback in time for it to be useful. Late feedback is a wasted effort.

Conclusion

In this chapter, I have tried to distill some guidelines for the effective use of written feedback. There is scarce research on this in the health professions. Ten guidelines are suggested by the literature, but they are not fool proof; the one thing the research suggests is that contexts vary to an extent that a strategy will work in one setting but not necessarily in all settings. Research in this area will pay large dividends.

Cross-References

- ▶ Conversational Learning in Health Professions Education: Learning Through Talk
- ▶ Debriefing Practices in Simulation-Based Education
- ▶ Focus on Theory: Emotions and Learning
- ▶ Measuring Performance: Current Practices in Surgical Education
- ▶ Medical Education: Trends and Context
- ▶ Programmatic Assessment in Health Professions Education
- ▶ Self-Regulated Learning: Focus on Theory

References

Abraham RM, Singaram VS. Third-year medical students' and clinical teachers' perceptions of formative assessment feedback in the simulated clinical setting. Afr J Health Prof Educ. 2016;8 (1Suppl 1):121–5.

Abraham RM, Singaram VS. Using deliberate practice framework to assess the quality of feedback in undergraduate clinical skills training. BMC Med Educ. 2019;19(1):105.

Agius NM, Wilkinson A. Students' and teachers' views of written feedback at undergraduate level: a literature review. Nurse Educ Today. 2014;34(4):552–9.

Ajjawi R, Boud D. Researching feedback dialogue: an interactional analysis approach. Assess Eval High Educ. 2017;42(2):252–65.

Archer JC. State of the science in health professional education: effective feedback. Med Educ. 2010;44:101–8.

Arluke A. Roundsmanship: inherent control on a medical teaching ward. Soc Sci Med. 1980;14A:297–302.

Awang Besar MN, Kamruddin MA, Siraj HH, Yaman MN, Bujang SM, Karim J, Jaafar AS. Evaluation of lecturer's feedback in mini clinical evaluation exercise assessment (Mini-CEX). Educ Med J. 2018;10(4):31–41. https://doi.org/10.21315/eimj2018.10.4.4.

Babovič M, Fu RH, Monrouxe LV. Understanding how to enhance efficacy and effectiveness of feedback via e-portfolio: a realist synthesis protocol. BMJ Open. 2019;9(5):e029173.

Barrett M, Georgoff P, Matusko N, Leininger L, Reddy RM, Sandhu G, Hughes DT. The effects of feedback fatigue and sex disparities in medical student feedback assessed using a minute feedback system. J Surg Educ. 2018;75(5):1245–9.

Bartlett M, Crossley J, McKinley R. Improving the quality of written feedback using written feedback. Educ Prim Care. 2017;28(1):16–22.

Bing-You R, Varaklis K, Hayes V, Trowbridge R, Kemp H, McKelvy D. The feedback tango: an integrative review and analysis of the content of the teacher–learner feedback exchange. Acad Med. 2018;93(4):657–63.

Bok HG, Jaarsma DA, Spruijt A, Van Beukelen P, Van Der Vleuten CP, Teunissen PW. Feedback-giving behaviour in performance evaluations during clinical clerkships. Med Teach. 2016;38 (1):88–95.

Boud D. Assessment and learning: contradictory or complementary? Chapter 2. In: Knight P, editor. Assessment for learning in higher education. London: Kogan Page; 1995.

Boud D, Molloy E, editors. Feedback in higher and professional education: understanding it and doing it well. London: Routledge; 2013.

Burch VC. The changing landscape of workplace-based assessment. J Appl Test Technol. 2019;20 (S2):37–59.

Canning J (2018) Feedback: a short academic literature review. Sharing Practice in Enhancing and Assuring Quality (SPEAQ) project. https://cpb-eu-w2.wpmucdn.com/blogs.brighton.ac.uk/dist/2/123/files/2014/11/Feedback-literature-review2-1hx2wyt.pdf. Accessed Jan 2020

Carless D, Salter D, Yang M, Lam J. Developing sustainable feedback practices. Stud High Educ. 2011;36:395–407.

Chertoff J, Wright A, Novak M, Fantone J, Fleming A, Ahmed T, Green MM, Kalet A, Linsenmeyer M, Jacobs J, Dokter C. Status of portfolios in undergraduate medical education in the LCME accredited US medical school. Med Teach. 2016;38(9):886–96.

Cheung WJ, Dudek N, Wood TJ, Frank JR. Daily encounter cards – evaluating the quality of documented assessments. J Grad Med Educ. 2016;8(4):601–4.

Chong I. Interplay among technical, socio-emotional and personal factors in written feedback research. Assess Eval High Educ. 2018;43(2):185–96.

Coleman E, O'Connor E. The role of WhatsApp® in medical education; a scoping review and instructional design model. BMC Med Educ. 2019;19(1):279.

Deeley SJ. Using technology to facilitate effective assessment for learning and feedback in higher education. Assess Eval High Educ. 2018;43(3):439–48. https://doi.org/10.1080/02602938. 2017.1356906.

Dekker H, Schönrock-Adema J, Snoek JW, van der Molen T, Cohen-Schotanus J. Which characteristics of written feedback are perceived as stimulating students' reflective competence: an exploratory study. BMC Med Educ. 2013;13(1):94.

Duijn CC, Welink LS, Mandoki M, ten Cate OT, Kremer WD, Bok HG. Am I ready for it? Students' perceptions of meaningful feedback on entrustable professional activities. Perspect Med Educ. 2017;6(4):256–64.

Dunworth K, Sanchez HS. Mediating factors in the provision of lecturers' written feedback to postgraduate taught students. Int J Educ Res. 2018;90:107–16.

Endacott R, Gray MA, Jasper MA, McMullan M, Miller C, Scholes J, Webb C. Using portfolios in the assessment of learning and competence: the impact of four models. Nurse Educ Pract. 2004;4(4):250–7.

Evans C. Making sense of assessment feedback in higher education. Rev Educ Res. 2013;83(1):70–120.

Fnais N, Soobiah C, Chen MH, Lillie E, Perrier L, Tashkhandi M, Straus SE, Mamdani M, Al-Omran M, Tricco AC. Harassment and discrimination in medical training: a systematic review and meta-analysis. Acad Med. 2014;89(5):817–27.

Gatewood E, De Gagne JC. The one-minute preceptor model: a systematic review. J Am Assoc Nurse Pract. 2019;31(1):46–57.

Gough S, Hamshire C. Supporting healthcare workforce development using simulation and ePortfolios. In Proceedings of E-Portfolio and identity conference (Epic). ADPIOS, Poitiers, France. 2012. http://epic.openrecognition.org/wp-content/uploads/sites/6/2018/02/ePIC-2012. pdf. Accessed 10 Dec 2020.

Graduate Careers Australia. Data from the course experience questionnaire 2010. 2012. http://www.graduatecareers.com.au/wp-content/uploads/2012/01/gca002524.pdf. Accessed 12 May 2012.

Gul RB, Tharani A, Lakhani A, Rizvi NF, Ali SK. Teachers' perceptions and practices of written feedback in higher education. World J Educ. 2016;6(3):10.

Halim UA, Riding DM. Systematic review of the prevalence, impact and mitigating strategies for bullying, undermining behaviour and harassment in the surgical workplace. Br J Surg. 2018;105 (11):1390–7.

Harvey P, Radomski N, O'Connor D. Written feedback and continuity of learning in a geographically distributed medical education program. Med Teach. 2013;35(12):1009–13.

Hattie J. Visible learning: a synthesis of 800+ meta-analyses on achievement. Oxford: Routledge; 2009.

Hattie J, Gan M. Instruction based on feedback. Chapter 13. In: Meyer RE, Alexander PA, editors. Handbook of research on learning and instruction. New York: Routledge; 2011.

Hattie J, Timperley H. The power of feedback. Rev Educ Res. 2007;77:81–112.

Heeneman S, de Grave W. Tensions in mentoring medical students toward self-directed and reflective learning in a longitudinal portfolio-based mentoring system–an activity theory analysis. Med Teach. 2017;39(4):368–76.

Hewson MG, Little ML. Giving feedback in medical education: verification of recommended techniques. J Gen Intern Med. 1998;13(2):111–6.

Hilton S, Rague B. Is video feedback more effective than written feedback? In 2015 IEEE frontiers in education conference (FIE) 2015. p. 1–6. IEEE.

Holmboe ES, Fiebach NH, Galaty LA, Huot S. Effectiveness of a focused educational intervention on resident evaluations from faculty: a randomized controlled trial. J Gen Intern Med. 2001;16:427–34.

Huxham M. Fast and effective feedback: are model answers the answer? Assess Eval High Educ. 2007;32:601–11.

Hyland K. Student perceptions of hidden messages in teacher written feedback. Stud Educ Eval. 2013;39(3):180–7.

Ion G, Cano-García E, Fernández-Ferrer M. Enhancing self-regulated learning through using written feedback in higher education. Int J Educ Res. 2017;85:1–0.

Jackson JL, Kay C, Jackson WC, Frank M. The quality of written feedback by attendings of internal medicine residents. J Gen Intern Med. 2015;30(7):973–8.

Jolly B, Boud D. Written feedback. In: Feedback in higher and professional education. London: Routledge; 2013. p. 104–24.

Lawson M, Nestel D, Jolly B. An e-portfolio in health professional education. Med Educ. 2004;38(5):569–70.

Lempp H, Seale C. The hidden curriculum in undergraduate medical education: qualitative study of medical students' perceptions of teaching. BMJ. 2004;329:770–3.

MacNeil K, Cuncic C, Voyer S, Butler D, Hatala R. Necessary but not sufficient: identifying conditions for effective feedback during internal medicine residents' clinical education. Adv Health Sci Educ. 2019;25:1–4.

Marbouti F, Mendoza-Garcia J, Diefes-Dux HA, Cardella ME. Written feedback provided by first-year engineering students, undergraduate teaching assistants, and educators on design project work. Eur J Eng Educ. 2019;44(1–2):179–95.

Molloy E, Ajjawi R, Bearman M, Noble C, Rudland J, Ryan A. Challenging feedback myths: values, learner involvement and promoting effects beyond the immediate task. Med Educ. 2020;54(1):33–9.

Morris C, Chikwa G. Audio versus written feedback: exploring learners' preference and the impact of feedback format on students' academic performance. Act Learn High Educ. 2016;17(2):125–37.

Nelson MM, Schunn CD. The nature of feedback: how different types of peer feedback affect writing performance. Instr Sci. 2009;37(4):375–401.

Nesbitt A, Pitcher A, James L, Sturrock A, Griffin A. Written feedback on supervised learning events. Clin Teach. 2014;11(4):279–83.

Nicol D. From monologue to dialogue: improving written feedback processes in mass higher education. Assess Eval High Educ. 2010;35:501–17.

Norcini JJ, Blank LL, Arnold GK, Kimball HR. The mini-CEX (clinical evaluation exercise): a preliminary investigation. Ann Intern Med. 1995;123(10):795–9.

O'Donovan BM, den Outer B, Price M, Lloyd A. What makes good feedback good? Stud High Educ. 2019;19:1–2.

Page M, Gardner J, Booth J. Validating written feedback in clinical formative assessment. Assess Eval High Educ. 2019;45:1–7.

Parappilly M, Woodman RJ, Randhawa S. Feasibility and effectiveness of different models of team-based learning approaches in STEMM-based disciplines. Res Sci Educ. 2019;4:1–5.

Pendleton D, Schofield T, Tate P, Havelock P. The new consultation. Oxford: Oxford University Press; 2003.

Price M, Handley K, Millar J, O'donovan B. Feedback: all that effort, but what is the effect? Assess Eval High Educ. 2010;35(3):277–89.

Rae AM, Cochrane DK. Listening to students: how to make written assessment feedback useful. Act Learn High Educ. 2008;9(3):217–30.

Rorty R. Contingency, irony, and solidarity. Cambridge, UK: Press Syndicate of University of Cambridge; 1989.

Rust C, O'Donovan B, Price M. A social constructivist assessment process model: how the research literature shows us this could be best practice. Assess Eval High Educ. 2005;30(3):231–40.

Ryan TA, Henderson M, Phillips MD. "Written feedback doesn't make sense": enhancing assessment feedback using technologies. In International conference of the Australian Association for Research in Education 2016: Transforming Educational Research 2016. p. 1–11. 2016. Australian Association for Research in Education.

Salerno SM, Jackson JL, O'malley PG. Interactive faculty development seminars improve the quality of written feedback in ambulatory teaching. J Gen Intern Med. 2003;18(10):831–4.

Sargeant J, Mcnaughton E, Mercer S, Murphy D, Sullivan P, Bruce DA. Providing feedback: exploring a model (emotion, content, outcomes) for facilitating multisource feedback. Med Teach. 2011;33(9):744–9.

Schillings M, Roebertsen H, Savelberg H, Whittingham J, Dolmans D. Peer-to-peer dialogue about teachers' written feedback enhances students' understanding on how to improve writing skills. Educ Stud. 2019;46:1–5.

Seabrook MA. Clinical students' initial reports of the educational climate in a single medical school. Med Educ. 2004;38:659–69.

Sellbjer S. "Have you read my comments? It is not noticeable. Change!" An analysis of feedback given to students who have failed examinations. Assess Eval High Educ. 2018;43(2):163–74.

Sharp P. Behaviour modification in the secondary school: a survey of students' attitudes to rewards and praise. Behav Approach Child. 1985;9:109–12.

Tai J, Ajjawi R, Boud D, Dawson P, Panadero E. Developing evaluative judgement: enabling students to make decisions about the quality of work. High Educ. 2018;76(3):467–81.

Telio S, Ajjawi R, Regehr G. The "educational alliance" as a framework for reconceptualizing feedback in medical education. Acad Med. 2015;90(5):609–14.

Tsui AB, Ng M. Do secondary L2 writers benefit from peer comments? J Second Lang Writ. 2000;9 (2):147–70.

Weller JM, Castanelli DJ, Chen Y, Jolly B. Making robust assessments of specialist trainees' workplace performance. Br J Anaesth. 2017;118(2):207–14.

Winstone NE, Nash RA. 11 developing students' proactive engagement with feedback. In: Innovative assessment in higher education: a handbook for academic practitioners, vol. 3. London/New York: Routledge, Taylor & Francis Group; 2019. p. 129.

Winstone NE, Nash RA, Rowntree J, Parker M. It'd be useful, but I wouldn't use it': barriers to university students feedback' seeking and recipience. Stud High Educ. 2017;42(11):2026–41.

Technology Considerations in Health Professions and Clinical Education

40

Christian Moro, Zane Stromberga, and James Birt

Contents

Introduction 744
Technology in Health Education 745
    Virtual and Augmented Reality 745
    Holograms and Mixed Reality 746
    Virtual Dissection Tables 747
    Social Media 748
    Mobile Applications/Devices 749
    3D Printing 750
    Online-Hosted Video 753
    Simulations with Technology-Enhanced Learning 754
    Serious Games 756
    E-Learning (Web Delivery) 758
    Audience Response 759
Conclusion 760
Cross-References 761
References 761

Abstract

Learning methods and pedagogy are shifting in clinical education. In particular, incorporating technology is increasingly important for training health professionals, where the necessary knowledge acquisition is typically much

---

C. Moro (✉) · Z. Stromberga
Faculty of Health Sciences and Medicine, Bond University, Gold Coast, QLD, Australia
e-mail: cmoro@bond.edu.au; zstrombe@bond.edu.au

J. Birt
Faculty of Society and Design, Bond University, Gold Coast, QLD, Australia
e-mail: jbirt@bond.edu.au

© Springer Nature Singapore Pte Ltd. 2023
D. Nestel et al. (eds.), *Clinical Education for the Health Professions*,
https://doi.org/10.1007/978-981-15-3344-0_118

more experiential, self-directed, and hands-on than many other disciplines. Virtual or mixed reality interventions are becoming more accessible and can be delivered through various modes in a way that integrates directly into learning environments. However, there are often limits to the capacity of the technology, leaving educators unclear of which technologies are useful, and how they can be integrated into the learning environment. This chapter provides an overview of virtual and augmented reality; holograms and mixed reality; virtual dissection tables; social media; mobile applications and devices; 3D printing; online hosted video; simulation with technology enhanced learning; serious games; e-learning; and audience response software. We provide insight into the use of technology in health professions and clinical education by defining the types of technologies and exploring published use-cases across disciplines.

Keywords

Virtual reality · Mixed reality · Augmented reality · Clinical education · Technology-enhanced learning · Medicine · Medical education · Blended learning

Introduction

Health professional educators are continuously incorporating technology in their pedagogical practices to enhance their ability to teach relevant, up-to-date content in an ever-changing environment. This chapter provides an overview of relevant research surrounding some of these technological interventions. This includes: virtual and augmented reality; holograms and mixed reality; virtual dissection tables; social media; mobile applications and devices; 3D printing; online hosted video; simulation with technology-enhanced learning; serious games; e-learning; and audience response software. We share published use-cases, research manuscripts, and reviews to highlight the breadth and depth of technology used in clinical health education. A literature search of different electronic databases was conducted using the following terms: (education OR training OR skills) AND (clinical OR health OR medical) AND (technology OR computer OR device OR simulation). As the focus of this chapter is on the current generation of educational technology, the search was limited to studies published between 2009 and 2019. This is not an exhaustive literature review but rather representational across different technologies and clinical education disciplines using qualitative synthesis. The core technologies identified include mobile applications/devices, 3D printing, video, simulation trainers with haptic devices, serious games, social media, e-learning, audience response, and XR (virtual reality, augmented reality, and mixed reality).

Technology in Health Education

Virtual and Augmented Reality

One of the primary concepts when learning physiology or anatomy is the relationships of structures in 3D space. Traditionally, cadavers or silicon models have been used to provide 3D representations as a supplement to textbook material. Developments in computing hardware and software can now allow the entire human body to be rendered in anatomically correct environments within virtual or augmented reality (Fig. 1). Both virtual and augmented reality applications have shown to be effective in enhancing the learning experience in various health profession courses (Birt et al. 2018; Moro et al. 2017a; Moro et al. 2017b) while also providing educators additional supplementary methods to engage students.

For clarity, the terminology in this review is adapted from Moro et al. (2017a):

- **Virtual reality**: The user's senses (sight, hearing and motion) are fully immersed in a synthetic environment that mimics the properties of the real world through high resolution, high refresh rate head-mounted displays, stereo headphones, and motion-tracking systems.
- **Augmented reality**: Using a camera and screen (i.e., smartphone or tablet), digital models are superimposed into the real-world. The user is then able to interact with both the real and virtual elements of their surrounding environment.
- **Three-dimensional tablet displays**: Using high resolution screens on tablets and smartphones to visualize 3D models and environments. The user interacts with digital aspects on the screen and manipulates objects using a mouse or finger gestures.

Virtual reality can be applied to help students learn and practice across in a variety of real-life scenarios. Virtual patients can be rendered on a screen, with cameras and

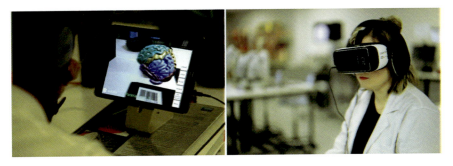

Fig. 1 Biomedical science students using augmented reality (left) and virtual reality (right) to explore regions of the human brain. (Photo: C. Moro)

microphones tracking the trainees' facial expressions, eye gazes, head poses, and vocal cues (Kuehn 2018). The virtual space is useful not only for learning but also for practising engagement, assessments of interpersonal interactions and real-world scenarios. In virtual reality, one limiting feature is that the learner is entirely immersed in the environment, making it difficult to take notes, ask questions, or be fully interactive with the teaching staff or other students in the area. In order to revise after the lesson, it is often difficult to get back into the same environment, and as such, some students do not find it as useful for learning as other methods (Moro et al. 2017b).

Augmented reality allows the opportunity to provide 3D interactive resources outside the classroom, such as that utilized in paramedic distance education (Birt et al. 2017) or enhance anatomy learning content (Moro et al. 2017a). It can also assist in training teachers (Sural 2018), create clinical scenarios (Sutherland et al. 2019), or enhance training for specific health professions such as radiation oncology (Jin et al. 2017). One benefit of augmented reality is the ability for consumer-level smartphones or tablets to render models in 3D. Therefore, students can learn from a range of readily available applications with no additional hardware requirements (Delello et al. 2015). However, augmented reality is limited by the capabilities of the smartphone/tablet and its built-in camera. In some cases, the mobile device camera does not recognize the objects correctly, and valuable in-class learning time is spent managing technological issues.

Holograms and Mixed Reality

A blending of virtual and augmented reality is possible through new devices such as the Microsoft HoloLens 2. This device enables virtual environments and models to be rendered as "holograms" within the user's visual space (Cowling and Moro 2019). Most of these products are still in the developer-level stage, and not yet widely available to consumers, although this technology does offer some potential benefits for future students in health education courses. The mixing of real and virtual worlds should reduce the levels of cybersickness or blurred-vision reported in many virtual reality applications (Moro et al. 2017b), while also allowing the learner to visualize components of the human body in complete 3D (Fig. 2).

While this technology is still relatively new, it shows a great promise in increasing the student's initiative to pursue learning and ability to understand abstract concepts and promotes academic performance (Liu et al. 2019). Holograms provide a new student-centered teaching model which can incorporate gestures, voice commands, interactions with models, and viewpoint tracking technology (Moro and Gregory 2019). While still new, and with only developer kits being used in universities at the moment, this holographic technology is poised to bridge the gap between augmented and virtual reality. The learner is free to take notes and interact with others in the class, as well as engage with the educator. Future research and published used-cases for these all-in-one holographic devices will provide more insights into the overall effectiveness of this mode for learning.

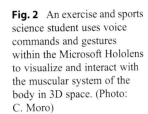
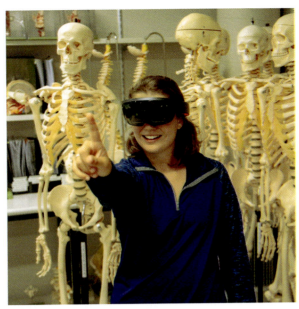

Fig. 2 An exercise and sports science student uses voice commands and gestures within the Microsoft Hololens to visualize and interact with the muscular system of the body in 3D space. (Photo: C. Moro)

Virtual Dissection Tables

While cadaveric dissection remains the primary method for teaching human anatomy, a range of hands-on digital multimedia devices are increasingly used to enhance the learning experience (Hosseini et al. 2018). A relatively new way to learn anatomy is in the form of virtual dissection tables. These tables have the potential to enhance the ability of learners to explore different anatomical components with ease (Moro and Periya 2019) and can significantly assist in the diverse cohort of life sciences students, including a mix of undergraduate and postgraduate students within nursing, physiotherapy, and dentistry courses (Narnaware and Neumeier 2019; Moro and Periya 2019). However, it is still uncertain if these technological supplements adequately prepare students for the workplace compared to traditional teaching methods (Moro and Mclean 2017).

The optimal methods appear to be for virtual tables to be used in conjunction with the cadaveric dissections (Ramsey-Stewart et al. 2010; Azer and Eizenberg 2007; Mathiowetz et al. 2016). Blending this technology with traditional teaching modes has provided educators with more options to facilitate learning. Virtual dissection tables have also shown great promise in many health professional courses. This includes where 94% of medical imaging students reported benefits from the use of a virtual dissection table for anatomy study (Custer and Michael 2015), and 90% of neuroanatomy students reporting the same (Anand and Singel 2017). In a review of 14 studies comparing different teaching approaches including dissection, prosection, and online computer-based teaching aids, the authors found that it remains unclear if the supplementary methods for learning anatomy are entirely useful, and commented that more sophisticated research designs are necessary before evidence-based teaching practices can occur (Winkelmann 2007).

Social Media

While social media is widely used by nearly all students studying within a higher education setting, it is not often integrated into curricula by educators (Chugh and Ruhi 2018). Therefore, there is a lack of research detailing the benefits of incorporating social media and its potential uses. Sterling et al. (2017) systematically appraised 29 peer-reviewed papers on the use of social media in medical education. The authors found that twitter, podcasts, and blogs were the most frequent social media strategies used to engage learners and enhance educational practice. YouTube and wikis were commonly used to teach skills and promote self-efficacy. Most studies were exploratory, highlighting privacy and online behavior within the professional context of health. However, the effect of social media in education was deemed mixed at best, with the quality of studies considered as modest. A systematic review of social media in nursing and midwifery education (O'connor et al. 2018) highlighted benefits of implementing social media in nursing curricula. For example, allowing information to be shared in real time, supporting a student-centered learning setting, and enhancing collaborative learning.

Hanson et al. (2011) assessed the use of social media as a means to improve health promotion using a survey ($n = 503$). The authors found that many health educators are using social media within education practice and highlight positive support of health education through social media. However, specific guidelines should be in place to attain best practice. In particular, four key constructions were recommended, including (1) performance expectancy or the degree to which an individual believes that using the system with help in job performance; (2) effort expectancy or ease associated with system use; (3) social influence or the perception of importance others believe in system use; and (4) facilitating conditions, or the degree to which an organization has the technical infrastructure to support use. It was found that the majority of individuals use social media personally, but few of them use it for work-related purposes because the business blocks social media use. The authors found that older educators lack the belief that using social media enhance job performance and those that perceive social media as positive are already users of social media themselves.

In medical education, Cheston et al. (2013) conducted a systematic review on the use of social media and found 14 studies that noted enhancement in knowledge (exam scores), attitudes (empathy), and skills (e.g., reflective writing). However, the authors pointed out that these studies were of low to moderate quality and that further investigations in this field are required. Overall, the use of social media in education offers an excellent medium for health-care professionals to share information and promote collaboration among its users. However, as information on social media can be added by anyone, the content should be monitored and assessed for quality (Moorhead et al. 2013). Furthermore, privacy and confidentiality should

40 Technology Considerations in Health Professions and Clinical Education

be considered, as the general public is generally unaware of the consequences of sharing personal information online (Adams 2010).

Mobile Applications/Devices

The potential of mobile devices, such as smartphones and tablets, to aid learning in a health profession education setting is clearly evident. These devices are capable of providing easy access to a wide variety of educational resources to support learning, such as virtual anatomy models and electronic books. Pimmer et al. (2016) provided a systematic review of 36 empirical papers that analyzed mobile and ubiquitous learning across disciplines in higher education to determine what types of mobile learning exist and explore the capabilities of mobile devices for facilitating practice and active learning. It was identified that health education and medicine are the dominant categories that have investigated the use of mobile learning.

Mobile devices can facilitate personalized, distributed, and more frequent practice allowing the hybrid design of education where learners can create multimodal representations of study material. This, in turn, can assist with reflective practice in both formal and informal learning situations leading to improved learning outcomes. The authors recommend more collaborative design between end-users and developers. Collaboration between learners that use social media allows for more informal education connecting prior knowledge, private lives, and formal didactic education design. In undergraduate nursing education, O'Connor and Andrews (2015) critically reviewed 24 studies on the use of mobile handheld technology to address challenges related to the theory-practice gap, lack of clinical supervision, and ad hoc learning in clinical environments. The authors found that most of the analyzed papers were exploratory adopting mixed methods to assess education effectiveness with most reporting improved efficiency, learning scaffolding, enhanced knowledge and skills, and decision making. However, the authors indicated that there was no clear definition of mobile technology across the literature making it difficult to make specific comparisons between the technological devices that can be hand-held.

A systematic review conducted by Kim and Park (2019) reviewed 11 randomized and non-randomized controlled trials published between 2011 and 2017 that evaluated the effects of smartphone-based mobile learning for nurses and nursing students and meta-analyzed 10 of them to analyze the effect sizes. Smartphone mobile learning was determined to be an effective tool that positively improved knowledge, skills, confidence, and attitude towards learning; however, it did not affect cognitive load and satisfaction with learning.

Using a survey of 29 questions on the Technology Acceptance Model, Briz-Ponce and García-Peñalvo (2015) recruited 124 participants to quantify acceptance of using mobile technology applications in medical education across both undergraduate medical students and practising clinicians. It was found that self-efficacy (ability to complete the tasks with the technology) and recommendation (a measure of mobile technology recommendation) are the strongest indicators of behavioral intention to use the technology. The authors concluded that as the number of mobile applications increases, the task of determining the effective use of these applications for medical education will become more challenging. It was recommended that future studies explore data using subgroups such as age, gender, and profile to gain deeper insights into the impact of these variables in the learning process.

Klímová (2018) reviewed 10 randomized controlled trials published between 2010 and 2017 that evaluated the use of mobile learning in medical education (those currently studying medicine, as well as doctors and other healthcare professionals). The author established that mobile learning is efficient and beneficial in the acquisition of new knowledge and skills and is perceived to be as an appropriate compliment to traditional learning methods. A qualitative systematic review conducted by Lall et al. (2019) sought out to determine the views of educators and learners on using mobile devices to aid learning and their perceived factors to enhance or hinder its implementation in medical and nursing education. The authors concluded that the portability of mobile devices can enhance interactions between the learners and the study material, fellow learners, and educators in various health professions. Some of the limitations of mobile devices are that they need to be implemented within the institution, as well as specialized training and support needed in order to fully comprehend the various options/functions of the devices

3D Printing

Three-dimensional (3D) printing is increasingly gaining recognition as a tool to enhance both healthcare education and practice (Fig. 3). Malik et al. (2015) analyzed 93 articles to highlight the uses of 3D printing in surgical practice and medical education. Specifically, 3D printing was identified as useful in education and clinical training across a number of disciplines, including orthopedics (to understand injuries of the musculoskeletal system), physiotherapy (to assess complicated anatomy), and for surgeons (to discuss deformity with patients). As anatomy is taught early-on in most health profession and clinical education curricula, means that the ability to 3D print human anatomical concepts and models can be of great use in a broad range of applications. It can be useful as a patient-learning device, such as to obtain informed consent for management of complex fractures, or for easing understanding in patients and their families before interventions or procedures. Physiotherapists can further explain concepts to their clients surrounding muscle and joint movements, or dentists can 3D print structures to show how fillings or alterations to the teeth can impact the jawline.

Virtual anatomical models can also be kept to create catalogues of pathology for educational purposes. These models can be used for anatomy learners and in training on rare complications or decision making for high-risk patients. Some of the

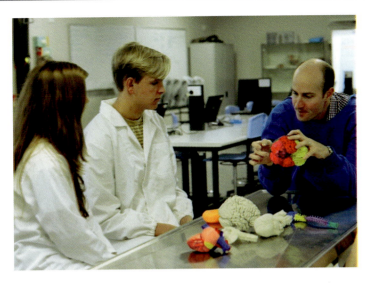

Fig. 3 An educator instructs Biomedical and Exercise Science students on central nervous system anatomy using 3D-printed models. (Photo: C. Moro)

limitations are related to a single type of material used in cheap 3D printing with an inability to simulate soft and hard tissues. Therefore, multi-material printers should be used to develop higher fidelity reproductions. Fine detailed structures are also challenging to create but, when designed correctly, can allow opportunities for complex visualizations used in neurosurgery training to allow for safe environments to practice operating on patients. 3D printing can also be used effectively to familiarize learners with surgical instruments. Malik et al. (2015) concluded that 3D printing allows for creative innovation within the surgical landscape, not just in training but also in practice with the future towards reconstruction and transplants.

To further assess the usefulness of 3D-printed models, Jones et al. (2016) used a qualitative survey on 51 medical students to explore the use of 3D-printed anatomical models to enhance surgical education and clinical practice. The fabricated models were created through a process of converting detailed MRI, CT, ultrasound, and mammogram data into printable 3D mesh models. Participants highlighted the usefulness of model integration into medical school curriculum but had concerns over the fabrication cost related to the model realism and the lack of sensory (haptic) feedback. It was highlighted by the authors that clinical use would require near-exact replicas of diseased human organs. To that end, it was suggested that future work needs to explore not only visual fidelity but also haptic fidelity. Future models should be fabricated with tactility by a combination of molds, printing, and materials.

There have been several research studies that have compared the use of 3D-printed anatomical models with more traditional learning methods, such as using cadavers and didactic lectures. In a double-blind randomized control trial where pre- and post-testing was used (Lim et al. 2016), the authors compared traditional external cardiac cadaveric anatomy with 3D-printed models to determine the effectiveness of 3D printing for self-directed anatomy learning. The 3D models were created using computed tomography (CT) and surface scanning of the heart anatomy, including vessels, vasculature, projections, and sulci. In this study, the authors split 52 participants across 3 groups to compare anatomy learning using cadaveric materials, 3D-printed models, and combined materials (cadavers with 3D-printed models). It was found that the group that used solely 3D-printed models scored significantly higher in the post-test that evaluated anatomy recall than the other two groups. The authors concluded that 3D-printed reproductions of anatomical structures have the potential to provide a readily available source of supplementary teaching materials. It was also noted that novice learners can be apprehensive when encountering cadaveric samples which promote the use of 3D-printed models as a useful primer to induce familiarity and break down inhibitions before use of cadavers which the authors identified as essential in anatomy learning.

A study conducted by Su et al. (2018) designed and produced 3D-printed models for congenital heart disease education. Sixty-three medical students participated in this study, where they were randomly allocated into two groups that participated in a medical seminar: the experimental group where 3D models were used and the control group without the 3D models. Assessment of the effectiveness of 3D-printed models was conducted using subjective (self-assessment using a Likert-style questionnaire) and objective (multiple-choice questions assessing knowledge acquisition and structural conceptualization) methods. The results from the questionnaire showed that the feedback from experimental group was significantly more positive than from the students in the control group. Students in the experimental group had significantly better test results in structural conceptualization when compared to the control group.

In Cai et al.'s (2018) study, 35 first-year medical students were recruited to evaluate the effectiveness of using 3D printed structures to assist in learning human anatomy. Students were assigned to two learning groups, namely the didactic learning group and simulation group. In didactic learning group, students learned about the locking-unlocking of the knee joint through a didactic lecture ($n = 18$) where they were also provided with lecture notes and skeleton models to explain the content related to the knee joint. The simulation group ($n = 17$) were provided with the same textual content as the didactic group; however, instead of using the skeletons to explain knee joint mechanisms, tutors used 3D-printed models. After 30 minutes, both groups were assessed using 11 multiple-choice questions, where students in the simulation group achieved significantly better results than the didactic learning group. There are some limitations of 3D printing, such as the lack of variety and tactile feedback compared using cadaveric material, or the fact that the plastic colors are not authentic when investigation anatomical body parts. However, as 3D printers increasingly enter the high school environment, more and more students entering health professional fields will have prior experience with this technology, and this will become a commonplace and easy technology to utilize in learning.

Online-Hosted Video

Another type of educational media that is capable of conveying information are videos. Tuong et al. (2014) conducted a systematic review from 1975 to 2012, looking at controlled clinical trials examining the effectiveness of video interventions in changing health behavior. Critical analysis was performed on 28 articles where the video had an effect on modifying health behavior. It was noted that videos are a less resource-intensive means of delivering educational content with the benefit of standardizing educational delivery. Video has the added benefit of being administered in many forms, such as being live-streamed, available for download, and having a physical copy of the material.

The downside of using videos as an educational tool is the lack of face-to-face counselling, which allows tailoring the content according to the needs of the patient. However, the benefits of easy content distribution offered by the use of videos can outweigh personalization based on patient needs. Tuong et al. (2014) concluded that the benefits of video instruction include both short- and long-term improvement to behavior, including a reduction in smoking, self-examination, and self-care. There is a plethora of educational videos readily available of video-sharing sites such as YouTube; however, the quality of those videos is unclear.

Duncan et al. (2013) assessed 100 YouTube sites and approximately 25 hours' worth of content across 10 common clinic skill-related topics. It is often expressed that YouTube and online video repository sites are perceived as "time wasters." The authors wanted to counter this argument by analyzing YouTube sites focusing on the integration of clinical skills delivered through YouTube videos. It was identified that topics with the most significant number of videos and user views were related to common skills across the nursing or health-related disciplines such as "cardiopulmonary resuscitation" and more specialized topics such as "pain assessment" with fewer user views. There were concerns regarding the quality of videos with only 1/100 videos analyzed were categorized as "good." The conclusion was that there was a need for more rigorous evaluation, and educators were encouraged to be more proactive in the recommendation of suitable materials as supplementary tools to learning. It was also noted that lecturers would often recommend YouTube videos from credible sources such as the World Health Organization, but independent and self-directed learners often stumbled across sources using the number of user views and likes as a guide to quality. Therefore, it could be said that YouTube is not about "time-wasting" but rather lack metrics that identify the quality of clinical education and learning.

To aid educators in integrating videos in their teaching practices, Dong and Goh (2015) compiled a list of 12 tips. In this article, advantages of using videos in teaching were discussed, as well as the requirements for teachers wishing to integrate this technology, namely knowledge about the technology and ability to make informed decisions on video use. Educators were able to choose between using existing videos that are compatible with their teaching strategy, as well as produce their content. However, there is an added difficulty in creating videos themselves, as it often requires professional guidance and technical skill. Strategies towards the successful implementation of this technology in the classroom and the promotion of student engagement were also discussed. In simulations, video-assisted debriefing can enable students to reflect upon their conduct and allows educators to provide individualized assistant to each member of a cohort. This is increasingly prevalent in health professional education such as physiotherapy and nursing, and there is an increasing body of literature surrounding this process (Ali and Miller 2018).

For educators, video content can be of great use when understanding which areas to focus on in teaching. For example, in physiotherapy students, a video-reflexive ethnography study identified the fact that students had only a limited ability to recognize errors during filmed clinical scenarios (Gough et al. 2016). As video equipment becomes cheaper and more accessible, and video content can be easily uploaded to learning management sites or online repositories, it is likely to see video becoming increasingly utilized in health profession courses.

Simulations with Technology-Enhanced Learning

Technology-enhanced simulation training is becoming increasingly prevalent health care education and adds to current simulation training used in disciplines such as physiotherapy since the 1980s (Owen 2016). Simulations provide a safe environment to practice skills before performing procedures in real life and are used in various scenarios, such as in postgraduate emergency on-call physiotherapists for their cardiorespiratory education (Gough et al. 2013). Simulated patients often work in real environments, but modern simulations are increasingly using technology-enhanced learning to create virtual patients, scenarios, or environments. Cook et al. (2011) analyzed 635 studies of simulation training in teaching laparoscopic surgery, gastrointestinal endoscopy, suturing skills, emergency resuscitation, team leadership, anatomical examination, and others. The authors implied that technology-enhanced simulation training is associated with improved outcomes in comparison with no intervention for health care professionals, with only 4% of the analyzed studies showing no increase in effect. Specifically, simulations lead to large positive gains with respect to knowledge use. The conclusion is that technology-enhanced simulation training has a large effect on knowledge, skills, and clinician behavior but less of an effect on patient care.

A bibliographic literature review of 24 high impact articles published between 2001 and 2011 identified four primary content areas of simulation use in medical education (Abraham et al. 2011): (i) background and history; (ii) procedural training and methods; (iii) quality and safety; and (iv) teamwork and communication. Simulations within health education can focus on a spectrum of activities, including skill training, learning procedures, clinical diagnoses, and facilitating clinical process and teamwork. Specifically, simulation gives users the ability to "hone their communication skills in a clinical setting" and provide "scenario experience."

40 Technology Considerations in Health Professions and Clinical Education   755

Table 1 Twelve features that highlight the best practice in simulation-based medical education

Feedback	Deliberate practice	Curriculum integration	Outcome measurement	Simulation fidelity	Skill acquisition and maintenance
Mastery learning	Transfer to practice	Team training	High-stakes testing	Instructor training	Educational and professional context

The ability to give and receive feedback while undertaking simulation training is invaluable in medical education. Simulation can be done individually or in teams through several different technologies available in both observation and interactive practice, and throughout its history has developed into an important learning method in contemporary health professions education (Owen 2016; Gough 2018). A qualitative systematic review covering literature between 2003 and 2009 identified which key variables were identified to inform on the best practices of using simulation-based practice in medical education teaching (Mcgaghie et al. 2010, Table 1).

The authors concluded that simulation-based medical education is maturing, but more specific thematic analysis of the research is required. This study was followed up by a revisit of the review in 2016 (Mcgaghie et al. 2016) looking at high impact work from 2010 to 2015. The authors identified that:

(i) Today's academic medical community educates twenty-first century physicians using nineteenth century thinking
(ii) The medical education community needs to understand how technology contributes to educational effectiveness
(iii) Difficult to define a definitive account of simulation-based education as the topic is a moving target
(iv) Simulation is the highest rated area of importance for medical education research
(v) Simulation technology is a key contributor to quality health professions education
(vi) Integration of simulation into existing curricula is challenging
(vii) Simulation with mastery learning can produce powerful educational interventions that yield immediate and lasting results
(viii) Cost-effective and efficient simulation is a challenge when educating and evaluating individuals

Cook et al. (2010a) analyzed 50 studies on the use of virtual patients across different health and clinical education professions. They concluded that virtual patients (patients coded and rendered using 3D modelling and animations) are associated with improved learning outcomes compared with no intervention for medical, dental, nursing, and other health-related professions. The authors indicated that there is no evidence that virtual patient simulation is superior to that of other training methods. However, it does assist with logistic barriers such as cost, distance learning, and self-direction. There is also evidence to support other beneficial impacts of using virtual reality for simulations in fields such as nursing, where it

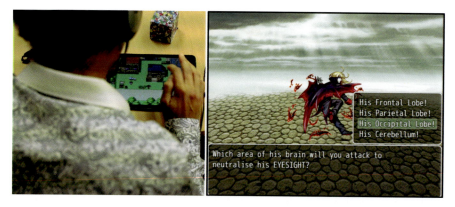

Fig. 4 A student revises using "The King's Request: Anatomy and Physiology Revision Game," a free game available online for learning within health professional education. (Images: C. Moro)

has helped to increase patient acuity, manage the high student-to-faculty ratios in some courses, while also minimizing the risks to patients from untrained students (Jenson and Forsyth 2012).

The quality and effectiveness of virtual patients or virtual worlds can vary in terms of their coding, design, and implementation, which can lead to different learning outcomes. However, this impact can be minimized in fields such as nursing, by using a multidisciplinary approach when developing these resources (Kilmon et al. 2010). It is difficult to answer questions regarding design bias through meta-analytic studies, and more work is required in direct qualitative comparisons of virtual patient design and user experience to better understand the effective use of virtual patients for training.

Serious Games

The development of computer technology and the accessibility of the internet has given rise to the use of serious games in higher education (Fig. 4). Serious games or "*games primarily focused on education rather than entertainment*" (Miller et al. 2011) are especially useful for simulated training, knowledge acquisition, skills development, and responsive narrative to convey meaning. Girard et al. (2013) explored the rapid growth of serious games by analyzing learning effect and engagement in serious games identifying that serious games might be powerful tools for learning, but more empirical studies were required to investigate the effectiveness in learning.

Boyle et al. (2016) analyzed 143 articles published between 2009 and 2014, identifying positive outcomes of games in education. The authors explored specific game outcomes concerning learning, knowledge acquisition, motivation, perception, behavioral change, and motor learning outcomes. The evidence indicated that there was a positive outcome from playing games. Simulation games were the most popular, allowing real-world replication and skills training. The most popular game genre was role-playing, followed by adventure games, strategy, problem solving, and puzzle games. It was identified that defining characteristics of a game was difficult when not classified as simulation and that constructs such as flow, engagement, and appeal should be used more when defining games research for education. Although the focus was on STEM subjects, health education was identified as the most popular for application of serious gaming and game-based learning.

Ricciardi and De Paolis (2014) examined serious games developed specifically for health professions and health-related fields including surgery, odontology, nursing, cardiology, first aid, dietetics, psychology, and more. They identified that serious gaming is a useful technology that improves learning and skills development, but the number of case studies was limited with first aid having the highest number of developed serious games given the importance around continuous training which serious games can achieve at a low cost. The cost factor was reiterated by Knight et al. (2010) in a pragmatic control trial that explored the use of serious games in the teaching of major incident triage and compared it to with traditional training methods. Learners ($n = 91$) were randomly assigned into two training groups: a traditional major incident triage card-sorting group and a serious game simulation group. Traditionally, learners are taught triage using a combination of quick physiological assessment using a mobile four state priority ranking in small practical workshops where they either work with live actors or mannequins. The problem is that reconstructing these live triage events are costly and unrepeatable.

Additionally, practical restrictions often limit the degree to which activities can reflect real world. In this study, a serious game case study was developed called triage trainer that allowed learners to play through a major incident scenario, triaging digital casualties. The results of the game showed that more causalities where triaged without an error using the serious game over the traditional card sort activity with no impact on time on task. It was recommended that feedback be improved in the serious game and that more involvement of the end-users is integrated earlier in the development process but that serious games are useful within medical education. Petit dit Dariel et al. (2013) examined the potential for serious games within nursing education, especially concerning clinical reasoning skills, complex problem solving, and pedagogical solutions to develop these within simulated safe environments.

Wang et al. (2016) conducted a more recent systematic review of serious games in training health care professionals with 42 games included in the review. Specific points were made about the cost associated with simulated mannequin delivery in terms of human resources and simulator costs and the cheaper costs associated with serious games. Gorbanev et al. (2018) provided a similar conclusion, stating that serious games have the potential to disrupt the industry, especially as it pertains not only to training costs but also to patient care. A serious games example of patient care can be seen in Robert et al. (2014) with serious games recommended as a treatment for Alzheimer's disease and related aging disorders. They have also been used widely in personal health care (Mccallum 2012) to prevent stress and manage pain and disease. What was noted by all articles was the complexity of building serious games, including the multidisciplinary teams required and the pilot nature of the studies. Additional concerns were raised by Gentry et al. (2019)

noting that most serious games research has been conducted in high-income countries with the cost of serious gaming and devices being a barrier for use in low and middle-income countries which are the most affected by a worldwide shortage of trained health workers. It was also noted that serious gaming is an emerging field and more rigorous research is required to compare serious games with controls including longitudinal patient outcomes, participant behavior, attitudes, and adverse effects.

E-Learning (Web Delivery)

Internet-based learning in health and medical education is rapidly growing. Being aware of the available technologies and how they are used to aid learning in a higher education setting is integral for understanding how the learner interacts with the study content (Moro and Kinash 2012). Cook et al. (2010b) conducted a systematic review to describe in detail the variations in configuration, instructional methods, and presentation elements in internet-based courses. Authors found that 89% of 266 studies included in this review used written text, and 55% used multimedia as a means to present educational content via web delivery. It was found that 24% of the studies used bot web-based and non-computer-based instructions. Specifically, in web-based courses, most employed specific instructional methods like patient cases self-assessment questions and feedback as a means to enhance learning. Authors suggested that educators wishing to incorporate web-based learning in the curriculum should consider a broad range of available web-based learning configurations and methods before choosing a specific approach.

Wong et al. (2010) conducted a qualitative systematic review of 249 research papers to produce a theory-based guide for developing and evaluating internet-based courses for clinical doctors and medical students. In this review, the authors sought to explain what type of internet-based education "works," produce a guideline for course developers, and extended the methodological knowledge base in medical education research. The review of the research articles presented two main findings: internet-based courses must be engaging to the user and interactivity is highly regarded. Additionally, while course design is a crucial factor in internet-based courses, special attention must also be paid to course-context interaction. One group might perceive a particular course as highly useful in one context, whereas a different group would find the same course much less useful in a different context. The authors suggest that educators wishing to implement internet-based learning should address a set of questions to increase the chances of their courses of being perceived and useful and provide an effective learning platform. These findings are consistent with similar studies demonstrating the benefits of e-books in facilitating learning in anatomy (Stirling and Birt 2014).

George et al. (2014) identified 60 randomized controlled trials published between 2000 and 2013 that focused on the learner's knowledge, skills, satisfactory, and attitudes towards e-learning in health education. The findings were based on the comparison between e-learning and traditional learning methods or between different modes of e-learning. The authors found that e-learning was found to be more effective than traditional learning in terms of knowledge and skills gained. Specifically, 29% of studies showed significantly higher knowledge acquisition, 40% showed significantly higher skill gain, and 14% showed higher satisfaction with e-learning when compared to traditional learning. The evidence from this review suggests that e-learning is equivalent and sometimes even more effective than traditional learning in terms of knowledge and skills acquisition. Furthermore, e-learning provides a convenient and cost-effective alternative to conventional learning. A systematic review conducted by Jayakumar et al. (2015) evaluating the use of e-learning in surgical education demonstrated that a variety of different learning material can be delivered through this medium, including case-based, theoretical knowledge, and surgical skills teaching. Out of the 38 articles included in this review, most reported significant knowledge gain from e-learning. However, two in three studies did not compare the knowledge gain to a control group. These studies can function as a proof of concept of using e-learning in surgical education. Nevertheless, future work in this area should focus on using appropriately designed studies.

Maertens et al. (2016) conducted a systematic review of e-learning in surgical training, 87 randomized controlled trials were critically evaluated to establish the evidence supporting e-learning as a teaching tool compared with either no intervention or alternative teaching methods. This review showed that e-learning is a useful tool in aiding the development of different surgical skills. However, evidence supporting the superiority of e-learning to traditional methods is limited. Indeed, only two of the randomized controlled trials demonstrated transfer of skills to the clinical environment; however, there was no evidence that showed improvement in patient outcomes.

Audience Response

Audience response technology has been widely used among educators to enhance student classroom involvement and active engagement. It usually consists of devices controlled by the learner (for example "clickers") which allows them to actively participate in the class by selecting responses to questions that are displayed of programs such as Microsoft PowerPoint and gaining instant feedback of the audience responses (for example, in a bar graph). Audience response can also be set up to allow students to provide questions as well as answers (Moro and Hensen 2017). An in-depth meta-analysis of 53 research articles (overall sample of 26,095 students) on the effects of audience response systems on cognition was conducted by Hunsu et al. (2016). The authors determined that clicker-based technology only produced a small but significant effect on different cognitive learning outcomes and a near-medium impact on non-cognitive learning outcomes. Furthermore, these effects were deemed as non-existent for course material recall or retention. The authors suggested that instructors should design questions that require critical thinking, knowledge application, and synthesis in order to meet higher order learning goals. However, these results should be interpreted with caution as 90% studies included in the analysis did not randomly assign participants into experimental and control groups as the studies were conducted on students in an already formed cohort. In addition, only 20% of the studies used measures of pre-test and post-test to establish the differences between participants at baseline. Indeed, a more substantial effect of using clicker-based technology was observed in studies where students were randomly assigned to experimental and control groups.

A systematic review and meta-analysis of 21 studies on the learning outcomes in health professional's education determined that 14 of the studies reported significant differences in knowledge scores in favor of the audience-response group. A meta-analysis of randomized-controlled trials revealed that there were no statistical differences in the knowledge scores between audience response and control groups, whereas non-randomized studies showed a significant difference (Nelson et al. 2012). Authors suggested that non-randomized studies over-estimated the impact of the audience response technology due to methodological limitations of their study design. Overall, the results obtained in this analysis were equivocal and more research with appropriate study design is required to draw definite conclusions. A follow-up systematic review conducted by Atlantis and Cheema (2015) 3 years after the publication of Nelson et al. (2012) review failed to support the hypothesis that audience response technologies have a significant effect on learning outcomes in health sciences and medical students and reiterated the need for more high-quality research in the area.

One primary benefit of audience response is that it allows students to respond in real time. In health education courses, the students are often presented with the theoretical content in the first few years, before experiencing the practical aspects (i.e., in the field or hospital environment). This means that after performing well in early years, students may still feel unprepared for practice by the time they are due to enter the practical years (Moro et al. 2019). Through allowing the students to be put on-the-spot, where they are able to answer questions or interact in real time, this may assist in their confidence to discuss learned content in front of a client, or patient, out in the field, clinical, or practical environment.

Conclusion

Technology use in health professional education is an exciting area of research. Educators face challenging decisions, such as which technology to incorporate in their teaching practices and which technology would work best for their students. It is apparent that further scholarship, research, and investigation in this area is essential, with the need for greater diligence in research methodology within studies. These developments in the education landscape do show a great promise for the future, and potential enhancements in learning outcomes for health profession students. Two major hurdles exist for educators wishing to adopt more technology in their curricula. The first is the requirement for skill training in technology, and the second is the often difficulty in finding evidence-based approaches and research specific to their areas. This chapter has outlined a variety of research surrounding the

40 Technology Considerations in Health Professions and Clinical Education

benefits, use-cases, and limitations of technologies used in an attempt to enhance learning within health profession and clinical education. Although not all approaches are available to all programs, due to limited funds, access to technology, or skilled staff, modern technology has introduced increasing options for educators wishing to enhance or alter their curriculum in a way that can improve student interactivity, engagement, and learning.

Cross-References

► Competencies of Health Professions Educators of the Future
► E-Learning: Development of a Fully Online 4th Year Psychology Program
► Future of Health Professions Education Curricula

References

Abraham J, Wade DM, O'connell KA, Desharnais S, Jacoby R. The use of simulation training in teaching health care quality and safety: an annotated bibliography. Am J Med Qual. 2011;26:229–38.

Adams SA. Blog-based applications and health information: two case studies that illustrate important questions for Consumer Health Informatics (CHI) research. Int J Med Inform. 2010;79: e89–96.

Ali AA, Miller ET. Effectiveness of video-assisted debriefing in health education: an integrative review. J Nurs Educ. 2018;57:14–20.

Anand M, Singel T. A comparative study of learning with "anatomage" virtual dissection table versus traditional dissection method in neuroanatomy. Indian J Clin Anat Physiol. 2017;4:177–80.

Atlantis E, Cheema BS. Effect of audience response system technology on learning outcomes in health students and professionals: an updated systematic review. Int J Evid Based Healthc. 2015;13:3–8.

Azer SA, Eizenberg N. Do we need dissection in an integrated problem-based learning medical course? Perceptions of first- and second-year students. Surg Radiol Anat. 2007;29:173–80.

Birt J, Moore E, Cowling M. Improving paramedic distance education through mobile mixed reality simulation. Australas J Educ Technol. 2017;33:69.

Birt J, Stromberga Z, Cowling M, Moro C. Mobile mixed reality for experiential learning and simulation in medical and health sciences education. Information. 2018;9:31.

Boyle EA, Hainey T, Connolly TM, Gray G, Earp J, Ott M, Lim T, Ninaus M, Ribeiro C, Pereira J. An update to the systematic literature review of empirical evidence of the impacts and outcomes of computer games and serious games. Comput Educ. 2016;94:178–92.

Briz-Ponce L, García-Peñalvo FJ. An empirical assessment of a technology acceptance model for apps in medical education. J Med Syst. 2015;39:176.

Cai B, Rajendran K, Bay BH, Lee J, Yen CC. The effects of a functional three-dimensional (3D) printed knee joint simulator in improving anatomical spatial knowledge. Anat Sci Educ. 2018;12:610–18.

Cheston CC, Flickinger TE, Chisolm MS. Social media use in medical education: a systematic review. Acad Med. 2013;88:893–901.

Chugh R, Ruhi U. Social media in higher education: a literature review of Facebook. Educ Inf Technol. 2018;23:605–16.

Cook DA, Erwin PJ, Triola MM. Computerized virtual patients in health professions education: a systematic review and meta-analysis. Acad Med. 2010a;85:1589–602.

Cook DA, Garside S, Levinson AJ, Dupras DM, Montori VM. What do we mean by web-based learning? A systematic review of the variability of interventions. Med Educ. 2010b;44:765–74.

Cook DA, Hatala R, Brydges R, Zendejas B, Szostek JH, Wang AT, Erwin PJ, Hamstra SJ. Technology-enhanced simulation for health professions education: A systematic review and meta-analysis. JAMA. 2011;306:978–88.

Cowling M, Moro C. Holographic teachers were supposed to be part of our future. What happened? The Conversation. 2019. https://theconversation.com/holographic-teachers-were-supposed-to-be-part-of-our-future-what-happened-108500.

Custer T, Michael K. The utilization of the anatomage virtual dissection table in the education of imaging science students. J Artic Radiat Sci Technol Educ. 2015;1:1–5.

Delello JA, Mcwhorter RR, Camp KM. Integrating augmented reality in higher education: a multidisciplinary study of student perceptions. J Educ Multimed Hypermed. 2015;24:209–33.

Dong C, Goh PS. Twelve tips for the effective use of videos in medical education. Med Teach. 2015;37:140–5.

Duncan I, Yarwood-Ross L, HAIGH C. YouTube as a source of clinical skills education. Nurse Educ Today. 2013;33:1576–80.

Gentry SV, Gauthier A, L'estrade Ehrstrom B, Wortley D, Lilienthal A, Tudor Car L, Dauwels-Okutsu S, Nikolaou CK, Zary N, Campbell J, Car J. Serious gaming and gamification education in health professions: systematic review. J Med Internet Res. 2019;21:e12994.

George PP, Papachristou N, Belisario JM, Wang W, Wark PA, Cotic Z, Rasmussen K, Sluiter R, Riboli-Sasco E, Tudor Car L, Musulanov EM, Molina JA, Heng BH, Zhang Y, Wheeler EL, AL Shorbaji N, Majeed A, Car J. Online eLearning for undergraduates in health professions: a systematic review of the impact on knowledge, skills, attitudes and satisfaction. J Glob Health. 2014;4:010406.

Girard C, Ecalle J, Magnan A. Serious games as new educational tools: how effective are they? A meta-analysis of recent studies. J Comput Assist Learn. 2013;29:207–19.

Gorbanev I, Agudelo-Londoño S, González RA, Cortes A, Pomares A, Delgadillo V, Yepes FJ, Muñoz Ó. A systematic review of serious games in medical education: quality of evidence and pedagogical strategy. Med Educ Online. 2018;23:1438718.

Gough S. Educating for professional practice through simulation. In: Delany C, Molloy E, editors. Learning and teaching in clinical contexts: a practical guide. Chatswood: Elsevier; 2018.

Gough S, Yohannes AM, Thomas C, Sixsmith J. Simulation-based education (SBE) within postgraduate emergency on-call physiotherapy in the United Kingdom. Nurse Educ Today. 2013;33:778–84.

Gough S, Yohannes AM, Murray J. Using video-reflexive ethnography and simulation-based education to explore patient management and error recognition by pre-registration physiotherapists. Adv Simul (Lond). 2016;1:9.

Hanson C, West J, Neiger B, Thackeray R, Barnes M, Mcintyre E. Use and acceptance of social media among health educators. Am J Health Educ. 2011;42:197–204.

Hosseini F, Oberoi V, Doroudi M, Vo L. A visual guide to foregut anatomy: using digital multimedia to enhance the learning of human gross anatomy. FASEB J. 2018;32:635.27.

Hunsu NJ, Adesope O, Bayly DJ. A meta-analysis of the effects of audience response systems (clicker-based technologies) on cognition and affect. Comput Educ. 2016;94:102–19.

Jayakumar N, Brunckhorst O, Dasgupta P, Khan MS, Ahmed K. e-Learning in surgical education: a systematic review. J Surg Educ. 2015;72:1145–57.

Jenson CE, Forsyth DM. Virtual reality simulation: using three-dimensional technology to teach nursing students. Comput Inform Nurs. 2012;30:312–8; quiz 319–20.

Jin W, Birckhead B, Perez B, Hoffe S. Augmented and virtual reality: exploring a future role in radiation oncology education and training. Appl Rad Oncol. 2017;6:13–20.

Jones DB, Sung R, Weinberg C, Korelitz T, Andrews R. Three-dimensional modeling may improve surgical education and clinical practice. Surg Innov. 2016;23:189–95.

Kilmon CA, Brown L, Ghosh S, Mikitiuk A. Immersive virtual reality simulations in nursing education. Nurs Educ Perspect. 2010;31:314–7.

Kim JH, Park H. Effects of smartphone-based mobile learning in nursing education: a systematic review and meta-analysis. Asian Nurs Res. 2019;13:20–9.

Klímová B. Mobile learning in medical education. J Med Syst. 2018;42:194.

Knight JF, Carley S, Tregunna B, Jarvis S, Smithies R, De Freitas S, Dunwell I, Mackway-Jones K. Serious gaming technology in major incident triage training: a pragmatic controlled trial. Resuscitation. 2010;81:1175–9.

Kuehn BM. Virtual and augmented reality put a twist on medical education. JAMA. 2018;319: 756–8.

Lall P, Rees R, Law GCY, Dunleavy G, Cotič Ž, Car J. Influences on the implementation of mobile learning for medical and nursing education: qualitative systematic review by the Digital Health Education Collaboration. J Med Internet Res. 2019;21:e12895.

Lim KHA, Loo ZY, Goldie SJ, Adams JW, Mcmenamin PG. Use of 3D printed models in medical education: a randomized control trial comparing 3D prints versus cadaveric materials for learning external cardiac anatomy. Anat Sci Educ. 2016;9:213–21.

Liu C, Chen X, Liu S, Zhang X, Ding S, Long Y, Zhou D. The exploration on interacting teaching mode of augmented reality based on holoLens. In: Cheung SKS, Jiao J, Lee L-K, Zhang X, Li KC, Zhan Z, editors. Technology in education: pedagogical innovations. Singapore: Springer; 2019. p. 91–102.

Maertens H, Madani A, Landry T, Vermassen F, Van Herzeele I, Aggarwal R. Systematic review of e-learning for surgical training. Br J Surg. 2016;103:1428–37.

Malik HH, Darwood ARJ, Shaunak S, Kulatilake P, El-Hilly AA, Mulki O, Baskaradas A. Three-dimensional printing in surgery: a review of current surgical applications. J Surg Res. 2015;199:512–22.

Mathiowetz V, Yu CH, Quake-Rapp C. Comparison of a gross anatomy laboratory to online anatomy software for teaching anatomy. Anat Sci Educ. 2016;9:52–9.

Mccallum S. Gamification and serious games for personalized health. Stud Health Technol Inform. 2012;177:85–96.

Mcgaghie WC, Issenberg SB, Petrusa ER, Scalese RJ. A critical review of simulation-based medical education research: 2003–2009. Med Educ. 2010;44:50–63.

Mcgaghie WC, Issenberg SB, Petrusa ER, Scalese RJ. Revisiting 'A critical review of simulation-based medical education research: 2003–2009'. Med Educ. 2016;50:986–91.

Miller LM, Chang C-I, Wang S, Beier ME, Klisch Y. Learning and motivational impacts of a multimedia science game. Comput Educ. 2011;57:1425–33.

Moorhead SA, Hazlett DE, Harrison L, Carroll JK, Irwin A, Hoving C. A new dimension of health care: systematic review of the uses, benefits, and limitations of social media for health communication. J Med Internet Res. 2013;15:e85.

Moro C, Gregory S. Utilising anatomical and physiological visualisations to enhance the face-to-face student learning experience in biomedical sciences and medicine. Adv Exp Med Biol. 2019;1156:41–8.

Moro C, Hensen D. Engaging timid students: backchannel as a tool to provide opportunities for interactivity and engagement within the university classroom. Educ Technol Solut. 2017;81:38–41.

Moro C, Kinash S. Developing online worksheets that work. Educ Technol Solut. 2012;52:52–54.

Moro C, Mclean M. Supporting students' transition to university and problem-based learning. Med Sci Educ. 2017;27:353–61.

Moro C, Periya S. Applied learning of anatomy and physiology: virtual dissection tables within medical and health sciences education. Bangkok Med J. 2019;15:121–7.

Moro C, Stromberga Z, Raikos A, Stirling A. The effectiveness of virtual and augmented reality in health sciences and medical anatomy. Anat Sci Educ. 2017a;10:549–59.

Moro C, Stromberga Z, Stirling A. Virtualisation devices for student learning: comparison between desktop-based (Oculus Rift) and mobile-based (Gear VR) virtual reality in medical and health science education. Australas J Educ Technol. 2017b;33:1.

Moro C, Spooner A, Mclean M. How prepared are students for the various transitions in their medical studies? An Australian university pilot study. MedEdPublish. 2019;8:25.

Narnaware Y, Neumeier M. Second-year nursing students' retention of gross anatomical knowledge. Anat Sci Educ. 2019. https://doi.org/10.1002/ase.1906.

Nelson C, Hartling L, Campbell S, Oswald AE. The effects of audience response systems on learning outcomes in health professions education. A BEME systematic review: BEME guide No. 21. Med Teach. 2012;34:e386–405.

O'connor S, Andrews T. Mobile technology and its use in clinical nursing education: a literature review. J Nurs Educ. 2015;54:137–44.

O'connor S, Jolliffe S, Stanmore E, Renwick L, Booth R. Social media in nursing and midwifery education: a mixed study systematic review. J Adv Nurs. 2018;74:2273–89.

Owen H. Simulation in healthcare education. An extensive history. Obstet Gynaecol. 2016;18:330.

Petit DIT Dariel OJ, Raby T, Ravaut F, Rothan-Tondeur M. Developing the serious games potential in nursing education. Nurse Educ Today. 2013;33:1569–75.

Pimmer C, Mateescu M, Gröhbiel U. Mobile and ubiquitous learning in higher education settings. A systematic review of empirical studies. Comput Hum Behav. 2016;63:490–501.

Ramsey-Stewart G, Burgess AW, Hill DA. Back to the future: teaching anatomy by whole-body dissection. Med J Aust. 2010;193:668–71.

Ricciardi F, De Paolis LT. A comprehensive review of serious games in health professions. Int J Comput Games Technol. 2014;2014:11.

Robert P, König A, Amieva H, Andrieu S, Bremond F, Bullock R, Ceccaldi M, Dubois B, Gauthier S, Kenigsberg P-A, Nave S, Orgogozo JM, Piano J, Benoit M, Touchon J, Vellas B, Yesavage J, Manera V. Recommendations for the use of serious games in people with Alzheimer's disease, related disorders and frailty. Front Aging Neurosci. 2014;6:54.

Sterling M, Leung P, Wright D, Bishop TF. The use of social media in graduate medical education: a systematic review. Acad Med. 2017;92:1043–56.

Stirling A, Birt J. An enriched multimedia eBook application to facilitate learning of anatomy. Anat Sci Educ. 2014;7:19–27.

Su W, Xiao Y, He S, Huang P, Deng X. Three-dimensional printing models in congenital heart disease education for medical students: a controlled comparative study. BMC Med Educ. 2018;18:178.

Sural I. Augmented reality experience: initial perceptions of higher education students. Int J Instr. 2018;11:565–76.

Sutherland J, Belec J, Sheikh A, Chepelev L, Althobaity W, Chow BJW, Mitsouras D, Christensen A, Rybicki FJ, La Russa DJ. Applying modern virtual and augmented reality technologies to medical images and models. J Digit Imaging. 2019;32:38–53.

Tuong W, Larsen ER, Armstrong AW. Videos to influence: a systematic review of effectiveness of video-based education in modifying health behaviors. J Behav Med. 2014;37:218–33.

Wang R, Demaria S Jr, Goldberg A, Katz D. A systematic review of serious games in training health care professionals. Simul Healthc. 2016;11:41–51.

Winkelmann A. Anatomical dissection as a teaching method in medical school: a review of the evidence. Med Educ. 2007;41:15–22.

Wong G, Greenhalgh T, Pawson RJBME. Internet-based medical education: a realist review of what works, for whom and in what circumstances. BMC Med Educ. 2010;10:12.

Role of Social Media in Health Professions Education

41

Victoria Brazil, Jessica Stokes-Parish, and Jesse Spurr

Contents

Introduction 766
What Is the Role of Social Media in Health Professions Education? 766
    Supporting Clinical Learning 766
    Supporting Clinical Teaching 767
    Supporting Faculty Development for Health Professional Educators 769
    Supporting Clinical and Educational Scholarship 769
    Other Roles 770
Contemporary Issues in Social Media Usage for Health Professions Education 771
    Managing Personal Social Media Reputation 771
    Defining Quality in Social Media 772
    Research into Social Media 772
    Patient/Consumer Perspectives and Interactions 773
    Ethical and Professionalism Issues 773
Conclusion 774
References 774

Abstract

Effective and safe use of social media in health professional education can represent both a *process* for learning and a *learning outcome* for learners,

---

V. Brazil (✉)
Faculty of Health Sciences and Medicine, Bond University, Gold Coast, QLD, Australia
e-mail: vbrazil@bond.edu.au

J. Stokes-Parish
Hunter Medical Research Institute, Hunter New England Local Health District, Newcastle, NSW, Australia
e-mail: jessica.stokesparish@gmail.com

J. Spurr
Intensive Care Unit, Redcliffe Hospital, Redcliffe, QLD, Australia
e-mail: jessespurr81@gmail.com

© Springer Nature Singapore Pte Ltd. 2023
D. Nestel et al. (eds.), *Clinical Education for the Health Professions*,
https://doi.org/10.1007/978-981-15-3344-0_119

teachers, and scholars. Achieving these goals requires specific skills and often new approaches for effective integration of social media.

This chapter considers health professionals' use of social media in education – the advantages, opportunities, and pitfalls – for learners, teachers, and scholars. We will consider some contemporary challenges including quality indicators, digital scholarship, ethics, and professionalism. A series of hypothetical case vignettes give readers tangible illustrations of our content.

Keywords

Social media · Health professional education · Online professionalism · Digital scholarship

Introduction

Social media "embraces a range of technologies that allow web-based and mobile applications to connect, create and engage user-generated content between individuals and organisations" (Roland et al. 2015). The term implies more than simply digital or online resources – sharing, interaction, collaboration, and dissemination are the "social" element of media that is broad ranging in scope – blogs, podcasts, and platforms such as YouTube, Twitter, Facebook, and Instagram.

The use of social media for personal and commercial purposes is global and growing, and the use for health professionals – as clinicians, educators, researchers, and advocates – also continues to grow and mature. Health professional learners and teachers have easy access to social media content that is global, comprehensive, and rapidly disseminated. There are opportunities to more rapidly close knowledge to practice gaps (Ng et al. 2019), but new knowledge and skills specific to the medium are required to realize this potential.

What Is the Role of Social Media in Health Professions Education?

Supporting Clinical Learning

Most health professionals will be *consumers* of social media, including reading/listening to materials on blogs, podcasts, and platforms like YouTube and Twitter, in practices similar to their personal use of social media. The "consumer use" for clinical learning is well established – for "just in time" clinical reference, within a structured undergraduate or postgraduate training program, or for continuing professional development (CPD). However, the use of social media-based resources for clinical learning is highly variable across professions and disciplines, levels of training, and there remains a paucity of evidence for impact or effectiveness.

In exploring medical residents' experiences with educational podcasts, Riddell et al. found that podcasts were "easy to use and engaging, enabling both broad exposure to content and targeted learning," and that learners were "often listening to podcasts while doing other activities, being motivated by an ever-present desire to use their time productively" (Riddell et al. 2019). At the CPD level, medical conferences and symposia now frequently leverage social media. "Tweeting the meeting" supports real-time scientific discussion among the physical audience, as well as immediate dissemination of potentially practice-changing information to a large global audience (Tanoue et al. 2018).

The volume and instant accessibility of social media resources means that learners (and their educators) need new skills – in *filtering* the volume of material available, *critically appraising* social media content, and *reconciling* use of social media resources with those considered more "traditional" (Roland and Brazil 2015).

Optimal searching for clinical updates or references may require more than just "Googling it," in an era of "information overload" (Glasziou 2008). Filtering relevant, quality content for clinical learning requires a strategy (Nickson 2019), including some technical skills (e.g., using web-based aggregators) and familiarity with contemporary (and emerging) platforms.

General principles of critical appraisal apply, and may be adapted to platforms like blogs and podcasts (Lin et al. 2015; Colmers et al. 2015). However, specific advice about sources and strategies may need to be discipline and/or learner context specific (Thoma et al. 2014; Weingart and Thoma 2015).

More active clinician participants are likely to engage in discussions and contribute opinion and/or content, fostering a sense of connection to peers, supervisors, and the larger professional community (Riddell et al. 2019). Chan (2018) describes a "critical clinician" role in social media – "skilled in the arts of critical appraisal and willing to interact with knowledge producers to provide thoughtful and meaningful critiques of their work." By joining online professional networks, clinicians may be encouraged toward new ways of learning, not just access to content, albeit with predictable challenges (Cadogan 2019). *(Case vignette Rafia)*

Case vignette 1: Rafia – Canadian Emergency Medicine Resident

Rafia consumes widely from the plethora of blogs and podcasts available for clinical learning in her speciality e.g., CandiEM, LITFL and Academic Life in EM. She has a specific interest in point of care ultrasound so subscribes to the "5-minute Sono" podcast. Rafia joins a team of co-residents (some based in the US and Australia) who decide to write a series of blog posts as part of their specialist exam preparation. She has just published a case report on lung ultrasound, so she establishes a Researchgate profile and promotes her publication on Twitter.

Supporting Clinical Teaching

Many health professional educators engage with social media as *curators* or "translational teachers" (Chan et al. 2018) where best practice, latest research, and leading concepts may be assimilated and presented for learners, colleagues, or patients. This group has access to an unprecedented volume of material on which to draw for their lessons, and a plethora of platforms on which to present their curated content. *(Case vignette Eric)*.

Case vignette 2: Eric – An Australian General Physician
Eric is looking for high quality continuing professional development, so listens to the "Pomegranate" podcast (produced by the Royal Australasian College of Physicians), and follows @RACP and a number of general physicians on Twitter. He develops a teaching session on polypharmacy for medical students by researching the topic using Google scholar and traditional database sources, and also by crowd sourcing key questions using Twitter polls. He shares notes from the talk via a wiki operating within the medical school intranet.

Health professional educators may create content related to clinical, research, or educational topics – producing blogs, podcasts, or even micro-blog discussion threads (Luo et al. 2019) for others consumption. Technology has enabled low barriers to entry for content creation – it is easy for health professionals to produce a blog, podcast or share created content on other platforms. *(Case vignette Michael)* This offers a "democratization" of the voices in health profession education, but amplifies concerns regarding quality and professionalism issues.

Case vignette 3: Michael – A US Based Emergency Medicine Educator
Michael has run a hugely successful emergency medicine (EM) educational blog for 10 years, with over a million unique visitors per year. His production team have recently partnered with an established EM journal and residency program organisation – for academic credibility and to leverage digital scholarship. Michael has just started posting brief summaries of key learning points from a clinical shift on Instagram ("Post it pearls"). He has sought advice from his hospital legal team about strategies to ensure patient confidentiality in doing this.

Social media–enabled teaching requires the same skills as for learners – in searching and critical appraisal – plus the ability to filter through a content expert perspective. New technical skills may be required for effective us of social media platforms – in communication, media, design, and/or information technology. *(Case vignette Mohammed)* Educators working in large teaching institutions may have access to specialist support, but the nature of social media "democratization" means that educators may now operate small-scale enterprises and ensuring quality and sustainability is a challenge. Many educational blogs and podcasts become defunct very quickly. There are sources of guidance – for example, specific technical and educational advice for podcasters (Cosimini et al. 2017), and for facilitating online journal clubs (Chan et al. 2015b).

Case vignette 4: Mohammed – An ICU RN with an Interest in Simulation-Based Education
Mohammed is an avid consumer of #FOAMed and #hcsim resources on social media, as a continuing professional development strategy for his clinical practice. He decides to create his own podcast and blog, working with a small

interprofessional production team. He spends hours each week recording, editing and writing free content for the blog, but finds the time spent is a fulfilling part of professional practice. The podcasts are promoted on Instagram, Twitter and LinkedIn. The podcast has a collaboration with an established simulation journal to feature articles on a regular basis.

Social media is not just accessing content online. Consistent with social learning theory (Bandura 1977) and network learning theories like connectivism (Goldie 2016), opportunities for interactivity, discussion, observation and questioning mean that social media also has the potential to enhance the educational *process* as much enhancing access to *content*. Siemens (2005) describes connectivism as a conceptual framework which views learning as a network phenomenon influenced by technology and socialization, with core principles:

- "Learning and knowledge rest in diversity of opinion
- Learning is a process of connecting specialised nodes or information sources
- Learning may reside in non-human appliances
- Capacity to know is more critical than what is currently known
- Nurturing and maintaining connections is needed to facilitate continual learning
- Ability to see connections between fields, ideas, and concepts is a core skill
- Accurate, up-to-date knowledge (currency) is the aim of all connectivist learning activities
- Decision-making is a learning process in itself" (Siemens 2005)

Educators should consider these principles in their pedagogical approach in order to fulfill the promise of social media.

Supporting Faculty Development for Health Professional Educators

Health professional educators are also likely to "consume" social media content and platforms related to their educational practice, and will find diverse options for their learning (Chan et al. 2015a). Social media also provides health professions educators with access to global virtual communities of educational practice (Yarris et al. 2019; Choo et al. 2015), including specific groups such as simulation educators (Thoma et al. 2018a) or discipline-based communities. Leveraging these online communities of practice for health professional educators can provide new opportunities for scholarship – for example, Natesan et al. (2019) presented a curated collection of feedback in medical education, selected via a social media call for papers.

Supporting Clinical and Educational Scholarship

Chan describes the *interactive investigator* role of health professionals using social media to generate (clinical or educational) research questions, collaborate with other researchers, and to disseminate results (Johannsson and Selak 2019). As an example,

Ng et al. (2019) reported a comprehensive social media strategy that was effective in disseminating recommendations from the National Tracheostomy Safety Project to front-line clinical staff.

Health professionals undertaking clinical or educational research may need new skills in using social media for study recruitment, intervention delivery (Arigo et al. 2018), and results dissemination (Widmer et al. 2019), and educators may need to incorporate these skills into curricula. Altmetrics are social media–based qualitative data that provides a measure of influence and impact of published articles, and are complementary to traditional, citation-based metrics. They may be used by researchers to demonstrate the breadth and diversity of dissemination (Chisolm 2017). *(Case vignette Frederick)*

Case vignette 5: Frederick – A Social Work Researcher Investigating Staff Wellbeing in the Paediatric Intensive Care Unit

Frederick is already part of an online community of practice on Twitter (#hcwellness.) He recruits health professionals to his studies via Twitter and Facebook. Frederick publishes papers in critical care journals, disseminates them via Twitter, and writes a guest blog post on wrapem.org. He is interviewed on a podcast about his research. When applying for academic promotion he is able to quote an Altmetric score of 79 for one of his papers.

Recognizing the value of social media contributions (i.e., blog posts, podcasts, microblogs) by health professionals as a measure of "digital scholarship" (Cabrera 2019) is relatively new. Institutions are developing criteria for incorporation into academic promotion and tenure decisions (Cabrera et al. 2017). In addressing this challenge, Sherbino et al. (2015) developed a consensus statement from 52 health professions educators in four countries, defining four key features of social media–based scholarship. "It must (1) be original; (2) advance the field of health professions education by building on theory, research or best practice; (3) be archived and disseminated; and (4) provide the health professions education community with the ability to comment on and provide feedback in a transparent fashion that informs wider discussion."

Other Roles

Health advocacy is regarded as a professional responsibility for healthcare providers, and is an increasing reason for social media use by health professionals (Moorhead et al. 2013). Supporting safe, effective, and ethically appropriate use of social media for this role requires skills and training, including knowledge of relevant legislative and professional society guidelines (Farnan et al. 2013).

Health professionals and their organizations may engage with social media for *organizational promotion* (Ventola 2014). In many countries, healthcare and health professions education is a marketplace, and a strong social media presence attracts patients and potential employees. The ethical issues inherent in this activity are not new, but may have specific considerations in practical application on social media.

Contemporary Issues in Social Media Usage for Health Professions Education

Managing Personal Social Media Reputation

Reputation is the public perception of an individual or organization (Horn et al. 2015), and health professionals indirectly or directly represent their employers. Social media can pose a threat, as much as a benefit, to the professional reputations of healthcare professionals and educators. The interconnection between faculty, students, and others has increased significantly with the rapid evolution of social media.

Identity, like reputation, is socially constructed through public appearance and interactions (Rambe 2013). Almost every Internet user has a social media/ online identity, and health professionals and educators will benefit from proactively managing their profile (Hanzel et al. 2018), to optimize career opportunities, learning collaborations, and for dissemination of clinical, educational, or research work.

Health professional learners need tools/advice on how to manage their online identity, including the style and content of social media platform profiles, and appropriate content and search engine optimization (SEO) of personal websites (Stiegler 2019). This may be especially relevant for undergraduate health professional learners who are often transitioning from purely personal use of social media to more professional use. *(Case vignette Brenton)* Delineating between professional and personal identities can pose a challenge to educators and health professionals alike. Attributes that should be central to the approach to social media use include maintaining privacy and confidentiality, and identifying the accepted behaviors for online conduct and professional boundaries (Au 2018). *(Case vignette Aleks)*

Case vignette 6: Brenton – A First Year Physiotherapy Student
Brenton learnt basic online safety at high school, and was peripherally involved in couple of incidents of online harassment in year 10. He is active on Facebook, Snapchat, and Instagram, with mostly personal use – party photos and travel. He now starts looking for online educational content and also develops a profile on LinkedIn and Twitter. One of his lecturers uses Twitter microblogs as a reflection adjunct. His university has a social media guide for students but Brenton is unaware of it.

Case vignette 7: Aleks – A Nursing Student Who Uses Snapchat for Video Blogging (Vlog)
Aleks is a final year nursing student with a large followership on Snapchat. She posts daily vlogs of "a day in the life of a nursing student," generally talking about how

mean a preceptor was or something "gross" she had to do. Aleks thinks she is being careful to avoid identifying details, but regularly posts while still wearing her university clinical placement uniform with visible logo. A concerned fellow student screen records a number of Aleks' posts and takes them to the clinical placement coordinator. Aleks was immediately withdrawn from clinical placement pending a review against the university's standards for placement and code of conduct.

Ultimately, health professional educators and learners should demonstrate behaviors online that they would be happy to emulate in real life, knowing that the behaviors might be amplified more rapidly.

Defining Quality in Social Media

Low barriers to entry in social media content creation and the rapid rise of online educational resources has meant there are few well-defined measures of quality. Mistakes occur even when resources are created by highly qualified clinicians and educators. Conflict of interest disclosures should apply, but are less frequently observed in practice (Niforatos et al. 2019). Without any overarching institutional responsibility, issues like version control, updating links, and managing intellectual property can be ignored.

In addition to relying on users' critical appraisal skills, there are suggested approaches and quality indicators (Lin et al. 2015; Thoma et al. 2018b; Colmers-Gray et al. 2019). One systematic review identified three core themes for quality – credibility (transparency, process, use of other resources, trustworthiness, and bias), content (professionalism, engagement, academic rigor, and orientation), and design (aesthetics, interaction, functionality, and ease of use) (Paterson et al. 2015).

Research into Social Media

Health professional use of social media provides a massive array of data and much of this can be categorized and explored as a product of use through social network data extraction and analytic engines. Much of the nascent literature about health professional social media use has focused on frequency data – reach or impressions generated from a conference – or comparisons of traditional citation metrics with volume of followership on social networks (Nomura et al. 2012). More recently, health professional researchers have looked to the social sciences and marketing disciplines for theoretical foundations to study social media. Roland et al. (2017) viewed the rapidly proliferating Twitter hashtag *#FOAMed* through the theoretical lens of communities of practice (CoP). They examined the interactions and connections of users – through social network analysis, the domain knowledge – through keyword and link frequency, and the social controls and application of knowledge to practice – through online ethnography, demonstrating that users of a network at the time comprising approximately 50,000 people were functioning as an online CoP.

Social media research provides an avenue to understand how technology is changing learning and how the learners are connected in an extensive and real time data set. With this great power, comes great responsibility, in ensuring rigor, where datamining lends support to almost any assertion. Roland et al. (2018) offered an initial standardized framework for reporting social media analytics research in healthcare, which may serve as a foundation for research design in this area.

Patient/Consumer Perspectives and Interactions

Patients are using social media for diverse needs – emotional, information, esteem, network support, social comparison, and emotional expression (Smailhodzic et al. 2016). Cocco et al. (2018) reported that online healthcare information is frequently sought before presenting to an emergency department and was found to have positive impact on the doctor–patient interaction. Healthcare professionals can optimize this through provision of high-quality online information, educating patients about resources and support groups, and helping to interpret information found online (Ventola 2014).

Healthcare professional learners may need guidance in managing professional boundaries on social media – for example "friend" requests – or being perceived as providing medical advice online.

Ethical and Professionalism Issues

Despite the transformational opportunity and nature of social media, issues surrounding professionalism and ethics persist. A number of representative bodies provide recommendations via policy and guides (Ventola 2014; Medical Board of Australia 2014). Using social media should be considered as an extension of professional behavior; workplace and governing body codes of conduct apply to all behaviors. Privacy and confidentiality are the most obvious challenges related to the use of social media. Health professionals and educators are legally and ethically bound to protect the data and individuals that we are privy to. Although this seems black and white, there are areas of gray. Rural areas benefit greatly from the accessibility of social media, where platforms such as WhatsApp® are used to share patient information for clinical review. Given the context, can this be considered a breach of professionalism or necessary for the care of patients? Most workplaces have guides or policies for social media use. Educators can provide health professional learners with general guidance and strategies for seeking advice in specific situations. *(Case vignette Shona)*

Case vignette 8: Shona – A Registered Nurse Working in Indigenous Health, and Aiming to Increase the Voice of the Nursing Profession

Shona uses Twitter and Facebook to engage with organisations and media outlets to identify the under-representation of the nursing profession in major public health debate. Shona leverages a network of academic and clinical nurses to call out and petition against major policy developments and mainstream media discussions around Indigenous health, primary healthcare and patient-centred care models for the absence of nursing professional engagement and voice. Shona is cautious in tone and has recently discussed her social media profile with her employers after being invited to speak at a national conference about professional advocacy. She was asked to shut down her profiles and could not get a clear reason. She is seeking support from the nursing union as she believes she has not breached any code or policy.

Conclusion

Social media offers learners and teachers new ways of accessing educational content, and new pedagogical approaches to learning. Realizing this potential requires specific skills in filtering and searching social media content, and awareness of available platforms. Scholars can increasingly use social media to facilitate, disseminate, and recognize their research. The use of social media in health professions education also brings risks, and learners and teachers need to consider personal and organizational strategies to manage ethical and professional challenges.

References

Arigo D, Pagoto S, Carter-Harris L, Lillie SE, Nebeker C. Using social media for health research: methodological and ethical considerations for recruitment and intervention delivery. Digit Health. 2018;4:2055207618771757.

Au A. Online physicians, offline patients: professional identity and ethics in social media use. Int J Sociol Soc Policy. 2018;38:474–83.

Bandura A. Social learning theory. Englewood Cliffs: Prentice-Hall; 1977.

Cabrera D. Danielcabrera [Internet] 2019. [cited 2019]. Available from: https://www.danielcabrera. org/resources/digitalscholarship/

Cabrera D, Vartabedian BS, Spinner RJ, Jordan BL, Aase LA, Timimi FK. More than likes and tweets: creating social media portfolios for academic promotion and tenure. J Grad Med Educ. 2017;9(4):421–5.

Cadogan M. 5 lessons learned. Life in the fast lane. September, 2019 https://litfl.com/5-lessons-learned/. Accessed 1st September, 2020.

Chan TM, Thoma B, Radecki R, Topf J, Woo HH, Kao LS, et al. Ten steps for setting up an online journal club. J Contin Educ Health Prof. 2015a;35(2):148–54.

Chan TM, Thoma B, Lin M. Creating, curating, and sharing online faculty development resources: the medical education in cases series experience. Acad Med. 2015b;90(6):785–9.

Chan T, Trueger NS, Roland D, Thoma B. Evidence-based medicine in the era of social media: scholarly engagement through participation and online interaction. CJEM. 2018;20(1):3–8.

Chisolm MS. Altmetrics for medical educators. Acad Psychiatry. 2017;41(4):460–6.

Choo EK, Ranney ML, Chan TM, Trueger NS, Walsh AE, Tegtmeyer K, et al. Twitter as a tool for communication and knowledge exchange in academic medicine: a guide for skeptics and novices. Med Teach. 2015;37(5):411–6.

Cocco AM, Zordan R, Taylor DM, Weiland TJ, Dilley SJ, Kant J, et al. Dr Google in the ED: searching for online health information by adult emergency department patients. Med J Aust. 2018;209(8):342–7.

Colmers IN, Paterson QS, Lin M, Thoma B, Chan TM. The quality checklists for health professions blogs and podcasts. Winnower. 2015;6:e144720.08769. https://doi.org/10.15200/winn.144720.08769.

Colmers-Gray IN, Krishnan K, Chan TM, Seth Trueger N, Paddock M, Grock A, et al. The revised METRIQ score: a quality evaluation tool for online educational resources. AEM Educ Train. 2019;3(4):387–92.

Cosimini MJ, Cho D, Liley F, Espinoza J. Podcasting in medical education: how long should an educational podcast be? J Grad Med Educ. 2017;9(3):388–9.

Farnan JM, Snyder Sulmasy L, Worster BK, Chaudhry HJ, Rhyne JA, Arora VM. Online medical professionalism: patient and public relationships: policy statement from the American College of Physicians and the Federation of State Medical Boards. Ann Intern Med. 2013;158(8):620–7.

Glasziou PP. Information overload: what's behind it, what's beyond it? Med J Aust. 2008;189 (2):84–5.

Goldie JGS. Connectivism: a knowledge learning theory for the digital age? Med Teach. 2016;38 (10):1064–9.

Hanzel T, Richards J, Schwitters P, Smith K, Wendland K, Martin J, et al. #DocsOnTwitter: how physicians use social media to build social capital. Hosp Top. 2018;96(1):9–17.

Horn IS, Taros T, Dirkes S, Hüer L, Rose M, Tietmeyer R, et al. Business reputation and social media: a primer on threats and responses. J Direct Data Digit Mark Pract. 2015;16(3):193–208.

Johannsson H, Selak T. Dissemination of medical publications on social media – is it the new standard? Anaesthesia. 2019. https://doi.org/10.1111/anae.14780.

Lin M, Thoma B, Trueger NS, Ankel F, Sherbino J, Chan T. Quality indicators for blogs and podcasts used in medical education: modified Delphi consensus recommendations by an international cohort of health professions educators. Postgrad Med J. 2015;91(1080):546–50.

Luo T, Shah SJ, Cromptom H. Using Twitter to support reflective learning in an asynchronous online course. Australas J Educ Technol. 2019;35(3). https://doi.org/10.14742/ajet.4124.

Medical Board of Australia. Social media policy: Australian Health Professional Regulation Authority. 2014. Available from: https://www.medicalboard.gov.au/Codes-Guidelines-Poli cies/Social-media-policy.aspx

Moorhead SA, Hazlett DE, Harrison L, Carroll JK, Irwin A, Hoving C. A new dimension of health care: systematic review of the uses, benefits, and limitations of social media for health communication. J Med Internet Res. 2013;15(4):e85.

Natesan SM, Krzyzaniak SM, Stehman C, Shaw R, Story D, Gottlieb M. Curated collections for educators: eight key papers about feedback in medical education. Cureus. 2019;11(3):e4164.

Ng FK, Wallace S, Coe B, Owen A, Lynch J, Bonvento B, et al. From smartphone to bed-side: exploring the use of social media to disseminate recommendations from the National Trache-ostomy Safety Project to front-line clinical staff. Anaesthesia. 2019. https://doi.org/10.1111/anae.14747.

Nickson C. Life in the fast lane [Internet] 2019 September 14, 2019. Available from: https://litfl. com/information-overload/

Niforatos JD, Lin L, Narang J, James A, Singletary A, Rose E, et al. Financial conflicts of interest among emergency medicine contributors on free open access medical education (FOAMed). Acad Emerg Med. 2019;26(7):814–7.

Nomura J, Genes N, Bollinger H, Bollinger M, Reed J. Twitter use during emergency medicine conferences. Am J Emerg Med. 2012;30:819–20.

Paterson QS, Thoma B, Milne WK, Lin M, Chan TM. A systematic review and qualitative analysis to determine quality indicators for health professions education blogs and podcasts. J Grad Med Educ. 2015;7(4):549–54.

Rambe P. Converged social media: identity management and engagement on Facebook Mobile and blogs. Australas J Educ Technol. 2013;29(3). https://doi.org/10.14742/ajet.117.

Riddell J, Robins L, Brown A, Sherbino J, Lin M, Ilgen JS. Independent and interwoven: a qualitative exploration of residents' experiences with educational podcasts. Acad Med. 2019. Publish Ahead of Print. https://doi.org/10.1097/ACM.0000000000002984.

Roland D, Brazil V. Top 10 ways to reconcile social media and 'traditional' education in emergency care. Emerg Med J. 2015;32(10):819–22.

Roland D, May N, Body R, Carley S, Lyttle MD. Are you a SCEPTIC? SoCial mEdia precision & uTility in conferences. Emerg Med J. 2015;32(5):412–3.

Roland D, Spurr J, Cabrera D. Preliminary evidence for the emergence of a health care online community of practice: using a netnographic framework for Twitter hashtag analytics. J Med Internet Res. 2017;19(7):e252.

Roland D, Spurr J, Cabrera D. Initial standardized framework for reporting social media analytics in emergency care research. West J Emerg Med. 2018;19(4):701–6.

Sherbino J, Arora VM, Van Melle E, Rogers R, Frank JR, Holmboe ES. Criteria for social media-based scholarship in health professions education. Postgrad Med J. 2015;91(1080):551–5.

Siemens G. Connectivism: a learning theory for the digital age. Int J Instruct Technol Distance Learn. 2005;3:3–10.

Smailhodzic E, Hooijsma W, Boonstra A, Langley DJ. Social media use in healthcare: a systematic review of effects on patients and on their relationship with healthcare professionals. BMC Health Serv Res. 2016;16(1):442.

Stiegler M. Marjorie Stiegler M.D. Physician leadership in a digital world. 2019. Available from: https://www.marjoriestieglermd.com/

Tanoue MT, Chatterjee D, Nguyen HL, Sekimura T, West BH, Elashoff D, et al. Tweeting the meeting. Circ Cardiovasc Qual Outcomes. 2018;11(11):e005018.

Thoma B, Joshi N, Trueger NS, Chan TM, Lin M. Five strategies to effectively use online resources in emergency medicine. Ann Emerg Med. 2014;64(4):392–5.

Thoma B, Brazil V, Spurr J, Palaganas J, Eppich W, Grant V, et al. Establishing a virtual community of practice in simulation: the value of social media. Simul Healthc. 2018a;13(2):124–30.

Thoma B, Chan TM, Kapur P, Sifford D, Siemens M, Paddock M, et al. The social media index as an Indicator of quality for emergency medicine blogs: a METRIQ study. Ann Emerg Med. 2018b;72(6):696–702.

Ventola CL. Social media and health care professionals: benefits, risks, and best practices. P T. 2014;39(7):491–520.

Weingart SD, Thoma B. The online hierarchy of needs: a beginner's guide to medical social media and FOAM. Emerg Med Australas. 2015;27(1):5.

Widmer RJ, Mandrekar J, Ward A, Aase LA, Lanier WL, Timimi FK, et al. Effect of promotion via social media on access of articles in an academic medical journal: a randomized controlled trial. Acad Med. 2019;94(10):1546–53.

Yarris LM, Chan TM, Gottlieb M, Juve AM. Finding your people in the digital age: virtual communities of practice to promote education scholarship. J Grad Med Educ. 2019;11(1):1–5.

E-learning: Development of a Fully Online 4th Year Psychology Program

42

F. J. Garivaldis, S. P. McKenzie, and M. Mundy

Contents

Introduction	778
A Fully Online 4th Year Program in Psychology: The Graduate Diploma of Psychology Advanced	780
The GDPA Course Structure	781
Course Content	781
GDPA Students and Student Support	783
Content Structure and Organization	784
Synchronous and Asynchronous Interaction	787
Academic and Work-Integrated Assessments	789
Student Satisfaction	790
Lessons Learnt and Recommendations	791
Concluding Remarks	792
Cross-References	793
References	793

Abstract

Traditionally, education and training has been restricted to major cities and centers in Australia, and the approach adopted to address the demands in remote areas has relied on migration incentives of already trained professionals to these locations. However, offering education and training directly to remote areas may provide better outcomes. This chapter describes the development of the Graduate Diploma of Psychology Advanced, a final (4th) year accredited program in psychology, which is the first in Australia to offer professional training in psychology in a fully online and flexible mode. The course aims to relieve the bottleneck of 4th year and expand access to education across Australia. The chapter describes the course's development and structure, and potentially

---

F. J. Garivaldis (✉) · S. P. McKenzie · M. Mundy
School of Psychological Sciences, Monash University, Melbourne, VIC, Australia
e-mail: filia.garivaldis@monash.edu

© Springer Nature Singapore Pte Ltd. 2023
D. Nestel et al. (eds.), *Clinical Education for the Health Professions*,
https://doi.org/10.1007/978-981-15-3344-0_56

transferable technological and online teaching and learning innovations. The chapter also presents learning analytic data on engagement with learning materials and course satisfaction, as well as provides key learnings as discussion points. It is anticipated that the chapter will aid in the design and development of other online courses that comprise both coursework and research components. The chapter shows that quality education can be made accessible online to those who are unable to enroll in traditional learning courses, due to location, work, and family commitments, or other personal reasons, to meet professional, personal, industry, and community needs.

Keywords

Online education · Psychology education · 4th year education bottleneck · Education innovation

Introduction

While the rate of mental health problems is similar Australia-wide, there are indicators that the mental health problem burden is greater in rural and remote areas. These indicators include 20% more hospitalizations due to mental illness (National Rural Health Alliance 2017) and a doubled rate of suicide in these areas compared with in major cities. Indicators also include a significant unmet demand for mental health services in rural and remote areas of the country (Australian Health Policy Collaboration 2019). According to the Australian Institute of Health and Welfare (2019), there are only around one third the number of psychologists available in remote Australia compared with in major cities and in 2015–2016 people in major cities were at least four times more likely to have accessed Medicare-funded mental health sessions than those in remote areas (National Rural Health Alliance 2017) (Medicare is the publicly funded healthcare system in Australia, operated by the Department of Human Services). A recent survey by the National Rural Health Alliance (2017) about the training needs of mental health service providers highlights a significant lack of availability of training in remote areas, largely due to the challenges of location, time, and cost (Littlefield 2016).

Exacerbating the lack of reach of the psychology profession in remote areas is an educational bottleneck in the training of psychology graduates that occurs when students are ready to progress to their 4th year of study, also known as the Honors year. This year is the culmination of undergraduate training in psychology and is a requirement for provisional professional registration as a psychologist. The 4th year of study in psychology is highly competitive due to its high demand for a limited number of places. As such, the 4th year is only available to students with the highest grades (Cruwys et al. 2015). This and other education bottlenecks are contributed to by the special education requirements of these and other courses, which includes a substantial research component, and the need for research supervisors.

The educational bottleneck in psychology is estimated to incur costs across various domains, including to the profession (Over 1991), teaching quality (Provost et al. 2010), the availability of services to the community (Franklin et al. 1996), and student well-being (Cruwys et al. 2015). Further, the traditional on-campus 4th year program is an intensive year of study, aiming to meet 4th year graduate attributes and employability skills standards, while at the same time balancing an emphasis on both content-knowledge acquisition as well as independent research. As a result, 4th year students typically experience high levels of psychological stress (Cruwys et al. 2015) as they strive to achieve a grade that will allow them to progress to a further limited selection of specialist postgraduate training.

Unfortunately, and despite the demand for registered practicing psychologists by industry and by psychology graduates, student numbers at the postgraduate level of training in Australia remain capped, with little growth in the number of places between 2008 and 2015. However, as the supply of registered psychologists via appropriate education and training remains a continuous need, it warrants solutions to be sought for barriers to the provision of such training, including the ongoing availability and capacity of academic teaching and research supervision, practice supervision, the use of campus resources, and facilities to deliver professional training within, and more importantly, the availability of all of these resources in remote parts of the country (Littlefield 2016).

To expand education including psychology education availability to more students, and further away, opportunities have arisen in recent years for educational programs to be developed and implemented that adopt an online mode of delivery. As such, the industry of online education, in Australia and abroad, has grown with the increased demand for flexible and modern methods of teaching and learning. Such programs are becoming increasingly popular (Aithal and Aithal 2016). Specifically, data from both the United States and Australia demonstrate that online learning enrolment is increasing steadily at approximately 5.6% per year (Allen and Seaman 2013; Australian Government Department of Education and Training 2018; Online Learning Consortium 2018).

Online courses of study open the door to a wider and more versatile use of space and time for teaching and learning. However, there are unprecedented demands faced by universities and academics unique to programs of this mode, such as the need to make good use of technological tools that allow and enhance content delivery, to invest in the skills and competencies of teachers and learners who use these tools (Bewane and Spector 2009; Oomen-Early and Murphy 2009), and to meet the demands of online learners for flexible learning (Bolliger and Martindale 2004). Additionally, online programs need to address new barriers to effective learning, which include perceived isolation of students and staff, poor motivation, and poor time management (Roddy et al. 2017) – all of which have more significant implications in the online mode than in the face-to-face mode. Finally, and in addition to these challenges, online courses of study are continuously striving to contest skepticism around the quality of education they offer (Geffen 1993), as well as meet expectations of growth and profitability rates set by universities.

This chapter discusses the development of a fully online 4th year program of study in psychology, the Graduate Diploma of Psychology Advanced (GDPA), delivered at Monash University in Australia since 2016. Given that the GDPA is delivered fully online, it allows access to quality psychology education in remote areas, which supports the development of a larger and more qualified mental health workforce to address issues including a lack of psychological services in rural and remote areas. The chapter presents key features of the course, innovations adopted to support its delivery of education excellence, preliminary data on the delivery model adopted, and a summary of key learnings. We show that online programs can offer educational benefits to students, involve challenging traditional or taken-for-granted methods of delivery using technological and educational innovations – all of which require substantial support to develop and deliver, including an investment of time and money that is equivalent, if not surpassing, that of the face-to-face mode.

A Fully Online 4th Year Program in Psychology: The Graduate Diploma of Psychology Advanced

Monash University has for many years delivered a competitive and highly regarded 4th year in psychology adopting a traditional on-campus mode of delivery. However, places in this course have always been limited by the capacity of teaching and research staff to supervise students one-on-one. In 2015, as part of the Monash University wide strategy for digital education, the Faculty of Medicine, Nursing, and Health Sciences expanded its repertoire of online courses to develop and deliver a fully online 4th year qualification in Psychology. This course is the GDPA and has been offered to students since March, 2016. Starting with an initial intake of 87 students, the course grew in enrolments sixfold in just 3 years.

The GDPA was envisaged to offer solutions to various restrictions faced by the on-campus 4th year program. The course was developed as part of a seven-year partnership between Monash University and Pearson Australia, under the Monash Pearson Alliance (MPA). Monash's choice of Pearson as a suitable collaborator to market and administer the GDPA was based on Pearson's history in designing flexible and efficiency modes of study; its expertise in digital marketing to achieve a broad reach to students across the country who may not otherwise have access to education; and the one-on-one pastoral care it provides to large and diverse student cohorts. Through the GDPA, the partnership has been able to meet the demand of students to enter the profession and the growing demand for psychologists in rural/ remote communities, by allowing students to remain in their community to study.

The GDPA was designed to be scalable, to support a theoretically unlimited number of students and engage a theoretically unlimited number of staff for the teaching and learning of these students. The course does not add a substantial strain to the on-campus facilities, despite that GDPA students have full access to all of the University's academic and non-academic services such as Careers and Employment, Student Counseling, and Research Ethics.

As such, the GDPA addresses the impact of the 4th year bottleneck, providing students with an alternative option to study at this level. The GDPA has alleviated some of the pressure of the 4th year, and the stress it produces for students, including in getting into the course, and addresses the need of industry to provide professional training to mental health service providers in remote parts of the country.

The GDPA offers the same opportunities for students studying 4th year to achieve psychological literacy (Cranney and Dunn 2011), the graduate attributes of the 4th year Australian Undergraduate Psychology Program (Cranney et al. 2009), as well as further employability skills needed at this level of professional training, and is fully accredited by the Australian Psychology Accreditation Council. Further, the course takes advantage of the online mode by offering a range of innovations to the on-campus 4th year program, including the capacity for students to complete a research project fully online, attention to student well-being and the development of resilience, and opportunities for work-integrated learning for the development of employability and transferrable skills using simulation-based education.

The GDPA Course Structure

The GDPA aims to provide equivalence to the on-campus 4th year in psychology training in terms of content, quality, and outcomes, with the exception of the time it takes to complete the course. Students of the GDPA study eight units one after the other, as opposed to concurrently, and hence they require a minimum of 1.4 years to complete the course, compared to the 1 year that it takes to complete the 4th year. The GDPA operates on a different academic calendar to the usual on-campus structure of two semesters. Rather, the GDPA is offered within an academic calendar comprising six 6-week teaching periods in a year, as opposed to two semesters. The first teaching period of the academic year of this calendar begins in early January, and the final teaching period ends in mid-December of that year. Students complete each unit in the GDPA within one 6-week teaching period, and each teaching period in the year (six altogether) currently alternates between coursework and research units. The course operates on a carousel model enabling six intakes of students per year, i.e., new students each teaching period.

Course Content

The course comprises 50% coursework and 50% research components. Of the five coursework units offered for the coursework component, students must complete three core units and one out of two electives. Some of the coursework units are adapted from the on-campus 4th year program. These units cover content on psychological assessment and intervention (core unit), ethical and professional issues (core unit), and clinical and developmental neuroscience (elective unit). The remaining units were units developed exclusively for GDPA students, and aim to address students' work readiness and employability (core unit), and familiarize students with contemporary applications of psychology (elective unit). These units expand GDPA students' career aspirations beyond just clinical psychology.

The remaining 50% of the course comprises undertaking a research project across four core research units. The main objective of the research units is to introduce students to the theoretical and methodological aspects of research under close supervision by an academic staff member, to introduce students to wider issues and disciplines in the practice and science of psychology, to provide training in both discipline-specific and generic research skills, and to prepare students for postgraduate study or employment. In addition to the research project dissertation, students must complete assessments designed to expand their knowledge of statistics, the ethics of psychological research and practice, research-related graduate attributes, and data analysis.

The Research Portal/Virtual Lab

The most significant innovation of the GDPA, enabling the course to deliver a substantial research component, and recently awarded for technological advancement to teaching and learning, is the Research Portal. The GDPA Research Portal, including the Virtual Lab (vLab), is a comprehensive online research environment, or one stop shop, which allows online and other users to conduct all stages of their research in an integrated and supported online environment. The Research Portal/vLab interface is structured to reflect a typical research sequence and provides users a range of research related information including on research topics, and research ethics submissions. The Research Portal/vLab also provides users online research capacities allowing fully online research participant acquisition, experiment and survey platforms, quantitative and qualitative data analysis, fully secured data storage, and one-on-one online supervision. The Research Portal/vLab allows all stages of the research process to be conducted, making it a valuable research tool for on-campus as well as online users. The Research Portal/vLab currently has over 1,200 users including over 600 non GDPA users, who are mainly on campus students and staff. Other important and potentially transferable GDPA innovations include its learning toolbox, which offers its students-structured and easily accessible academic revision and support material, and also non-academic success-enhancing materials including student well-being-related materials, and other whole student success-enhancing features including mindfulness course components.

The GDPA delivers content to students grouped in cohorts of up to 35 during the coursework units, which are each supported by a dedicated Instructor. Similarly, students are organized in groups between 4 and 6 per research project, supported by a dedicated project Supervisor. Similarly, to the on-campus program, each coursework and research unit in the GDPA is coordinated, refined, and kept up to date by a unit coordinator, who provides all academic oversight of the content, and the marking and moderation of assessments. In the research units, supervisors are supported by senior supervisors, who provide mentoring and guidance, and oversee the ethical and practical feasibility of a set of research projects that fall within the senior supervisors' areas of expertise and research interests.

The course content is delivered via the learning management system – Moodle, and comprises the following resources and activities; weekly module eWorkbooks with activities, weekly one-hour online class and consultation hour with a dedicated instructor, prescribed readings, discussion forums, and assessments, including quizzes.

GDPA Students and Student Support

In the first three years of the course, 532 students were actively enrolled, with 347 students graduating from the GDPA. In addition, 240 students were on intermission, and 257 students had discontinued.

Online courses of study have characteristically higher rates of attrition compared to on-campus equivalents (Oomen-Early and Murphy 2009). The attrition of students appears to increase slightly over time, but this occurs alongside course growth, as shown in Fig. 1. On average, the course-wide attrition rate is approximately 12%, with a slight increase in attrition during the unit on statistics, and a slight decrease during units of the research project. The main reason why students withdraw from a unit relates to changes in student circumstances or challenges that pop up and which may compromise the academic performance of students during that teaching period. Discontinuation, on the other hand, which is when a student withdraws from the course indefinitely, is less common at this level of study, but most likely to occur during the first three units into the course. The

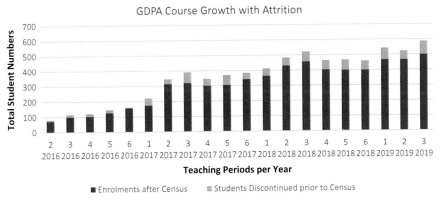

Fig. 1 Total number of GDPA students including attrition across each teaching period of the first 3 years of course delivery

main reason why students may discontinue from the course relates to the realization that they are unable to keep up with its intense study mode.

Student support services exclusively available to GDPA students are provided by Pearson Australia, under the Monash Pearson Alliance partnership. Pearson Australia's student engagement and retention team provides ongoing support through personalized coaching, as well as 24/7 technical support, to ensure student retention through to graduation. To illustrate, using learning analytics, students identified as at risk of falling behind or discontinuing are proactively engaged and provided additional guidance so they can successfully complete their course. Even when a student takes a break from their study, contact is maintained with them to ensure they are prepared to return to study when they choose. This level of pastoral care for students studying online is critical, primarily because most of them are new to the experience of studying online, and many have not studied at university for several years, or have to manage additional commitments such as working full time or taking care of family. In addition, this level of pastoral care allays the stress experienced by this cohort of students, enabling them to work optimally towards achieving grades to maintain eligibility for further study, and reducing rates of attrition and discontinuation.

Of the 532 active students in June 2019, 84% are female, and 16% are male. These percentages reflect those in the profession, as well as the online mode of study, both of which attract more females than males (Price 2006). Current GDPA students have a mean age of 32 years, which also reflects the tendency for online courses of study to attract mature-aged students (Moore and Kearskey 2005).

The majority of GDPA students reside in Victoria (42%) and New South Wales (27%). Up to 26% ($N = 240$) of GDPA students have been located in rural or remote locations, and less than 3% are located internationally. Figure 2 shows the number of students located across the country that form the 26% that are based rurally or remotely.

Content Structure and Organization

Developing a course requires careful consideration of the learning and support needs of its learners. As such, the GDPA has needed to consider the intrinsic

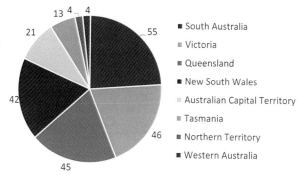

Fig. 2 Number of GDPA students living in rural or remote areas across Australia. (Listed in the figure in order of highest to lowest)

needs of both 4th year students as well as the needs of online learners in general, in the design of teaching and learning. A seminal study on 4th year students has shown that students at this level of study report poor well-being compared to student norms (Cruwys et al. 2015). Almost half of these students in this study reported depression scores in the clinical range, with symptoms persisting if their achievement aspirations were not met. The study also showed that students bounce back in terms of their well-being after completing the 4th year, which suggests that the cause of the stress during the 4th year is the 4th year itself. Buffers to the stress experienced by 4th year students that were identified in this study related to feelings of control over academic outcomes, social connection, and group membership. These buffers could be seen as inherent needs of this group of students, and these needs mirror those of online students. It is, however, more challenging to address these needs in online courses of study, which may contribute to the higher rates of attrition within equivalent capstone courses such as the GDPA, compared to the on-campus program.

Online students have additional needs, the most important concerning flexibility as they are often juggling multiple roles and responsibilities (Johnson 2015). Being older than on-campus students, online students are usually working or caring for family full time. Similar to their on-campus peers, online 4th year students are career driven, most often striving to enter the psychology profession.

As such, to provide structure and context to the student's learning experience, and meet need for control, flexibility, and convenience (Bollinger and Martindale 2004; Roddy et al. 2017), all of the material of a unit is presented in the form of a downloadable weekly eWorkbook. The eWorkbook addresses various intangibles prevalent of online courses, including the *what*, *why*, *when*, and *how* students need to learn. The eWorkbook is all-inclusive and comprehensive and is especially important considering the intense nature of the units being delivered in the GDPA. The eWorkbooks need to pre-empt and address student questions and concerns from the outset, and offer additional support for student needs that arise (Roddy et al. 2017), such as supplementary learning resources.

There are six eWorkbooks that students complete per unit, one corresponding to each week of a teaching period, and dedicated to one module of content. The eWorkbooks are created using the "Book" resource in Moodle, and contain up to 10 pages of learning material, including an overview page and a references page at the end. The overview page offers a snap shot of that week's learning plan. Specifically, this page displays a summary table of the lectorial topics to be covered, the prescribed readings relating to the module content on these topics, the videos students will watch, and the activities they will complete.

Cohesion is achieved between these resources in the rest of the eWorkbook by a narrative, written by an academic or subject expert. The narrative provides a context to the learning material that is equivalent to what on-campus students would receive during a lecture. For example, students may be introduced to a particular topic via the narrative, where the significance and relevance of that topic is emphasized, and where the most up-to-date information on that topic is summarized. Students may then be asked to read a journal article on a specific element of this topic, before they complete a learning activity to consolidate their learning. This topic may be required to be covered prior to that week's synchronously delivered online class, to enable discussion during the online class. The prescriptive nature of the eWorkbooks means that in the limited time that students have dedicated to study, they can focus on actively learning the materials, using meta-cognitive skills to reflect on, plan, and self-regulate their learning experience (Khiat 2015), rather than try to make sense of what goes where.

Moreover, the eWorkbooks contain opportunities for learner-learner interaction, and learner-instructor interaction, all of which promote student success online (Pascarella and Terenzini 2005). Specifically, these opportunities engage students outside of a synchronous online class, which is argued to promote active learning and the practice of higher order and transferrable skills (Khan et al. 2017). For example, during these interactions, students can develop interpersonal skills, communication skills, team and group work skills, and networking skills, depending on the content of the interaction. Overall, the broad repertoire of learning resources offered in the eWorkbooks facilitates student engagement and meets the needs of different learning preferences (Khan et al. 2017).

A further ingredient for student engagement is meaningful interaction with the institution (Pascarella and Terenzini 2005). As such, the eWorkbooks of all units contain content that has direct links with on-campus. This content is included to foster a sense of belongingness and connectedness with the institution, and buffer the perceived isolation of studying online. For example, each unit contains a series of "focus interviews" of key researchers in the School of Psychological Sciences of the university, extracts of recorded on-campus lectures and special seminars delivered by on-campus academics, and special feature learning material created exclusively for the course by on-campus experts. The formatting of the eWorkbooks also adheres to the Monash University marketing and communications strategy, whereby university icons and images are used.

The content of two eWorkbook at a time is assessed via a 45 minute quiz, containing 30 multiple choice questions. As such, a total of three quizzes assess eWorkbook content for each of the six modules of a unit. The quizzes are delivered using the Respondus Lockdown Browser, a software that creates a secure online test environment for online exams and prevents access to other browsers at the time of testing.

Qualitative evidence suggests that the eWorkbooks are effective in delivering the course materials. Specifically, course evaluation surveys administered soon after the course had launched yielded unsolicited student comments around the usefulness and comprehensiveness (60% of comments), enjoyableness (33% of comments), and novelty of the eWorkbooks, in the way they presented information (27% of comments). Of all positive qualitative comments received in the first few course evaluations, 42% referred to the word "workbook."

Similarly, the academic staff that instruct on the course have stated that the eWorkbooks offer equity in accessibility, provide a standardized learning approach in place of serendipitous learning, overcome differences in socioeconomic status of students unlike the use of textbooks that require purchasing, enable self-paced learning and flexibility, offer sustainability in use and re-use, and accommodate a variety of learning styles, offering written material, multi-media, individual, and group-based activities. Indeed, the GDPA was the first course in the School of Psychological Sciences to develop and utilize eWorkbooks – a resource that has since been taken up by the other two online/flexible mode undergraduate courses in the School.

Interestingly, the way the eWorkbooks are completed by students changes throughout the teaching period, in what appears in learning analytics data to look like drops in completion. The completion of an eWorkbook is operationalized in the learning analytics as having "viewed" all of the pages of an eWorkbook from first (overview page) to last (references page). The proportion of students who reached the last page of the first module eWorkbook, i.e., the references page, ranges between 30% and 44%, with an average of 36.47% completion rate across all units. The proportion of students completing the sixth/final module eWorkbook ranges between 0% and 33%, with an average of 17.33%. These rates do not capture study behavior such as skipping the references page, nor does the data capture how long students spent in the eWorkbook, or whether they accessed readings of videos from alternative links. Despite this apparent drop in eWorkbook completion during a unit, students receive consistent quiz scores throughout the unit, reflecting consistent levels of learning throughout the unit. As such, the analytics around rates of eWorkbook completion between the first to the last eWorkbook reflect more so a change in students' study approaches, rather than engagement.

Synchronous and Asynchronous Interaction

The GDPA affords various opportunities for students to engage with each other, via both synchronous and asynchronous platforms. For example, discussion forums and weekly online classes are offered to students throughout their unit. These forums are places for students to discuss unit content with peers, and vary in their level of guidance offered, i.e., from structured and specific questions to open-ended opportunities for reflection. They encourage active engagement with the course materials and social interaction: both of which are core components of student success online (Muilenburg and Berge 2005; Pascarella and Terenzini 2005). In addition, these platforms may help reduce perceived isolation, which is a key contributor to student attrition (Oomen-Early and Murphy 2009).

Online classes are delivered weekly through the teleconferencing software Zoom (and previously BlackBoard Collaborate) and offer the opportunity for synchronous interaction between students in a cohort and their Instructor. The classes are structured like tutorials, in that they provide some theoretical background upon which group activities are built and facilitated. The classes are recommended to students, but recordings are made for students who cannot attend. Students attend the classes virtually, from their location of study, most often their home.

To assess engagement with the online classes, the attendance for each class in each week was recorded and a percentage of the total students who attended a class in each week was calculated. Attendance at the online classes has been observed to differ within the teaching period, with attendance dropping as the teaching period progresses. Figure 3 shows the trend in attendance across Weeks 1–6 for each of the coursework units. The values are the percentage of students who attended the online class for Statistics (PSY4401), Ethics (PSY4405), Psychological Assessment (PSY4406), Psychology in Industry (PSY4407), and Clinical and Developmental Neuroscience (PSY4408). In summary, less than half of students attend classes after the first 2 weeks, but slight differences in trends can be observed between units, which depend on the nature of content in that unit and the weekly online class. It is also noteworthy that assessment deadlines in these teaching periods occur in weeks 3 and 5, which impact on online class attendance.

These results reflect trends in lecture attendance or non-attendance that can be observed in on-campus courses (Oldfield et al. 2019), and which pose a general concern for universities. Oldfield et al. (2019) have identified that predictors of on-campus non-attendance at lectures and seminars include a low sense of belongingness to the university, being engaged in paid employment, having social life commitments, facing coursework deadlines, and experiencing mental health issues. All of these factors sound like likely predictors of non-attendance for online courses as well, although future research could compare, specifically, the reasons for non-attendance between on-campus and online courses, and the impact this has on psychological outcomes, such as promoting the sense of belongingness, and other academic outcomes, such as grades.

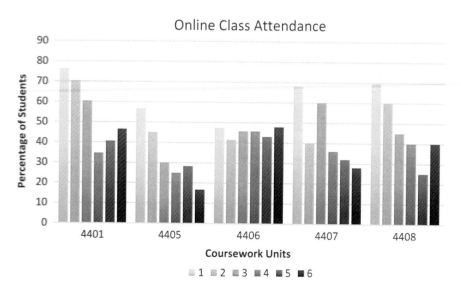

Fig. 3 Percentage of students attending the weekly online class across each of the 6 weeks of a teaching period and across each of the coursework units

Academic and Work-Integrated Assessments

Each course unit of the GDPA contains three types of assessment. The coursework units comprise an academic assignment, such as an essay or oral presentation, a work-integrated learning assignment such as a psychological report, research symposium presentation, case study analysis, or critical review, and a series of three multiple choice quizzes. This variety of assessments is intended to address a variety of skills, discipline-related and generic skills, to enhance the employability of GDPA graduates.

Work-integrated learning is the process of integration between workplaces, higher education institutions, industry, and government (Cooper et al. 2010) and is fuelled by the growing need of industry for work-ready graduates. Work-integrated assignments, in particular, are intended to increase the work readiness of students. Work readiness skills include non-technical, non-clinical, generic, and transferable skills, such as teamwork, communication, and problem solving. Additional skills may include organizational acumen, social intelligence, personal characteristics, and work competence, all of which are desirable of graduates (Caballero et al. 2011). The work-integrated assignments in the GDPA, listed above, aim to provide an authentic experience to students in terms of what to expect in the workplace.

In addition to the coursework unit assessments, the three research project units each require students to submit a whole of research thesis component – introduction, method, results, and discussion. Students have the opportunity to improve their thesis components on the basis of summative feedback before combining them to produce a whole thesis of 9,000–12,000 words based on their independent research project, equivalent to that completed in the on-campus 4th year course. In addition to the research thesis-related assessment, GDPA research project unit assessments comprise an oral thesis proposal, research ethics application, data analysis plan, and graduate research attributes reflection.

Due to the intense nature of the course, GDPA coursework unit students are provided with guidance in preparing their assessments via formative feedback on one draft on the assignment that is a hurdle requirement (worth $>40\%$ of the total unit grade). Formative feedback is effective when offered in a timely manner, when it focuses on attainable changes needed to be made, and encourages deeper thinking. Formative feedback can enhance the motivation and engagement of the learner, and improve the learner-instructor relationship (Regan 2010).

Indeed, personalized and timely feedback is provided for all assessment tasks in the course. This type of feedback, whether formative or summative, promotes student success online and offline (Li and Beverly 2008; Lee 2010). Specifically, students in the GDPA receive detailed summative feedback (annotations on their submission, a completed rubric, and overall comments), as well as a grade, 1 week after submission. Timely feedback ensures that this feedback has optimal impact on student learning and enables the implementation of all types of feedback to subsequent assignments in the same unit, and subsequent units, considering the fast-paced nature of the course.

Student Satisfaction

Data on student satisfaction of the course have been derived from the Student Evaluation of Teaching Units (SETUs); specifically, the responses to the question "Overall, I was satisfied with this unit." SETU surveys are advertised to students enrolled in any unit at Monash University at the end of their teaching period. Students rate a number of areas on a five-point Likert scale, from Strongly Disagree (1) to Strongly Agree (5), with point 3 representing a neutral response. To calculate a median, these ratings are assumed to be evenly distributed on a continuous scale. For example, scores of 4 are assumed to be evenly distributed between 3.5 and 4.49. The SETUs from all 27 coursework and research units of the GDPA delivered between the second teaching period of 2016 and the final teaching period of 2017 were used to produce Fig. 4.

Response rates for evaluations ranged between 12% and 56% of enrolled students, with an average of 33.37%. Only one unit received less than 20% response rate. Figure 4 shows that satisfaction fluctuates between teaching periods, and that there is a clear pattern of average satisfaction by unit.

In addition to the SETU question around overall satisfaction presented in Fig. 4, students rated their engagement with the learning materials consistently high across each of the teaching periods. Qualitative feedback from the SETUs highlights the course's strengths in the teaching and supervision of research, and notably the Instructors and Supervisors and their relationships with the students. Additional consistent strengths commented on were the feedback provided and the course materials, namely the eWorkbooks and their contents. These results align with previous literature, which has identified that a key predictor of online course satisfaction is the timeliness of feedback, social presence, course flexibility, and the availability of support services, including technical support (Barnes 2017).

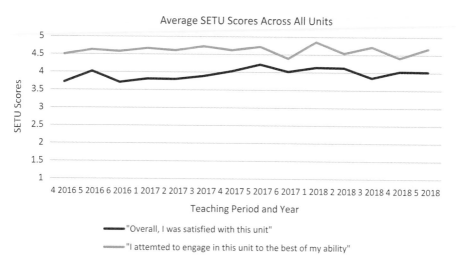

Fig. 4 Average SETU scores across each teaching period

Lessons Learnt and Recommendations

Since the GDPA was first launched in early 2016, it has been developed and delivered following a carousel model, with each teaching period involving the delivery of a one unit as well as the development of the upcoming unit. Since early 2018, the course and its staff have transitioned from a development phase to a 100% delivery and unit refinement phase. Crucial to this transition, and the growth of the course to over 500 students, has been the facilitation of close working relationships between academic and educational design staff. In addition, the leadership of the course during the development phase involved close monitoring of activities, the prescription of tight processes and procedures, centralized decision making, as well as the adoption of a unit style guide to achieve consistency in course materials, and coherence between units. In the current delivery and refinement phase, communication and decision making has been decentralized, to enable greater autonomy among Unit Coordinators such that continual refinements can take place efficiently at this large scale.

The specific lessons learnt since the course was launched, however, include the following:

1. *Allow for adequate time to plan the entire course, before the planning of individual units.*
   While the carousel model of the course enabled the concurrent development and delivery of units, and a process of student feedback to be obtained during this development, compromises were made that added to the costs of the development of the course. We assert that there is a need to decide on the assessment strategy per unit, distinct learning outcomes per unit, the structure and format of the delivery of resources which need to be uniform per unit, and the method of course development as early as possible. Upon establishing these details, a needs approach to recruiting educational designers and learning management system experts can be adopted, there can be a development of clear guidelines in development activities, such as templates, standards, and curriculum maps, and agreement can be obtained by everyone involved.
2. *Take a systemic approach to course development, recognizing the dynamic relationship between learning and teaching, and the impact of the whole, rather than the parts, on student outcomes:*
   Adequate variety has been achieved in the GDPA already, with a good balance of reading and viewing material, information from researchers and practitioners, 4th year on-campus content as well as new advancements in the field. However, upon delivering the course, it has been apparent that the way some resources are used impacts on how other resources are used. For example, weekly online class attendance is relatively low in the course, despite that these classes are the only opportunity students have to meet and interact with peers and the class Instructor. This outcome, however, should not be attributed to the nature of the material covered in these classes, or the scheduling of the classes, as these change each teaching period, and yet the trend remains the same. Rather, an investigation

needs to occur as to why the online classes have low attendance. An obvious reason could relate to the busy lives of students, who are often juggling study with work and family commitments, although the sizable majority of students on our course are in their twenties. A less obvious reason, however, could relate to the comprehensive nature of the eWorkbooks, offering students many opportunities for asynchronous engagement, and which students have commented explicitly about. Indeed, a reliance on asynchronous modes of communication between students in online courses is the norm (Hung et al. 2010). However, this reliance could be to the detriment of synchronous activities in the course. If some asynchronous activities were removed, such as the provision of formative feedback, students may consider attendance at the online classes more necessary. Instead, perhaps learning opportunities that cannot be gained elsewhere in the units could attract students to the online classes, and particularly material that addresses the interpersonal skills that are so important for the profession of psychology, and often left out of online courses.

3. *Deliver the course with competent and technologically trained academic staff.* Online courses of study require the appointment of staff that possess all of the knowledge and curricula equivalent to on campus courses, but with additional skills and competencies unique to the online mode. Specifically, instructors of online courses need to effectively communicate, manage technology, and develop rapport and relationships with students to overcome the obstacles often faced in the online mode, such as the limitations around face-to-face interaction (Roddy et al. 2016). When a course has a substantial research component, in particular, such as the GDPA, it is also important that staff possess adequate experience and competence in conducting research and in supervision. Finally, for an online 4th year course of study to be equivalent to its on-campus counterpart, it also requires equivalence in staff competence and qualifications, as well as the professional development opportunities that help retain this staff.

Concluding Remarks

What seems to be currently working well in the GDPA is the blend of rich and engaging learning material, the clear schedule and structure of this learning material which comes in the form of an eWorkbook, the flexible nature of the course that enables students to study at times convenient to them, and the availability and accessibility of both support staff and academic staff to address any student concerns or issues.

To achieve this combination of online educational practice, including the innovations of the Psychology Research Portal and student well-being material such as mindfulness practices, there has been a substantial investment in time, money, expertise, and the coming together of various professionals at the university. This approach to building resources not only meets the needs of online students, but offers the benefits of the multi modal nature of online study, which has not yet been fully realized, to benefit all higher education students.

Cross-References

▶ Self-Regulated Learning: Focus on Theory

References

Aithal PS, Aithal S. Impact of on-line education on higher education system. Int J Eng Res Mod Educ. 2016;1:225–35.

Allen E, Seaman J. Changing course: ten years of tracking online education in the United States. Babson Survey Research Group. 2013

Australian Government, Department of Education and Training. Selected higher education statistics – 2018 student data. 2018. Retrieved from https://www.education.gov.au/selected-higher-educa tion-statistics-2018-student-data

Australian Health Policy Collaboration. Deaths from suicide – remoteness. 2019. Retrieved from http://www.atlasesaustralia.com.au/ahpc/remoteness_graph/deaths-suicides.html

Australian Institute for Health and Welfare. 2019. Retrieved from https://www.aihw.gov.au/reports/ mental-health-services/mental-health-services-in-australia/report-contents/mental-health- workforce/registered-psychologists

Barnes C. An analysis of student perceptions of the quality and course satisfaction of online courses. J High Educ Theory Pract. 2017;17(6):92–8.

Bewane J, Spector JM. Prioritization of online instructor roles: implications for competency-based teacher education programs. Distance Educ. 2009;30:383–97. https://doi.org/10.1080/015879 10903236536.

Bolliger DU, Martindale T. Key factors for determining student satisfaction in online courses. Int J e-Learn. 2004;6:61–7.

Caballero CL, Walker A, Fuller-Tyszkiewicz M. The work readiness scale (WRS): developing a measure to assess work readiness in college graduates. J Teach Learn Grad Employ. 2011;2(2):41–54.

Cooper L, Orrell J, Bowden M. Work integrated learning: a guide to effective practice. Oxon: Routledge; 2010.

Cranney J, Dunn DS. Psychological literacy and the psychologically literate citizen: new frontiers for a global discipline. In: Cranney J, Dunn DS, editors. The psychologically literate citizen: foundations and global perspectives. New York: Oxford University Press; 2011. p. 3–12.

Cranney J, Turnbull C, Provost SC, Martin F, Katsikitis M, White FA, Varcin KJ. Graduate attributes of the four-year Australian undergraduate psychology program. Aust Psychol. 2009;44:253–62. https://doi.org/10.1080/00050060903037268.

Cruwys T, Greenaway KH, Haslam SA. The stress of passing through an educational bottleneck: a longitudinal study of psychology Honours students. Aust Psychol. 2015;50:372–81.

Franklin J, Gibson D, Merkel-Stoll JAN, Neufelt M, Vergara-Yiu H. Trends in the advertised demand for psychology graduates. Aust Psychol. 1996;31(2):138–43.

Geffen GM. The scientist-practitioner model: what is the role of the fourth year in psychology? Aust Psychol. 1993;28(1):35–8. https://doi.org/10.1080/00050069308258863.

Hung ML, Chou C, Chen CH, Own ZY. Learner readiness for online learning: scale development and student perceptions. J Comp Educ. 2010;55:1080–90. https://doi.org/10.1016/j.comped u.2010.05.004.

Johnson GM. On-campus and fully-online university students: comparing demographics, digital technology use and learning characteristics. J Univ Teach Learn Pract. 2015;12:11–51.

Khan A, Egbue O, Palkie E, Madden J. Active learning: engaging students to maximize learning in an online course. Electron J e-Learn. 2017;15(2):107–15.

Khiat, H. Measuring self-directed learning: a diagnostic tool for adult learners. Journal of University Teaching and Learning Practice; 2015. 12. Available at: http://ro.uow.edu.au/jutlp/vol12/iss2/2

Lee JW. Online support service quality, online learning acceptance, and student satisfaction. Internet High Educ. 2010;13:277–83. https://doi.org/10.1016/j.iheduc.2010.08.002.

Li CS, Beverly I. An overview of online education: attractiveness, benefits, challenges, concerns, and recommendations. Coll Stud J. 2008;42:449–58.

Littlefield L. Psychology education and training: a future model. InPsych. 2016;38(2). Retrieved from https://www.psychology.org.au/inpsych/2016/april/feature

Moore MG, Kearskey G. Distance education: a system's view. Belmont: Wadsworth Publishing; 2005.

Muilenburg LY, Berge ZL. Student barriers to online learning: a factor analytic study. Distance Educ. 2005;26:29–48. https://doi.org/10.1080/01587910500081269.

National Rural Health Alliance. 2017. Retrieved from https://ruralhealth.org.au/sites/default/files/publications/nrha-mental-health-factsheet-dec-2017.pdf

Oldfield J, Rodwell J, Curry L, Marks G.A face in a sea of faces: exploring university students' reasons for non-attendance to teaching sessions, Journal of Further and Higher Education, 2019;43(4):443–452.

Online Learning Consortium. Grade increase: tracking distance education in the United States. 2018. Retrieved from https://onlinelearningconsortium.org/read/grade-increase-tracking-distance-education-united-states/

Oomen-Early J, Murphy L. Self-actualization and e-learning: a qualitative investigation of university faculty's perceived barriers to effective online instruction. Int J e-Learn. 2009;8:223–40.

Over R. Impending crises for psychology departments in Australian universities? Another look. Aust Psychol. 1991;26(2):112–5. https://doi.org/10.1080/00050069108258846.

Pascarella ET, Terenzini PT. How college affects students. San Francisco: Jossey-Bass; 2005.

Price I. Gender differences and similarities in online courses: challenging stereotypical views of women. J Comput Assist Learn. 2006;22:349–59. https://doi.org/10.1111/j.1365-2729.2006.00181.x.

Provost SC, Hannan G, Martin FH, Farrell G, Lipp OV, Terry DJ, Wilson PH. Where should the balance be between "scientist" and "practitioner" in Australian undergraduate psychology? Aust Psychol. 2010;45(4):243–8. https://doi.org/10.1080/00050060903443227.

Regan PJ. Read between the lines; the emancipatory nature of formative annotative feedback on draft assignments. Syst Pract Action Res. 2010;23:453–66. https://doi.org/10.1007/s11213-010-9168-2.

Roddy C, Amiet DL, Chung J, Holt C, Shaw L, McKenzie S, Garivaldis F, Lodge JM, Mundy ME. Applying best practice online learning, teaching, and support to intensive online environments: an integrative review. Front Educ. 2017;2(59). https://doi.org/10.3389/feduc.2017.00059.

Teaching Diversity in Healthcare Education: Conceptual Clarity and the Need for an Intersectional Transdisciplinary Approach

43

Helen Bintley and Riya E. George

Contents

Introduction 796
Diversity: How It Is Conceptualized, Theorized, and Taught in Healthcare Education 797
    Conceptual Clarity: The Journey from Cultural Competence to Diversity 797
    Theoretical Clarity: The Journey from "Other" to "Self" 801
    Evaluation and Curriculum: The Mismatch Between Theory and Practice 805
Intersectional Transdisciplinarity in Healthcare Education: Thinking Beyond Models and
Frameworks 806
    Transdisciplinarity: Theory, Application, and Challenges of Using this Concept in
    Healthcare Education 806
    Intersectional Transdisciplinarity: An Alternative Approach to Diversity Education 807
    BRAIDE: An Example of Intersectional Transdisciplinary Diversity Education in
    Medicine 809
Conclusion 810
References 810

Abstract

In this chapter, we explore the complexity of difference and the implications of this complexity for diversity education in healthcare. Drawing on fundamental ontology and epistemology from philosophy, education, and healthcare, we explore the importance of concepts, theories, and vocabularies in the

---

H. Bintley (✉) · R. E. George
Barts and The London, School of Medicine and Dentistry, Queen Mary University of London, London, UK
e-mail: h.bintley@qmul.ac.uk; r.george@qmul.ac.uk

© Springer Nature Singapore Pte Ltd. 2023
D. Nestel et al. (eds.), *Clinical Education for the Health Professions*,
https://doi.org/10.1007/978-981-15-3344-0_57

development and delivery of diversity education in healthcare. We discuss the need for conceptual and theoretical clarity in many areas of diversity education, the importance of intersectionality in this respect, and the discord that exists between theory and practice in this context.

With this in mind, we then go on to consider solutions to the challenges of teaching and researching diversity education by evaluating the importance of transdisciplinarity as a vector for transforming understandings of complexity. With reference to the work of others as well as our own, we conclude by exploring the possibility of using an intersectional transdisciplinary approach to teaching and researching diversity education in healthcare. The implications of such an approach are considered in relation to institutional commitment and holistic working practices, thereby suggesting that conflict, debate, and subjective experience are important for bridging the divide between theory and practice.

Keywords

Diversity · Education · Healthcare · Intersectionality · Transdisciplinarity · Complexity · Difference · Self

Introduction

Concepts of diversity challenge global, historical, and political understanding of identity, power, and belonging. The UK population is richly diverse and ever developing. However, changes in the demographic landscape of the UK (Census Data 2017) present complex challenges for healthcare professionals and policy makers in achieving equitable care (Napier et al. 2014). Diversity education is designed to address these challenges by attempting to improve the knowledge, skills, and attitudes of healthcare professionals in serving culturally diverse populations (General Medical Council (GMC) 2009; Nursing and Midwifery Council 2015; Department of Health. Success Measures 2012). However, beyond broad agreements, how to teach diversity education has become a conundrum with questions about how, when, where, and why it should take place (George et al. 2019a, b).

In this chapter, the authors critically disentangle the vocabulary used in diversity education providing conceptual clarity about terms such as diversity. An overview of landmark theoretical frameworks is presented, highlighting the range of educational and political influences that have permeated our evolving understanding of diversity in healthcare education. Using examples from our practice and that of others, we discuss the discord between theoretical and practical applications of diversity education and the need for an intersectional, transdisciplinary approach in the future.

Diversity: How It Is Conceptualized, Theorized, and Taught in Healthcare Education

Conceptual Clarity: The Journey from Cultural Competence to Diversity

Understanding of self and others is important for constructions of identity and social norms and through debate and subversion, questioning of those social norms. As Butler discusses, "the terms by which we are recognised as human are socially constructed and changeable" (Butler 2004, p. 2). Although changeable, categorization of people through terms such as gender, race, ethnicity, and sexual orientation can make some individuals appear more socially desirable than others. If we are able to dismantle these categories, we open the possibility of difference, but if not, it is difficult for individuals to recognize themselves within these categories and live their lives to the fullest (Butler 2004). Definitions related to diversity are therefore important to critically understand in order to avoid simplistic categorization.

Relating this to healthcare, diversity education is a term synonymous with labels such as "cultural competence"; "equality, diversity, and inclusion"; and "unconscious bias." The assortment of vocabulary for these types of educational teaching reveals the lack of consensus concerning the "correct" terminology. These terms also vary across healthcare contexts with "diversity" being used more in the UK (Dogra et al. 2015), "culture" and "ethnicity" frequently applied across Europe (Sorensen et al. 2019), and "cultural competence" remaining prominent in the USA (Betancourt and Cervantes 2009). Definitions of diversity are complex, nuanced, and varied depending on the context and discipline in which they are utilized. The considerable variation and lack of conceptual clarity of these terms results in different diversity educations with differing intentions and educational objectives. Therefore, to better challenge our understanding and use of diversity in healthcare education, the terms cultural competence, culture, and equality must first be explored.

Early diversity education in healthcare proceeded within the remit of cultural competency training. The literature demonstrates several descriptions of cultural competence, the most commonly cited being "a set of congruent behaviours, attitudes and policies that come together to enable that system, agency or those professionals to work effectively in cross-cultural situations" (Cross et al. 1989, p. 1). The concept of cultural competence became prominent in healthcare as increasing numbers of studies showed significant disparities in health outcomes among minority ethnic groups. Initial healthcare training followed the premise that particular races and ethnicities had certain cultural beliefs and attitudes that impacted the delivery of healthcare services. Based on this early conceptualization, learners were expected to acquire knowledge about "other" cultures, i.e., their history, traditions, and core beliefs.

This traditional notion of cultural competence was reflected in definitions of culture, which favored group-based distinctions, categorizing people based on factors such as religion, race, or ethnicity, with an assumption of homogeneity in their healthcare needs (Bhui et al. 2012). However, cultural competence models attracted negative criticisms about their assumptions that a healthcare professional can learn all they need to know about any one cultural group (Shen 2016). Criticisms were made of the disregard for the complexity of culture and that one could become "culturally competent" by learning a "shopping list" of generalized facts pertaining to assumed homogenous groups.

Culture is a highly debated concept with no single agreed definition. One definition of culture defined by Diversity in Medicine and Health is, "culture is a socially transmitted pattern of shared meanings by which people communicate, perpetuate and develop their knowledge and attitudes about life. An individual's cultural identity may be based on heritage as well as individual circumstances and personal choice and is a dynamic entity" (Dogra et al. 2015, p. 323). The manner and variation upon which shared meanings of culture are understood and practiced by individuals give rise to differences in understanding of health and illness. While values, beliefs, and practices can be shared in a "culture," "diversity" recognizes the heterogeneity among cultures and identifies characteristics that are autonomous and distinct. This acknowledgment of difference is vital in avoiding categorization that can create imbalances of power within shared social systems and stops the "undoing" (Butler 2004) of dominant discourses.

For instance, categorization of the gendered body in many shared cultures encompasses a compulsory heterosexuality (Butler 1990). This is congruent with heteronormativity (a societal understanding of relationships in which the perceived dominant structure is heterosexuality (Jeppesen 2016)) and heterosexual discourse, discourse being "bodies of ideas that produce and regulate the world in their own terms, rendering some things commonplace and other things non-sensical" (Youdell 2006, p. 36). However, this does not reflect the range of difference present in peoples' conceptions and expressions of gender and reveals the fiction of gender categorization (Butler 1990).

Many cultures inherently use such categorization in part because it creates the illusion of stability and understanding. However, those whose discursive gender performativity (the construction, rehearsal, and expression of gender within discourse (Butler 1990)) means they lie outside of heteronormative discourse can be othered. This creates a *dominant* heterosexual discourse in which categories of normal and pathological (Foucault 1969) based on sexual orientation and gender identity are made possible and nonheterosexual identities are seen as deviant.

In its broadest sense, any "difference" can be regarded as diversity and can include "all facets that define the way individuals perceive themselves" (Dogra et al. 2015, p. 323). Diversity is a term often associated with the concept of "equality" a widely acknowledged notion, which aims to ensure fairness in the distribution of healthcare services and practice, and describes "treating all individuals the same" (Bogg 2010, p. 2). Hand in hand with these concepts of difference and equality is legislation. The first cohort of equality legislation included the Sex

Discrimination Act (1975) and was centered on the concept of "formal equality," meaning "likes must be treated alike" (Hepple 2010, p. 2), which referred to the need for identical clinical practices and heath provision to all individuals irrespective of their diversity.

Gradually, a growing transition toward the concept of "substantive equality" was reflected in legislation, which describes the need for practical adjustments within public bodies to cater for the diverse needs of individuals. The Equality Act (2010) streamlined all previous discrimination Acts and attempted to codify the numerous array of Acts and regulations, which formed the foundation of anti-discrimination laws in the UK. It provides a single Act, which draws attention to a variety of differences and aims to strengthen the protection of individuals. However, the Equality Act (2010) is not without its criticisms. For instance, in an important and necessary move, transgender identity was included in the protected characteristics of the Equality Act in 2010. However, there is evidence to suggest that despite this change, people who identify as transgender continue to experience significant discrimination in many areas including healthcare (Hudson-Sharp and Metcalf 2016). In a parliamentary report on transgender equality (House of Commons Women and Equality Committee 2016), it was stated that the definitions used in the Act were unclear and included outdated language such as "transsexual." This created confusion and contributed to certain individuals being left outside of legal protection.

Many authors in the field have acknowledged that diversity education is driven by political motives associated with equality legalization as opposed to clinical and educational need, resulting in diversity education being perceived as a legal "tickbox" requirement. The strong political influence on the development of diversity education has resulted in many unintended consequences, one being the compartmentalization of diversity characteristics such as race or sexual orientation as single, static facets of identity. This compartmentalization discounts the importance of the *interplay* between different facets and contextual, sociohistorical factors.

As equality legislation became broader in scope, the concept of "diversity" originated and new ways of conceptualizing "equality" began. It is widely acknowledged the "one-size-fits-all approach" is not appropriate for most clinical groups. "Diversity" became a favorable concept as it broadened the notion of "cultural competence" and was articulated in a manner that did not minimize racial inequalities but drew focus on the health needs of the entire population. Diversity and equality therefore became more inclusive of the complexity of identity and attempted to identify the intersections of diversity issues.

Intersectionality (Crenshaw 1990) is a term borne out of third-wave feminist and antiracist movements and is acknowledged in diversity education literature, although more emphasized in social identity theories and health inequalities literature. Collins and Blige describe intersectionality as "a way of understanding and analysing complexity in the world, in people and in human experiences. The events and conditions of social and political life and the self can seldom be understood as shaped by one factor. They are shaped by many factors in diverse and mutually influencing ways" (Collins and Blige 2016, p. 2).

As Crenshaw comments in her seminal article on intersectionality, "When the [antiracist and feminist] practices expound identity as 'woman' or 'person of colour' as an either/or proposition, they relegate the identity of women of colour to a location that resists telling" (Crenshaw 1990, p. 1242). Collins (1998) developed this theory further, arguing that diversity is experienced to differing degrees at different times and because race, gender, and socioeconomic status are more visible, this visibility disproportionately compounds their impact. In this way, issues of diversity have the potential to enable layers of oppression that are not additive but multiplied. These layers of oppression are related to hierarchy and access to power and create specific social locations for those affected, which in turn are dynamic and constantly changing.

Intersectionality has strongly pushed against the notion of *blaming the victim* referring to the simplicity of attributing healthcare disparities to cultural or social behaviors alone. Instead, it recognizes healthcare disparities as part of a reciprocal web of problems associated with inequality, inequity, and oppression. It illuminates the *convergence* of experiences in a given sociohistorical and situational landscape.

Intersectionality draws upon a range of disciplines and overtly discusses social determinants of health. This is in contrast to decontextualized biomedical approaches present in healthcare education, which have influenced traditional notions of cultural competence and emphasize the behaviors of groups of patients as a source of healthcare disparities. This biomedical approach also has the propensity to create a power imbalance in favor of the healthcare professional. In Foucault's (1975) discussion on the subject in *The Birth of the Clinic*, a doctor's medical gaze strips away non-biomedical patient information and creates a power relationship that for the healthcare professional is doctor, and not patient, orientated.

This is in part because the biomedical model "assumes that all illness is secondary to disease" (Wade and Halligan 2004, p. 1398) and can therefore be treated by members of the medical profession. This has implications for patient care including an underappreciation of the patient's experience of illness, body-mind dualism, and a perceived priority of cure over care (Crowley-Matoka et al. 2009). Foucault argues that the power imbalance created by this approach affects communication, decision-making processes, and the treatment and labelling of different diseases. This, Canales (2010) argues, leads to exclusionary othering, where power relationships between people (in this instance patients and healthcare professionals) lead to subordination, which creates the potential for discrimination.

Various theoretical frameworks have been used in healthcare curriculums to teach diversity. While the authors describe their theoretical models or frameworks, the literature describing diversity education infrequently refers to a clear theoretical position, which is attributable to the lack of conceptual clarity of key terms. In the next section, we build upon the conceptual clarity of the term diversity and its key associated concepts to provide theoretical clarity on the purpose of diversity education in healthcare.

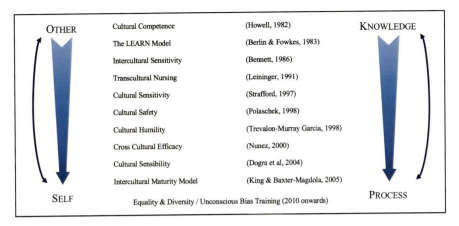

Fig. 1 Overview of theoretical frameworks used to teach diversity in healthcare, developed by R.E. George, 2017 (2017)

Theoretical Clarity: The Journey from "Other" to "Self"

We have seen so far how conceptual confusion has enabled discrepancies in how diversity education should be understood, theoretically framed, and delivered. However, by critically exploring theoretical frameworks used in diversity in healthcare, we can see how and why there has been a movement from traditional notions of cultural competence to process-oriented models, where understanding the self takes precedence over gaining expertise about others (Fig. 1).

The notion of cultural competence stemmed from evidence suggesting racial and ethnic disparities in healthcare. Howell's model of cultural competence (Howell 1982) was one of the earliest theoretical frameworks in the 1980s. It defines a developmental four-stage approach of consciousness and competence that individuals progress through in becoming culturally competent, through the delivery of knowledge about "other" cultural groups. This model was influential in illustrating the need for staged learning in the development of cultural competence, which was later inherited by the frameworks developed by other authors (Campina-Bacote 2000; Bennet 1986). The structure of this theoretical framework suggests that achieving cultural competence is a linear process, failing to consider that individuals may regress back to previous stages or advance forward to the latter stages and that some may not transition through all stages.

The theoretical frameworks during the 1980s attempted to operationalize the stages in which cultural competence is developed (Bennet 1986); however they are abstract in their descriptions of the types of educational strategies and materials to achieve the proposed stages of development. The theoretical frameworks during the 1990s to 2000 illustrate the distinct fusion between cultural competence models and the emerging frameworks eliciting the importance of self-awareness.

Transcultural nursing emerged in 1991 (Leininger 1991) and was centered on culturally based care, values, and practices. Leininger's 'theory acknowledges the cultural dynamics that influence the nurse-client relationship, with the goal of providing culturally congruent holistic care. Care modalities are re-patterned toward the specific cultural needs of the patient and require co-participation and working together. However, it does not specify the skills necessary to elicit culturally relevant information from the patient nor does it stipulate how to work cooperatively to achieve culturally congruent care. Furthermore, the model appears to pay an unbalanced attention to the cultural aspects of the patient as opposed to the healthcare professional. These criticisms were raised by other authors, including the lack of significance about the influence of the provider's cultural background in their understanding of the patient's cultural needs (Duffy 2001). Duffy argued that "greater critical self-reflection and acknowledgement of self" (Duffy 2001, p. 2) should be included.

Cultural sensitivity (Stafford et al. 1997) begins to advance the notion of "cultural competence" and proceeds by accepting the fact that there are cultural differences and similarities between individuals and those cultural differences are of equal value. Stafford defines cultural sensitivity as "being aware that cultural differences and similarities exist and have an effect on values, learning and behaviour" (Stafford et al. 1997, p. 78). In contrast to theoretical frameworks in the 1980s, it does not advocate a staged developmental continuum to achieving cultural competence and appears closely compatible with the notions of transcultural nursing.

Cultural safety (Polaschek 1998) developed as a subsidiary model of transcultural nursing, specifically addressing nursing practices toward different ethnicities and the needs of indigenous minority communities. The term "safety" had not been mentioned previously in theoretical frameworks concerning culture and sheds light on the status of certain groups and how they are perceived and treated in society. It argues that no healthcare interaction is ever simply objective. Rather a health professional operates from their own cultural mind-set, which influences how they relate to those they care for. This model is unique in explicitly drawing attention to the clinical relevance and safety of acknowledging cultural factors and the consequence of failing to do so for incorrect diagnoses, poorer quality of care, and unsuitable care plans. Nonetheless, it is developed specifically for indigenous populations, and although it may allude to the diversity within specific ethnic groups, it appears to assume that attitudes and practices may be culturally similar.

Cultural humility (Tervalon and Murray-Garcia 1998) is a theoretical model, which challenges the concept of learning finite bodies of knowledge about "other" cultural groups, which are typically expected in cultural competence models. Cultural humility proposes that "self-humility" allows professionals to engage in a lifelong commitment toward self-learning, evaluation, critique, and understanding of the power dynamics involved in the practitioner-patient relationship. It echoes the principles of patient-centered care and challenges professionals to grasp the importance of learning with and from patients. In comparison to models of cultural competence, cultural humility is a philosophy and an approach to practice and continual professional development.

More recent theoretical frameworks developed in the twentieth century demonstrate a move toward broader conceptualizations of culture and the introduction of the term "diversity." For example, the cross-cultural efficacy model (Nunez 2000) asserts that neither the caregiver's nor the patient's culture offers a preferred view. Nunez describes clinical encounters as a "tri-cultural" interaction, where the culture of the patient, healthcare provider, and the organization coexists. Nunez actively recognizes the shared, multidimensional dynamics involved in clinical practice, allowing for a broad appreciation of differences at play rather than a knowledge-based approach.

The cultural sensibility model (Dogra 2004) focuses on encouraging healthcare professionals to understand their own sense of self and how this affects their perceptions of others. Akin to the cultural humility framework (Tervalon and Murray-Garcia 1998), it begins with professionals developing self-reflection and humility in order to help them make sense of their interactions with others. The cultural sensibility model is one of the few models where the approach is framed within a sound educational background. However, it does not explicitly address the necessity of interpersonal skills in cross-cultural interactions. Although it acknowledges the significance of context, it pays little attention to the cultural dynamics involved in clinical interactions. In comparison with the cultural humility model, both the cross-cultural efficacy and cultural sensibility models place less emphasis on the importance of the relationship between practitioners and their colleagues and the organizational/institutional factors influencing their personal and professional identity.

The intercultural maturity model (King and Baxter Magolda 2005) was developed shortly after the cultural sensibility model and adopts a constructive development approach (Kegan 1994; Piaget 1952). This refers to an individual's ability to internalize, interpret, and make sense of an experience. It is also developmental in accounting for the growth of increased capacity in one's ability to construct meaning in a more adaptive way over time. This model recognizes that achieving competence in cross-cultural settings is not an endpoint but a developmental process that adopts a continual cyclic practice. As with its predecessors, this model also emphasizes the importance of continual self-reflection, awareness, critique, and evaluation of one's understanding of personal culture and that of others. It emphasizes the impact of power, privilege, and oppression (issues highlighted in the concept of intersectionality), which affect the construction of knowledge, images of self, and interactions with others.

The different theoretical frameworks suggest a more pluralistic way of thinking about cultural differences than was originally proposed in cultural competence models. There is also inevitably some borrowing and cross-fertilization as understanding grows and frameworks develop. This cross-fertilization can be useful in developing ideas from multiple theoretical traditions and adds perspectives about the sociopolitical-historical context in which they are being produced. This departure from other to self and knowledge-based to process-oriented models can be seen in institutional requirements and healthcare expectations concerning diversity education (Fig. 2).

Despite theoretical frameworks related to diversity education gravitating toward the importance of the self, the concept of intersectionality has not been exploited and

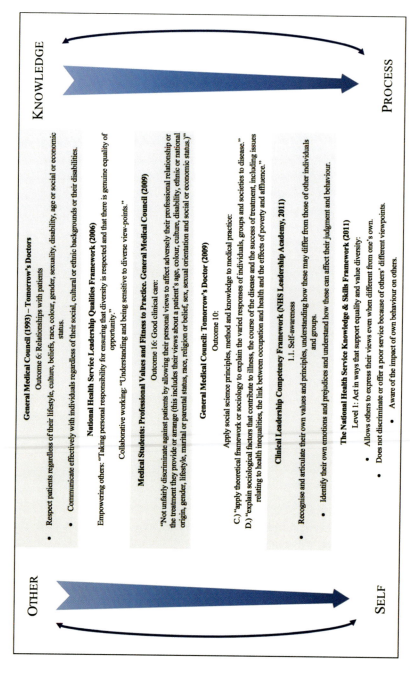

Fig. 2 Overview of institutional requirements and policies in healthcare education for diversity teaching (developed by R.E George, 2017) (George 2017)

is challenging to identify in diversity education literature in healthcare. While the principles associated with intersectionality have been acknowledged in some theoretical frameworks, they are not overtly addressed. Furthermore, categorical approaches to identity continue to prevail in diversity education, and models such as transcultural nursing and cultural safety superficially address these issues (often only in a political manner by providing reference to equality legislations) despite commendable theoretical underpinnings to the contrary. This results in applications of these models unintentionally perpetuating dehumanizing stereotypes among patient groups and highlights the discord between theory and practice.

Evaluation and Curriculum: The Mismatch Between Theory and Practice

Despite progress in diversity education, learning objectives remain unclear and the associated literature remains limited. Price et al. (2005) conducted a systematic review of the methodological rigor of studies exploring healthcare-related diversity education and found studies were of low to moderate quality and of small value for the development of approaches in this field. In the UK (as well as the USA, Canada, and in certain parts of Europe), the quality of the literature does not appear to be consistently improving, and although an increasing number of healthcare guidelines encourage diversity education, there is little consistency in terms of delivery.

Diversity education has few robust evaluative mechanisms that appropriately capture the experiences of those involved and rarely includes long-term effects on patient outcomes. There is limited evidence to indicate whether the impact of diversity education is known or even being measured (Anderson et al. 2003). This is in part because of the heterogeneity of curriculum designs, which makes evaluation complex. There are no two studies that could evaluate the same diversity education experience (Price et al. 2005), and the lack of uniformity in educational designs makes it challenging to identify specific knowledge, attitudes, and skills, which should be measured.

Furthermore, many of the theoretical frameworks used in diversity teaching in healthcare are challenging to translate into an educational setting. Authors have criticized diversity education for oversimplifying identity, perpetuating categorization, stereotyping, and assuming homogeneity of people within diverse groups (Dogra et al. 2015; Sorensen et al. 2019). In addition, the lack of senior institutional support in establishing diversity curriculums remains an ongoing issue. Institutional buy-in without meaningful commitment runs the risk of enabling tokenistic, politically driven diversity interventions something, which could perpetuate simplistic understandings of diversity issues (George et al. 2015).

This is compounded by the educational philosophy on which higher education bases its understanding of health, illness, and education. Biomedical approaches remain deeply entrenched in healthcare education, which posit the idea of absolute truths and that there are "fixed truths about cultural groups that can be learned" (Dogra et al. 2015, p. 324). Driven by a positivist approach, these fixed truths give the illusion of objectivity through the separation of subject and object. Debates about the complex nature of subject and object, subjectivity, and their relationship to the self are considerable, ongoing, and beyond the remit of this chapter. However, a subject can be defined as an embodied entity (i.e., a human) and is used to differentiate subject from object, where the object is the entity, which is observed (i.e., reality). However, Foucault discusses how the representation of the object, the dynamic nature of the subject, and the influence of power on the relationship between these entities make simplistic categorization of the subject and object problematic (Foucault 1983); as we have seen above, simplistic categorizations can be destructive.

Furthermore, Nicolescu (2014) argues that the separation of subject and object (in this context humans from reality) is artificial, causing simplification and categorization of reality. Therefore, the complexity of the space between the subject and object is something that intersectionality and transdisciplinarity can provide educators and researchers with an opportunity to reconsider.

Intersectional Transdisciplinarity in Healthcare Education: Thinking Beyond Models and Frameworks

Transdisciplinarity: Theory, Application, and Challenges of Using this Concept in Healthcare Education

Transdisciplinarity is often described in relation to research methodologies and sustainability science and was first discussed by social reformers and education scholars in the 1970s, including Piaget. The concept has gone through several periods of popularity and subsequent obscurity, each peak of activity coinciding with sociopolitical events including the end of the cold war, changes in global communication, and climate change (Bernstein 2015). Generally, there appear to be two schools of thought concerning transdisciplinarity. Nicolescu, a theoretical physicist and leading scholar in this area, described it as transcending the constraints of disciplinary silos, thereby enabling people to look beyond the essentialism of subject and object and embrace the philosophical complexity of the space in between these entities (Nicolescu 2002, 2006, 2014). He describes transdisciplinarity as, "That which is at once between the disciplines, across the disciplines and beyond the disciplines ... one of the imperatives is the unity of knowledge" (Nicolescu 2014, p. 187).

Another school of thought emerged at a similar time to Nicolescu and is arguably more practical as it concentrates on directly answering real-world problems using experience across a range of disciplines. Gibbons et al. (1994) worked collaboratively using their "Mode 2" transdisciplinary framework to solve context-specific issues of the day. The Mode 2 framework utilizes a range of transdisciplinary perspectives to formulate key research questions and associated research agendas. Their concept was highly analytical and helped in the establishment of transdisciplinarity in research methodologies and policy production (Bernstein 2015) and is associated with the Zurich approach to transdisciplinarity (Klein et al. 2001).

McGregor (2015) argues that the Zurich approach that emerged from Gibbons et al.'s (1994) work assumes that scientific knowledge creation is the highest in terms of academic value and that a transdisciplinary research approach is designed to use stakeholder expertise to enhance *scientific* knowledge creation. Nicolescu (2014) also argues that Gibbons et al.'s (1994) understanding of transdisciplinarity constrains the approach to the interaction of disciplines within social limits in part because of its concentration on transdisciplinary problem-solving and because it limits understanding of people to within social systems.

Due to the complex nature of this approach, like intersectionality, the term transdisciplinarity is used interchangeably with interdisciplinarity and multi-disciplinarity, which are often ambiguously defined. Choi et al. (Choi and Pak 2006) describe these terms as being on a spectrum of multiple disciplinary approaches with overall aims being to resolve complex issues, create multiple perspectives on issues, and provide excellent healthcare through research and guidelines. However, transdisciplinary approaches do this in a holistic manner, drawing on expertise inside and outside of academia.

Transdisciplinary approaches have been used in healthcare for decades (Kessel and Rosenfield 2008) in areas such as population science, curriculum development, and HIV medicine. However, limitations exist that constrain the use of transdisciplinarity in this context. As Gehlert et al. (2010) discusses, transdisciplinary approaches often represent an ideal as opposed to a reality in medicine and medical research. Challenges in using a transdisciplinary approach include people having to work outside of their comfort zones and conflict between individuals. The value placed on the knowledge created by different collaborating disciplines was also identified as a challenge, as was the rigid nature of higher education and funding structures for individuals and groups. We argue that another challenge with using transdisciplinary approaches in *diversity* education and research is the considerable disagreement that exists within disciplines. If single discipline cannot find agreement (even to disagree) about how to discuss the complexity of diversity and difference, how can we expect those in different disciplines and those outside of the academy to do so either.

Intersectional Transdisciplinarity: An Alternative Approach to Diversity Education

The simultaneous acknowledgment of an intersectional transdisciplinary approach addresses the aforementioned limitations in these two schools of thought. In making this argument, it is not our intention to artificially combine these two concepts in a hope to find a solution to all of the challenges described. Instead, using a range of theories, models, and practical examples, we aim to reconsider difference as both a philosophical and practical issue. We define intersectional transdisciplinarity in diversity education as a way of challenging illusions of stability related to understanding and categorization of difference within human experience. Intersectional transdisciplinarity strives for unity of knowledge about existence that utilizes perspectives from across, between, and beyond disciplines in relation to inequality, inequity, and oppression outside of the constraints of isolated social systems.

Intersectionality and transdisciplinarity are complementary in approach and application. Both consider the complexity of human experience and the multilayered factors that play a part in this multifaceted experience. Both have also been applied to global issues such as social injustice and climate change, respectively. However, the relationship between intersectionality and transdisciplinarity is less linear than it initially appears. Authors have argued that intersectionality is a transdisciplinary theory (Blige 2010), but it is arguably true that intersectionality explores issues within social systems, something which transdisciplinarity would encourage moving beyond (Nicolescu 2014). There have therefore been discussions about the need to reconsider understandings of "systems" within intersectionality and how this reconsideration could apply to the complexity of difference (Walby 2007).

This debate is complex and ever-evolving, and therefore we argue that a theoretically driven combination of these two approaches can enable a reconsideration of difference outside of social limits. We also argue that this could help us rethink assumptions about the space between the subject and object (Nicolescu 2014). This creates the opportunity for transformation: the creation of new theory and methodologies that are borne out of the conflicting and complementary elements of both approaches.

This combination also enables a reconsideration of the self as contiguous with time, space, and place and in so doing re-evaluates the value of co-constructing knowledge using experience spanning history, space, and sociopolitical contexts. This fundamental approach also leaves room for conflict and disagreement and the exploration of inequality within micro, meso, and macro levels in, for instance, higher education institutions. In higher education, both intersectionality and transdisciplinarity also face difficulty with institutional commitment bought about by conflicting educational priorities and challenging funding structures. However, through an intersectional transdisciplinary approach, the individuals involved would represent a range of people, some of whom will be in powerful institutional and political positions, making it more likely that interventions would be valued.

Examples from the healthcare literature illustrating a similar combination of approaches are limited. In one example, Clark et al. (2015) argue that intersectionality and critical reflexivity provide the methodological and theoretical basis on which transdisciplinarity can be developed as a source of knowledge creation in their discipline, addiction research. They discuss the utility of transdisciplinarity for researching "real-world problems," and using examples from their own practice, they illustrate the gaps in care that are made clear when applying this approach, most notably institutional and governmental policy development. How our approach differs from Clark et al. (Clark et al. 2015) is that we include intersectionality and transdisciplinarity within one approach that encompasses all three of ontology, logic, and epistemology (Nicolescu 2014) relating them to the complexity of difference. We argue that this approach needs to include debate, providing a space to discuss uncomfortable issues and through this debate transform our understanding about the issues. With this in mind, our main aim is not knowledge production and transdisciplinary problem-solving but a collaboration that takes all those involved to a new, holistic understanding of the complexity of diversity.

BRAIDE: An Example of Intersectional Transdisciplinary Diversity Education in Medicine

An example of using intersectional transdisciplinarity from our own practice is BRAIDE (Bringing Resources and Awareness In Diversity Education). BRAIDE is an eLearning platform designed to explore diversity with staff and students and feeds into existing diversity curriculum content in the medical degree in our institution. Multimodal teaching approaches were used to challenge the biomedical model and enable those accessing the site to explore and discuss the "self" more generally in relation to diversity.

We worked with collaborators such as BARC (Building the Anti-Racist Classroom (BARC) Collective 2019) using their Student Journey Game. This can be played by both academics and members of professional services staff and has been developed for UK university staff that are committed to or involved in developing interventions that address racial discrimination and inequalities in higher education. The BARC Student Journey Game has been designed in collaboration with BARC artist in residence Maria D'Amico and Student Consultants, specifically the undergraduate students of color leading the Re-imagining Attainment For All 2 (RAFA2), Higher Education Funding Council for England/Office for Students project. The game was commissioned in 2019 by RAFA2 teams based at Queen Mary University of London and University of Roehampton. We also worked with an academic and documentary filmmaker (Fong 2016) to explore the complexity of identity through her film exploring the lives of transgender people in the UK. The film was used as part of face-to-face and self-directed learning sessions, and students were encouraged to discuss their subjective experience of watching and reflecting on the film in a discussion forum on BRAIDE.

As well as forming part of the core curriculum in clinical and communication skills, BRAIDE formed part of a special study component for first-year medical students in our institution. Within this, poetry and conceptual art workshops were used to encourage students to challenge their understanding about diversity. In one workshop, students were asked to use colored ribbons to weave a creative piece as a platform to talk about intersectionality, complexity, subject, and object. Students fed back that this workshop helped them think about diversity in relation to their professional and personal identity and enabled them to relate diversity to themselves, others, and the implications of healthcare inequalities in different contexts.

With internal funding and crucially senior management commitment, we were able to integrate diversity education into our medical curriculum in years 1 and 3. However, internal funding also limited us to using the platform within our institution only. The majority of content development and delivery was therefore undertaken by us as leads for the project, which was challenging with our other professional commitments. Kessel et al. (Kessel and Rosenfield 2008) advocate a "heterarchy" to overcome an overreliance on central researchers, which they define as a flattening out of hierarchical structures that can be used both as an analytical tool and the application of transdisciplinary approaches. To employ heterarchy, they suggest flexibility not just in terms of roles but also methodology and communication between stakeholders.

Another challenge was coordinating a transdisciplinary team and ensuring multiple perspectives on diversity were heard and valued. This was influenced by the support we received during the project, and Kessel et al. (Kessel and Rosenfield 2008) suggest to approach funders that appreciate the complexity of transdisciplinary projects to overcome this. They use the example of the National Institute of Health, discussing guidelines and supportive mechanisms that they have in place to make a transdisciplinary project possible. Therefore, looking forward it will be important to take account of the policy of funders in relation to the unique challenges of intersectional transdisciplinary projects.

Conclusion

We have seen that diversity is a complex term, understandings of which depend on perspective, history, and context. Diversity is a term that is defined by and defines other terms and the way in which these terms interact and influence policy, practice, and curriculum design. We have also seen that there are a multitude of conflicting and complementing theories that demonstrate the complexity of diversity and its impact on stakeholders of higher education and healthcare. Teaching diversity is challenging and needs consideration beyond politically driven, superficial interventions, and the authors argue this necessitates an intersectional transdisciplinary approach.

References

Anderson LM, Scrimshaw SC, Fullilove MT, Fielding JE, Normand J. Task force on community preventive services. Culturally competent healthcare systems: A systematic review. Am J Prev Med. 2003;24(3):68–79.

Bennet MJ. A developmental approach to training for intercultural sensitivity. Int J Intercult Relat. 1986;10(2):179–96.

Bernstein JH. Transdisciplinarity: a review of its origins, developments and current issues. J Res Pract. 2015;11(1):Article R1. http://jrp.icaap.org/index.php/jrp/article/view/510/412. Accessed 6 June 2019.

Betancourt JR, Cervantes MC. Cross cultural medical education in the United States; key principles and experiences. Kaohsiung J Med Sci. 2009;25(9):471–8.

Bhui K, Ascoli M, Nuamh O. The place of race and racism in cultural competence: what can we learn from the English experiences about the narratives of evidence and argument? Transcult Psychiatry. 2012;49(2):185–205.

Blige S. Recent feminist outlooks on intersectionality. Diogenes. 2010;225:58–72.

Bogg D. Values and ethics in mental health practice. In: Brown K, editor. Post qualifying social work practice series. Exeter: Learning Matters; 2010.

Building the Anti-Racist Classroom (BARC) Collective. Student journey game. In: Roehampton University and Queen Mary University of London. Reimagining Attainment for All 2 Project, 2019. https://barcworkshop.org/resources/student-journey-game/. Accessed 12 June 2019.

Butler J. Gender trouble: feminism and the subversion of identity. New York: Routledge; 1990.

Butler J. Undoing gender. New York: Routledge; 2004.

Campina-Bacote J. A model and instrument for addressing cultural competency in health care. J Nurs Educ. 2000;38:203–7.

Canales MK. Othering: difference understood? A 10-year analysis and critique of the nursing literature. Adv Nurs Sci. 2010;33(1):15–34.

Census Data. Office for National Statistics: census data report, United Kingdom. 2017. https://www.ons.gov.uk/census. Accessed 16 June 2019.

Choi BCK, Pak AWP. Multidisciplinarity, interdisciplinarity and transdisciplinarity in health research, services, education and policy. 1: Definitions, objectives, and evidence of effectiveness. Clin Invest Med. 2006;2(9):351–64.

Clark N, Handlooky I, Sinclair D. Using reflexivity to achieve transdisciplinarity in nursing and social work. In: Greaves L, Poole N, Boyle E, editors. Transforming addiction: gender, trauma, transdisciplinarity. London: Routledge; 2015. p. 120–37.

Collins PH. It's all in the family: intersections of gender, race and nation. Hypatia. 1998;13(3):62–82.

Collins PH, Blige S. Intersectionality. Malden: Polity Press; 2016.

Crenshaw K. Mapping the margins: intersectionality, identity politics, and violence against women of color. Stanford Law Rev. 1990;43(6):1241–99.

Cross TL, Bazron BJ, Isaacs MR, Dennis KW. Towards a culturally competent system of care. A monograph on effective services for minority children who are severely emotionally disturbed. Washington, DC: Georgetown University Centre Child Health and Mental Health Policy, CASSP Technical Assistance Center; 1989. http://csmha.umaryland.edu/how/cultural_compe tency_2001. Accessed 16 June 2019.

Crowley-Matoka M, Saha S, Dobscha SK, Burgess DJ. Problems of quality and equity in pain management: exploring the role of biomedical culture. Pain Med. 2009;10(7):1312–24.

Department of Health. Success Measures. In: Equality objectives action plan. 2012. https://www.gov.uk/government/publications/department-of-health-equality-objectives-2012-to-2016. Accessed 16 June 2019.

Dogra N. Cultural competence or cultural sensibility? A comparison of two ideal type models to teach cultural diversity to medical students. Int J Med. 2004;5(4):223–31.

Dogra N, Bhatti F, Ertubey C, Kelly M, Rowlands A, Singh D, Turner M. Teaching diversity to medical undergraduate; curriculum development, delivery and assessment. AMEE guide no. 103. Med Teach. 2015;38(4):323–37.

Duffy ME. A critique of cultural education in nursing. J Adv Nurs. 2001;36(4):487–95.

Fong R. Deconstructing Zoe: performing race. Zapruder World. 2016; 4. http://zapruderworld.org/journal/archive/volume-4/deconstructing-zoe-performing-race/. Accessed 18 June 2019.

Foucault M. The archaeology of knowledge. London: Routledge; 1969.

Foucault M. The birth of the clinic: an archaeology of medical perception. New York: Vintage Books; 1975.

Foucault M. The subject and power. In: Dreyfus H, Rabinow P, editors. Beyond structuralism and hermeneutics. Chicago: The University of Chicago Press; 1983. p. 208–26.

Gehlert S, Murray A, Sohmer D, McClintock M, Conzen S, Olopade O. The importance of transdisciplinary collaborations for understanding and resolving health disparities. Soc Work Public Health. 2010;25(3–4):408–22.

General Medical Council (GMC). Medical students: professional values and fitness to practice. London: General Medical Council; 2009.

George RE. Doctoral thesis: how to better teach and evaluate diversity education in the National Health Service and health educational institutions in the United Kingdom. University of Leicester; 2017. https://ethos.bl.uk/OrderDetails.do?uin=uk.bl.ethos.733702. Accessed 16 June 2019.

George RE, Dogra N, Thornicroft G. Exploration of cultural competency training in UK healthcare settings. A critical interpretive review of the literature. Divers Equal Health Care. 2015;12(3):104–15.

George RE, Haque E, Choudry B. How can we improve health and healthcare experiences of Black, Asian and Minority Ethnic (BAME) communities? In: Tackling healthcare inequalities: a practical guide. CRC Press Taylor and Francis: FL: USA; 2019a.

George RE, Smith K, O'Reily M, Dogra N. Perspectives of patients with mental illness on how to better teach and evaluate diversity education in the National Health Service. J Contin Educ Health Prof. 2019b;39(2):92–102.

Gibbons M, Limoges C, Nowotny H, Schwartzman S, Scott P, Trow M. The new production of knowledge. London: SAGE; 1994.

Hepple B. The new single equality act in Britain. Equal Rights Rev. 2010;5:11–23.

House of Commons Women and Equality Committee. Transgender equality. London: The Stationary Office Limited; 2016.

Howell WS. The empathetic communicator. Belmont: Wadsworth Publishing; 1982.

Hudson-Sharp N, Metcalf H. Inequality among lesbian, gay, bisexual and transgender groups in the UK: a review of evidence. London: NIESR; 2016.

Jeppesen S. Heteronormativity. In: Goldberg AE, editor. The SAGE encyclopedia of LGBTQ studies. Thousand Oaks: SAGE; 2016. p. 493–6.

Kegan R. In over our heads; the mental demands of modern life. Cambridge, MA: Harvard University Press; 1994.

Kessel F, Rosenfield PL. Toward transdisciplinary research: historical and contemporary perspectives. Am J Prev Med. 2008;35(2S):S225–34.

King PM, Baxter Magolda MB. A developmental model of intercultural maturity. J Coll Stud Dev. 2005;46(6):571–92.

Klein JT, Grossenbacher-Mansuy W, Häberli R, Bill A, Scholz R, Welti M. Transdisciplinarity: joint problem solving among science, technology, and society. Berlin: Birkhäuser Verlag; 2001.

Leininger MM. Culture care diversity & universality: a theory of nursing. New York: National League for Nursing Press; 1991.

McGregor SLT. The Nicolescuian and Zurich approaches to transdisciplinarity. Integral Leadersh Rev. 2015;15(2). http://integralleadershipreview.com/13135-616-the-nicolescuian-and-zurich-approaches-to-transdisciplinarity/. Accessed 18 June 2019.

Napier AD, Ancarno C, Butler B, Calabrese J, Chater A, Chatterjee H, Woolf K. Culture and health. Lancet. 2014;384(9954):1607–39. https://doi.org/10.1016/S0140-6736(14)61603-2.

Nicolescu B. Manifesto of transdisciplinarity. New York: SUNY Press; 2002.

Nicolescu B. Transdisciplinarity – past, present and future. In: Haverkroft B, Rejintjes C, editors. Moving world- views – reshaping sciences, policies and practices for endogenous sustainable development. Amsterdam: COMPAS Editions; 2006. p. 142–66.

Nicolescu B. Methodology of transdisciplinarity. J New Paradigm Res. 2014;70(3–4):186–99.

Nunez AE. Transforming cultural competence into cross-cultural efficacy in women's health education. Acad Med. 2000;75:1071–80.

Nursing and Midwifery Council. Prioritise people. In: The code: professional standards of practice and behaviour for nurses and midwives. London: Nursing and Midwifery Council; 2015. https://www.nmc.org.uk/globalassets/sitedocuments/nmc-publications/nmc-code.pdf. Accessed 16 June 2019.

Piaget J. The origins of intelligence in children. New York: International University Press; 1952.

Polaschek NR. Cultural safety: a new concept nursing people of different ethnicities. J Adv Nurs. 1998;27:452–7.

Price E, Beach MC, Gary TL, Robinson KA, Gozu A, Palacio A, Smarth C, Jenckes M, Feuerstein C, Bass EB, Powe N, Cooper LA. A systematic review of the methodological rigor of studies evaluating cultural competence training of health professionals. Acad Med. 2005;80(6):578–86.

Shen Z. Cultural competence models and cultural competence assessment instruments in nursing: A literature review. J Transcult Nurs. 2016;26(3):308–21.

Sorensen J, Norredam M, Surrmond J, Carter-Pokras O, Garcia-Ramirez M, Krasnik A. Need for ensuring cultural competence in medical programmes of European Universities. BMC Med Educ. 2019;19(21):1–8.

Stafford JR, Bowman R, Ewing J, Lopez-De Fede A. Building cultural bridges. Bloomington: National Educational Service; 1997.

Tervalon M, Murray-Garcia J. Cultural humility versus cultural competence: a critical distinction in defining physician training outcomes in multi-cultural education. J HealthCare Poor Underserved. 1998;9:117–25.

Wade DT, Halligan PW. Do biomedical models of illness make for good healthcare systems? BMJ. 2004;329(7479):1398–401.

Walby S. Complexity theory, systems theory, and multiple intersecting social inequalities. Philos Soc Sci. 2007;37:449–70.

Youdell D. Diversity, inequality, and a post-structural politics for education. Discourse: Stud Cult Polit Educ. 2006;27(1):33–42.

Planetary Health: Educating the Current and Future Health Workforce

44

Michelle McLean, Lynne Madden, Janie Maxwell,
Patricia Nanya Schwerdtle, Janet Richardson, Judith Singleton,
Kristen MacKenzie-Shalders, Georgia Behrens, Nick Cooling,
Richard Matthews, and Graeme Horton

> *Health professionals have leading roles to play in addressing
> climate change ... The pervasive threats to health posed by
> climate change demand decisive actions from health
> professionals and governments to protect the health of current
> and future generations.*
> *Haines and Ebi (2019, p. 271)*

Contents

Introduction: A Changing Planet and the Impact on Human Health	817
Recognizing the "Environment" as a Determinant of Health	818
Planetary Health Becoming Mainstream	819
Health Professionals' Roles	820
Environmental Footprint of Health Care	821
Responding to the Challenges: Preparing the Current and Future Health Workforce	821

M. McLean (✉) · R. Matthews
Faculty of Health Sciences & Medicine, Bond University, Gold Coast, QLD, Australia
e-mail: mimclean@bond.edu.au; rmatthew@bond.edu.au

L. Madden · G. Behrens
School of Medicine, Sydney, University of Notre Dame, Sydney, NSW, Australia
e-mail: lynne.madden@nd.edu.au; georgia.behrens@my.nd.edu.au

J. Maxwell
Nossal Institute of Global Health, University of Melbourne, Melbourne, VIC, Australia
e-mail: jane.maxwell@unimelb.edu.au

P. N. Schwerdtle
Nursing and Midwifery, Faculty of Medicine, Nursing and Health Sciences, Monash University Melbourne, Melbourne, VIC, Australia

Institute of Global Health, Heidelberg University, Heidelberg, Germany
e-mail: patricia.schwerdtle@monash.edu

J. Richardson
School of Nursing and Midwifery, University of Plymouth, Plymouth, UK

© Springer Nature Singapore Pte Ltd. 2023
D. Nestel et al. (eds.), *Clinical Education for the Health Professions*,
https://doi.org/10.1007/978-981-15-3344-0_121

International Action 822
    Professional Organizations and Associations 822
    Medical Student Organizations 823
National Action 823
    Professional Bodies 823
    Accreditation Standards 823
    Student Associations 824
Higher Education Action: Health Professions Education 825
From Theory to Practice: Case Studies from Medicine, Nursing, Pharmacy and Dietetics:
Integrating Planetary Health and Sustainability into Health Professions Education 827
Conclusions 833
Cross-References 834
Appendix 1. Position Statements and Declarations From National Health Professional
Organizations and Postgraduate Medical Colleges 834
    National Professional Bodies 834
    Postgraduate Medical Colleges 834
Appendix 2. International and Country-Based Organizations Providing Resources and/or
Case Studies Relating to Sustainability in Health Care and Health Care Education
(Alphabetical) 836
Appendix 3. Features of an Environmentally Accountable Medical School (Applicable to All
Health Professions) (Boelen et al. 2016) 839
Appendix 4. Ethical Framework (With Questions) Relating to Large Infrastructural
Projects 840
References 841

Abstract

Human health and well-being are inextricably linked to the environment, but human development in Western countries has been at the expense of the natural environment, largely through our reliance on fossil fuels. As we may have already reached "tipping points" in terms of some global environmental changes (e.g., climate change, biodiversity loss, air pollution), threatening human health and well-being, health professionals must respond urgently through mitigation, adaptation, and advocacy. Many are, however, not sufficiently informed to feel

---

J. Singleton
School of Clinical Sciences (Pharmacy), Faculty of Health, Queensland University of Technology, Brisbane, QLD, Australia
e-mail: judith.singleton@qut.edu.au

K. MacKenzie-Shalders
Master of Nutrition & Dietetic Practice, Faculty of Health Sciences & Medicine, Bond University, Gold Coast, QLD, Australia
e-mail: kmackenz@bond.edu.au

N. Cooling
School of Medicine, College of Health & Medicine, University of Tasmania, Hobart, TAS, Australia
e-mail: nick.cooling@utas.edu.au

G. Horton
Faculty of Health and Medicine, University of Newcastle, Newcastle, NSW, Australia
e-mail: graeme.horton@newcastle.edu.au

44 Planetary Health: Educating the Current and Future Health Workforce

confident to do so. There is thus an imperative to upskill and educate practicing health professionals and current health professional students to practice environmentally sustainable health care and to take action to protect the environment to ensure human health. This chapter sets the scene in terms of the importance of the environmental determinants of health for individuals and for populations. It also provides health professionals and health professions educators with a resource list and case studies to guide the integration of planetary health and sustainable health care into the curriculum.

> **Keywords**
>
> Environmental determinants of health · Planetary health · Climate change · Global environmental changes · Environmentally sustainable health care · Health professions education

Introduction: A Changing Planet and the Impact on Human Health

The burning of fossil fuels such as coal, oil, and gas has led to a steady rise in the average global temperature (*global warming*) through the generation of greenhouse gases (GHGs), and with this, an increase in the frequency of extreme weather events such as heat waves, cyclones, and floods. Over the past decade, the global health risks associated with climate change such as heat stress, vector-borne diseases, and threatened food and water security have been well documented (Whitmee et al. 2015; Myers 2017; Intergovernmental Panel on Climate Change (IPCC) 2018; Ebi et al. 2018; Watts et al. 2018; Haines and Ebi 2019), with Haines and Ebi (2019) in particular providing a comprehensive guide to the health risks individuals are likely to experience (https://www.nejm.org/doi/full/10.1056/NEJMra1807873).

While Costello and colleagues (2009) warned that the impact of climate change on human health could potentially reverse the health gains of the last 50 years, Whitmee and colleagues (2015) viewed responding to climate change as a health opportunity – "*Given the potential of climate change to reverse the health gains from economic development, and the health co-benefits that accrue from actions for a sustainable economy, tackling climate change could be the greatest global health opportunity of this century*" (p. 1861). The authors, however, highlighted the need for urgent action, noting that the health care professions were only just *beginning to rise* to the challenge. While almost all countries have committed to reduce carbon emissions and limit temperature increase to 2 °C but preferably 1.5 °C (United Nations Climate Change Paris Agreement 2015), the transition to a low carbon economy has been slow. The 2018 *Lancet* Countdown Report paints a bleak picture, concluding that trends in climate change impact, exposure, and vulnerabilities indicate a high risk for the current and future health of all populations as well as threatening the viability of national health systems (Watts et al. 2018). Authors of the

2019 Countdown Report concluded that the published indicators suggest that warming is happening more rapidly than governments are able or willing to respond, with opportunities being missed. They have advocated for bold new approaches in terms of policy, research, and business to change course, stating that it will require all 7.5 billion people on the planet to ensure that a child born today is not defined by climate change (Watts et al. 2019).

Climate change is but one of several global environmental changes (GECs) impacting human health. In addition to climate change, planetary boundaries relating to the Earth's finite resources that may have already been crossed include biodiversity loss and disruption to the global nitrogen cycle (Rockström et al. 2009; Gupta et al. 2019), while changing patterns of land use, fresh water depletion, ocean acidification, stratospheric ozone depletion, atmospheric aerosol loading, and chemical and other forms of pollution continue to place pressures on the environment and its capacity to support human life (Prüss-Ustün et al. 2016; Myers 2017; United Nations Environment Program (UNEP) 2019; Frumkin and Haines 2019; Haines and Ebi 2019; Tong and Ebi 2019; Gupta et al. 2019).

The World Health Organization (2016) estimates that 23% of all annual global deaths (approximately 12.6 million) are linked to environmental risks such as air, water, and soil pollution, chemical exposure, climate change, and ultraviolet radiation. "*Air pollution and climate change*" topped the WHO's 2019 list of global threats to human health (WHO 2019). Particulate matter from burning fossil fuels compromises the health of millions of people, with death caused by poor air quality highest in low- and middle-income countries (Prüss-Ustün et al. 2016; Myers 2017; Cohen et al. 2017; Watts et al. 2018; Frumkin and Haines 2019; Gupta et al. 2019). In addition, the Health Effects Institute (2019) estimates that 93% of the world's children under the age of 15 years breathe air that endangers their health and places them at serious risk of death.

Recognizing the "Environment" as a Determinant of Health

Although framed within the context of urban planning, Barton and Grant's (2006) *Settlement Health* Map, modified from Dahlgren and Whitehead's (1991) "main determinants of health" model, captures the overarching importance of the global ecosystem on human health and well-being (Fig. 1). As health and well-being are inextricably linked to a healthy planet, intact ecosystems, clean air, and a stable climate are important determinants of individual and population health. Since the industrial revolution, however, improvement in the social determinants of health (i.e., the conditions under which we are born, grow, work, live, and age) in Western countries has been at the expense of our natural environment (Whitmee et al. 2015; Myers 2017; Frumkin and Haines 2019):

> ... we have been mortgaging the health of future generations to realise economic and development gains in the present. By unsustainably exploiting nature's resources, human civilisation has flourished but now risks substantial health effects from the degradation of nature's life support systems in the future. (Whitmee et al. 2015, p. 1973)

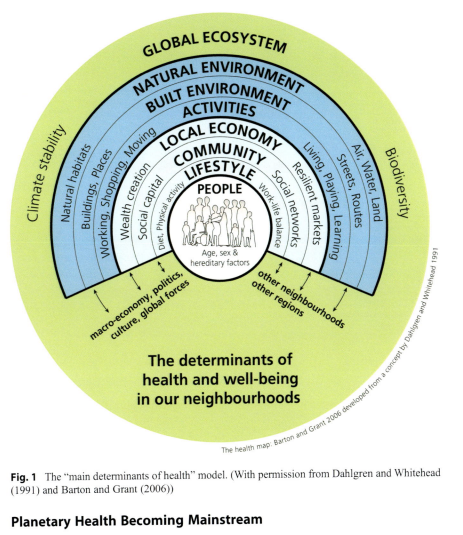

Fig. 1 The "main determinants of health" model. (With permission from Dahlgren and Whitehead (1991) and Barton and Grant (2006))

Planetary Health Becoming Mainstream

To safeguard the health and well-being of current and future generations, it is essential to protect the natural environment (Rockström et al. 2009; Whitmee et al. 2015; Prüss-Ustün et al. 2016; Myers 2017; Gupta et al. 2019). The United Nations (UN), through the 2030 Sustainable Development Goals (SDGs), recognizes the need to protect the planet to ensure that all people can enjoy a healthy future (Fig. 2).

Considering the link between a healthy environment and human health, planetary health is now becoming mainstream (Horton et al. 2014; Horton and Lo 2015; Horton 2016; Whitmee et al. 2015; Myers 2017; Capon et al. 2018; Prescott et al. 2018). Recent planetary health contributions include the following:

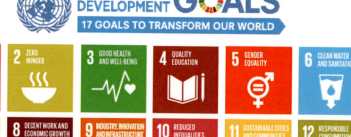
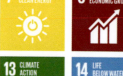

Fig. 2 The UN 2030 Sustainable Development Goals (http://www.un.org/sustainabledevelopment/sustainable-development-goals/)

- **2015:** Described as "*the achievement of the highest attainable standard of health, wellbeing, and equity worldwide through judicious attention to the human systems – political, economic, and social – that shape the future of humanity and the Earth's natural systems that define the safe environmental limits within which humanity can flourish. Put simply, planetary health is the health of human civilization and the state of the natural systems on which it depends.*" (Whitmee et al. 2015, p. 1978).
- **2017:** *Lancet Planetary Health* and an infographic website launched to promote inquiry into sustainable human civilizations at a time when humankind faces unprecedented dangers and threats such as poverty, malnutrition, fresh water contamination, industrialization, population growth, inequities, urbanization, climate change, declining ocean health, unsustainable land use, war, conflict, and social injustice: https://www.thelancet.com/infographics/planetary-health.
- **2017:** The University of Sydney developed a Planetary Health platform: https://sydney.edu.au/research/centres/planetary-health-platform.html.
- **2018**: The Canmore Declaration: Statement of Principles for Planetary Health published (Prescott et al. 2018).

Health Professionals' Roles

As frontline witnesses to the toll of climate change (and other GECs) on the health of individuals and communities, health professionals are ideally positioned to advocate for collective action to protect the environment to ensure the health and well-being of current and future generations. Health professionals have thus been urged to take a lead in tackling the current and future health challenges (e.g., through mitigation, adaptation, and advocacy) caused by a changing climate and disruptions to the natural environment (Mortimer 2010; Ramanathan and Haines 2016; Capon et al. 2018; Kreslake et al. 2018; Watts et al. 2018; Singleton 2019; Haines and Ebi 2019; Clark 2019; Shelton et al. 2019). The need for action is urgent as we approach (and may already have exceeded) environmental "tipping" points beyond which damage is irreversible (Rockström et al. 2009; Gupta et al. 2019). In some contexts, health professionals may also need to be the "voice" of the marginalized, vulnerable, or disempowered, such as Indigenous populations, children, women, and the elderly, who are often at greatest risk (Myers 2017; Kreslake et al. 2018; Tong and Ebi 2019).

Environmental Footprint of Health Care

Health care is a contributor to climate change and environmental degradation as it has a relatively large footprint in terms of resource usage, GHG emissions, and waste (McGain and Naylor 2014; Eckelman and Sherman 2016; Pencheon 2018; Malik et al. 2018; Pichler et al. 2019; Shelton et al. 2019; Health Care Without Harm/ ARUP 2019). Australia's healthcare services, for example, contribute 7% of the national carbon emissions (Malik et al. 2018). The UK's National Health Service (NHS) has demonstrated that a health system can reduce its environmental footprint and is currently on track to become carbon neutral by the earliest possible point in line with the UK's 2008 National Climate Change Act. Between 2007 and 2017, the NHS reduced its carbon emissions by 18.5%, water usage by 21%, and diverted 85% of waste from landfill despite some NHS activity indicators increasing by 27.5% (Pencheon 2018; Sustainable Development Unit 2018). A concomitant £90 million annual financial savings was reported, mainly in terms of energy, waste, and water (SDU 2018). For the health care sector to reduce its carbon emissions to zero within 30 years requires a more sustainable service delivery (Charlesworth and Jamieson 2017, 2018; Coughlin et al. 2018). Well-informed, proactive, and committed health professionals are vital to achieve the transition to sustainable practice.

Responding to the Challenges: Preparing the Current and Future Health Workforce

As physicians (and other health professionals) are *"society's go-betweens"* (Gómez et al. 2013, p. 169) and because they hold public trust, they are well placed to educate their patients and society about the environment and health (Gómez et al. 2013; Myers 2017). Many health practitioners are, however, not sufficiently informed and are unprepared for this role (Charlesworth et al. 2012; Purcell and McGirr 2014, 2018; Hathaway and Maibach 2018).

Developing a more informed and proactive current and future health workforce should thus be a priority. In the next section, we describe the response and actions of various health professions education stakeholders (e.g., professional bodies, students, health professionals, educators) both internationally and in some countries to prepare the health workforce to meet the health challenges of a changing planet as well as mitigate further environmental degradation and warming. Further information is available in Appendix 1, while Appendix 2 lists a range of organizations offering resources and/or supportive membership.

International Action

Many health professionals and health professional students and their representative organizations and associations have taken a stand on environmental issues that impact on human health. An example of a global health professional call to action was the Consensus Statement *Doctors for Climate Action* initiated by the Royal Australasian College of Physicians (RACP) immediately prior to the 2015 Conference of the Parties 21 (COP21) in Paris. This Statement was signed by 68 health, medical, and student organizations and 1500 individual health professionals from 46 countries (https://www.racp.edu.au/docs/default-source/advocacy-library/pa-dfca-global-consensus-statement.pdf?sfvrsn=1a6d311a_12). Another example is the September 2018 call to action on climate change by five million doctors, nurses, and public health professionals and 17,000 hospitals in 120 countries prior to COP24 (WHO 2018).

Examples of position statements and declarations from international professional and student organizations and associations are listed below. They highlight the urgent need for health practitioners to become more informed and to practice environmentally sustainable health care.

Professional Organizations and Associations

- *World Organisation of Family Doctors (WONCA):* Declaration calling for family doctors of the world to act on planetary health: https://www.wonca.net/site/DefaultSite/filesystem/documents/Groups/Environment/2019%20Planetary%20health.pdf
- *World Medical Association (WMA):* World Medical Association Resolution on Climate Emergency: https://www.wma.net/policies-post/wma-resolution-on-climate-emergency/
- *International Council of Nurses (ICN):* Position statement: Nurses, climate change and health: https://www.icn.ch/sites/default/files/inline-files/ICN%20PS%20Nurses%252c%20climate%20change%20and%20health%20FINAL%20.pdf
- *International Pharmaceutical Federation (FIP):* Position statement: Environmentally sustainable pharmacy practice: Green pharmacy: https://www.fip.org/file/1535

Medical Student Organizations

The International Federation of Medical Students' Associations (IFMSA), which represents 1.3 million medical students, has been active in advocating for action on climate change:

- Student Climate Change and Health Training manual with WHO support (2016): https://ifmsa.org/wp-content/uploads/2017/03/Final-IFMSA-Climate-and-health-training-Manual-2016.pdf.
- Climate Change and Health Policy (2018). https://ifmsa.org/wp-content/uploads/2018/09/GS_AM2018_Policy_Climate-Change-and-Health_final.pdf.
- 2020 Vision for Climate Health in Medical Curricula document, calling on all medical schools to include an element of climate health in their curricula by 2020 and to integrate climate health in all aspects of medical school life by 2025. A Working Group is formulating a Climate Change and Health Education Framework to equip its members with tools to implement this 2020 vision, in addition to creating an Assessment Scorecard for members to score their medical universities in terms of climate change and health education (https://phreportcard.org/our-metrics/).

National Action

At a national level, drivers of change influencing education, training, and practice in the health professions include professional bodies, accreditation standards, postgraduate colleges, health professions educators, and students.

Professional Bodies

National professional bodies such as the Australian Medical Association (AMA) and postgraduate medical colleges such as the UK's Academy of Medical Royal Colleges (AMRC) and the Council of Presidents of Medical Colleges in Australia have published position statements and declarations (Appendix 1). Recent ones include the AMA's 2019 Position Statement on *Environmental Sustainability* and the 2019 Royal Australasian College of General Practitioners' *Climate change and human health* Position Statement.

Accreditation Standards

Despite these declarations and position statements, health professional education providers have been slow to incorporate planetary health and environmentally sustainable health care concepts into curricula. Introducing these into accreditation standards for the regulated health professions is a systematic way to achieve change as courses and their education providers must meet these standards. For example, the accreditation standards for primary medical programs as Graduate Outcome Statements (GOSs) are published in the UK by the General Medical Council (GMC) and in Australasia by the Australian Medical Council (AMC). The GOSs establish what medical students "must know and be able to do" at graduation:

- *GMC (UK):* By the summer of 2020, all UK medical schools must ensure that graduating doctors are able to apply the principles of sustainable health care to their practice through Graduate Outcome 25 – *"Newly qualified doctors must be able to apply the principles, methods and knowledge of population health and the improvement of health and sustainable healthcare to medical practice."* An example of a learning objective for this Outcome is: *"They must be able to c) evaluate the environmental, social, behavioural and cultural factors which influence health and disease in different populations"* (GMC 2018).
- *AMC (Australasia):* Current accreditation standards and GOSs for medical programs in Australasia do not reference climate change, planetary health, or environmentally sustainable health care. Consequently, in 2016, the Medical Deans of Australia and New Zealand (MDANZ), the peak body for professional medical education in Australia and New Zealand, commissioned a Climate Change and Health Working Group to collaboratively develop learning objectives and curriculum resources (Madden et al. 2018). Proposed amendments to the AMC GOSs (with Learning Objectives) were circulated to all medical schools in 2018. This work will also inform a forthcoming review of AMC Accreditation Standards.

Student Associations

National student associations are influencing the direction of health professions education (Tun 2019). The Australian Medical Students' Association (AMSA) has developed several resources and called for all Australian medical school curricula to include the impacts of climate change (Behrens et al. 2018). Students for Global Health UK has also called on its members to campaign for greater inclusion of planetary health and air pollution in medicine and health sciences curricula. The New Zealand Medical Students' Association (NZMSA), with nine other New Zealand Health Students' Associations, independently made a submission to their Government relating to the 2019 Zero Carbon Bill Amendment. The Canadian Federation of Medical Students (CFMS), through its Health and Environment Adaptive Task Force, are developing core environmental health competencies for Canadian medical curricula (Hackett et al. 2020).

Medical student resources include:

- **AMSA:** Online climate change and health short course (text): https://docs. google.com/document/d/1YTVuk8IKGphi0oOFd1TeEhltGEAU_UUiV_NmX cGHgyM/edit

- **AMSA:** Sustainable events guide: https://amsa.org.au/blog/amsa-sustainable-events-guide
- **NZMSA:** Position statement on climate change: https://docs.google.com/document/d/1l_qog9T5IDM4e2zLGtKuyysDT9AcawSs8vy_tSbwB8M/edit
- **CFMS:** Planetary Health competencies for Canadian medical students: https://www.cfms.org/what-we-do/global-health/heart-competencies.html and https://www.cfms.org/what-we-do/global-health/heart.html

Students in other health professions have also been active. For example, a recent American National Student Nurses Association conference unanimously accepted a resolution entitled *Increased Nursing Student Action on and Awareness of the Effects of Climate Change on Health* (Jackman-Murphy et al. 2018).

Higher Education Action: Health Professions Education

Although accreditation bodies overseeing health professions education have been slow to incorporate sustainability into accreditation standards, concerned health professions educators have identified learning outcomes and activities, for example, Gómez et al. (2013), Walpole and colleagues (2016, 2017, 2019), Maxwell and Blashki (2016), Grose et al. (2017), Teherani et al. (2017), Wellbery et al. (2018), and Singleton (2019).

Ideally, *environmental accountability* should be included in the health professions school and college mission statements and activities (Boelen et al. 2016; Walpole et al. 2017). In a 2016 Association for Medical Education in Europe (AMEE) Guide on socially accountable medical schools, Boelen and colleagues wrote under *Future Challenges* that "*Foremost amongst the global priorities is the threat to the planet from environmental changes, including but not limited to our climate*" (p. 1087; Appendix 3). Many of these principles have now been included in AMEE's ASPIRE Awards criteria for Social Accountability Excellence (https://aspire-to-excellence.org/Areas+of+Excellence/).

In the next section, we present case studies, mainly from Australia, showcasing how different health professions are incorporating, planetary health and environmental sustainability in their curricula. We would, however, like to offer some initial guidance in the form of Schwerdtle and colleagues' (2019) tips relating to the *Why? What?* and *How?* of integrating environmental sustainability into health professional programs (Table 1).

In addition, Tun's (2019) recent research has identified enablers and barriers with respect to this integration. Enablers included:

- Demand from students
- International momentum in higher education to include sustainability in training

Table 1 Twelve tips for embedding environmental sustainability in health professions curricula (Schwerdtle et al. 2019)

Steps	Tips
Why?	1. Highlight the role of health professionals and the urgency to act while contextualizing climate change in the broader field of planetary health 2. Connect environmental sustainability content to broader education and professional practice objectives
What?	3. Prepare students for the health impacts of climate change by exploring adaptation and mitigation strategies 4. Inspire students with the health co-benefits of mitigation 5. Embrace broad conceptualizations of professionalism by incorporating environmental ethics, advocacy, and leadership 6. Expand the biomedical approach to health by routinely incorporating environmental determinants of health in sessions
How?	7. Collaborate through sharing resources, publishing and evaluating interventions 8. Prioritize content for local relevance and professional utility 9. Integrate environmental sustainability into the core curriculum with increasing complexity and reinforcement throughout the course 10. Instill knowledge, skills, and attitudes about environmental sustainability 11. Assess students using formative, portfolio-based, and student-led tasks that promote reflection 12. Strive for progress with positivity and persistence

- A new accreditation legitimacy, for example, the GMC mandate for all medical curricula
- Leadership from other stakeholders such as postgraduate colleges which might already require students and trainees to manage resources and minimize waste in clinical practice

Barriers included:

- A shortage of educators who are sufficiently knowledgeable about sustainable health care
- An already overcrowded curriculum
- Uncertainty about where to introduce sustainability into the curriculum
- Need for learning resources
- Difficulty assessing the associated learning
- The emotional impact which requires resilience, that is, sustainability is complex and emotional and so training and support is required to maintain a positive outlook.

Finally, the 2030 Sustainable Development Goals (SDGs) provide a framework for integrating sustainability into health professions curricula. Increasingly, universities are becoming signatories to the SDGs, often in line with a strengthening of their social (and environmental) accountability (http://sdg.iisd.org/news/reports-focus-on-role-of-universities-in-achieving-sdgs/). In April 2019, the *Times Higher Education* (*THE*) published its first-ever University Impact Ratings to recognize institutions tackling global issues based on how universities committed to 11 of the 17 SDGs (https://www.timeshighereducation.com/student/best-universities/top-universities-world-global-impact).

From Theory to Practice: Case Studies from Medicine, Nursing, Pharmacy and Dietetics: Integrating Planetary Health and Sustainability into Health Professions Education

This section begins with a case study describing how Australian medical college staff and students' personal experiences of recent catastrophic bushfires and floods stimulated additional climate change and sustainability inclusions in the curriculum.

University of Tasmania (Australia) – Preparing medical students for climate-induced disasters (Nick Cooling)

Why is it important? Personal experiences of the 2018 Tasmania floods and 2019 bushfires prompted students to reflect on the causes and effects of these extreme environmental events.

What was done? Using a "students as partners" approach, the existing education program on sustainability across the five-year undergraduate curriculum was reviewed. Already in place was an integrated lecture and workshop series (biodiversity, sustainable health care, public health, global health, planetary health) supplemented by optional capstone experiences including research projects, international electives, peer to peer online learning with international partner medical schools (e.g., Nusa Cendana University, Indonesia) and participation with non-governmental groups such as Doctors for the Environment, Fossil Free Tasmania, IMPACT and The ISSUE Foundation. Curriculum reform in partnership with students included additional sessions by external community activists, integration with the AMC's *Health & Society* theme, and integrating sustainability into the clinical consultation.

Outcomes: Students became more aware that vulnerable individuals suffer the most, compounding existing poverty, mental health, or marginalization. They also developed skills in advocacy and activism and learnt ways to bring about change in macro- (the community) and micro- (the consultation) contexts. Examples of student "activism" include:

- Political lobbying, for example, fossil fuel divestment by the university (Years 1–2)
- Creating patient education tools explaining climate change (Year 3)
- Student-led curriculum reform in climate change (Year 3)
- Responding to natural disasters, for example, floods and bushfires (Year 3)
- Implementing an equipment reuse and recycling program in the teaching hospital (Years 3–5)
- Undertaking research projects with aerobiology, climate change, and ocean sustainability groups (Years 4–5)

Table 2 Two case studies showcasing integration of sustainability at a curriculum level. Medicine and nursing

	Medicine: *Bond University (Australia) – Integrating planetary health and sustainable health care into the undergraduate medical program (Michelle McLean)*	**Nursing:** *University of Plymouth (UK) – Integrating sustainability into the Nursing and Midwifery curriculum (Janet Richardson)*
Why is it important?	Medical students have a responsibility to reduce the environmental footprint of health care by practicing sustainability individually and professionally	Sustainability education needs to be relevant to clinical practice
What was done?	1. *Years 1–2:* Problem-based learning cases reviewed and, where appropriate, a non-drug intervention added using the RACGPs' evidence-based Handbook of Non-Drug Interventions: HANDI – https://www.racgp.org.au/clinical-resources/clinical-guidelines/handbook-of-non-drug-interventions-handi. HANDI also included in the Year 3 and Year 5 General Practice syllabus 2. *Year 2:* Over several weeks, students engage in a series of activities incorporating Global Health, Planetary Health and sustainable health care: *Presentations:* Groups of 8–9 students present key definitions and concepts, e.g., 2030 UN SDGs, epidemic, pandemic, syndemic, etc. Presentations become student resources *Workshop:* Students identify historic, current, and future health issues globally and locally. Climate change is identified as a current health issue which is then discussed, including the environmental footprint of health care *Assignment:* Using the 2030 SDGs (SDG13 + others), teams of 4–5 students identify a "problem" impacting on health and well-being, submit a proposal, receive feedback, then work on their "product" for about five weeks *Conference:* Best 6–8 "products" selected by faculty assessors invited to present. Cohort selects "People's Choice" winners. Certificates and environmentally sustainable prizes awarded	A scenario-based learning approach to integrating sustainability, climate change, and health into the nursing and midwifery undergraduate curriculum: *Year 1:* Importance of climate change and nursing practice introduced through a case study supported by readings and resources. In a family with a child suffering from asthma (providing links to air pollution), a pregnant mother who goes into labor and is unable to reach the hospital due to flooding. She suffers renal failure and her care is compromised as an earthquake disrupts the supply of essential renal consumables *Year 2:* Students explore resources used and the manufacture of common clinical items made from potentially scarce (or energy-intensive and environmentally damaging) natural resources (e.g., oil and cotton). To encourage an interdisciplinary approach, product design students participate, providing opportunities for innovative discussion about possible solutions to challenges health practitioners will face when items such as plastic intravenous infusions sets are no longer available. Waste management and recycling using research evidence involving financial and environmental costs of hospital waste are also discussed. *Resource:* https://www.youtube.com/watch?v=zlFT2Dbg08o *Year 3:* In a public health module, students explore a scenario of an *Escherichia coli* outbreak linked to a heat wave, followed by excessive rain

(continued)

44 Planetary Health: Educating the Current and Future Health Workforce

Table 2 (continued)

	Medicine: *Bond University (Australia) – Integrating planetary health and sustainable health care into the undergraduate medical program (Michelle McLean)*	**Nursing:** *University of Plymouth (UK) – Integrating sustainability into the Nursing and Midwifery curriculum (Janet Richardson)*
		causing run-off from agricultural land adjacent to an estuary *Year 3:* In the leadership and management module, students complete a "green ward challenge," discussing how they can use resources and manage waste more sustainably. They also consider opportunities for promoting the health co-benefits of living more sustainably, e.g., how eating less meat is good for the environment and reduces heart disease and stroke and the dual health and environmental benefits of exercising and hence less driving *Year 3:* Final year student projects address the sustainability implications of their research, competing for the sustainability prize
What are/ were the outcomes?	Well received. This is work in progress as curriculum coordinators and leads work to integrate additional sessions into the five-year program	Evaluation suggests that these educational interventions changed awareness and knowledge of sustainability in nurse education and clinical practice. Several alumni are making significant changes in their workplace practice

Below, in Tables 2 and 3, we offer a series of case studies showcasing the inclusion of planetary health and sustainability into medical, nursing, pharmacy, and dietetics curricula. Table 4 then presents two examples of how the ethics relating to climate change and environmental issues and health can be incorporated into the curriculum.

These case studies all reflect a uni-professional approach to integrating planetary health and sustainability into the curriculum. We recognize, however, that the delivery of environmentally sustainable health care benefits from an interprofessional approach (Grose et al. 2017). A starting point for planning interprofessional learning opportunities would be to use one or more of Stone and colleagues' (2018) twelve cross-cutting (transdisciplinary) principles for planetary health education, e.g. (1) a planetary health lens, (2) urgency and scale, (3) policy, (4) organizing and movement-building, (5) communication, and (6) systems thinking

Table 3 Case studies showcasing integration of sustainability at a curriculum level: Pharmacy and dietetics

	Pharmacy: *Queensland University of Technology (Australia) – Integrating sustainability in the Bachelor of Pharmacy (Hons) curriculum (Judith Singleton)*	**Dietetics:** *Bond University (Australia) – Integrating sustainability in the Masters of Dietetics (Kristen MacKenzie-Shalders)*
Why is it important?	The pharmaceutical industry is responsible for about 19% of Australia's health care carbon footprint (Malik et al. 2018). Pharmacists thus have a moral obligation to deliver more sustainable pharmaceutical practice. As the International Pharmaceutical Federation (2015) states that pharmacists have a responsibility to minimize the environmental impact of pharmaceuticals, the "One Health" approach involves educating future pharmacists to be "green"	Several 2030 SDGs relate to our food system. Bond University dietitians recognize the need for dietary goals that promote environmental sustainability
What was done?	Environmental aspects of pharmaceutical care included across the four-year degree using the 2030 SDG framework. Highlights include: *Year 2:* Sustainability concepts introduced in depth in the *"Quality Use of Medicines"* (QUM) subject. QUM is a key objective of Australia's National Medicines Policy, which aims to optimize treatment options judiciously, appropriately, safely and efficaciously (Australian Government 2000). By considering first if a medicine is required (judicious), then ensuring the patient receives the appropriate dose (appropriate), medicine waste and medicines entering the environment may be reduced, aligning with sustainability principles. Students also learn about entry pathways of pharmaceuticals into the environment, appropriate disposal of unwanted pharmaceuticals, including the federally funded take-back program for unwanted pharmaceuticals, the Return Unwanted Medicines (RUM) program (Australian Government, National Return & Disposal of Unwanted Medicines Limited 2019).	Several sustainability activities introduced in a two-year Master of Nutrition and Dietetic Practice: *Visit:* Farmers' market and supermarket. Activities include completing a food miles activity to compare transit requirements between local and international produce, completing a related pricing activity and questions related to the transparency of packaging on the environmental cost of the food and discussing the concept of Food Citizenship *Visit:* Commercial farm, followed by a workshop and debate exploring "paddock to plate" concepts and principles of organic farming compared with conventional farming practices *Cooking exercise:* Learn core culinary/food literacy skills in *"Nutrition and Food Science"* workshops *Visit:* Local hospital with a Room-Service-on-Demand food service system; complete additional learning activities related to the benefits, e.g., model minimizes plate and production waste and as a cook-fresh system, there is more capacity to decrease packaging, tailor the menu to be more sustainable and shop locally *Lecture and workshop:* Future of food and environmental sustainability in *"Nutrition Issues and Priorities."*

(continued)

44 Planetary Health: Educating the Current and Future Health Workforce

Table 3 (continued)

	These principles are embedded across all patient-integrated care subjects in the degree. *Year 4:* Students introduced to sustainable business practices in the Business Management subject, highlighting that sustainable practices can have health and financial co-benefits	*Workshop: "Food Service Dietetics"* provides a global context for environmental sustainability in food service, the practicality of applying core food sustainability principles in a commercial foodservice, assessment of sustainable recommendations to a rural hospital *Food service placements:* Explore issues related to environmental sustainability, e. g., measuring plate and production waste, recycling practices, conducting a needs assessment related to environmental sustainability for placement sites. Findings communicated to key stakeholders and other students *Readings:* Environmental sustainability in dietetics
What are/ were the outcomes?	Although specific outcomes have not been measured, assessment relating to sustainability includes summative online quizzes and sustainability considerations in their Year 4 business management assignment	Ninety-five percent of students were confident or very confident to make dietary recommendations regarding environmental sustainability, 100% believed sustainability should be within a dietitian's scope of practice, and 100% agreed that sustainability is a global issue that needs to be addressed

and transdisciplinary collaborations, etc. The next case study presents an Australian example of cross-disciplinary collaborative research to investigate the integration of sustainability across several health professions.

Monash University (Australia) – Researching the feasibility of integrating sustainability into the Nursing and Midwifery curriculum: From a uni-professional to a multiprofessional approach (Patricia Nayna Schwerdtle)

Why is this important? Health care practitioners work in multiprofessional teams and, as sustainable health care is the responsibility of all health professionals, it makes sense that health professional students learn together about sustainability.

What was done previously? In Nursing and Midwifery, environmental sustainability, the health impacts of climate change, and the role of nurses and midwives in terms of mitigation, advocacy, and adaptation were integrated into an undergraduate global health module (i.e., a uni-professional approach).

What is currently being done? An interdisciplinary research study is underway to explore factors that influence the capacity to provide environmental sustainability and climate change education across 12 health professions. The mixed methods approach involves an online survey, followed by a facilitated "hackathon" to illuminate challenges and opportunities. Actionable recommendations will inform the Faculty of Medicine, Nursing and Health Sciences' proposal for interdisciplinary learning.

Table 4 Ethics case studies in medicine

	Notre Dame University (Australia) – Ethics of climate change (Lynne Madden)	*Bond University (Australia) – An ethical framework for exploring the consequences of large infrastructural projects (Richard Matthews)*
Why is it important?	Health care delivery in high income countries has a large carbon footprint. To ensure a stable global climate, protect biodiversity, and reduce harm, the environmental footprint of health care must be reduced. Achieving sustainable health care presents moral challenges and the study of bioethics can help practitioners develop the capacity to recognize and examine these challenges (Zaidi 2017) UNESCO's 2017 *Declaration of Ethical Principles in Relation to Climate Change* commits member states to providing the appropriate professional education	When considering the potential harm and risks in terms of public health, environmental sustainability, and health and well-being when large infrastructural projects such as mines are proposed, it is important to explore more than the downstream costs such as air and water pollution. Unnoticed and often invisible upstream production costs must also be discussed
What was done?	A bioethics course was introduced into Year 1 of the four-year medical program in 2017. The course includes a series of case studies comprising a one-hour lecture and a one-hour facilitated small group discussion. One case study examines the ethical issues posed by climate change and the responses, particularly as they relate to health and health care. Students consider the multiple health care decision perspectives in a hospital and the ethical issues associated with the introduction of an anesthetic gas with a GHG emission 1000 times greater than a gas currently in use	Using X coal mine in Australia as an example, students can explore: *Ecological consequences* *Health consequences* *Cultural consequences* *Legal considerations* *Gender and age considerations* *Economic considerations* **Appendix 4** provides a series of questions for each of these considerations or consequences
What are/ were the outcomes?	Requires students to consider ethical issues in the delivery of health care that extend beyond individual patients to the community, including other countries and future generations. The case study illustrates how decisions they make as health practitioners affect the environmental sustainability of health care and how ethics can guide their decision-making	Framework was provided to Year 2 groups working on relevant Planetary Health assignments. It will be used in 2020 in an ethics session on environmental justice

Outcomes: Expected to be implemented in 2020.

The final case study describes institutional collaboration to develop a nursing toolkit in several languages. It has also been used by nonhealth disciplines (Richardson et al. 2016; Mukonoweshuro et al. 2018).

NurSus (Nursing Sustainability) Toolkit (three European and one UK university collaboration) – Enhancing nursing and health professional education for sustainability and climate change (Janet Richardson).

Why is it important? Sustainability literacy and competency are important outcomes in nursing and other health professions education.

What was done? Funded by the European Union, the *NurSusTOOLKIT* was developed with content based on research across Europe in terms of what nurses need to know about sustainability and climate change. The Toolkit provides free teaching and learning resources in several languages, using a range of pedagogical approaches (e.g., lecture notes; activities) and draws on theories from education for sustainable development trailed with students and educators (Alvarez et al. 2018). Guidance is provided in terms of where in the curriculum specific topics could be integrated as well as recommendations for assessment.

Outcomes: Materials have been used by educators in all health professions education and in business and accounting.

NurSusTOOLKIT: http://nursus.eu/uk/

Conclusions

The need to address climate change and other environmental threats to protect the health of our planet and human survival is urgent. It is our responsibility as educators of current and future health professionals to enable them to rise to these challenges. This chapter has described several approaches to prepare health professionals to practice environmentally sustainable health care to reduce the sector's environmental footprint, be prepared for the rapidly changing patterns of morbidity and mortality, and to anticipate when extreme weather events may compromise the capacity of the health system to respond to the urgent needs of populations and individuals. We must, however, also prepare current and future health professionals to advocate for change in the health and education sectors and society in general. We also need to foster their sense of global citizenship in terms of planetary health. Health professionals should, in line with many of their professional organizations' statements and declarations, become stewards of the planet's limited resources as well as actively advocate for the vulnerable and marginalized who are and will suffer the most from environmental disturbances – *"The rich will find their world to be more expensive, inconvenient, uncomfortable, disrupted, and colourless – in general, more unpleasant and unpredictable, perhaps greatly so. The poor [and the young and elderly] will die"* (Smith 2008, p. 1).

The window of opportunity for successful mitigation of increasing global temperatures and environmental degradation is closing. Beyond this, our responses may be limited to adapting to the consequences of our inaction. Health professions education is currently not doing enough to create an informed and skilled workforce. The pace of change needs to accelerate. We hope that the case studies and resources provided in this chapter inspire educators and health professionals to implement change both within their curricula and in educational workplaces.

Cross-References

▶ Interprofessional Education (IPE): Trends and Context

Appendix 1. Position Statements and Declarations From National Health Professional Organizations and Postgraduate Medical Colleges

National Professional Bodies

Australian Medical Association (AMA): Recently published several position statements addressing climate change, resource stewardship, and sustainability include:
- *Health Care and Climate Change* (2015): https://ama.com.au/position-statement/ama-position-statement-climate-change-and-human-health-2004-revised-2015
- *Doctor's Role in Stewardship of Health Care Resources* (2016): https://ama.com.au/position-statement/doctors-role-stewardship-health-care-resources-2016
- *Environmental Sustainability in Health Care* (2019): https://ama.com.au/position-statement/environmental-sustainability-health-care-2019

Postgraduate Medical Colleges

Academy of Medical Royal Colleges (AMRC, UK): The UK's AMRC is a good example of how collectively medical colleges are promoting sustainability, not just in terms of travel, procurement, building, and divestment from fossil fuel companies, but also in terms of community engagement (AMRC 2014). Relevant AMRC documents include:

- *Facing the Future: Sustainability for Medical Royal Colleges:* https://www.aomrc.org.uk/wp-content/uploads/2016/05/Facing_the_Future_Sustainabilty_for_MRC_1014.pdf
- *Protecting Resources Promoting Value. A Doctor's Guide to Cutting Waste in Clinical Care:* https://www.aomrc.org.uk/reports-guidance/protecting-resources-promoting-value-1114/

Council of College Presidents (CPMC, Australia): Following a Roundtable Forum on climate change and health, the CPMC released a 2018 Communique recognizing the need for more sustainable health care and evidenced-based strategies for the management of climate change and extreme weather-related risks to health and health care infrastructure, operations, and personnel: https://cpmc.edu.au/communique/managing-and-responding-to-climate-risks-in-healthcare/

Royal College of Physicians (RCP, UK): Has a health care sustainability program that aims to reduce the environmental, social, and financial impacts of the health service. The College has produced a series of policy position papers:

44 Planetary Health: Educating the Current and Future Health Workforce

- *Every Breath We Take: The Lifelong Impact of Air Pollution (2016)*: https://www.rcplondon.ac.uk/projects/outputs/every-breath-we-take-lifelong-impact-air-pollution
- *Breaking the Fever: Sustainability and Climate Change in the NHS (2017)*: https://www.rcplondon.ac.uk/projects/outputs/breaking-fever-sustainability-and-climate-change-nhs
- *Less Waste, More Health: A Health Professional's Guide to Reducing Waste (2018)*: https://www.rcplondon.ac.uk/projects/outputs/less-waste-more-health-health-professionals-guide-reducing-waste

Royal Australasian College of Physicians (RACP): In June 2015, the RACP announced that it would divest from fossil fuels due to the health impacts of climate change. At the same time and in the lead up to COP21, the RACP mobilized health professional organizations and health professionals around the world in Doctors for Climate Action, a petition calling for strong commitments for global action in Paris. In 2016, a series of position papers were published that have informed policy and advocacy initiatives:

- *Climate change and health* (2016): https://www.racp.edu.au/docs/default-source/advocacy-library/climate-change-and-health-position-statement.pdf
- *Environmentally sustainable health care* (2016): https://www.racp.edu.au/docs/default-source/advocacy-library/environmentally-sustainable-healthcare-position-statement.pdf
- *Health benefits of mitigating climate change* (2016): https://www.racp.edu.au/docs/default-source/advocacy-library/health-benefits-of-mitigating-climate-change-position-statement.pdf

Royal Australasian College of General Practitioners (RACGP):

- *Climate change and human health* Position Statement (2019): https://www.racgp.org.au/FSDEDEV/media/documents/RACGP/Position%20statements/Climate-change-and-human-health.pdf

American College of Physicians (ACP): In addition to a position statement, the ACP website provides several resources for physicians:

- *Position statement on climate change and health:* https://annals.org/aim/fullarticle/2513976/climate-change-health-position-paper-american-college-physicians?resultClick=3&_ga=2.114596612.2038160052.1556863397-358539027.1556863397.
- *A Climate Change Toolkit:* https://www.acponline.org/advocacy/advocacy-in-action/climate-change-toolkit
- Medical Society Consortium (physicians in medical societies representing over half of the nation's doctors) member report on the health impacts of climate change: https://medsocietiesforclimatehealth.org/reports/medical-alert/

Royal Australasian College of Surgeons (RACS): Recommends that surgeons and hospitals reduce the impact of surgery on the environment.

- *Environmental Impact of Surgical Practice* Position Paper (2018): https://www.surgeons.org/news/advocacy/2018-06-18-environmental-impact-of-surgical-practice.

Appendix 2. International and Country-Based Organizations Providing Resources and/or Case Studies Relating to Sustainability in Health Care and Health Care Education (Alphabetical)

Alliance of Nurses for Healthy Environments: https://envirn.org/
A wealth of resources available from this US-based Alliance with a range of work group offering free resources: Education, research, practice, policy and advocacy, climate change, safer chemicals, food sustainability, and energy and health.

Canadian Association of Physicians for the Environment (CAPE): https://cape.ca/
CAPE works to better human health by protecting the planet. The Guiding Principles relate to evidence-based and ethics-driven education, collaboration, advancement off human health by addressing environmental issues, and advocacy in terms of healthier environments and ecosystems. A toolkit is available: https://cape.ca/campaigns/cli mate-health-policy/climate-change-toolkit-for-health-professionals/

Centre for Disease Control (CDC): https://www.cdc.gov/climateandhealth/default. htm. A range of resources available, including the BRACE – Building Resistance Against Climate Effects – framework.

Centre for Sustainable Healthcare Education (CHE): https://networks.sustaina blehealthcare.org.uk/network/sustainable-healthcare-education

A network for those interested in educating health professionals for planetary health in terms of understanding the links between human health and the environment and developing skills for creating a sustainable health service. An example of an available case study is *Driving sustainable healthcare education through the development of assessment practices:* https://networks.sustainablehealthcare.org.uk/networks/sustain able-healthcare-education/driving-sustainable-healthcare-education-through

Climate and Health Alliance (CAHA): https://www.caha.org.au/
A coalition of health care stakeholders advocating for strong policy action to reduce the threat climate change poses to human health. Offers an opportunity for different health professions to collaborate and collectively advocate. CAHA further strengthens Australian campaigns by building on global initiatives, for example, CAHA's Healthcare Climate Challenge represents the Australian arm of Global Green and Healthy Hospitals. CAHA endeavors to link its energy projects with the international Healthy Energy Initiative. The CAHA campaign for a National Strategy

on Climate Health and Wellbeing has developed a framework for the federal government to take leadership on climate change and to meet its Paris Agreement obligations.

Doctors for the Environment, Australia (DEA): https://www.dea.org.au/
Represents medical professionals, researchers, and students. Aims to promote human health through environmental health. Has a broad national network with each state liaising with local and state governments, and universities, providing climate change and health presentations, political briefings and making policy submissions. DEA convenes an annual national conference which is a crucial opportunity for health professional education. The conference regularly includes workshops to upskill health professionals and students in media, public speaking, policy submissions, and practice sustainability. DEA encourages students to join state committees and regularly supports students to provide further education for their university peers. DEA works closely with medical associations such as the AMA and AMSA, medical training colleges and state and local government.

Environmental Justice Australia: https://www.envirojustice.org.au/
Nature's legal team. Uses technical expertise and practical understanding of the law to protect nature and defend communities' rights to a healthy environment. For cases and publications: https://www.envirojustice.org.au/publications/

Global Consortium on Climate and Health Education: https://www.mailman.columbia.edu/research/global-consortium-climate-and-health-education
Hosted by Columbia University School of Public Health, the mission of this Consortium is to advance global health security and educate professionals on the effects of climate change. A range of resources, online courses and MOOCs as well as learning outcomes are available.

Global Green and Healthy Hospitals Network: https://www.greenhospitals.net/
Comprises health organizations dedicated to reducing their ecological footprint and promoting public and environmental health, with sharing of best practice models and strategies such as operating theatre waste reduction, anesthetic GHG reductions, parking lot lighting energy savings and transport action plans. A Green Challenge award recognizes innovation in meeting environmental challenges: https://www.greenhospitals.net/case-studies/#clima.

Healthcare without Harm: https://noharm.org/
Works to transform health care worldwide to reduce its environmental footprint, becoming a community anchor for sustainability and a leader in the global movement for environmental health and justice. Programs include medical waste, toxic materials, safer chemicals, green building and energy, healthy food, pharmaceuticals, green purchasing, climate and health, transportation, and water.

Healthcare Environmental Resource Center: http://www.hercenter.org/
A US-based center with the website maintained by the National Center of Manufacturing and funded by the Environmental Protection Services. Provides pollution

prevention and environmental compliance assistance information for the healthcare sector. Intended to be a comprehensive resource, covering all the varieties of hospital wastes and the rules that apply, including both federal regulations and the specific rules that apply in different states. HERC also includes environmental compliance information for dental offices and assisted living/nursing care communities.

MedAct (UK): https://www.medact.org/project/divestment/
The Mission is to support health professionals from all disciplines to work together towards a world in which everyone can truly achieve and exercise their human right to health. The Organization's campaigns include Fossil Fuel Divestment, Healthy Planet Healthy World, Hospital Food, Sustainable Food Systems, Diets & Health.

Menus of Change Initiative: http://www.menusofchange.org/
Initiative from The Culinary Institute of America and Harvard T.H. Chan School of Public Health that strives to realize a long-term, practical vision integrating optimal nutrition and public health, environmental stewardship and restoration as well as social responsibility concerns within the foodservice industry and the culinary profession. Resources and case studies are available.

Pharmacists for the Environment, Australia: https://www.facebook.com/ PharmEnviroAus/?ref=br_rs
Pharmacists for the Environment Australia (PEA) is committed to advocacy and promotion of sustainable pharmacy practices for better human and planet health. The website is currently under construction: http://www.pea.org.au/?fbclid=IwAR1Inp-P_bX3ndnuIGwmE8s8ctO8KhAjzsjukGT3OTfHkGeZ_SYpuAeh7OM

Planetary Health Alliance: https://planetaryhealthalliance.org/planetary-health; https://planetaryhealthalliance.org/education
Consortium of universities, NGOs, and partners committed to advancing planetary health. Educational resources include planetary health syllabi, workshops, videos, etc.

Practice Greenhealth: https://practicegreenhealth.org/
The leading US membership and networking organization for sustainable health care, delivering environmental solutions to hospitals and health systems across the United States. A range of toolkits are on offer, for example, anesthetic gas toolkit, greenhouse gas reduction toolkit.

Sustainable Development Unit (UK): https://www.sduhealth.org.uk/
Funded by and accountable to NHS England and Public Health England to work across the NHS, public health and social care system. Supports the NHS, public health, and social care to embed and promote the three elements of sustainable development: Environmental, social, and financial. Helps organizations across health and care embed and promotes sustainable development in order to reduce emissions, save money, and improve the health of people and communities. Involved in the long-term needs of the health system including adaptation of health service

44 Planetary Health: Educating the Current and Future Health Workforce

delivery, health promotion, tackling the wider determinants of health, corporate social responsibility, and developing new sustainable models of care.

- Case studies from various NHS units and hospitals: https://www.sduhealth.org.uk/resources/case-studies.aspx
- Tool for sustainable planning: https://srp.digital/
- 2018 Sustainable Development Report: https://www.sduhealth.org.uk/policy-strategy/reporting/natural-resource-footprint-2018.aspx

World Bank: https://www.worldbank.org/en/topic/climatechange
Keeping global temperature rise to below 2 °C will require co-ordinated global action at an unprecedented scale and speed. The World Bank Group is committed to helping countries meet their national climate targets. Three relevant links are:

- Climate change and health: http://www.worldbank.org/en/topic/climatechangeandhealth

One of the resources includes a document entitled Climate-Smart Healthcare: Low-Carbon and Resilience Strategies for the Health: https://openknowledge.worldbank.org/handle/10986/27809

- Climate-smart agriculture: http://www.worldbank.org/en/topic/climate-smart-agriculture
- Disaster risk management: http://www.worldbank.org/en/topic/disasterriskmanagement

World Health Organization (WHO)
More than 7000 people working in 150 country offices in six regional offices, with headquarters in Geneva. The World Health Assembly is the governing body. Its list of programs is long, from Accountability for women's and children's health to Zoonoses and Veterinary public health. Some useful resources include:

- Healthy hospitals, healthy planet, healthy people: Addressing climate change in healthcare settings: https://www.who.int/globalchange/publications/healthcare_settings/en/
- Operational framework for building climate resilient health systems:https://en.unesco.org/themes/education-sustainable-development
- 2030 Sustainable Development Goals (SDGs), Global Action Plan: https://www.who.int/sdg/en/

Appendix 3. Features of an Environmentally Accountable Medical School (Applicable to All Health Professions) (Boelen et al. 2016)

An *environmentally accountable* medical school or HP college should be:

1. *Environmentally responsible*: Aware of GECs facing society and recognizes its impact on future students, staff, and populations served by the school. Responsibility includes tracking the school's carbon footprint and other resource usage such as water.

2. *Environmentally responsive*: Aware of requirements to reduce the school's impact on local and global environment, having policies and priorities for saving water, raw materials and energy, for example, through amending building and travel policies, reducing, recycling, encouraging sustainability initiatives, and individual champions.

3. *Environmentally accountable:* Has clear, effective policies to reduce the school's environmental impact and through education, research and service to ensure health systems are sustainable for future generations. Includes linking awareness and responsiveness to challenges with clear, evidence-based action plans, working with local communities so the school and the communities it serves can reduce their environmental impact and minimize damage where impact is unavoidable. Has measurable outcomes.

Appendix 4. Ethical Framework (With Questions) Relating to Large Infrastructural Projects

Ecological consequences
- What ecosystems will be affected? What flora and fauna will be affected?
- What are the potential impacts on water (e.g., usage, pollution, run-off)?
- What are the potential pollutants? What measures are required to prevent or minimize them?
- In the event of an accident, what species will be affected by the failure?
- Are measures in place to ensure that a clean-up happens in the event of bankruptcy, abandonment or at the end of the life of the project?

Health consequences
- Whose health and well-being are likely to be negatively affected?
- What specific physical and mental health impacts are foreseeable?
- In the event of an accident, which communities will be affected?

Cultural consequences
- What happens to burial grounds, ceremonial places and other spiritual locations and other cultural centers?
- In the event of a disruption, what are the physical and mental health consequences?

Legal considerations
- What are the health and other consequences of undermining the laws of a local community?

Gender and age considerations

- How might the establishment of the project increase the suffering and poor health of impacted women, children, and the elderly?

Economic considerations

- Which communities and individuals benefit from the mine and which are harmed?
- Within those communities, how are benefits and harms distributed?
- Who bears the costs of damage to personal property or impacts on physical and mental well-being as a result of the project's activities?

References

Alvarez NC, Richardson J, Parra-Anguita G, Linares-Abad M, Huss N, Grande Gascón ML, et al. Developing digital educational materials for nursing and sustainability: the results of an observational study. Nurse Educ Today. 2018;60:139–46.

Australian Government. National medicines policy. Department of Health and Ageing. 2000. https://www.health.gov.au/internet/main/publishing.nsf/Content/National%20Medicines%20 Policy-1. Accessed 16 Apr 2019.

Barton H, Grant M. A health map for the local human habitat. J Royal Soc Prom Health. 2006;126(6):252–3.

Behrens G, Zhang Y, Beggs P. Lancet countdown 2018 report: briefing for Australian policymakers. http://www.lancetcountdown.org/media/1394/2018-lancet-countdown-australia-policy-brief-final-for-upload.pdf. Accessed 20 Apr 2019.

Boelen C, Pearson D, Kaufman A, Rouke J, Woollard R, Marsh D, Gibbs T. Producing a socially accountable medical school: AMEE Guide No. 109. Med Teach. 2016;38(11):1078–91.

Capon T, Talley NJ, Horton R. Planetary health: what is it and what should doctors do? MJA. 2018;208(7):296–7.

Charlesworth KE, Jamieson M. New sources of value for health and care in a carbon-constrained world. J Pub Health. 2017;39(4):691–7. https://academic.oup.com/jpubhealth/article/39/4/691/ 2918119?searchresult=1

Charlesworth KE, Jamieson M. Healthcare in a carbon-constrained world. Aust Health Rev. 2018;43(3):241–5. https://www.publish.csiro.au/AH/AH17184

Charlesworth KE, Ray S, Head F, Pencheon D. Developing an environmentally sustainable NHS: outcomes of implementing an educational intervention on sustainable health care with UK public health registrars. NSW Pub Health Bull. 2012;23:1–2. https://doi.org/10.1071/NB11018.

Clark C Sustainable nursing: putting environmental stewardship to practice. 2019. https://nursing.wisc.edu/sustainable-nursing-putting-environmental-stewardship-to-practice/. Accessed 23 June 2019.

Cohen AJ, Brauer M, Burnett R, Anderson HR, Frostad J, Estep K, et al. Estimates and 25-year trends of the global burden of disease attributable to ambient air pollution: an analysis of data from the Global Burden of Diseases Study 2015. Lancet. 2017;389:1907–18.

Costello M, Abbas A, Allen S, et al. Managing the health effects of climate change. Lancet. 2009;373:1693–733.

Coughlin S, Roberts D, O'Neill K, Brooks P. Looking to tomorrow's healthcare today: a participatory perspective. Intern Med J. 2018;48:92–6.

Dahlgren G, Whitehead M. "The main determinants of health" model. 1991. In: Dahlgren G, Whitehead M, editors. European strategies for tackling social inequities in health: levelling up Part 2. Copenhagen: WHO Regional Office for Europe; 2007. http://www.euro.who.int/__data/ assets/pdf_file/0018/103824/E89384.pdf.

Ebi K, Campbell-Lendrum D, Wyns A. The 1.5 health report. Climate Tracker. 2018. IPCC Report. https://www.who.int/globalchange/181008_the_1_5_healthreport.pdf

Eckelman MJ, Sherman J. Environmental impacts of the U.S. health care system and effects on public health. PLoS One. 2016;11(6):e0157014. https://doi.org/10.1371/journal.pone.0157014.

Frumkin H, Haines A. Global environmental change and noncommunicable disease risks. Ann Rev Public Health. 2019;40:261–82.

General Medical Council (United Kingdom). 2018. Tomorrow's Doctor. https://www.gmc-uk.org/-/media/documents/dc11326-outcomes-for-graduates-2018_pdf-75040796.pdf. Accessed 28 Apr 2019.

Gómez A, Balsari S, Nusbaum J, Heerboth A, Lemery J. Environment, biodiversity, and the education of the physician of the future. Acad Med. 2013;88:168–72.

Grose J, Doman M, Kelsey J, Richardson J, Woods M. Integrating sustainability education into nursing using an interdisciplinary approach. Local Econ. 2017;30(3):342–51.

Gupta J, Hurley F, Grobick A, et al. Communicating the health of the planet and its links to human health. Lancet Planet Health. 2019;3(5):e204–6.

Hackett F, Got T, Kitching GT, MacQueen K, Cohen A. Training Canadian doctors for the health challenges of climate change. Lancet Planet Health. 2020; early online https://www.thelancet.com/journals/lanplh/article/PIIS2542-5196%2819%2930242-6/fulltext

Haines A, Ebi K. The imperative for climate action to protect health. NEJM. 2019;380:263–73.

Hathaway J, Maibach EW. Health implications of climate change: a review of the literature about the perception of the public and health professionals. Curr Environ Health Rep. 2018;5:197–214.

Health Care Without Harm/ARUP. Health care's climate footprint. Green Paper Number 1. 2019. https://noharm-global.org/content/global/reducing-healthcares-environmental-footprint. Accessed 4 Oct 2019.

Health Effects Institute. State of global air. 2019. https://www.stateofglobalair.org/. Accessed 6 May 2019.

Horton R. Offline: planetary health – gains and challenges. Lancet. 2016;388:2462.

Horton R, Lo S. Planetary health: a new science for exceptional action. Lancet. 2015;386:1921–2.

Horton R, Beaglehole R, Bonita R, Raeburn J, McKee M, Wall S. From public to planetary health: a manifesto. Lancet. 2014;383:847.

Intergovernmental Panel on Climate Change (IPCC). Global warming of 1.5 °C. 2018. https://www.ipcc.ch/sr15/. Accessed 5 May 2019.

International Pharmaceutical Federation (FIP). FIP statement of policy: environmentally sustainable pharmacy practice: green pharmacy. 2015. https://www.fip.org/www/uploads/database_file.php?id=376&table_id=. Accessed 27 Apr 2019.

Jackman-Murphy KP, Uznanski W, McDermott-Levy R, Cook C. Climate change: preparing the nurses of the future. Deans Notes. 2018;39(2):1–3.

Kreslake JM, Sarfaty M, Roser-Renouf C, Leiserowitz AA, Maibach EW. The critical role of health professionals in climate change prevention and preparedness. Am J Public Health. 2018;108(S2):S68–9. https://ajph.aphapublications.org/doi/full/10.2105/AJPH.2017.304044

Madden DL, McLean M, Horton G. Preparing medical graduates for the health effects of climate change: an Australasian collaboration. MJA. 2018;208(7):291–2. https://www.mja.com.au/journal/2018/208/7/preparing-medical-graduates-health-effects-climate-change-australasian

Malik A, Lenzen M, McAlister S, McGain F. The carbon footprint of Australian health care. Lancet Planet Health. 2018;2:e27–35.

Maxwell J, Blashki G. Teaching about climate change in medical education: an opportunity. J Pub Health Res. 2016;5(1):673. https://www.jphres.org/index.php/jphres/article/view/673

McGain F, Naylor C. Environmental sustainability in hospitals – a systematic review and research agenda. J Health Serv Res Policy. 2014;19(4):245–52.

Mortimer F. The sustainable physician. Clin Med. 2010;10(2):110–1.

Mukonoweshuro R, Richardson J, Grose J, Tauringana V, Suchanging C. Accounting undergraduates' attitudes towards sustainability and climate change through using a sustainability scenario-based intervention within curriculum to enhance employability attributes. Int J Bus Res. 2018;18(4):81–90.

Myers SS. Planetary health: protecting human health on a rapidly changing planet. Lancet. 2017;390:2860–8.

Pencheon D. Developing a sustainable health care system: the United Kingdom experience. MJA. 2018;2018(5):284–5. https://www.mja.com.au/system/files/issues/208_07/10.5694mja17.01134.pdf

Pichler P-P, Jaccard IS, Weisz U, Weisz H. International comparison of health care carbon footprints. Environ Res Lett. 2019;14:064004. https://doi.org/10.1088/1748-9326/ab19el.

Prescott SL, Logan AC, Albrecht G, et al. The Canmore declaration: statement of principles for planetary health. Challenges. 2018;9:31. https://www.mdpi.com/2078-1547/9/2/31

Prüss-Ustün A, Wolf J, Corvalán C, Bos R, Neira M. Preventing disease through healthy environments. A global assessment of the burden of disease from environmental risks. 2016. World Health Organization. https://apps.who.int/iris/bitstream/handle/10665/204585/9789241565519 6_eng.pdf;jsessionid=B0C830DB53BDC6660A1A55BDAAE071CD?sequence=1. Accessed 27 Apr 2019.

Purcell R, McGirr J. Preparing rural general practitioners and health services for climate change and extreme weather. Aust J Rural Health. 2014;22:8–14.

Purcell R, McGirr J. Rural health service managers' perspectives on preparing rural health services for climate change. Aust J Rural Health. 2018;26:20–5.

Ramanathan V, Haines A. Healthcare professionals must lead on climate change. BMJ. 2016;355: i5245. https://doi.org/10.1136/bmj.i5245.

Richardson J, Grose J, Allum P. Can a health and sustainability scenario session change undergraduate paramedic students' attitudes towards sustainability and climate change? J Paramed Pract. 2016;8(3):130–6.

Rockström J, Steffen W, Noone K, Persson A, et al. A safe operating space for humanity. Nature. 2009;461(7263):462–75. https://doi.org/10.1038/461472a.

Schwerdtle PN, Maxwell J, Horton G, Bonnamy J. 12 tips for teaching environmental sustainability to health professionals. Med Teach 2019. https://doi.org/10.1080/0142159X.2018.1551994. (early online).

Shelton CL, McBain SC, Mortimer F, White SM. A new role for anaesthetists in environmentally-sustainable healthcare. Anaesthesia. 2019;74:1091–4. https://doi.org/10.1111/anae.14647.

Singleton JA. On our watch: It is time for the profession to take responsibility for its environmental impact. Pharmacy GRIT, 2019;Autumn:4–6. https://eprints.qut.edu.au/129484/

Smith KR. Introduction: mitigating, adapting, and suffering: how much of each? Ann Rev Pub Health. 2008;29(32). https://www.annualreviews.org/doi/full/10.1146/annurev.pu.29.031708.100011

Stone SB, Myers SS, Golden CD, et al. Cross-cutting principles for planetary health education. Lancet Planet Health. 2018;2:192–3.

Sustainable Development Unit, UK National Health Service. Sustainable development in the health and care system e Health Check 2018. Cambridge: SDU; 2018. https://www.sduhealth.org.uk/policy-strategy/reporting/sustainable-development-in-health-and-care-report-2018.aspx. Accessed 20 Feb 2019.

Teherani A, Nishimura H, Apatira L, Newman T, Ryan S. Identification of core objectives for teaching sustainable healthcare education. Med Educ Online. 2017;22:1. https://doi.org/ 10.1080/10872981.2017.1386042.

Tong S, Ebi K. Preventing and mitigating health risks of climate change. Environ Res. 2019;174:9–13.

Tun MS. Fulfilling a new obligation: teaching and learning of sustainable healthcare in medical education curriculum. Med Teach. 2019;41(10):1168–77. https://doi.org/10.1080/0142159X. 2019.1623870.

United Nations Climate Change. The Paris Agreement. https://unfccc.int/process-and-meetings/the-paris-agreement/the-paris-agreement. Accessed 5 May 2019.

United Nations Environment Programme. GEO-6: summary for policymakers. 2019. https:// wedocs.unep.org/bitstream/handle/20.500.11822/27652/GEO6SPM_EN.pdf?sequence=1&is Allowed=y. Accessed 5 May 2109.

Walpole SC, Pearson D, Coad J, Barna S. What do tomorrow's doctors need to learn about ecosystems? – A BEME systematic review: BEME Guide No. 36. Med Teach. 2016;38 (4):338–52.

Walpole SC, Vyas A, Maxwell J, Canny BJ, Woollard R, Wellbery C, et al. Building an environmentally accountable medical curriculum through international collaboration. Med Teach. 2017;39(10):1040–50.

Walpole SC, Barna S, Richardson J, Rother H-A. Sustainable healthcare education: integrating planetary health into clinical education. Lancet Planet Health. 2019;3:e6–7.

Watts N, Amann M, Arnell N, Ayeb-Karlsson S, Belesova K, Bery H, et al. The 2018 report of the *Lancet* countdown on health and climate change: shaping the health of nations for centuries. Lancet. 2018;392:2479–514.

Watts N, Amann M, Arnell N, Ayeb-Karlsson S, Belesova K, et al. The 2019 report of the *Lancet* countdown on health and climate change: ensuring that the health of a child born today is not defined by a changing climate. Lancet. 2019;394:1836–78.

Wellbery C, Sheffield P, Timmireddy K, Sarfaty M, Teherani A, Fallar R. It's time for medical schools to introduce climate change into their curricula. Acad Med. 2018;93:1774–7.

Whitmee S, Haines A, Beyrer C, Boltz F, Capon AG, de Souza Diaz BF, Ezeh A, et al. Safeguarding human health in the Anthropocene epoch: report of the Rockefeller Foundation-*Lancet* Commission on planetary health. Lancet. 2015;386:1973–2028.

World Health Organization (WHO). An estimated 12.6 million deaths each year are attributable to unhealthy environments. 2016. https://www.who.int/news-room/detail/15-03-2016-an-estimated-12-6-million-deaths-each-year-are-attributable-to-unhealthy-environments. Accessed 5 May 2019.

World Health Organization (WHO). COP24 special report. Health & climate change. Geneva: WHO; 2018. https://www.who.int/globalchange/publications/COP24-report-health-climate-change/en/. Accessed 27 Apr 2019.

World Health Organization (WHO). Ten threats to global health in 2019. https://www.who.int/emergencies/ten-threats-to-global-health-in-2019. Accessed 20 Apr 2019.

Zaidi AA. The "Buy One, Get One Free" ethics of investing public and philanthropic funds in health and climate. AMA J Ethics. 2017;19(12):1193–201.